Occupational Health

Occupational Health
Recognizing and Preventing Work-Related Disease

Second Edition

Edited by
Barry S. Levy, M.D., M.P.H.
Program Officer, Occupational and Environmental Health, Management Sciences for Health, Boston, Massachusetts

David H. Wegman, M.D., M.S.
Professor and Head, Department of Work Environment, College of Engineering, and Director, Work Environment Laboratory, Center for Productivity Enhancement, University of Lowell, Lowell, Massachusetts

Foreword by
J. Donald Millar, M.D.,
Director, National Institute for Occupational Safety and Health

With 36 photographs by Earl Dotter, Photographer, American Labor Education Center

Little, Brown and Company
Boston/Toronto

To our wives and our children
Nancy, Laura, and Benjamin Levy
Peggy, Marya, and Jesse Wegman
for their never-ending
encouragement and support

Contents

III. Hazardous Workplace Exposures

IV. Occupational Disorders by System

Foreword to the Second Edition

The Occupational Safety and Health Act of 1970 enunciated a historically unprecedented vision when it expressed the will of Congress to "assure so far as possible, every working man and woman in the Nation safe and healthful working conditions." To make this vision a reality is the goal of the professional in occupational safety and health. Achieving this goal involves the coordinated dedication of the skills of several different scientific disciplines. It is not an easy task. A broad spectrum of hazards must be addressed in the varied and ever-changing American workplace.

Early in the development of occupational health, the "company fence" became a convenient boundary for defining the scope of occupational risks and the adverse health effects related to work. In recent years, however, it has become clear that work-related diseases and injuries have important consequences for the family of the worker and the general community. In short, today's oc-

cupational health problem is all too quickly a community public health problem as well.

We continue to face the traditional occupational diseases and injuries within traditional and non-traditional settings. But we must also contend with new problems created by new technologies. A clear understanding of the nature and extent of occupational hazards and consequent health effects is critically necessary to their prevention. In this book, the authors share their comprehensive knowledge of both the science of occupational health and the political and social milieu in which it must be practiced. Much credit is due to Barry S. Levy and David H. Wegman for bringing forward this excellent resource, which will prove useful to all who daily strive to recognize and prevent occupational diseases and injuries.

J. Donald Millar, M.D.

Foreword to the First Edition

The medicine and the science of occupational health are universal. A discovery made in a distant part of the world will be valid here. Basic knowledge enhanced by other branches of medical science will help explain occupational disease. The pathology, physiology, chemistry, physics, and toxicology that help to form the scientific base for occupational medicine are not unique to occupational medicine.

However, unlike other medical specialties that deal with a single organ or system or have a special diagnostic or therapeutic approach, occupational medicine is a part of preventive medicine. It is distinguished by its focus on environmental determinants of diseases and methods of disease prevention.

Occupational medicine is finally attracting the interest and attention it deserves. This field has the potential to contribute more to human welfare than any other health specialty. Occupational hazards are the most preventable cause of disease, disability, and death. Unlike many other public health problems, we often know who is exposed to what. When the effect of an exposure can be measured, it is often possible to construct an exposure-effect curve. Thus, good epidemiology can describe causal relationships. And because the exposures are in the workplace, they are by definition preventable.

Although the science of occupational medicine is universal, the economic, political, and social environments determine whether and how we make progress and prevent occupational disease. *Occupational Health* is unusual because it consciously places the science of occupational medicine in the current United States economic, political, and social context. It will provide the reader with far more than basic science. It presents information on how to succeed with the prime task: protecting the health of workers.

To be an effective occupational health professional, one must understand five basic points concerning occupational health in the United States today:

1. The occupational health laws are strong.
2. The ethics of the field need strengthening.
3. Prevention must be the underlying objective of all activities.
4. Control technology and substitution are the critical strategies for prevention.
5. To prevent disease effectively, we must rely on laboratory tests for the data on which to base public health policy rather than waiting for epidemiology to count human bodies.

These five points need to be expanded.

1. We have very strong occupational safety and health statutes. The Coal Mine Safety and Health Act of 1969, the Occupational Safety and Health Act of 1970, and the Federal Mine Safety and Health Act of 1977 require the employer to provide every worker with a safe and healthful workplace. With the burden placed squarely on the employer, the laws give strong enforcement powers to the government. Complaints from workers may trigger inspections. This powerful rule means that

worker knowledge of occupational safety and health is important, and that worker education efforts are especially effective ways to prevent disease and injury. The enforcement agency has a right of entry to any workplace to carry out inspections. Criminal penalties are provided for willful violations and violations that lead to a worker's death. The strength of the statutes should not mislead one to believe that the laws work effectively or that the federal government has always wanted them to work. Under a government not committed to protecting workers, only the language is strong.

2. There is an ethical tradition in American medicine that physicians' and other health professionals' first responsibility is to their patients. There is a cloud over this great tradition in the field of occupational health. Physicians, industrial hygienists, and others have failed at times to serve their patients, choosing instead to serve their employers (often the employer of their patients). Examples exist where health professionals informed the employer of hazards in the factory that were causing disease in workers without telling the workers, or, worse, while reassuring workers of the safety of the workplace. This dilemma does not arise with every patient or every encounter, but there is frequently a conflict between the interests of the worker or patient and that of the health professional's employer. If occupational medicine and industrial hygiene are ever to gain the respect of other medical and public health professionals, it is clear that a consistent policy must resolve these conflicts in favor of the patient.

3. As it is important for occupational health professionals to serve the workers whom they see as patients, the same professionals must be able to assure that occupational disease is prevented. In the United States system, that means that they must be able to influence the behavior of the employer. They must convince management to correct the problems. They must teach workers. Or, they must call in enforcement agencies.

Occupational medicine can benefit only a relatively few patients as a purely clinical specialty. Many problems are chronic and progressive, and most can be remedied only by avoiding exposure. Thus, the effectiveness of occupational physicians hinges almost entirely on their ability to prevent disease. Occupational health research must also lead to prevention, with the understanding that basic science advances may have to precede preventive programs. Eventually, both clinical practice and research in occupational medicine will be judged by their ability to prevent disease.

4. At one time, it may have been sufficient to diagnose an occupational disease and describe the exposure that caused it. With a new emphasis on prevention, all occupational health professionals must have an understanding of the approaches to prevention, especially engineering controls, or control technology, and substitution. Since the health professional's role is to assure that workers are protected, to assist in the promulgation of new standards, and to convince management to act to protect workers, it is not sufficient to link the disease to the exposure. It has become critical that we demonstrate that engineering controls are possible or that safer materials can be used. For example, studies of aluminum reduction have centered on coal tar pitch volatiles released in pot-room operations. Precision in describing the carcinogenic effects will be edifying, but either enclosing the pot-room or isolating the worker holds the key to prevention. Substitution is an accepted approach in manufacturing processes. When one raw material is too expensive, another is substituted, often requiring modification in the process. Similar attention is now required to substitute safer for more hazardous materials or chemicals. The dye industry, for example, is being asked to find substitutes for benzidine and related dyes that have been found to cause cancer. Thus, effectiveness in occupational health requires an awareness of production technology.

5. Epidemiology is the basic science of all public health, but we are confronted with problems that defy the epidemiologist. How can we prevent diseases that have a long latent period between exposure and manifestation if we must wait for the epidemiologist to warn us? With many new chem-

icals introduced into the workplace each year, occupational health today must rely on laboratory tests to help set public policy. Both animal studies and in vitro tests for toxicity, mutagenicity, teratogenicity, and carcinogenicity will have to suffice for many major decisions about what exposures are likely to be dangerous and therefore must be avoided. Similar results will have to guide decisions about the safety of industrial processes and the desirability of substitution and other preventive measures. A clear understanding of the uses and limitations of toxicology and laboratory medicine is now essential to practice occupational medicine. With more experience, scientists will no longer be concerned that predictive tests are misunderstood or misused in public health decisions.

We will realize that the certainty required to take a protective and conservative public health action is generally less than that required to prove a basic research hypothesis.

In conclusion, occupational health is the application of biology, medicine, epidemiology, engineering, economics, education, politics, the law, and other disciplines to protect workers from diseases of the workplace. With this diversity of disciplines, the challenge will always be exciting and intellectually stimulating.

Anthony Robbins
Former Director, National
Institute for Occupational
Safety and Health

Preface

Although work-related disease is common and preventable, health professional schools in the United States seldom provide instruction in its recognition and prevention. Because one reason for this oversight is the absence of adequate curricular and resource materials in occupational health, we developed this textbook. Although we planned this second edition of *Occupational Health* for medical students, we also designed it to be useful to practicing physicians and students or practitioners in other health disciplines.

We believe that the most important distinguishing feature of occupational diseases and injuries is that, in principle, they are preventable. We therefore emphasize throughout this book the crucial role that health professionals can play both in recognizing work-related medical conditions and in taking appropriate measures to prevent them. Too often, health professionals have believed that work-related medical problems are part of progress and advanced industrial development, that therefore they will always be with us, and that whatever we do will make little difference. Our text is intended to facilitate a shift in this belief. Work-related medical problems, in fact, can be substantially decreased or eliminated, and health professionals have vital roles to play. But to do so health professionals must change their orientation about occupational disorders from after-the-fact treatment to early recognition and prevention. While participating in the prevention and control of work-related disorders, health professionals must recognize that occupational health deals with a body of scientific information in a complex po-

litical, social, and economic arena. This arena is filled with often-conflicting interests, perspectives, assumptions, and approaches to recognizing, defining, treating, and preventing problems. For example, in the United States, the occurrence of occupational diseases or injuries often implies that some individual or group has been at fault and is therefore legally responsible for damages. We therefore also deal with a wide range of nonmedical subjects that are relevant to occupational health.

Part I focuses on general concepts and data concerning occupational health in the United States and aspects of work in America. Part II is devoted to various approaches to recognizing and preventing occupational disease, regulating the work environment, and evaluating and compensating diseased and injured workers. Part III addresses hazardous workplace exposures and their effects. In contrast, Part IV describes occupational disorders by organ system. Part V examines occupational health and women, minorities, and agricultural workers. Part VI considers the perspectives of occupational health professionals in management and labor in the United States and issues of occupational health in selected other countries. Finally, three appendixes provide detailed information on workplace toxins, training and career opportunities in occupational health, and other sources of information in this field.

The variety of perspectives is also reflected by the diversity in contributors. Their backgrounds, viewpoints, and current activities vary widely. They include primary care and specialty physicians who work or have worked in academia, industry, labor, and government. They also importantly include professionals in industrial hygiene, safety and ergonomics, psychology, labor, economics, law, and sociology. In developing and editing this text, we did not attempt to present a single point of view because in occupational health there is no such thing.

There is also diversity in format of presentation of material in the text, which reflects the diversity and excitement in this field. We have used case studies, tables, photographs, drawings, boxes, and other materials to make the book not only informative but also explanatory, interesting, and readable. Bibliographies in each chapter, appendixes to some chapters, and the appendixes at the end of the text are designed to lead the reader with interest in a particular subject to further sources of information. This book is designed to be used primarily as a textbook, not a reference book; therefore, references are kept to a minimum, many of the tables are not comprehensive but rather illustrative, and technical detail on diagnosis, treatment, and prevention is not included.

A comment on the use of the term *health professional* is in order. Although the physician or nurse has traditionally been the provider of health care for work-related disorders, we often refer to the health professional. This term recognizes the increasing roles and responsibilities in this field of nurse practitioners, physician's assistants, industrial hygienists, and occupational safety and ergonomics specialists.

In sum, our primary intent is to present basic information that we believe is valuable to all health professionals. Ultimately, the recognition, treatment, control, prevention, and compensation of occupational diseases and injuries must be made as objectively and compassionately as possible. It should necessarily be based on good science and medicine and the recognition of the health rights of workers, including the right to a safe and healthy workplace. *Occupational Health* is intended to contribute to this end.

B.S.L.
D.H.W.

Acknowledgments

The development of the second edition of *Occupational Health* has required the assistance and support of many people, for which we are most appreciative. We acknowledge the contributions of the many chapter authors whose work is appropriately credited within the text. However, there were many other "behind-the-scenes" people to whom we express our deep gratitude and appreciation.

A number of individuals in the Medical Division of Little, Brown and Company deserve much credit for their outstanding work. We are particularly grateful for the help of our editor, Chris Davis, and our production editor, Elizabeth Willingham; the continued support of Lynne Herndon, Publisher; the secretarial help of Kristina Johnson; the encouragement of our original editor, Curtis Vouwie, who is now publishing a periodical on occupational health; and the work of our first edition production editor, Robert M. Davis.

We hope that the illustrative materials throughout the book offer understanding and insights not easily gained from the text alone. We wish to call special attention to the work of Earl Dotter, who provided many outstanding photographs of workers and workplaces. We are grateful to him for sharing his photographic genius in this manner. We were also provided with excellent photographs by Marilee Caliendo, David Christiani, Christer Hogstedt, Nicolas Kaufman, Ken Light, and Gustavo Molina. We also thank artist Nick Thorkelson for sharing his talent and perspective in a series of creative drawings that convey concepts difficult to capture in words or photographs.

We are grateful to the following individuals who critically reviewed draft chapters and made helpful comments that were incorporated into the final text: Edward L. Baker, Leslie Boden, William A. Burgess, Alexander Cohen, Janet Fleetwood, Martin Horowitz, Alan McLean, and Michael Silverstein. We also note that Chapter 9 was derived from Chapter 17 in *Maxcy-Rosenau Public Health and Preventive Medicine* (12th ed.) edited by John M. Last.

We wish to thank Deana Fowler for the excellent work in developing a practical and functional index and Marcia Knoll, June Pearson, Karen Shimahara, Nell Switzer, Maureen Wall, and Evalon Witt for their substantial assistance in helping us and the contributing authors to meet the many deadlines.

While the second edition of this textbook is different and improved over the first edition by updating and some expansion, it draws heavily on the first in content and style. We again express our appreciation to the many people who made important contributions to the first edition.

Finally, B.S.L. acknowledges his parents Bernice and Jerome Levy, Department of Family and Community Medicine Chairman N. Lynn Eckhert, and Occupational Health Program Administrator Beverly Johnson; and D.H.W. acknowledges his parents Isabel and Myron Wegman for their long-term and dedicated support.

B.S.L.
D.H.W.

Contributors

Kenneth A. Arndt, M.D.
Professor of Dermatology, Harvard Medical School;
Dermatologist-in-Chief, Beth Israel Hospital,
Boston, Massachusetts
Chapter 23

Nicholas A. Ashford, Ph.D., J.D.
Associate Professor of Technology and Policy, Center
for Technology, Policy and Industrial Development,
Massachusetts Institute of Technology,
Cambridge, Massachusetts
Chapter 10

Dean B. Baker, M.D., M.P.H.
Associate Professor of Community Medicine, Division
of Environmental and Occupational Medicine, Mount
Sinai School of Medicine of the City University of
New York, New York, New York
Chapter 20

Edward L. Baker, Jr., M.D., M.P.H.
Deputy Director, National Institute for Occupational
Safety and Health, Atlanta, Georgia
Chapter 25

Michael Bigby, M.D.
Research Associate, Harvard Medical School;
Associate Dermatologist, Beth Israel Hospital,
Boston, Massachusetts
Chapter 23

Duane L. Block, M.D.
Consulting Professor of Health Sciences, Oakland
University, Rochester, Michigan; Corporate Medical
Director (Retired), Ford Motor Company,
Dearborn, Michigan
Chapter 34

Leslie I. Boden, Ph.D.
Associate Professor, Environmental Health Section,
Boston University School of Medicine and School of
Public Health, Boston, Massachusetts
Chapter 11

Marianne Parker Brown, M.P.H.
Occupational Health Program Coordinator,
University of California at Los Angeles Labor Center,
Los Angeles, California
Appendix C

Marilee A. Caliendo, R.B.P.
Director, Biomedical Media Center,
University of Massachusetts Medical Center,
Worcester, Massachusetts
Photographs

David C. Christiani, M.D., M.P.H., M.S.
Assistant Professor of Occupational Medicine, Harvard
School of Public Health, Boston, Massachusetts;
Director, Occupational Health Service, Massachusetts
Respiratory Hospital, South Braintree, Massachusetts
Chapters 21 and 36

Molly Joel Coye, M.D., M.P.H.
Commissioner of Health, New Jersey Department of
Health, Trenton, New Jersey; Associate Clinical
Professor, Department of Environmental and
Community Medicine, University of Medicine and
Dentistry of New Jersey-Robert Wood Johnson
Medical School, Piscataway, New Jersey
Chapter 33

Robert I. Davis, Ph.D.
Assistant Professor of Hearing and Speech Science,
State University of New York at Plattsburgh,
Plattsburgh, New York
Chapter 17

Charles D. DelTatto, B.S., P.T.
Program Specialist, The Return to Work Center,
Industrial Rehabilitation Associates,
Easthampton, Massachusetts
Box, Chapter 12

Peter Dooley
United Automobile Workers Health and
Safety Department, Detroit, Michigan
Box, Chapter 35

Earl Dotter
Photographer, American Labor Education Center,
Washington, D.C.
Photographs

Ellen A. Eisen, Sc.D.
Assistant Professor of Occupational Health, Harvard
School of Public Health, Boston, Massachusetts
Chapter 5

Richard Fenske, Ph.D.
Assistant Professor of Environmental Science, Rutgers
University, New Brunswick, New Jersey
Chapter 33

Lawrence J. Fine, M.D., Dr.P.H.
Chief, Division of Surveillance, Hazard Evaluations,
and Field Studies, National Institute for Occupational
Safety and Health, Cincinnati, Ohio
Chapter 22

Howard Frumkin, M.D., M.P.H.
Assistant Professor of Medicine, University of
Pennsylvania School of Medicine,
Philadelphia, Pennsylvania
Chapters 14 and 15 and Appendixes A and B

Nelson M. Gantz, M.D., F.A.C.P.
Professor of Medicine and Microbiology and Clinical
Director of Infectious Diseases, Department of
Medicine, University of Massachusetts Medical School;
Hospital Epidemiologist, University of Massachusetts
Medical Center, Worcester, Massachusetts
Chapter 19

Bernard D. Goldstein, M.D.
Professor and Chairman, Department of
Environmental and Community Medicine, University
of Medicine and Dentistry of New Jersey-Robert Wood
Johnson Medical School, Piscataway, New Jersey
Chapter 28

William E. Halperin, M.D., M.P.H.
Chief, Industrywide Studies Branch, Division of
Surveillance, Hazard Evaluations, and Field Studies,
National Institute for Occupational Safety and Health,
Cincinnati, Ohio
Chapter 6

Roger P. Hamernik, Ph.D.
Professor, Physics and Speech and Hearing
Departments, and Director, Auditory Research
Laboratories, State University of New York at
Plattsburgh, Plattsburgh, New York
Chapter 17

Maureen C. Hatch, Ph.D.
Assistant Professor of Epidemiology, Columbia
University School of Public Health, New York,
New York
Chapter 26

Jay Himmelstein, M.D., M.P.H.
Assistant Professor of Family and Community
Medicine, University of Massachusetts Medical School;
Associate Director, Occupational Health Program,
University of Massachusetts Medical Center,
Worcester, Massachusetts
Chapter 12

Howard Hu, M.D., M.P.H., M.S.
Research Fellow, Departments of Epidemiology and
Occupational Health, Harvard School of Public
Health; Clinical Instructor, Department of Medicine,
Boston City Hospital, Boston, Massachusetts
Chapter 18 and Appendix B

Daniel E. Kass, M.S.P.H.
Trainer, Hunter-Montefiore Health and Safety Training
Program, Department of Community Health
Education, Hunter College, New York, New York
Appendix C

Nicolas Kaufman, B.A.
Filmmaker, Nick Kaufman Productions,
Newtonville, Massachusetts
Photographs

W. Monroe Keyserling, Ph.D.
Assistant Professor of Industrial and Operations
Engineering, University of Michigan,
Ann Arbor, Michigan
Chapters 8 and 9

Howard M. Kipen, M.D., M.P.H.
Assistant Professor of Environmental and Community
Medicine, University of Medicine and Dentistry of
New Jersey-Robert Wood Johnson Medical School,
Piscataway, New Jersey; Attending Physician,
Department of Medicine, Robert Wood Johnson
University Hospital, New Brunswick, New Jersey
Chapter 28

Philip J. Landrigan, M.D., M.S.
Professor of Community Medicine and Pediatrics,
Mount Sinai School of Medicine of the City University
of New York, New York, New York
Chapter 30

Charles Levenstein, Ph.D., M.S.(O.H.)
Professor, Department of Work Environment, College
of Engineering, University of Lowell,
Lowell, Massachusetts
Chapter 2 and Box, Chapter 1

Barry S. Levy, M.D., M.P.H.
Professor and Director, Occupational Health Program,
Department of Family and Community Medicine,
University of Massachusetts Medical Center,
Worcester, Massachusetts
Chapters 1, 3, 4, 6, and 15

Ken Light, B.G.S.
Vallejo, California
Former Photographer and Filmmaker, Labor
Occupational Health Program, University of California
at Berkeley, Berkeley, California
Photographs

Ruth Lilis, M.D.
Professor, Department of Community Medicine,
Mount Sinai School of Medicine of the City University
of New York; Attending Physician, Mount Sinai
Hospital, New York, New York
Chapter 30

Marian Marbury, Sc.D.
Environmental Epidemiologist, Minnesota Department
of Health, Minneapolis, Minnesota
Appendix to Chapter 31

James Melius, M.D.
Division of Environmental Health Assessment, New
York State Department of Health, Albany, New York
Appendix A

René Mendes, M.D., Dr.P.H.
Professor of Occupational Health, School of Medical
Sciences, State University of Campinas, Campinas,
Brazil; Regional Adviser on Occupational Safety and
Health, International Labor Office, São Paulo, Brazil
Chapter 36

David Michaels, Ph.D., M.P.H.
Assistant Professor, Department of Epidemiology and
Social Medicine, Albert Einstein College of Medicine
of Yeshiva University; Director, Program in
Occupational Health, Montefiore Medical Center,
Bronx, New York
Chapter 36 and Appendix to Chapter 3

Larry M. Miller, Ph.D.
Associate Professor and Chair, Department of
Sociology and Anthropology, Southeastern
Massachusetts University, North Dartmouth,
Massachusetts
Chapter 2

**Gustavo E. Molina, M.D., M.Occ.H.,
M.P.H.**
Epidemiologist, Pan American Center for Human
Ecology and Health, Pan American Health
Organization, World Health Organization, Metepec,
Mexico
Photographs

John M. Peters, M.D.
Professor of Preventive Medicine, University of
Southern California School of Medicine,
Los Angeles, California
Box, Chapter 1

Glenn S. Pransky, M.D., M.Occ.H.
Assistant Professor, Department of Family and
Community Medicine, University of Massachusetts
Medical School, Worcester, Massachusetts
Chapters 12 and 29

Laura Punnett, Sc.D.
Assistant Professor, Department of Work Environment,
College of Engineering, University of Lowell,
Lowell, Massachusetts
Box, Chapter 31

Margaret M. Quinn, M.S., M.I.H.
Chief, Industrial Hygiene Services, Occupational
Health Program, University of Massachusetts Medical
School, Worcester, Massachusetts
Chapters 31 and Box, Chapter 4

Kathleen M. Rest, M.P.A.
Pew Fellow, Health Policy Institute, Boston University,
Boston, Massachusetts
Chapter 13

Cathy Schwartz, R.N.
Women's Committee, Massachusetts Coalition
of Occupational Safety and Health,
Boston, Massachusetts
Box, Chapter 31

Barbara A. Silverstein, Ph.D.
Assistant Research Scientist, Department of
Environmental and Industrial Health, University
of Michigan School of Public Health,
Ann Arbor, Michigan
Chapter 22

Michael Silverstein, M.D., M.P.H.
Assistant Director, Health and Safety Department,
International Union, United Automobile Workers,
Detroit, Michigan
Chapter 35

David H. Sliney, M.S.
Chief, Laser Branch, Laser Microwave Division,
United States Army Environmental Hygiene Agency,
Aberdeen Proving Ground, Maryland
Chapter 24

Thomas J. Smith, Ph.D.
Professor of Family and Community Medicine and Co-
director, Environmental Health Sciences Program,
University of Massachusetts Medical School,
Worcester, Massachusetts
Chapter 7

Stover H. Snook, Ph.D.
Project Director, Ergonomics, Liberty Mutual
Insurance Company, Hopkinton, Massachusetts;
Lecturer on Ergonomics, Harvard School of Public
Health, Boston, Massachusetts
Chapter 22

**Corinne J. Solomon, R.N., M.P.H.,
C.O.H.N.**
Assistant Professor, Occupational Health, Department
of Nursing, Graduate Program, Simmons College,
Boston, Massachusetts; President and Consultant, CJ
Associates, Hopkinton, Massachusetts
Box, Chapter 34

Frederick P. Sperounis, Ph.D.
Associate Professor of Sociology, University of Lowell;
Vice President of University Relations and
Development, University of Lowell,
Lowell, Massachusetts
Chapter 2

Zena A. Stein, M.A., M.B., B.Ch.
Professor of Public Health (Epidemiology), Columbia
University School of Public Health, New York,
New York
Chapter 26

Edward C. Swanson, M.B.A., P.T.
Program Specialist, The Return to Work Center,
Industrial Rehabilitation Associates, Easthampton,
Massachusetts
Box, Chapter 12

Gilles P. Thériault, M.D., Dr.P.H.
Associate Professor and Director, School of
Occupational Health, McGill University, Attending
Physician, Department of Community Medicine,
Montreal General Hospital, Montreal,
Quebec, Canada
Chapter 27

Nick Thorkelson, B.A.
Graphic Artist, Somerville, Massachusetts
Drawings

**Patricia Hyland Travers, M.S., R.N.,
C.O.H.N.**
Director, Occupational Health Nursing Program,
Educational Resource Center, Harvard School of
Public Health, Boston, Massachusetts
Appendix B

Arthur C. Upton, M.D.
Professor and Director, Institute of Environmental
Medicine, New York University School of Medicine,
New York, New York
Chapter 16

Paul F. Vinger, M.D.
Assistant Clinical Professor of Ophthalmology,
Harvard Medical School, Boston, Massachusetts
Chapter 24

Bailus Walker, Jr., Ph.D., M.P.H.
Professor of Environmental Health, School of Public
Health Sciences, State University of New York at
Albany, Albany, New York
Chapter 32

James L. Weeks, Sc.D., C.I.H.
Deputy Administrator for Occupational Health,
Occupational Health and Safety Department, United
Mine Workers of America, Washington, D.C.
Boxes, Chapters 10 and 35

David H. Wegman, M.D., M.S.
Professor and Head, Department of Work
Environment, College of Engineering, and Director,
Work Environment Laboratory, Center for
Productivity Enhancement, University of Lowell,
Lowell, Massachusetts
Chapters 1, 3, 4, 5, and 21

Susan R. Woskie, M.S.
Research Industrial Hygienist, Department of Family
and Community Medicine, University
of Massachusetts Medical School,
Worcester, Massachusetts
Chapter 31

Gu Xue-qi, M.D., M.P.H.
Professor, Department of Occupational Health,
Shanghai Medical University, Shanghai, People's
Republic of China
Chapter 36

Richard A. Youngstrom, M.S., M.S.(IH)
IUE Local 201 Health and Safety Coordinator,
Lynn, Massachusetts
Box, Chapter 35

Stephen Zoloth, Ph.D., M.P.H.
Associate Professor, Hunter College School of Health
Sciences, New York, New York; Program in
Occupational Health, Department of Epidemiology
and Social Medicine, Montefiore Medical Center,
Bronx, New York
Appendix to Chapter 3

1
Occupational Health in the United States: An Overview

Barry S. Levy and David H. Wegman

A pregnant woman who works as a laboratory technician asks her obstetrician if she should change her job or stop working because of the chemicals to which she and her fetus are exposed.

A middle-aged man visits his orthopedic surgeon and states that he is totally disabled from chronic back pain, which he attributes to lifting heavy objects for many years as a construction worker.

A long-distance truck driver asks his cardiologist how soon after his recent myocardial infarction he will be able to return to work and what kinds of tasks he will be able to perform.

A former asbestos worker with lung cancer asks his surgeon if he can submit a claim for workers' compensation for his disease.

An oncologist observes an unusual cluster of bladder cancer cases among middle-aged women in a small town.

The vice-president of a small tool and die company asks a local family physician to advise his company regarding prevention of occupational disease among his employees.

A pediatric nurse practitioner diagnoses lead poisoning in a young child and wonders if the source of the lead may be dust brought home on the workclothes of the father, who works in a battery plant.

And three women who work for a plastics company, all complaining of severe rashes on their hands and forearms, consult an internist, who believes their problems may be work-related.

These are but a few examples of the numerous occupational health challenges facing health professionals. Virtually all health professionals need to be able to deal with these challenges effectively. They therefore need to be able to recognize, manage, and prevent work-related injuries and diseases.

THE UNITED STATES WORKFORCE

Before discussing various aspects of work-related medical problems in the United States, it is useful to consider the "at risk" group: the American workforce. Work and the work ethic are basic to life in the United States. Most adults spend almost one-fourth of their time at work, and despite the high degree of automation and computerization of American industry, many workers are exposed to dust, chemicals, noise, and other workplace hazards. Table 1-1 categorizes the almost 110 million workers in the United States by industry, and Table 1-2, by occupation (Fig. 1-1). Over 40 percent of the U.S. workforce consists of women (Fig. 1-2). These statistics overlook full-time homemakers, who are usually not included in data on the U.S. workforce. Approximately 18 percent of American workers belong to unions, a lower percentage than in most industrialized nations. Most U.S. workers are employed by small or moderate-size firms that do not employ physicians or other health professionals to provide health and safety programs.

Only about 1,000 occupational health physicians who have been certified by the American

3

**Table 1-1. Employed persons
in the United States, by industry (1986)**

Industry	Size of workforce (in millions)
Agriculture	3.2
Mining	0.9
Construction	7.3
Manufacturing	21.0
Transportation, communications, and public utilities	7.7
Wholesale trade	4.4
Retail trade	18.4
Finance, insurance, real estate	7.4
Private services	34.3
Public administration	5.1
Total	109.6*

*Because of rounding, the sum of the components does not
add up to the total.
Source: Employment and earnings. Bureau of Labor Statistics, U.S. Department of Labor, 1987.

**Table 1-2. Employed persons in the
United States, by occupational category (1986)**

Occupational category	Number of workers (in millions)
Executive, administrative, and managerial workers	12.6
Professional workers	13.9
Technicians and related support workers	3.4
Sales workers	13.2
Administrative support workers, including clerical workers	17.7
Precision production, craft, and repair workers	13.4
Operators, fabricators, and laborers, except transport	12.5
Transport equipment operators	4.6
Service workers	14.7
Farming, forestry, and fishing industry workers	3.4
Total	109.6*

*Total slightly greater than sum of above because of rounding off numbers.
Source: Employment and earnings. Bureau of Labor Statistics, U.S. Department of Labor, 1987.

Board of Preventive Medicine practice in the United States. Therefore, most workers with work-related medical problems are treated by physicians who have little or no training in occupational health. Similar shortages exist for qualified occupational health nurses and other personnel in the field.

MAGNITUDE OF THE PROBLEM

Workers in the United States and elsewhere are exposed to a wide range of occupational health and safety hazards (Figs. 1-3, 1-4, and 1-5). An estimated 20 million work-related injuries and 390,000 new work-related illnesses occur each year in the United States. However, the number of occupational diseases and injuries reported each year is much lower. Analyses of reported injuries by industry and reported illnesses by category are shown in Tables 1-3 and 1-4. In addition, it is estimated that there may be 100,000 or more work-related deaths in the United States each

year. According to the NIOSH National Traumatic Occupational Fatality data base, approximately 7,000 *traumatic* occupational fatalities occur in the United States each year; the highest rates are in mining (30 per 100,000 workers per year), construction (23 per 100,000), and agriculture (20 per 100,000). While these statistics provide some idea of the scope and types of occupational medical problems, they grossly underestimate the role of the workplace in causing new diseases and injuries and exacerbating existing ones. In addition, statistics do not represent the relative distribution of various work-related diseases. For example, because skin disorders are easy to recognize and to relate to working conditions, their representation in Table 1-4 (33 percent of all work-related disorders) exaggerates their relative importance. As indicated in the box on page 10, myths about

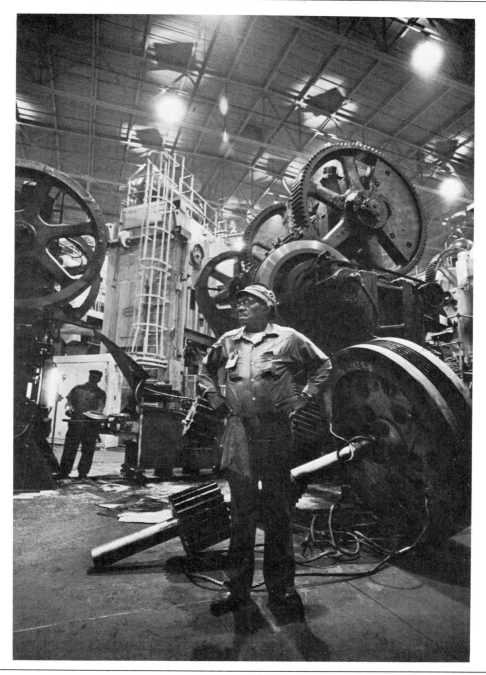

Fig. 1-1. While a declining percentage of workers in the United States work in heavy manufacturing, it still represents a major part of the economy and a source of many occupational health and safety hazards.
(Photograph by Earl Dotter.)

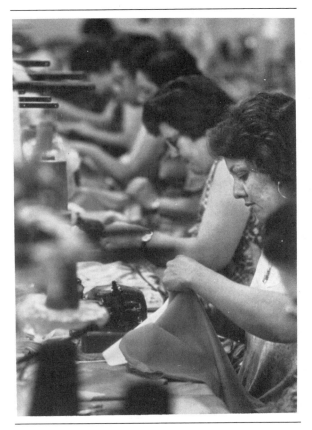

Fig. 1-2. The garment industry, largely unchanged in this century, is a major employer of women, who constitute over 40 percent of the U.S. workforce. (Photograph by Earl Dotter.)

work-related disease impede the identification of occupational health problems.

The difficulty in obtaining accurate estimates of the frequency of work-related diseases is due to several factors:

1. Many problems do not come to the attention of health professionals and employers and, therefore, are not included in data collection systems. A worker may not recognize a medical problem as being work-related, but even when the connection is obvious, a variety of disincentives may deter the worker from reporting such a problem, the greatest being fear of losing a job. Training workers about both occupational hazards and legal rights has been helpful.

2. Many occupational medical problems that do come to the attention of physicians and employers are not recognized as work-related. Recognition of work-related disease is often difficult because of the long period between initial exposure and onset of symptoms (or time of diagnosis), making cause-effect relationships difficult to assess. It is also difficult because of the many and varied occupational and nonoccupational hazards to which most workers are exposed. Training of health professionals in occupational health has begun to reverse this trend.

3. Some medical problems recognized by health professionals or employers as work-related are not reported because the association with work is equivocal and because reporting requirements are not strict. The initiation of occupational disease surveillance activities by federal and state governments has begun to address this problem.

4. Because many occupational medical problems are preventable, their very persistence implies that some individual or group is legally and economically responsible for creating or perpetuating them.

Two important aspects of occupational disease distinguish it from other medical problems:

Recognition of work-related medical problems is almost totally dependent on obtaining occupational information in the medical history. The health professional must know when to suspect a work-related medical problem and what questions to ask in an occupational history to evaluate the work-relatedness of that problem (see Chap. 3).

In contrast to many nonoccupational diseases, occupational diseases can almost always be prevented. Most occupational medical problems can be alleviated by a variety of preventive approaches in which professionals in health, safety, and other fields play vital roles (see Chap. 4).

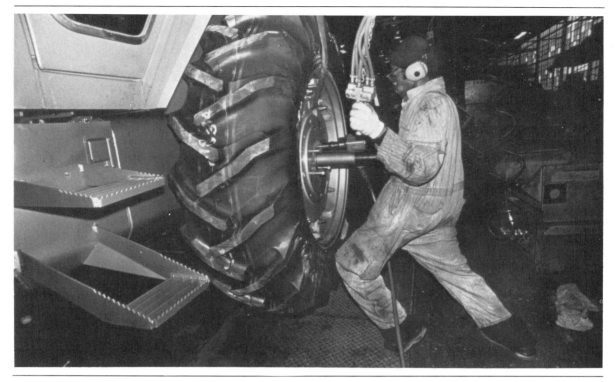

Fig. 1-3. Mixed occupational hazards occur in many jobs. This worker is exposed to loud noise and risk of low back injury.
(Photograph by Earl Dotter.)

CURRENT CONCERNS WITH OCCUPATIONAL HEALTH ISSUES

Although occupational health in the United States has a long history (see box on page 11), legislation, social activism, educational activities, and other developments have contributed to increased interest in work-related medical problems in recent years. Some of these developments are summarized below.

Governmental Role

With the passage of the Federal Coal Mine Safety and Health Act of 1969 and the Occupational Safety and Health Act (OSHAct) of 1970, the federal government began taking a more active role in the creation and enforcement of standards for a safe and healthful workplace (see Chap. 10). In addition, the OSHAct established the National Institute for Occupational Safety and Health (NIOSH), which has (1) greatly expanded epidemiologic and laboratory research into the causes of occupational diseases and injuries and the methods of preventing them; and (2) begun to strengthen the training of occupational health and safety professionals.

Occupational Safety and Health Education

A variety of factors have contributed to a recent growth in education and training opportunities for workers, employers, health professionals, and others. Unions have recently directed more attention to occupational health and safety through

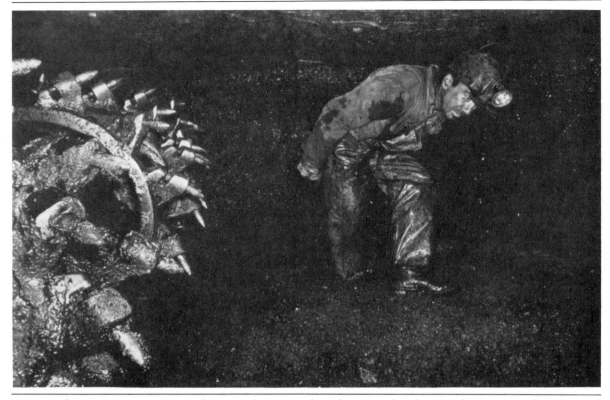

Fig. 1-4. The continuous mining machine greatly increased productivity of underground mines as well as dust and noise exposure.
(Photograph by Earl Dotter.)

collective bargaining agreements, hiring of health professionals, workplace health and safety committees, educational programs, and support of epidemiologic studies. Worker education has been facilitated by Right-to-Know laws and regulations, independent coalitions for occupational safety and health (COSH groups) (see Appendix C), employer-sponsored programs, and academic institutions concerned with occupational health and safety. When available, government funds for medical student, resident, and other professional training programs in occupational health have improved existing professional training opportunities and created new ones. Furthermore, alerted to the critical problems associated with asbestos, lead,

pesticides, and ionizing radiation, the mass media have made the public aware of many workplace hazards.

Concern with Social and Ethical Questions
Serious social and ethical problems have arisen in recent years concerning such subjects as allegiance of occupational physicians who are employed by management, workers' "Right to Know" about job hazards, confidentiality of workers' medical records kept by employers, and restricting female workers of childbearing age from certain jobs. Controversies relating to such subjects will eventually be settled by labor-management negotiations and by the deliberations of the courts and

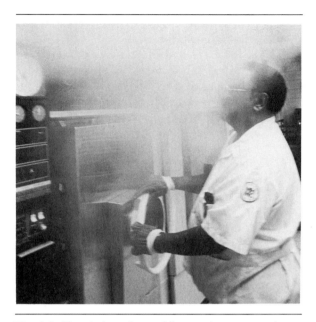

Fig. 1-5. Hospital worker, while opening an autoclave, is exposed to carcinogenic ethylene oxide gas. Hospital workers are exposed to chemical, biologic, and physical hazards as well as psychological stress at work. (Photograph by Earl Dotter.)

legislative and executive bodies of government. As an example, in 1980 the United States Supreme Court upheld a worker's right to refuse hazardous work; it ruled that he or she could not be discharged or discriminated against for exercising the right not to work under conditions he or she reasonably believed to be very dangerous.

Workplace-Related Health and Medical Programs

Health care is increasingly available in or near the workplace. Increasingly the emphasis is on prevention programs focused on education and screening. Some programs deal not only with specific occupational medical problems but also with problems such as hypertension and smoking that may be a function of the personal lifestyles of workers. In recent years, there has been substantial

Table 1-3. Occupational injury incidence rates in the United States, by industry, private sector, 1985

Industry	Number of injuries per 100 full-time workers
Construction	15.0
Agriculture, forestry, and fishing	11.0
Manufacturing	10.0
Transportation and public utilities	8.5
Mining	8.3
Retail trade	7.5
Wholesale trade	7.1
Services	5.3
Finance, insurance, and real estate	1.9
Average	7.7

Source: Bureau of Labor Statistics, U.S. Department of Labor, 1987.

Table 1-4. Distribution of occupational illnesses in the United States, by category of illness, private sector, 1985

Category of illness	Estimated number[a]	Percent
Skin diseases or disorders	41,800	33
Disorders associated with repeated trauma	37,000	30
Respiratory conditions due to toxic agents	11,600	9
Disorders due to physical agents	9,000	7
Poisoning	4,200	3
Dust diseases of the lungs	1,700	1
All other occupational illnesses	20,100	16
Total	125,400	99[b]

[a]Excludes firms with fewer than 11 employees.
[b]Sum is slightly less than 100 percent because numbers above are rounded off.
Source: Bureau of Labor Statistics, U.S. Department of Labor, 1987.

growth in both academic-oriented occupational health clinics and free-standing or hospital-based community clinics providing occupational medicine services. A number of hospital-based programs have been designed primarily for financial reasons; the impact of these on occupational disease and injury prevention is not yet clear.

Liability

An extremely controversial force in occupational health is the product liability suit. Workers, barred from suing their employers under workers' compensation laws and unhappy about deregulation of the workplace, have increasingly turned to "third party," or product liability, suits as a means of getting redress for occupational disease. Liability suits are not a particularly effective way to ensure compensation on a general scale because of the uncertainty of the jury system. However, the fear of liability suits has driven many employers to preventive activity. Although such suits currently play an important role in directing attention to prevention of some diseases, the method is cumbersome and inequitable. Most recently, some jurisdictions have turned to criminal prosecution of the most egregious health and safety offenders. It is hoped that in the future these problems can be dealt with in a more rational way.

Advances in Technology

Recent advances in technology have facilitated the identification of workplace hazards and potential hazards. Most notable are in vitro assays to determine mutagenicity (and to suspect carcinogenicity) of substances, improvements in ways of determining the presence and measuring the levels of workplace hazards, and new methods of monitoring concentrations of hazardous substances in body fluids and the physiologic impairments they cause.

The Environmental Movement

Public concern for a safe and healthful environment, from protecting air, soil, and water from contamination to ensuring safety in consumer products, extends to the workplace. It is increas-

---

12 MYTHS ABOUT WORK-RELATED DISEASE—John M. Peters

1. "It can't be a bad place to work. Joe has been working here for 45 years and there is nothing wrong with him."
2. "It is only statistical, so it is of no clinical significance."
3. "Our working population is healthier than the average population."
4. "There is no problem—the exposure level is below the standard."
5. "It will cost too much to control the problem; it will put us out of business."
6. "It is only a mortality study and you know how inaccurate death certificates are."
7. "Okay, there is a problem, but it is not the occupational exposure. It is all the smoking and drinking the workers do."
8. "Exposures are good for people because they keep up their defenses. If we stop exposing them, their defenses will break down."
9. "If there is a problem, it is because of all the old exposures that do not exist any longer."
10. "We have this party for retired people and they all look great."
11. "Don't tell the workers; they will only worry."
12. "If there is a problem, the nurses and doctors in the clinic would know about it because the workers would tell them."

---

ingly recognized that, when considering asbestos or pesticides, noise or radiation, there is a continuum of exposures that extends from the workplace to the general environment.

CONCLUSION

Some readers of this text will at some time work with management, labor, or government, and a few will become full-time occupational health professionals. However, almost all health professionals who read it will at times have to deal

A BRIEF HISTORY OF OCCUPATIONAL HEALTH IN THE UNITED STATES
—Charles Levenstein

Only rarely in United States history has occupational health received substantial attention from the public. The reason for this may be that our nation has been so deeply committed to progress through industrial and technical advance that we have not wanted to acknowledge some of the more tragic human costs involved. Or it may be that the fairly grim struggle of workers simply to make a living has made attention to the health hazards of employment seem secondary. Or it may be that the American labor movement has not been strong enough to drive home the point to society at large that, in fact, work in the United States has often been dangerous to health.

Occupational medicine in Europe has a much larger tradition. As early as the sixteenth century Paracelsus studied occupational problems of miners and foundry and smelter workers. Agricola's work on mining and metallurgy, *De re metallica*, was also written in the sixteenth century. However, Bernardino Ramazzini (1633–1714) is generally accepted as the parent of industrial medicine; his compendium of health hazards of the medieval crafts is harked back to even today.

In the United States the onset of the Industrial Revolution brought with it some public concern, particularly for safety problems. In 1867 Massachusetts created the first department of factory inspection in the country, and ten years later enacted the first job safety law, which required guards for textile spinning machinery. The Knights of Labor, the leading labor organization in the 1870s and 1880s, demanded "the adoption of measures providing for the health and safety of those engaged in mining and manufacturing, building industries, and for indemnification . . . for injuries." By 1900 most heavily industrialized states had minimal legislation dealing with employment hazards. In addition, more than 200 publications concerning occupational diseases appeared before 1900.

The real burst in activity and concern for occupational safety and health, however, occurred after 1900. By then, the shaping of the modern industrial economy was proceeding at full steam, and labor unrest was expressed in union activity and political and social protest. Factories then used much lead and many other toxic materials. The chemical industry was confronting workers with new dangers, and the introduction of machinery, the use of lifting tackle and conveyors, and the sheer increase in the size of manufacturing operations were causing serious problems for worker safety.

At earlier stages of industrial development employers had successfully avoided financial responsibility for injuries to employees, but by 1900 workers were winning court suits against negligent firms. In 1910 the National Association of Manufacturers and the National Civic Federation, whose members included large corporations, began to lobby extensively for state workers' compensation laws. These laws provided a limited, insurable, no-fault liability system that would assure injured workers some economic protection without subjecting employers to unpredictable and conceivably larger payments.

At about the same time, Dr. Alice Hamilton, then living among immigrant working people in Chicago, began her long career studying toxic exposures in industry. Her work on lead received national attention and in 1919 she became the first female Harvard faculty member when she was appointed to the recently organized industrial hygiene program. Also, in 1910, the Joint Board of Sanitary Control of the Cloak, Suit, and Skirt Industry of Greater New York was established as a result of a massive strike of garment workers; the first National Conference on Industrial Diseases was held; Cornell Medical College established an occupational disease clinic in New York; the U.S.

Bureau of Mines was created; and the U.S. Public Health Service began its studies in industrial health.

During the next decade, occupational health concern and activity accelerated, especially with the onset of World War I and the accompanying increase in federal government attention to labor for the war effort. In 1913 the National Safety Council was organized and began its "safety first" educational activities. In 1916 the predecessor organization to the American Occupational Medical Association was established. Although virtually all of the leading figures in the group were company physicians, Joseph W. Schereschewsky, M.D., head of the federal office of industrial hygiene, was elected its first president. Two years later, Harry Mock, M.D., medical director for a large retail sales company, became the second president. His motto was "Physical qualifications, plus occupational qualifications, equal a job," an indication of his focus on physical examination for job placement rather than on industrial hygiene. By 1920 the workers' compensation legislative effort had largely succeeded, although the American labor movement expressed serious reservations about its adequacy. Trade unionists also were not happy about the company physician focus on pre-employment physical examinations rather than on occupational health hazards.

Although Dr. Hamilton and others continued their studies, and occasional "scandals" like cancer among young radium watch dial painters did reach the public eye, it was not until the resurgence of the labor movement in the 1930s that national attention was again directed to occupational health problems. Passed in 1936, the Walsh-Healey Public Contracts Act required compliance with health and safety standards by employers receiving federal contracts over $10,000. Then, as war became imminent, the federal government provided funds to states for industrial health and safety programs, and the Bureau of Mines was authorized to inspect and investigate mine hazards.

Despite the Walsh-Healey Act, the 1940s, 1950s, and 1960s were decades without substantial new attention directed to occupational health problems. Workers' compensation legislation was thought to have dealt with the key problems by providing income security to injured workers and an economic incentive to employers to maintain safe working conditions. Attention to occupational disease was placed on a back shelf; workers only rarely received compensation for disabilities resulting from the less obvious industrial health problems such as occupational cancer with its long period between exposure and onset of symptoms. An exception to the general neglect of the field was the establishment of radiation safety standards with passage of the Atomic Energy Act in 1954.

Labor's political and economic strength had been severely depleted in the postwar period, and it was not until the beginning of the environmental movement in the 1960s that concern about the polluted working environment again became widespread. The 29 percent increase in industrial accident rates that occurred between 1961 and 1970 stirred up great concern in the trade union movement. The new era of struggles over occupational health problems really began, however, with the death of 78 miners in a 1968 coal mine explosion in Farmington, West Virginia. This tragedy placed industrial health and safety on the political agenda of the nation in a way that day-to-day human damage could not. In 1969 the Coal Mine Health and Safety Act was passed, and a year later the Occupational Safety and Health Act was made federal law. In 1972 the Black Lung Benefits Act was passed. The Toxic Substances Control Act, enacted in 1976, provided for extensive restriction of the hazards of the chemical industry. In addition to regulatory efforts, some firms took individual initiatives in dealing with hazards; also, labor and management developed joint schemes for hazard investigation and control.

By the end of the 1970s, however, the political impetus that had put occupational health high on the nation's agenda was being undercut by the economic crisis and powerful opposition.

During the 1980s, conservative backlash has resulted in federal deregulation of occupational safety and health, weakening OSHA and increasing reliance on voluntary compliance with standards. Progress in the development of new standards has come to a virtual halt and the NIOSH budget has suffered. Important new initiatives have developed on a local level, however, that have sometimes forced national attention. Grassroots coalitions of occupational health activists, local trade unions, and environmental groups (sometimes called COSH groups) have been able to get "Right-to-Know" laws passed in many states and cities and ultimately pushed a reluctant OSHA to promulgate the Hazard Communication Standard. Workers' increasing reliance on product liability suits and most recently on criminal prosecutions is evidence, however, of the failure of the federal government to pursue seriously the fulfillment of its duty to ensure safe and healthful workplaces to all American workers.

After 14 years of legal struggle, farm workers finally won a field sanitation standard—only because the courts insisted that OSHA take action. In occupational health as in many other socially progressive fields, political attention focused on the role of the courts and the ideological position of judges, as a conservative presidential administration attempted to consolidate its victories in deregulating the workplace. The rise of company "worksite health promotion" and fitness campaigns drew employer attention away from controlling environments and aimed at altering individual employee behavior.

The 1980s are demonstrating that occupational safety and health have taken a permanent place of high priority to American workers, but that significant ideological and powerful political (and economic) forces oppose realization of a safe and healthful workplace for all.

with work-related medical problems. Pulmonary disease specialists see asbestosis and occupational asthma; ophthalmologists diagnose and treat work-related conjunctivitis and foreign bodies in the eye; orthopedic surgeons frequently evaluate work-related musculoskeletal disorders; and providers of primary care are confronted with a wide range of medical problems that either are work-related—such as trauma, back and skin problems, and toxic reactions—or have a critical impact on the patient's capacity to work. Clearly, all types of health professionals have a vital role in recognizing and preventing work-related disease.

BIBLIOGRAPHY (suggested books for beginning an occupational health library)

Ashford NA. Crisis in the workplace. Cambridge: MIT Press, 1976.
An in-depth analysis of the technical, legal, political and economic problems in occupational health and safety.
Brodeur P. Expendable Americans. New York: Viking, 1974.
A detailed account of the sociopolitical forces that have worked against dissemination of research information on occupational hazards and effective enforcement of occupational health and safety laws. Focus on asbestos.
Burgess W. Recognition of health hazards in industry: A review of materials and processes. New York: Wiley, 1981.
An excellent summary of industrial hazards.
Hamilton A. Exploring the dangerous trades; an autobiography. Boston: Little, Brown, 1943.
A classic historical reference.
Hunter D. The diseases of occupations. 6th ed. London: Hodder & Stoughton, 1978.
A comprehensive but uncritical review of the history and related literature of occupational health.

Proctor NH, Hughes JP. Chemical hazards of the work-place. Philadelphia: Lippincott, 1978.
Brief summaries on 386 chemical hazards, including basics about their chemical, physical, and toxicologic characteristics; diagnostic criteria, including special tests; and treatment and medical control measures.

Rom W. ed. Environmental and occupational medicine. Boston: Little, Brown, 1983.
An excellent in-depth textbook.

Schilling RSF. ed. Occupational health practice. 2nd ed. London: Butterworths, 1981.
A general overview of occupational disease and health services with a British orientation.

Zenz C. ed. Occupational medicine: Principles and practical applications. 2nd ed. Chicago: Year Book, 1988.
Broad and detailed review designed for physicians with responsibility for occupational medical departments in industry and occupational physicians in general.

Zenz C. ed. Developments in occupational medicine. Chicago: Year Book, 1980.
A good complement to Zenz's other book, covering different topics as well as sections on epidemiology and health considerations for women at work.

SELECTED PERIODICAL PUBLICATIONS IN OCCUPATIONAL HEALTH DISCIPLINES

Occupational Health and Occupational Medicine

American Journal of Industrial Medicine, published monthly by Alan R. Liss, Inc., 41 E. 11th Street, New York, NY 10003.

British Journal of Industrial Medicine, published monthly by the British Medical Association, Tavistock Square, London WC1H 9JR (U.S. address: 1172 Commonwealth Avenue, Boston, MA 02134).

Journal of Occupational Medicine, published monthly by the American Occupational Medical Association, 55 West Seegers Road, Arlington Heights, IL 60005.

Scandinavian Journal of Work, Environment, and Health, published bimonthly by occupational health agencies and boards in Finland, Sweden, Norway, and Denmark; address: Haartmaninkatu 1, SF-00290, Helsinki 29, Finland.

Seminars in Occupational Medicine, published quarterly by Thieme Inc., 381 Park Avenue South, New York, NY 10016.

State of the Art Reviews: Occupational Medicine, published quarterly by Hanley & Belfus, Inc., 210 S. 13th Street, Philadelphia, PA 19107.

Occupational Health Nursing

American Association of Occupational Health Nurses Journal, published monthly, 50 Lenox Pointe, Atlanta GA 30324.

Industrial Hygiene

American Industrial Hygiene Association Journal, published monthly by the American Industrial Hygiene Association, 475 Wolf Ledges Parkway, Akron, OH 44311-1087.

The Annals of Occupational Hygiene, published quarterly by Pergamon Journals, Maxwell House, Fairview Park, Elmsford, NY 10523 (alternate address: Headington Hill Hall, Oxford OX3 0BW, United Kingdom).

Applied Industrial Hygiene, published bimonthly by Applied Industrial Hygiene, Inc., a subsidiary of the American Conference of Governmental Industrial Hygienists, 6500 Glenway Avenue, Building D-7, Cincinnati, OH 45211-4438.

Occupational Safety

Journal of Occupational Accidents, published quarterly by Elsevier, Journal Information Center, 52 Vanderbilt Avenue, New York, NY 10017.

Professional Safety, published monthly by the American Society of Safety Engineers, 1800 E. Oakton Street, Des Plaines, IL 60018-2187.

Safety and Health, published monthly by the National Safety Council, 444 N. Michigan Avenue, Chicago, IL 60611.

General News and Scientific Update Publications

BNA Reporter, published weekly by the Bureau of National Affairs, 1231 25th Street N.W., Washington, D.C. 20027.

Occupational and Environmental Health Report, published monthly by Curtis Vovwie, 12 Marshall Street, Boston, MA 02108.

Occupational Health and Safety Letter, published biweekly by ENVIRONEWS, INC., 1331 Pennsylvania Avenue N.W., Washington, D.C. 20004.

2
The American Workplace:
A Sociological Perspective

Frederick P. Sperounis, Larry M. Miller, and Charles Levenstein

"... we must first of all recall a principle that has always been taught by the Church: the principle of the priority of labor over capital. *This principle directly concerns the process of production: in this process labor is always a primary* efficient cause, *while capital, the whole collection of means of production, remains a mere* instrument *or instrumental cause. This principle is an evident truth that emerges from the whole of man's historical experience."*
Pope John Paul II, *On Human Work* (1981)

To be effective in recognizing and preventing work-related diseases and injuries, health and safety professionals need an understanding of workplaces and an appreciation for the nature of work. This chapter presents a perspective that can enable one to have a clearer understanding of work and workplaces in the United States today.

THE DIFFERENCE BETWEEN WORK AND LABOR

Work is a necessary human activity. People work to survive. Even those who do not work rely on others working. Many of those whose work returns much more to them than mere survival could not survive without it. Still, the experience of work is very different from person to person and from situation to situation. The word *work,* as it is commonly used, blurs important distinctions that are not often noticed but are acknowledged all the time in our use of the terms *work* and *labor.* Hard work is thought of as healthy; hard labor is puni-

tive. Workers are a general category; laborers are those who engage in the most back-breaking and mindless chores. This distinction between work and labor is neither trivial nor accidental; it is ancient and found in every European language.

Originally, this linguistic distinction was rooted in a clear practical difference. Work and labor were distinct activities carried on by different groups of people. Labor described the activity of slaves, serfs, and peasants. It was enforced, directed by others, menial, and brutalizing. Work referred to the activities of artists and artisans. It was autonomous, self-directed, creative, and fulfilling. Such technical precision is unnecessary in everyday language, but the concepts involved are important and remain embodied in common English usage to a degree. We may sometimes say *work* when we are referring to labor; we never say *labor* when we are referring to work.

CONFLICT BETWEEN THE PROFIT MOTIVE AND INDIVIDUAL FULFILLMENT

The single most important fact about work in America is that there is little of it. Of the 110 million Americans in the workforce, approximately 92 percent work as employees of others. Approximately one quarter have professional, managerial, or supervisory employment, with varying degrees of partial autonomy and control over their own jobs. These people both work and labor. Most American workers, though, only labor. They find what jobs they can and, by and large, do what they need to do to keep them. They do not choose what they will make, under what conditions they will make it, or what will happen to it afterwards. These choices are made for them by their employers, the sales and labor markets, and the workings of the economy as a whole. Whatever control most Americans have over how much they receive in return for their labor, how long they labor, how hard they labor, and the quality of the workplace environment is acquired in a contractual situation in which the workers' desire for comfort, income, safety, and leisure is continually counterbalanced by the employers' need for profit.

The U.S. government report *Work in America* reviewed a wide range of studies on the attitudes and problems of American workers [1]. The fact that work—in the broad sense—is necessary for physical survival tends to obscure the degree to which work is important to people for its own sake. For example, several studies indicate that most people would continue to work even if they did not need the money. Reasons for this finding include the importance of the social interactions of the workplace, the desire to feel needed, and the desire to contribute to the common good. In addition, industrial sociology studies have shown that workers with high morale and some ability to control the amount of their output often respond to these conditions not by increasing their leisure but by devoting more attention to details of craftsmanship. This reaction, interestingly, often frustrates employers and managers, who see increased craftsmanship as of little economic value compared to increased productivity.

Most workers have profound ambivalence about their jobs. They seek both income and less tangible satisfactions from their work (Fig. 2-1). An unemployed miner reflected [2]:

Some no doubt will find this a sad thing, the fact of me not having any work I mean. Others simply won't notice, while still others, with a more fundamental way of looking at things and sadly lacking a working-class consciousness, will utter some such expression as "Lucky bastard!" . . . Frankly, I hate work. Of course I could

also say with equal truth that I love work; that it is a supremely interesting activity; that it is often fascinating; that I wish I did not have to do it; that I wish I had a job at which I could earn a decent wage. . . .

The contradictions in this statement cannot be written off as the contrariness of human nature; they correspond to contradictions in the real situation. What workers love about work is the opportunity to guide their own lives, to do meaningful things, or "to get back from the activity not only the physical means to live, but also a confirmation of significance, of the process of being oneself and alive in this unique way" [3]. On the other hand workers oppose their work being made meaningless by the ways it is organized by others and bleached of integrity, autonomy, and creativity for reasons of efficiency, productivity, and profit.

THE CONTEMPORARY WORKPLACE

What is the experience of work actually like? First of all, more and more Americans are working for large employers [4]. The process of economic concentration, the absorption of ever larger fractions of the economy into a small number of economic entities, appears inexorable. Of the 1.75 million corporations that existed in 1971, 2,800 held 68 percent of all corporate assets and employed about 38 percent of all private sector employees. In manufacturing, where economic concentration is most advanced, only 11 percent of the nation's manufacturing corporations had more than 100 manufacturing employees. These corporations employed 75 percent of the manufacturing workforce and accounted for 79 percent of all the value added* in manufacturing. A mere 4 percent of manufacturing employers had 250 or more workers; they employed 57 percent of the manufacturing workforce that produced 63 percent of the total value added. It was in such workplaces that work was most fractionated. By 1983, when al-

---

*The value of sales minus the value of material inputs.

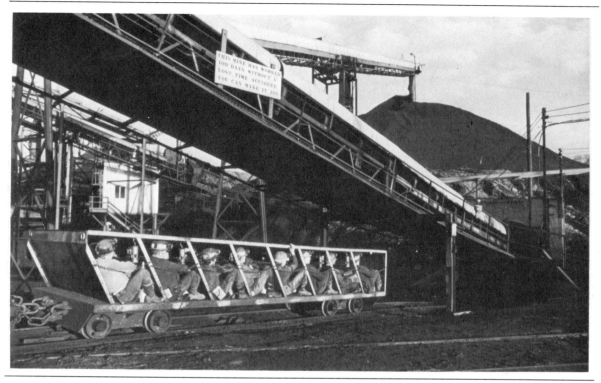

Fig. 2-1. Coal miners on their way to work.
(Photograph by Earl Dotter.)

most 3 million corporations filed tax returns in the United States, the 3,000 largest owned almost 75 percent of corporate assets. The 500 largest industrial concerns owned $1.4 trillion in assets and employed over 14 million workers. The largest 100 companies in this group owned 68 percent of the top 500's assets and employed 59 percent of their workers. The situation had not changed substantially in the 12 years since the 1971 data, noted above, were compiled.

The general tendency in management theory from Adam Smith in 1776 to the present has been to divide work into ever more discrete units to increase productivity, cheapen the cost of labor, and increase management's control over the labor process (Fig. 2-2). This quest for efficiency became more self-conscious and explicit in the early twentieth century with the work of such partisans of scientific management as Taylor and Gilbreth. In their view the worker should be treated not as a whole person but rather as a collection of machine-like movements: walk, bend, grasp, sit, depress typewriter key. Such motions can be analyzed, timed, and reassembled into a program for maximum productivity.

The implementation of such a mechanical conception required that the worker's relationship to work be reduced to the status of a tool. The redesign of production in the twentieth century has consistently aimed at completely separating the conception of work—thinking about what needs to be done, planning, and organization—from its performance. Conception became concentrated in the hands of managers and engineers. Performance

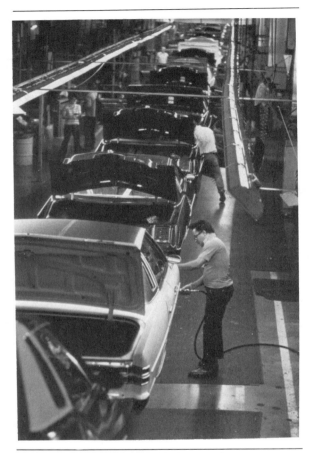

Fig. 2-2. Automobile assembly line workers. (Photograph by Earl Dotter.)

became, by design, necessarily thoughtless. This is well illustrated by the following comment by an automobile assembly line worker [5]:

My father worked in auto for 35 years and he never talked about the job. What's there to say? A car comes, I weld it; a car comes, I weld it; a car comes, I weld it. One hundred and one times an hour. . . . There is a lot of variety in the paint shop . . . you clip on the color hose, bleed out the old color, and squirt. Clip, bleed, squirt, think; clip, bleed, squirt, yawn; clip, bleed, squirt, scratch your nose. Only now the [company has] taken away the time to scratch your nose.

A spot-welder at another automobile assembly plant gave this comment [6]:

I stand in one spot, about [a] two or three feet area, all night. The only time a person stops is when the line stops. We do about 32 jobs per car, per unit. Forty-eight units an hour, eight hours a day. Thirty-two times 48 times eight. Figure it out. That's how many times I push that button. The noise, oh, it's tremendous. You open your mouth and you're liable to get a mouthful of sparks. . . . It don't stop. It just goes and goes and goes and goes. I bet there's men who have lived and died out there, never seen the end of that line. And they never will—because it's endless. It's like a serpent. It's just all body, no tail. It can do things to you. . . . Repetition is such that if you were to think about the job itself, you'd slowly go out of your mind. . . . I don't like the pressure, the intimidation. How would you like to go up to someone and say, "I would like to go to the bathroom?" If the foreman doesn't like you, he'll make you hold it, just ignore you. Should I leave this job to go to the bathroom I risk being fired. The line moves all the time. . . . You really begin to wonder. What price do they put on me? Look at the price they put on the machine. If that machine breaks down, there is somebody out there to fix it right away. If I break down, I'm just pushed over to the other side till another man takes my place. The only thing they have on their mind is to keep that line running.

The fragmentation and simplification of individual tasks in the interest of overall productivity have wide-ranging implications for the quality of work life. With the separation of conception from performance and the division of performance into multiple repetitive tasks, the intrinsic satisfactions of "work," craftsmanship, and the ability to take pride in the whole finished product necessarily diminish. In the absence of such motivation, employers are forced to rely on supervisory hierarchies and monetary rewards and punishments, such as piece rates and bonuses, to motivate workers in carrot-and-stick fashion. The degree to which a rigid shop-floor discipline is imposed can be oppressive, as illustrated by the following quotation from a worker [6]:

You're too busy to talk. Can't hear. They got these little guys coming around in white shirts and if they see you running your mouth, "This guy needs more work." A lot of guys who've been in jail they say you don't work as hard in jail. They say, "Man, jail ain't never been this bad."

An automobile assembly plant worker described the situation as follows [5]:

I'll tell you what it's like, it's like the army. They even use the same words like *direct order*. Supposedly you have a contract so that there are some things they just can't make you do. Except, if the foreman gives you a direct order, you do it, or you're out ... fired or else they give you a DLO—disciplinary layoff. Which means you're out without pay for however long they say. . . . Last week someone up the line put a stinkbomb in a car. I do rear cushions and the foreman says, "You get in that car." We said, "If you can put your head in that car we'll do the job." So the foreman says, "I'm giving you a direct order." So I hold my breath and do it. My job is every other car so I let the next one pass. He gets on me and I say, "Jack, it ain't my car. Please, I done your dirty work and the other one wasn't mine." But he keeps at me and I wind up with a week off. Now, I got a hot committeeman who really stuck up for me. Do you know what? They sent him home too. Gave the committeeman a DLO!

Formally, unionized workers try to regain some control over the labor process through the collective bargaining procedure: through the negotiation of work rules and grievance mechanisms, the institutionalized process for adjudicating individual complaints. However, only 18 percent of workers in the United States are unionized, and, as we have seen above, even where grievance mechanisms exist, they are not always respected. Informally, workers seek what escapes they can find or fabricate. They sneak a surreptitious cigarette, they fantasize, they horse around, and they fight. "Anything so that you don't feel like a machine" is a common refrain. Small acts of sabotage like the stinkbomb occur as vengeance or simply as letting off steam.

In the United States, trade unions have never achieved the power, recognition, and social standing of labor movements in other Western industrial countries. In Great Britain, 55 percent of workers are in unions and, although not currently in power, labor governments have ruled the country. In Sweden, more than 95 percent of blue-collar workers are organized, and approximately 75 percent of white-collar employees are in unions. For most of the past 45 years, Sweden has had a labor government and the labor laws reflect that power [7]. By way of contrast, in the United States about 18 percent of workers are in unions and, except for a brief period during World War II, the unions have had to struggle for their existence. In such a labor relations setting, occupational health and safety issues give way to the effort to establish and keep the right to organize and to have a voice in wage determination, seniority rules, promotions, layoffs, and a host of other "bread-and-butter" issues. Some unions have been successful and militant about health and safety, but employers frequently view such labor efforts as infringements on management's right to control technology. The failure of an important segment of American industry to accept collective bargaining as a legitimate means for workers to express their concerns—and, sometimes, their anger—has resulted in individual informal acts of resistance. It may also have resulted in some workers turning their anger inward and resorting to alcohol or drugs to make it through the day.

THE DRIVE FOR GREATER PRODUCTIVITY

The capital expense involved in modern production leads employers to seek the highest possible rates of productivity. The normal social interactions among workers, which in a less mechanized and fragmented work process appear as part of the rhythm of work itself, are seen as disruptive of production, and attempts on the part of workers to establish some level of control and sociability in the workplace are often misconstrued. Employers and managers who see such acts as threats to productivity and efficiency consider them to be indications of laziness. Workers may view them in a similar way or as efforts to protect themselves against the requirements of a fragmented division of labor that treats them as tools rather than as people. These attempts at greater control actually represent, consciously or unconsciously, the individual's desire to replace labor with work. But the structure of the contemporary workplace undercuts such acts of rebellion and assertion.

This experience of work is not confined to the assembly line; it is typical, if not in detail then certainly in general outline, of most manual work in contemporary America—mining, construction, large-scale agriculture (Fig. 2-3). Furthermore, the assembly line has become the model for organizing many other types of workplaces. As the United States government report *Work in America* noted [1]:

The office today, where work is segmented and authoritarian, is often a factory. For a growing number of jobs, there is little to distinguish them but the color of the worker's collar: computer keypunch operations and typing pools share much in common with the automobile assembly line. Secretaries, clerks, and bureaucrats were once grateful for having been spared the dehumanization of the factory. White-collar jobs were rare; they had higher status than blue-collar jobs. But today the clerk, and not the operative on the assembly line, is the typical American worker, and such positions offer little in the way of prestige. Furthermore, the size of the organizations that employ the bulk of office workers has grown, imparting to the clerical worker the same impartiality that the blue-collar worker experiences in the factory. The organization acknowledges the presence of the worker only when he makes a mistake or fails to follow a rule, whether in factory or bureaucracy, whether under public or private control.

Innovations like word-processing technology and computerized recordkeeping have turned large offices into so many paper-pushing assembly lines. One study cited in the U.S. government report found that clerical office work is routinized and subdivided to such an extreme that, for example, one insurance company had over 350 job titles for its 2,000 clerical employees. The creation of typing pools and the like has broken the close personal tie that frequently existed between secretaries and their employers, and new technology has downgraded the skills required. With these changes, clerical work becomes subject to the same kind of machine-like analysis and control as factory work.

One typist at an insurance company described the oppressiveness of her job this way [8]:

Everything is time-rated. On a particular time rate you're supposed to be able to put out X number of pieces of paper a day. Each sheet has a number that automatically goes on the tape when you push the button. So you can't cheat. . . . The people that sit next to me have been there five, six years. There is no way they're going to go anywhere. I don't want to sit there and type. I think I'm smarter than that. The biggest promotion is, if you're lucky, they might make you a secretary. That's on top of the totem pole. . . . And the petty regulations. You have to ask permission to leave the floor to get a box of cigarettes. You have to ask permission to do just about everything that involves leaving your desk. . . . Very few men in this company have any conception of what it's like to sit and type all day, or ask permission to go to the bathroom.

Or consider the following description of monotony and domination during a working day by the operator of a check-sorting machine at a large bank [8]:

You have to stand on your feet constantly. When you're feeding the machine, you're moving to empty the pockets at the same time and turning around to fill up the tray and putting the tray when it's full to the other side. . . . They don't have any fresh air circulating and you're breathing in dust all the time with sixty people and thirty or forty machines going. There's a lot of dirt because the checks give off a lot of dust. . . . It's like the machine is running you. You're like a computer.

Similar situations are often found in service, retail, distributive, and other types of work. What is

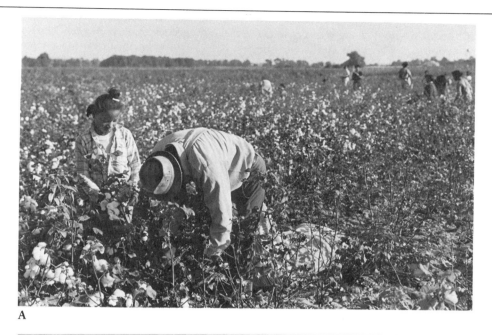

A

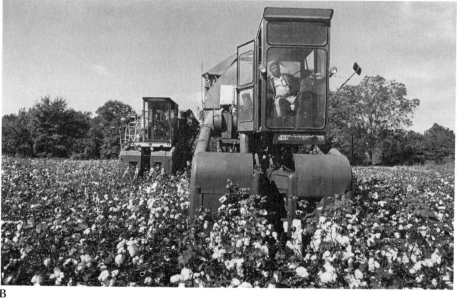

B

Fig. 2-3. A. Handpicking of cotton. B. Mechanized picking. Mechanized picking results
in more trash content in cotton. Trash is believed to contain the agent responsible for
byssinosis (see Chap. 21).
(Photographs by Earl Dotter.)

true for the autoworker, the word processor, and the keypunch operator is increasingly the case for the short-order cook, the checkout clerk, and the telephone operator. One young woman described to us her sense of powerlessness and alienation as a grocery store cashier [9]:

It was extremely repetitive work. Pushing numbers all day sort of got to me. I used to have dreams, or should I say nightmares, all night long of ringing up customers' orders when it was after closing time. I have even woken up and found myself sitting up in bed talking to customers. That job ended when the whole building exploded one night because of some faulty electrical work.

The summer of my senior year in high school. I got another job as a cashier in a discount department store, doing the same thing, pushing numbers again. My nightmare of talking to customers in my sleep began again. . . . This was a job that was an extremely strict one. There was no leeway about anything. They had cameras above the registers watching us to see if we were polite, if we checked inside of containers for any hidden merchandise, checked the tags to see if they were switched, etc. If we failed to do something we were given a written warning. . . .

Everyone who worked there, with the exception of the management, was part-time. The schedules were made so that no one had exactly forty hours. I worked for three months, 35 to 38 hours per week. By not giving us those few extra hours, they saved themselves a lot of money by not having to give their employees benefits, insurance, etc. Of course, their hiring, firing, quitting went on week after week. There weren't too many loyal employees.

An office worker describing her job used the same military metaphor heard at the automobile assembly plant [9]:

[My boss] was one of those people who wear their position. She was the manager so she believed she had the right to overpower me. Working for her reminded me of the days I was in boot camp. You're not an individual, you're just one of the troops, or in this case just another employee. . . . You had to look right, smile and do a good job so Mr. So-and-So could make a lot of money. After a while you feel more like a piece in a money machine rather than a person.

Fig. 2-4. There is a surprising amount of isolation in today's work environment. (Photograph by Earl Dotter.)

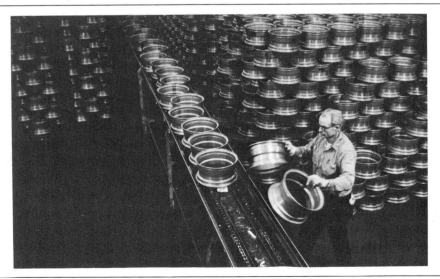

A fractionated division of labor and "scientific" work discipline are ways of exerting managerial control in the interests of efficiency and profit (Figs. 2-4, 2-5). But the experience of alienation and powerlessness on the part of the workers is not limited to workplaces where this type of organization is imposed. Many jobs in small shops—particularly in the service and retail sectors, which employ the largest number of women and youth—are equally unattractive despite their lack of specialization. This powerlessness on the job is exemplified in the following account by a waitress [9]:

The owner of the restaurant I waitress at was quoted as saying, "Waitresses come a dime a dozen." You can see what kind of respect he has for his employees, none. I often think about quitting. They never tell you when you're doing your work well, but they are right there ready to jump on your back when something goes wrong. Once I said to my partner, "I'm going to quit, it's not worth the aggravation." She replied, "Well, you better not unless you've got another job . . . just relax, you'll get over it." But I never really do get over it.

They don't care about your personal life. Last Sunday I was on for a double shift. I had worked Friday night, Saturday night, and now it was Sunday and like always I work a double shift. It's almost mandatory and almost everyone does.

Well, I'm a college student and it's finals week and my mind is overloaded. And to top it off my boyfriend woke up with a 103 temperature. I hated to leave him home sick and alone for 12 hours. I went up to the manager after the first 6 hours and explained the situation to her and said, "It's slow, why don't you let me go home?" Finally after much persuasion, she let me go. The clincher was she said, "If anything goes wrong, it's your fault. I don't want the owner to blame me for not having enough workers." Management always blames the waitress.

Another thing about the job that really interferes with my personal life is that you never know when you're working—the schedule isn't put up until Saturday and Sunday is the first day on it. So you can only make plans for the following week after you've seen the schedule.

Fig. 2-5. Monotony characterizes many jobs. (Photograph by Earl Dotter.)

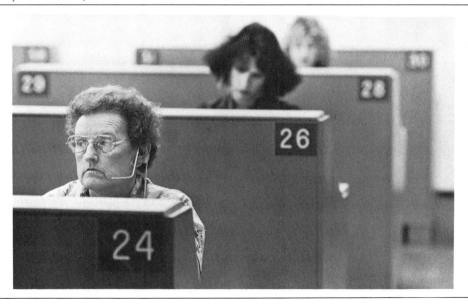

Sometimes I'm on call. If this isn't trying to manipulate your life! I'm supposed to stay home and if it gets busy she'll call me in and I'm supposed to drop everything and run to work. When I was called in three weeks in a row on the same day I asked her, "Why don't you put me on the schedule in the first place?" She didn't reply. I knew it was because the owner only wants to pay as few employees as possible.

UNEMPLOYMENT

It is striking that, even given the unsatisfying nature of most jobs and the hostility that this produces in many workers, almost all workers would rather have a job than no job at all. One worker says of unemployment [8], "Lovely life if you happen to be a turnip. . . . One does not willingly opt for near-the-bone life on the dole. My personal problem is easily solved. All I need is work."

Unemployment is more destructive to physical and mental health than all but the most dangerous jobs. Recent studies have even suggested a correlation between unemployment and mortality from heart disease, liver disease, suicide, and other stress-related ailments. Interestingly, changing levels of unemployment have an impact not just among unemployed workers themselves but also within their families. For example, households in which the husband is unemployed or underemployed show rates of domestic violence two to three times greater than households of fully employed men.

One of the most striking research findings on unemployed workers is the near unanimity with which workers internalize the experience of joblessness as one of personal lack of worth. This sense of worthlessness appears completely unrelated to a worker's actual degree of responsibility in losing his or her job.

In the contemporary American economy, the unemployed, like the poor, are always with us. In the last decade, the unemployment rate has fluctuated between 6 and 11 percent. (Some economists have proposed that a 5 percent unemployment rate should be considered "full

employment.") Furthermore, this focus is only on those actively seeking work; by excluding those jobless who, through discouragement, have stopped looking or never began, the official data understate the magnitude of the problem.

THE FUTURE OF WORK

We continue to wrestle not only with a refractory unemployment problem but also with other difficult problems for workers created by changes in the structure of the economy. Manufacturing industry in the United States, while remarkably productive, has been declining as a source of employment for American workers. Some, forced out of relatively high-paying unionized jobs in manufacturing, have had to take minimum wage service industry employment. Years of building up skill and experience have evaporated and with them, the "middle-class lifestyle" that manufacturing employment supported. Much of the service industry is unorganized, so the labor movement has suffered as its manufacturing bulwark declined and workers moved into small nonunion firms with low pay, few benefits, and few rights. The service industry includes a wide array of firms, from fast-food outlets to high-tech consulting companies. The health care industry falls in this category, and some of its problems are illustrative of the new issues facing workers.

Hospitals developed a tradition of operating like businesses early in this century, but with the establishment of Medicare and Medicaid in the mid-1960s, the combination of private and public insurance and subsidy enabled medical care to expand and become big business. Investor-owned chains grew substantially in the 1970s, partly by acquiring existing hospitals, and to some extent, by building new ones. Soaring medical care costs have attracted the unhappy eye of government, employers (who pay for fringe benefits), and the public. The chains have been criticized for cutting back on the quality of health care by cutting back on staff. In addition, occupational health professionals understand that understaffing may cause injuries and mental stress among hospital employees.

Management in the service industry may make the same mistakes about labor that we have seen in manufacturing. A recent study comparing computerized manufacturing in Japan and the United States faults American managers for underutilizing labor, incurring extraordinary "technology" costs because of their unwillingness to trust workers and to grant them more control of the work process [10]. Similar problems will emerge in the service industry, including in health care, if employers fail to appreciate the importance—and creativity—of American workers.

A CASE FOR GREATER WORKER AUTONOMY

It is worth remembering that the workers' situation was not always so dissatisfying. Historically, most of the parameters that shape the meaning of work have been more frequently controlled by the workers themselves rather than imposed on them by others.

For 95 percent of human history the social unit consisted of classless foraging bands whose limited needs were easily satisfied. Individual men and women had considerable control over how hard they worked and what they worked at. One anthropologist has graphically described such bands as the "first affluent society" [11]. A study of the !Kung, a contemporary foraging society in the Kalahari Desert in Namibia, found that !Kung men and women each worked a maximum of 40 hours a week, including all food preparation, housework, and child care [12].

In both foraging and simple agricultural societies people worked to satisfy their own needs and the needs of their families; decisions about the amount, pace, and duration of work were subordinated to the perceived needs of the workers not only for subsistence but also for leisure, recreation, and intimacy. To a lesser extent this ordering of priorities is also seen among self-employed craftspersons and family farmers; however, their involvement in a more complex extended society (for example, participation in market production and the need to pay taxes) limits their ability to subordinate production to other aspects of life (leisure, recreation, and intimacy).

Control of the work process remained in the hands of the workers until the early days of industrial factory production. Up to that time, skilled workers controlled the technical knowledge necessary for production and passed it along from worker to worker in the form of craft secrets that employers were often ignorant of. Thus, nineteenth century skilled workers—and even some twentieth century workers such as master machinists—were able to control or significantly influence the organization and pace of the production process. The introduction of new technologies has undermined and largely eliminated this control. Now it is not the workers but engineers, supervisors, and employers who control both what happens to the product and the organization of work.

The last 7,000 years have been marked by two contradictory phenomena. From the invention of agriculture through the invention of the microprocessor, the capacity of humans to produce goods and services capable of promoting and enriching well-being and the enjoyment of life has vastly increased. However, this process has been accompanied and in many ways produced by changes in the nature of work that led to the loss of self-control over the labor process. Since work-related disease is often a by-product of the conditions in which many workers now labor, only by changing those conditions can occupational disease be minimized. A preventive approach to work-related disease requires, in part, restoring control over the labor process and work conditions to those who are at risk.

REFERENCES

1. O'Toole J, ed. Work in America (report of a special task force to the Secretary of Health, Education, and Welfare). Cambridge: MIT Press, 1973: 38–39.
2. Keenan J. On the dole. In: Fraser R, ed. Work:

Twenty personal accounts. Harmondsworth, England: Penguin, 1968.

3. Williams R. The meanings of work. In: Fraser R, ed. Work: Twenty personal accounts. Harmondsworth, England: Penguin, 1968.

4. U.S. Bureau of the Census. Statistical abstract of the United States. 107th ed. Washington, D.C.: U.S. Government Printing Office, 1986.

5. Garson B. All the livelong day: the meaning and demeaning of work. New York: Penguin, 1977.

6. Terkel S. Working. New York: Pantheon, 1974.

7. Elling RH. The struggle for workers' health. Farmingdale, NY: Baywood Publishing, 1986: 72–73.

8. Tepperman J. Not servants, not machines: office workers speak out. Boston: Beacon Press, 1976.

9. Miller L. Unpublished interview. Southeastern Massachusetts University, 1980.

10. Jaikumar R. Postindustrial manufacturing. Harvard Business Review 1986; Nov–Dec 69–76.

11. Thompson EP. The making of the English working class. New York: Vintage, 1963.

12. Lee R. The !Kung San: men, women, and work in a foraging society. Cambridge, England: Cambridge University Press, 1980.

BIBLIOGRAPHY

Braverman H. Labor and monopoly capital: the degradation of work in the 20th century. New York: Monthly Review Press, 1974.
Study of the role and impact of scientific management, which revolutionized labor process studies. No other single book on work in contemporary America combines breadth of empirical range with analytical rigor quite like this one.

Fraser R, ed. Work: twenty personal accounts. Harmondsworth, England: Penguin, 1968, 1969 (2 vols.).
A remarkable set of first-person accounts of work and its meaning. The contributors range from factory and office workers to engineers, architects, and a croupier. Includes Raymond Williams' fine essay.

Garson B. All the livelong day: The meaning and demeaning of routine work. New York: Penguin, 1977.
A well-written journalistic account of the work lives of ordinary Americans by a fine interviewer and an insightful commentator.

Maurer H. Not working. New York: Holt Rinehart Winston, 1979.
Inspired by Studs Terkel, this young journalist produced an uneven, but irreplaceable, record of the unemployed worker in the late 1970s.

O'Toole J. ed. Work in America. Cambridge, MA: MIT Press, 1973.
This U.S. government report is valuable reading for anyone interested in the quality of work life in contemporary America.

Pfeffer R. Working for capitalism. New York: Columbia University Press, 1979.
This political scientist spent his sabbatical year as a forklift operator in a large Baltimore factory. He combines a pithy first-person account with a thorough command of contemporary labor process scholarship.

Terkel S. Working. New York: Pantheon, 1974.
Ordinary working people say extraordinary and insightful things about themselves and their work.

Zimbalist A. Case studies on the labor process. New York: Monthly Review Press, 1979.
A collection of essays that deals with recent changes in the labor process in factory work, building trades, and office work. David Noble's essay is "must" reading.

II
Approaches to Recognizing and Preventing Occupational Disease

3
Recognizing Occupational Disease

Barry S. Levy and David H. Wegman

Recognition of work-related disease is crucial in establishing the correct diagnosis and approach to treatment in affected individuals, preventing recurrence of disease, determining whether other workers are at risk of the same disease, assuring that affected workers receive economic compensation legally due them, and finally, discovering new relationships between work exposures and disease. This chapter deals with recognizing occupational disease in individual patients by taking an occupational history and in groups or populations of workers by conducting surveillance of occupational disease.

THE OCCUPATIONAL HISTORY

Consider the following four cases.

A woman who worked in a high-tech manufacturing plant had numbness in her distal arms and legs that her physician attributed to her diabetes.

A machinist was noted by his supervisor to have loss of balance on the job and was diagnosed at a nearby urgent care center as being acutely intoxicated with alcohol.

A garment worker was told by her primary care physician that the numbness and weakness in some of her fingers were due to her rheumatoid arthritis.

A man working at a bottle-making factory was told by his internist that the worsening of his chronic cough was due to cigarette smoking.

In each of these situations the physician made a reasonable and considered evaluation and diagnosis. The facts fit together and resulted in a coherent story, leading each physician to recommend a specific therapeutic and preventive regimen. In each of the cases, however, the physician made an incorrect diagnosis because of a common oversight—failure to take an occupational history.

The first patient had a peripheral neuropathy and the second, acute central nervous system (CNS) intoxication, both caused by exposure to solvents at work. The garment worker had carpal tunnel syndrome, possibly caused by some combination of her rheumatoid arthritis and the strenuous repetitive movements she performed with her hands and wrists hundreds of times an hour. The man working in the bottle-making factory had worsening of his chronic cough and other respiratory tract symptoms due to exposure to hydrochloric acid fumes at work.

This is not to say that the associations noted by the physicians were unrelated to the conditions diagnosed. They were probably contributory in at least the first, third, and fourth cases, but without the occupational history, proper therapy and prevention could not be planned.

The identification of work-related medical problems depends most importantly on the occupational history. Physical examination findings and laboratory test results may sometimes raise suspicion or help confirm that a disease or injury is work-related, but ultimately it is information obtained from an occupational history that determines the likelihood that a medical problem is work-related (see first box on p. 30). A phrase or two in the psychosocial section of the medical history is not enough; the physician should obtain

WORLD HEALTH ORGANIZATION
DISTINCTION BETWEEN
OCCUPATIONAL AND
WORK-RELATED DISEASES

The World Health Organization (WHO) recently advocated the following use of the terms *occupational* and *work-related* diseases. Although we use these terms interchangeably in this book, we expect that this new distinction will become increasingly useful in understanding the full range of the impact of work on health, and could have important implications in the future for diagnosis and treatment of workers, as well as for research.

WHO has stated:

Occupational diseases . . . stand at one end of the spectrum of work-relatedness where the relationship to specific causative factors at work has been fully established and the factors concerned can be identified, measured, and eventually controlled. At the other end [are] diseases [that] may have a weak, inconsistent, unclear relationship to working conditions; in the middle of the spectrum there is a possible causal relationship but the strength and magnitude of it may vary.*

Work-related diseases may be partially caused by adverse working conditions. They may be aggravated, accelerated, or exacerbated by workplace exposures, and they may impair working capacity.

Personal characteristics and other environmental and sociocultural factors usually play a role as risk factors in work-related diseases, which are often more common than occupational diseases.

*World Health Organization: *Identification and Control of Work-Related Diseases.* Technical Report No. 174. Geneva: WHO, 1985.

OUTLINE OF THE OCCUPATIONAL
HISTORY
1. Descriptions of all jobs held
2. Work exposures
3. Timing of symptoms
4. Epidemiology of symptoms or illness among other workers
5. Nonwork exposures and other factors

---

data on the current and the two major past occupations for all patients. The extent of detail will depend largely on the physician's level of suspicion that work may have caused or contributed to the illness. (See box for suggested questions on current work.) The history should be recorded with great care and precision so that the data may be used for legal or research purposes.

What Questions to Ask

The occupational history has five key parts (see box above): (1) a description of all of the patient's pertinent jobs—past and present, (2) a review of exposures faced by the patient in these jobs, (3) information on the timing of symptoms in relation to work, (4) data on similar problems among co-workers, and (5) information on nonwork factors, such as smoking and hobbies, that may cause or contribute to disease.

Some hospitals or clinics have standardized forms for recording the occupational history, which can expedite taking and recording this information. Ideally, such forms should include a grid, with column headings for job, employer, industry, major job tasks, dates of starting and stopping jobs, and major work exposures. (Asking questions about whether the patient has had any exposures to hazardous substances or physical factors, such as noise or radiation, from a list prepared in advance may be helpful.) On such an occupational history form (Fig. 3-1), the rows of the grid should be completed with information on

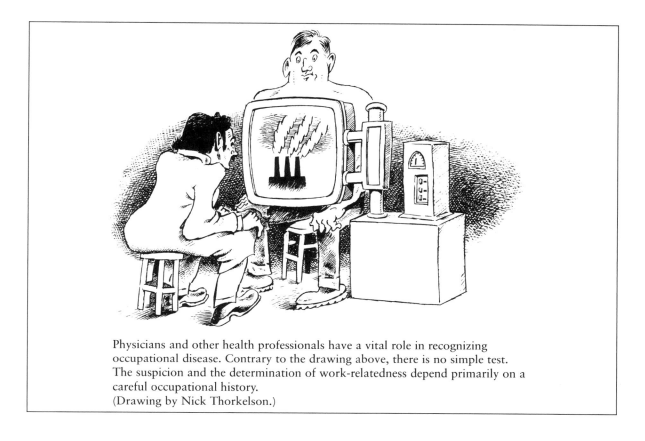

Physicians and other health professionals have a vital role in recognizing occupational disease. Contrary to the drawing above, there is no simple test. The suspicion and the determination of work-relatedness depend primarily on a careful occupational history.
(Drawing by Nick Thorkelson.)

each job, starting with the current or most recent job.

Further elaboration on each of the key parts of an occupational history may be helpful.

Descriptions of All Jobs Held
The history should include descriptions of all jobs held by the patient; in some cases it may be important also to obtain information on summer and part-time jobs held while attending school. (Generally, details of these jobs are sought only on second interviews.) Job titles alone are not sufficient: an electrician may work in a plant where lead storage batteries are manufactured, a clerk may work in a pesticide-formulating company, or a physician may perform research with hepatitis B virus. It is important to remember that workers in heavy industry are not the only ones prone to occupational diseases—so are clerks, electronic equipment assembly workers, domestic workers, food service employees, and virtually all other types of workers. To learn exactly what the patient does at work, it may be useful to have the patient describe a typical work shift from start to finish and simulate the performance of work tasks by demonstrating the body movements associated with them. A visit to the patient's workplace by the physician may be necessary and is always informative.

The history should describe routine tasks (unless the job title is self-explanatory); unusual and over-time tasks such as cleaning out tanks should also be noted, since they may be the most hazardous in

1. Please provide the following information on your work history.

Job	Employer	Industry	Major job tasks	Dates of starting stopping		Major work exposures*
Military?						
Part-time work?						

2. Have you had any possibly hazardous exposures outside of work? _____ If yes, complete the following.

Major exposures	Associated activity	Location	Dates of starting stopping	

3. Have you ever smoked cigarettes? _____ If yes, please answer the following questions.
How old were you when you started smoking? _____
On average, how many packs have you smoked a day? _____
Do you currently smoke? _____ If no, how old were you when you stopped smoking? _____

*Such as chemicals, fumes, dusts, vapors, gases, noise, and radiation.

Fig. 3-1. Sample occupational history form. (From BS Levy, DH Wegman. The occupational history in medical practice: What questions to ask and when to ask them. Postgrad Med 1986; 79:301.)

which a patient is involved. It is important to ask about second or part-time jobs, the patient's work in the home as a homemaker or parent, and service in the military.

Work Exposures
The patient should be carefully questioned about working conditions and past and present chemical, physical, biologic, and psychologic exposures. As in other parts of a medical history, to avoid limiting the responses, initially use open-ended questions such as, "What have you worked with?" Then ask more specific questions such as, "Were you ever exposed to lead? Other heavy metals? Solvents? Asbestos? Dyes?" Some knowledge of the most likely exposures in the jobs listed can help

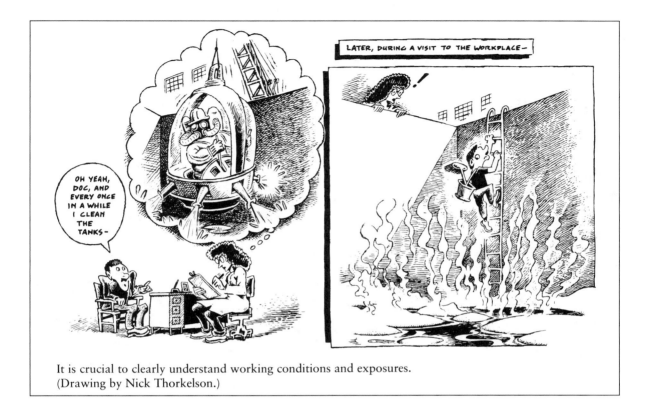

It is crucial to clearly understand working conditions and exposures.
(Drawing by Nick Thorkelson.)

focus additional questions, and it is important to remember that tasks performed in adjacent parts of the workplace can also contribute to a worker's exposures. It is often worthwhile to repeat these questions in a somewhat different manner at two points in the interview because patients will sometimes recall, on repeat questioning, exposures that they initially overlooked. Also inquire about unusual accidents or incidents such as spills of hazardous material that may be related to the patient's problem; work in confined spaces (Fig. 3-2); and new substances or changed processes at work.

Many workplace chemicals and other substances are referred to only by brand names, slang terms, or coded numbers. It should be possible, however, for a physician to obtain the ingredients of most chemicals and to determine the nature of any hazard (see the appendix to this chapter). In many states and localities, Right-to-Know laws facilitate the process whereby workers and their physicians, with only limited information, can determine the toxic effects of these substances. The federal Hazard Communication Standard is also helpful (see Chap. 10).

It is important to quantify these exposures as accurately as possible. Clinicians can estimate the degree of exposure by determining the duration of exposure and route of entry. Large amounts of volatile substances, such as solvents, can be inhaled unknowingly, especially if they do not irritate the upper respiratory tract or if they do not have a strong odor. Large amounts of certain substances—again, solvents are a good example—can be absorbed through the skin with the worker un-

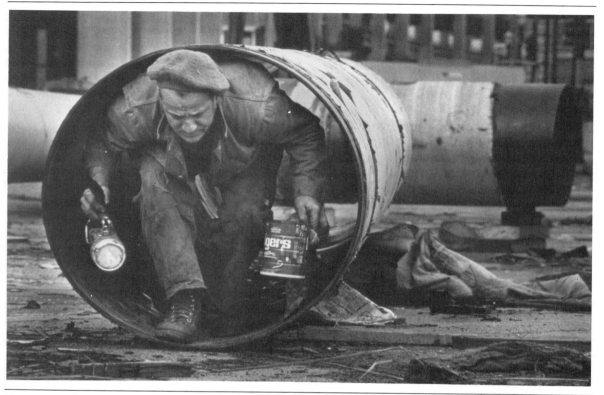

Fig. 3-2. Work in confined spaces.
(Photograph by Earl Dotter.)

aware of the degree of this exposure. The patient should be asked to describe the amount of a potentially hazardous material that contacts skin or clothes or is inhaled, on a typical workday. The patient should also provide information on eating, drinking, and smoking in the workplace (contamination of hands can lead to inadvertent ingestion of toxic materials) (Fig. 3-3); hand-washing and showering at work; changing work-clothes; and who cleans the workclothes.

It should be determined if personal protective equipment (such as gloves, workclothes, masks, respirators, and hearing protectors) has been provided, and if, when, and how often the worker has used this equipment. If personal protective equip-

ment is not being used, it is important to determine the reasons. Masks and respirators are frequently not worn because of poor fit, discomfort in hot weather, and difficulty in communicating. In addition, masks and respirators that are not properly maintained are ineffective. If personal protective equipment is being used, determine if it appears to fit and work properly. Ask whether protective engineering systems and devices such as ventilation systems are present in the workplace and whether they seem to function adequately.

Timing of Symptoms
Information on the time course of the patient's symptoms is often vital in determining if a given

these and related questions the physician can determine if the period from the start of exposure to the onset of symptoms and the time course of the patient's symptoms are consistent with those of the suspected illness. For example, certain irritants with low water solubility will produce severe pulmonary damage and even fatal pulmonary edema with onset about 12 to 18 hours after work ceases. Symptoms of byssinosis ("brown lung") are characteristically worse on returning to work on Monday morning. Nitroglycerin workers, whose blood vessels have dilated due to work exposure to nitrates, may suffer "withdrawal" angina while away from work. Thus, since latent periods vary, occupational etiologies should not be ruled out because timing of symptoms does not initially correlate with time at work.

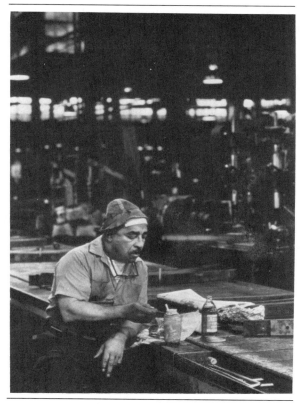

Fig. 3-3. Workers eating in the workplace may ingest toxic substances.
(Photograph by Earl Dotter.)

Epidemiology of Symptoms or Illness Among Other Workers

The patient's knowledge of other workers at the same workplace or in similar jobs elsewhere who are suffering from the same symptoms or illness may be the most important clue to recognizing work-related disease. The physician should inquire further what the affected workers share in common such as similar job, exposure, physical location in the workplace, age, or sex. Ask about birth defects among offspring, fertility problems, cancer incidence, and high turnover of workers or their early retirement for health reasons. Workers and then their physicians linked the pesticide DBCP (dibromochloropropane) to male sterility and the catalyst DMAPN (dimethylaminopropionitrile) to bladder neuropathy by recognizing that similarly exposed workers had the same medical problems. Unfortunately, workers may not always be aware of symptoms present in coworkers.

Nonwork Exposures and Other Factors

Sometimes there is a synergistic relationship between occupational and nonoccupational factors in causing disease. The physician should ask if the patient smokes cigarettes or drinks alcohol; if so,

disease or syndrome is work-related or not. The following questions are often useful: "Do the symptoms begin shortly after the start of the workday? Do they disappear shortly after leaving work? Are they present during weekends or vacation periods? Are they time-related to certain processes, work tasks, or work exposures? Have you recently begun a new job, worked with a new process, or been exposed to a new chemical in the workplace?"

Questions on recent changes at work are often critical in suspecting or proving that a disease is work-related. On the basis of the responses to amount and duration should be quantified. For skin problems, questions should be asked regarding recent exposure to new soaps, cosmetics, and clothes. The physician should also ask: Does the patient have hobbies (such as woodworking or gardening) or other non-work activities that involve potentially hazardous chemical, physical, biologic, or psychologic exposures that may account for the symptoms? Does the patient live near any factories, waste dump sites, or contaminated sources of water? Does the patient live with someone who brings hazardous workplace subtances home on workclothes, shoes, or hair? The same suggestions noted in the Work Exposures section apply here: repeated questioning, quantification of exposure to the degree possible, and obtaining generic names of substances. Questioning should be aimed at determining both current and past exposures.

Other information the physician obtains may supplement the occupational history. It is useful to know whether the patient has had preplacement or periodic physical and laboratory examinations at work. For example, preplacement audiograms or pulmonary function test results may be helpful in determining if hearing impairment or respiratory symptoms are work-related or not. Since OSHA regulations mandate periodic screening of workers with certain exposures (such as asbestos and coke oven emissions), and since many employers are voluntarily providing health screening in the workplace, it is increasingly likely that such information may be available to a physician, if the worker approves of its release.

Finally, it is often useful to ask the patient whether there is some reason to suspect that the symptoms may be work-related.

WHEN TO TAKE A COMPLETE OCCUPATIONAL HISTORY

A work history should always contain information on past and present jobs of the patient to provide a good understanding of how the patient spends the workday and what potential health hazards may exist. Of course, however, it is impossible to obtain a detailed, 20-minute or longer occupational history on every patient seen. But every medical history should include the individual's two major previous jobs and current job.

In the following situations the physician should have a strong suspicion of occupational factors or influences on the development of the problem and take a detailed, complete occupational history. Many symptoms appear to be nonspecific but may well have their origin in an occupational exposure.

Respiratory Disease
Virtually any respiratory symptoms can be work-related. It is all too easy to diagnose acute respiratory symptoms as acute tracheobronchitis or viral infection when the actual diagnosis may be occupational asthma, or chronic symptoms as chronic obstructive pulmonary disease (COPD) when the actual diagnosis may be asbestosis. Viruses and cigarettes are too often assumed to be the sole agents responsible for respiratory disease. Adult-onset asthma is frequently work-related but often not recognized as such. In addition, patients with preexisting asthma may have exacerbations of their otherwise quiescent condition when exposed to workplace sensitizers. Less commonly, pulmonary edema can be caused by workplace chemicals such as phosgene or oxides of nitrogen; a detailed work history should therefore be obtained for anyone with acute pulmonary edema when no likely nonoccupational cause can be identified (see Chap. 21).

Skin Disorders
Many skin disorders are nonspecific in nature, bothersome but not life-threatening, and self-limited. Diagnoses are often nonspecific, and all too often a brief occupational history that may identify the offending irritant, sensitizer, or other factor is not taken. Contact dermatitis, which accounts for about 90 percent of all work-related skin disease, does not have a characteristic appearance. Determination of the etiologic agent and work-relatedness depends on a carefully obtained work history (see Chap. 23).

Hearing Impairment

Many cases of hearing impairment are falsely attributed to aging (presbycusis) or other nonoccupational causes. In the early 1970s it was estimated that as many as one-sixth of American workers were exposed to hazardous noise at work; thus, a detailed occupational history should be obtained from anyone with hearing impairment. Recommendations for the prevention of future hearing loss should also be made (see Chap. 17).

Back and Joint Symptoms

Much back pain is at least partially work-related in etiology, but there are no tests or other procedures that can differentiate work-related from non-work–related back problems; the determination of likelihood depends on the occupational history. A surprising number of cases of arthritis and tenosynovitis are caused by unnatural repetitive movements associated with work tasks. Ergonomics, the study of interactions between worker and machine, helps prevent some of these problems (see Chaps. 9 and 22).

Cancer

A significant percentage of cancer cases is known to be caused by work exposures, and each year more occupational carcinogens are discovered. Initial evidence that a workplace substance is carcinogenic has come more often from individual clinicians' reports than from large-scale epidemiologic studies. This effort would be facilitated if occupational histories were obtained on all patients with cancer. Of importance in considering occupational cancer is that exposure to the carcinogen may have been 20 or more years before diagnosis of the disease, and the exposure need not have been continued over the entire time interval (see Chap. 15).

Exacerbation of Coronary
Artery Disease Symptoms

Exposure to stress and to carbon monoxide and other chemicals in the workplace may increase the frequency or severity of the symptoms of coronary artery disease (see Chap. 27).

Liver Disease

As with respiratory disease, it is all too easy to give liver ailments common diagnoses such as viral hepatitis or alcoholic cirrhosis rather than less common diagnoses of work-related toxic problems. It is always important to take a good occupational history with liver disease. Hepatotoxins encountered in the workplace are discussed in Chapter 29.

Neuropsychiatric Problems

The possibility of relating neuropsychiatric problems to the workplace is often overlooked. Peripheral neuropathies are more frequently attributed to diabetes, alcohol abuse, or "unknown etiology"; central nervous system depression to substance abuse or psychiatric problems; and behavioral abnormalities (which may, in fact, be the first sign of work-related stress or less frequently a neurotoxic problem) to psychosis or personality disorder. More than 100 chemicals (including virtually all solvents) can cause central nervous system depression, and several neurotoxins (including arsenic, lead, mercury, and methyl n-butyl ketone) can produce peripheral neuropathy. Carbon disulfide exposure can cause symptoms that mimic a psychosis (see Chap. 25).

Illnesses of Unknown Cause

A detailed complete occupational history is essential in all cases where the cause of illness is unknown or not certain, or the diagnosis is obscure.

In many other situations, a fairly complete work history is useful. For example, in determining the appropriate timing and type of work for a patient recuperating from an acute myocardial infarction, the physician should have a very good understanding of the patient's past work history, particularly in terms of any physical and psychologic stresses. In addition, it is important to inquire about the impact a patient's nonoccupational medical problem may be having on work.

In conclusion, despite modern technology, the occupational history is the essential factor in raising the suspicion of and ultimately proving the work-relatedness of a medical problem.

It is surprising how current the following advice still is:

If the recording interne would only treat the poison from which the man is suffering with as much interest as he gives to the coffee the patient has drunk and tobacco he has smoked, if he would ask as carefully about the length of time he was exposed to the poison as about the age at which he had measles, the task of the searcher for the truth about industrial poisons would be made so very much easier.*

SURVEILLANCE OF OCCUPATIONAL DISEASE

As we have seen, the occupational history determines the work-relatedness of medical problems of the individual worker. *Surveillance*—the systematic collection, analysis, and dissemination of disease data on groups or populations—is required to identify occupational disease at the group or population level. It can be performed in an open-ended manner or focused on a particular disease or group of workers.

Surveillance can be used to monitor either the occurrence of diseases (or physiologic abnormalities) or the presence of hazardous substances and worker exposures to them. This section focuses on its use in monitoring the occurrence of disease. For chronic diseases caused by workplace exposures, monitoring of *exposures,* however, may be more useful. This possibility exists because a number of exposure-effect relationships are sufficiently well described that long-term exposure to known levels of a material can be said to predictably result in the chronic illness. Furthermore, the long latency period between exposure and onset of chronic work-related disease makes it difficult to associate the exposure with the disease in an individual case. For diseases of shorter latency, direct disease surveillance may be very useful.

In occupational health, surveillance proceeds in two different ways. First, data can be used to monitor trends in the occurrence of selected disorders. These trends often indicate the effectiveness of control programs and guide public health measures to improve them. Second, surveillance can be used to identify individual workers with occupational disease so that they receive appropriate medical care and their coworkers and workplaces can be evaluated. This latter use of surveillance, known as active case identification and follow-up, is the focus of a NIOSH-sponsored program, the Sentinel Event Notification System for Occupational Risks (SENSOR).

Surveillance of any disease depends on its recognition (diagnosis). Because occupational disease is difficult to diagnose, surveillance for occupational disease is not well developed, and consequently the available data on work-related medical problems, as cited in Chapter 1, are assumed to be underestimates and skewed reflections of actual occupational disease incidence. Surveillance for occupational disease requires the collection of data from several different sources.

Bureau of Labor Statistics Data

Annual surveys of a sample of employers, performed by the Bureau of Labor Statistics (BLS) of the U.S. Department of Labor in cooperation with OSHA, provide data for the projection of the incidence of work-related disease and injury. However, NIOSH has questioned the usefulness of these surveys, citing their analyses of only broad categories of disease, the absence of specific criteria for determining the occupational relationship of disease, the absence of a state-level response mechanism for surveillance findings, and the lateness of reports and their failure to analyze data by size, type, and geographic location of workplaces.

Workers' Compensation Data

In most states, workers' compensation data represent the most readily available information on work-related *injuries.* However, these data exclude affected workers who do not file, are biased

*Alice Hamilton. *Industrial Poisons in the U.S.* (1925)

to the more severe injuries and illnesses, exclude most cases of chronic work-related *disease,* and are limited by adjudication procedures and diagnostic criteria that vary from state to state (see Chap. 11).

Surveying Workers

Interviews and examinations of workers can be a more effective surveillance approach than the two mentioned above. One survey of small industries found that 98 percent of cases of probable occupational disease found by the survey were not recorded in the employer's OSHA log or in workers' compensation claim data. For a variety of reasons, cases of occupational disease may not be identified even where specific guidelines are available.

Union Records

Unions may have morbidity or mortality data, often related to medical or death benefit programs, that can be used for surveillance. Even without this information, union records can define the exposed, or at-risk population, of workers whose names can be cross-checked against health effects data from, for example, a state health department division of vital records (see Chap. 35).

Employer Records

Employer records can be helpful for morbidity data, although such data are likely to be underestimates of the incidence of disease; such records may also provide valuable information on exposure (see Chap. 34).

Vital Events

Information on death or birth certificates is often relevant to surveillance. For example, cause of death and limited occupational data can be abstracted from death certificates, and in some states birth defect information and some occupational data on parents are included on birth certificates.

Disability Records

Disability records can be examined as a potentially useful source of surveillance data (see Chap. 12).

Cancer Registries

Hospital-based, regional, or statewide cancer incidence registries can be useful sources of surveillance data on cancer.

Physician Reporting

In some states and elsewhere (for example, Alberta, Canada, and West Germany) the law requires physicians to report all work-related diseases and injuries or certain specified ("scheduled") conditions. In the United States these laws have up to now not been generally very effective and reporting has been minimal; however, NIOSH is attempting to improve the quality of physician reporting through its SENSOR program, focusing on common, easily diagnosed, short-latency occupational diseases, such as lead poisoning and occupational asthma.

Emergency Department Visits

A recently begun system developed by NIOSH focuses on emergency department visits for surveillance of occupational injuries. Data are obtained from a representative sample of emergency departments in the United States.

Sentinel Event Approaches

Morbidity and mortality data from physicians, hospitals, and vital statistics bureaus may show certain sentinel events that can be used as markers of specific occupational exposures. For example, cases of or deaths from mesothelioma and asbestosis are markers of asbestos exposure.

Surveillance for communicable disease in the United States has been very helpful in identifying high-risk groups for disease, recognizing disease outbreaks and providing clues to the etiology of diseases and effectiveness of control measures. With time, it is likely that improved surveillance of occupational disease will yield additional useful information. It is incumbent on physicians to cooperate with existing surveillance systems and to utilize available surveillance data in identifying and preventing cases of work-related disease.

More information on surveillance of occupational disease can be obtained from:

Surveillance Coordinating Activity, NIOSH, Centers for Disease Control, Atlanta, GA 30333

Workers' compensation system agencies in most states

Bureau of Labor Statistics, U.S. Department of Labor, Washington, D.C.

BIBLIOGRAPHY

Goldman RH, Peters JM. The occupational and environmental health history. *JAMA* 1981; 246:2831.
An excellent article with more detail on the occupational history.

Baker EL Jr. Surveillance of occupational illness and injury in the United States: current perspectives and future directions. July 15, 1987. (Copies available from Edward L. Baker, Jr., M.D., NIOSH, Centers for Disease Control, Atlanta, GA 30333.)
An excellent review article on occupational disease surveillance in the U.S.

Bureau of Labor Statistics, U.S. Department of Labor. Towards improved measurement and reporting of occupational illness and disease. (Symposium Proceedings, Albuquerque, NM, 1985.) Washington, DC: U.S. Department of Labor, 1987.
State-of-the-art review of practical issues in occupational disease surveillance and proposals for the future.

Froines JR, Dellenbaugh CA, Wegman DH. Occupational health surveillance: a means to identify work-related risk. *Amer J Pub Health* 1986; 76:1089.
Introduction to the concept of hazard surveillance.

Halperin WE, Frazier TM. Surveillance and the effects of workplace exposure. *Ann Rev Pub Health* 1985; 6:419.
An excellent review on the subject.

Rutstein DD, Mullan RJ, Frazier TM, et al. Sentinel health events (occupational): a basis for physician recognition and public health surveillance. *Amer J Pub Health* 1983; 73:1054.
Adaptation of the general concept of sentinel health events to occupational disease.

APPENDIX

How to Research the Toxic Effects of Chemical Substances

David Michaels and Stephen Zoloth

In taking work histories, you are likely to discover that many of your patients are exposed to one or more substances whose toxic properties are unknown or unfamiliar to you. It is necessary to investigate the potential toxicity of these products. The following is a systematic approach to important resources in this area. These are resources with which you should become familiar, since they will be useful in providing information necessary for determining if your patients' health problems are work-related.

STEP 1: SET PRIORITIES

It is often impractical to research every substance and process to which your patients are exposed. A few common-sense guidelines may help focus your efforts on the more important exposures—those most likely to cause disease.

Ask the patient for guidance. Workers are usually well aware of the most potentially toxic substances to which they are exposed; the products they are particularly concerned about warrant your attention. In many cases, workers have themselves obtained useful information about chemical hazards, often from labels on containers, their union, or other sources, and they will share it with you.

Furthermore, by observing health and disease patterns among themselves, workers are often able to identify clusters of work-related disease. While this is especially true for acute health problems that occur shortly after exposure, it is often the case for chronic disease as well. Inquire if your patients suspect that their health problems, or those of other workers, are job-related.

Consider the magnitude of exposure. If your patient has more intensive or prolonged exposure to two or three substances, these should be investigated first. It is vital to remember, however, that even low-dose exposure to a carcinogen is cause for concern (see Chap. 15).

Consider toxicologic information. Your background reading will alert you to the toxicity of certain classes of chemicals; it should help you be "selectively suspicious" and to direct your research accordingly. For example, you will learn that halogenated hydrocarbons, organochlorine pesticides, and heavy metals should generally be given priority in your research, since they may be extremely toxic.

Consider clinical-toxicologic correlations. If the onset of symptoms in your patient dates from the introduction of a new chemical in the workplace, this product certainly deserves further investigation.

Consider epidemiologic correlations. If your patient and his or her coworkers share the same symptoms or diseases, discover what exposures they have in common.

STEP 2: OBTAIN THE GENERIC NAME
Many chemicals used in the workplace are known by their trade names. It can be extremely difficult to investigate a substance without knowing its generic, or chemical, name or ingredients.

Use Right-to-Know laws and regulations. Now most U.S. workers employed in the private sector have the right, under the OSHA Hazard Communication Standard, to obtain information about the chemicals they work with from their employer (see Chap. 10). In addition, many public sector workers have similar rights under Right-to-Know laws in effect in 25 states. Under these regulations, employers must provide workers with information on all hazardous chemicals used in the workplace through labeling containers, distributing Material Safety Data Sheets (MSDSs) and conducting training programs. The MSDS for a product, generally prepared by its manufacturer, is of particular importance to health care providers since it lists the product's generic ingredients, their toxic properties, recommendations for safe use, and other important information.

If your patient is working with a product under suspicion, he or she can request the MSDS from the employer and provide you with it. Your patient has the right to make this request—you do not, and your contacting the employer may jeopardize your patient's job. *Never* contact your patient's employer without his or her permission.

It is important to remember, however, that MSDSs can be incomplete or out of date. While MSDSs are valuable as sources of generic names and chemicals, the toxicity information they contain should be confirmed in other sources, when possible; do not rely on MSDSs alone. In addition, if your patient is no longer employed or no longer working with the substance, it may be difficult to obtain the appropriate MSDS.

Finally, it should be noted that in many states and localities, community residents, firefighters, and others have the same rights to information about chemicals used by local employers under community Right-to-Know regulations.

Contact the manufacturer. You should not call your patient's employer, but you may decide to contact the manufacturer of the substance in question. Product labels usually contain the manufacturer's name and often an address as well. If the address is not listed, use *Thomas' Register of American Manufacturers* (Thomas Publishing Co., New York, 1987), available at many public libraries. In contacting a manufacturer, request the MSDSs on the substances of interest. Calls from physicians and other health care providers generally receive quick responses from manufacturers, who may be concerned about potential liability.

Contact the poison control center. Poison control centers are a vital source of data on both the generic ingredients and acute toxic properties of chemical substances, and there is one in every region of the United States.

Contact NIOSH. NIOSH has a computerized data bank of the ingredients of trade name substances from the National Occupational Hazard Survey. While this data bank is incomplete, NIOSH continues to update it and is able to provide the generic names of approximately one-third of the trade name products requested. Contact Hazard Surveillance Section, NIOSH, Mailstop R-19, 4676 Columbia Parkway, Cincinnati, Ohio 45226. The phone number is (513) 841-4491.

Check reference books. Several are useful sources of generic ingredient information. For example, the *Clinical Toxicology of Commercial Products* (5th ed.) (R. Gosselin, R. Smith, and H. Hodge, Williams & Wilkins, Baltimore, 1984), available in all medical libraries, lists the ingredients of over 17,500 trade name products. If you encounter what may be a synonym or trade name of a chemical, use the *NIOSH Registry of Toxic Effects of Chemical Substances,* commonly known as RTECS (1983–84 Cumulative Supplement to the 1981–82 edition, NIOSH publication No. 86-103). If neither of these is sufficient, try one of the several chemical dictionaries or collections of synonyms that list common trade names.

STEP 3: RESEARCH THE CHEMICAL
Information provided on a MSDS or a label on the toxic effects of the chemical is often incomplete. It is important to obtain the most accurate and current toxicologic information. There are many sources that provide detailed toxicity data. Several chapters of this book review the effects of chemicals on specific organ systems and their bibliographies are good starting points. In addition, major textbooks of industrial hygiene, toxicology, and pharmacology generally have chapters devoted to specific chemicals or families of chemicals (see Bibliography, Chap. 14). In addition to these sources, the following approaches may be useful to researching the toxic effects of chemicals.

Chemical Fact Sheets
Toxicologic data on specific chemicals can be found in chemical fact sheets. Similar to MSDSs, chemical fact sheets are brief summaries of toxicologic data. For example, NIOSH published *Occupational Health Guidelines for Chemical Hazards* (NIOSH publication No. 81-123). This three-volume set of fact sheets covers more than 300 substances for which there are federal occupational safety and health regulations. Among the topics included for each chemical are a description of symptoms and signs of exposure, recommended medical surveillance protocols, and a summary of the toxicology data.

In addition, many state health and labor departments also publish chemical fact sheets or serve as resources for information on hazardous chemicals. For example, the New Jersey and New York state health departments both provide well-researched fact sheets on industrial chemicals, and the California health department has a Hazard Evaluation Surveillance and Information System, which provides assistance in researching chemical exposures and effects.

In addition to these sources, two NIOSH publications also provide summaries of chemical toxicity. The *Pocket Guide to Chemical Hazards* (NIOSH publication No. 85-114) lists major industrial chemicals and provides a statement on their toxicity, protective equipment, and exposure limits. The RTECS is much more extensive, covering more than 80,000 chemicals, and provides a gateway into the toxicologic literature. The entries in RTECS are telegraphic and unevaluated summaries of recent toxicology data. RTECS is best used to identify references to the toxicologic literature. RTECS can be a useful reference and is available from the U.S. Government Printing Office in two paperbound volumes. These volumes are updated every five years; on microfiche, it is updated quarterly. It also can be accessed as a computer data base.

Using Computers to Research Chemicals
The rapid growth of the microcomputer industry, telecommunications, and public and private data bases provides another method of researching toxic properties of chemicals. Bibliographic data bases, such as the National Library of Medi-

cine's (NLM) MEDLINE and TOXLINE, contain references to the published medical and toxicologic literature. MEDLINE contains references to approximately 500,000 citations from 3,000 biomedical journals and provides health professionals rapid access to the most recently published information on any biomedical subject. MEDLINE is searched using key words or names to scan the data base. When the search is completed, references to articles in the data base that contain the key words or names will be listed. The author, title, journal name, and abstract for each reference can be printed out immediately or printed off-line and mailed to you from NLM.

Occupational and environmental health references are also accessible through TOXLINE. This data base contains references to more than 400,000 published human and animal toxicity studies, effects of environmental chemicals and pollutants, adverse drug reactions, and analytical methods.

Finally, TOXNET is a comprehensive data base containing both factual information and references covering several thousand chemicals. One advantage of TOXNET is that statements on toxicity and biomedical effects undergo scientific peer review.

Until recently, searching these computerized data bases had to be done at a medical library. The reference librarian developed a search strategy and consulted the data base while you waited. While most medical libraries still provide this service and reference librarians are the best source of information on how to use the data bases, it is now possible to use microcomputers and telecommunication packages to search NLM and other data bases from your home or office.

If you have a personal computer and a modem, access to the NLM can be accomplished using the NLM's inexpensive software package, *Grateful Med*. The *Grateful Med* package, which is extremely easy to use, formats the search with your prompting. The results of the search can be printed directly, downloaded to your diskette, or mailed to you from the NLM. Information about *MEDLINE, TOXLINE, TOXNET,* and *Grateful Med* can be obtained from the Medlars Management Section, National Library of Medicine, Building 38, Room 4N421, 8600 Rockville Pike, Bethesda, MD, 20894; phone: (800) 638-8480.

In addition to *Grateful Med,* several commercial telecommunications networks provide access to the NLM data bases. For example, *BRS Colleague, Compuserve,* and *Dialog Information Systems* all allow on-line access to NLM as well as to a wide range of other data bases. Generally, billing is a combination of an hourly connect-time charge and a print fee. Information about these and other privately run networks is available in most personal computing magazines.

4
Preventing Occupational Disease

Barry S. Levy and David H. Wegman

Occupational diseases are in principle preventable. Prevention is facilitated by awareness of occupational health problems by workers and employers, by research on hazards and their control, and by government regulations. In addition, physicians and other health professionals can play a vital role in preventing work-related disease if they recognize an obligation to go beyond the individual patient they may be treating and take appropriate action to prevent occurrence of the disease in other workers.

METHODS OF PREVENTION

Measures to prevent occupational disease and injury can be arbitrarily divided into two categories: those that primarily impact the workplace and those that primarily impact the worker. These are described below and illustrated in many places in this text.

The three methods of prevention described below directly reduce or remove potential hazards in the workplace by changing the workplace environment or production processes (see also Chap. 7):

Installation of engineering controls and devices, such as exhaust systems that remove hazardous dusts (Fig. 4-1), soundproofing materials that reduce loud noise, and enclosures that isolate hazardous processes. The major impediments to installation of engineering controls are cost and lack of awareness that such solutions are available.

Changed work practices, such as wetting asbes-

tos before removing it from a building, rather than removing it dry.

Substitution of a nonhazardous substance for a hazardous one. An example is the frequent substitution of fibrous glass for asbestos. Substitution carries with it, however, certain risks because substitute materials have often not been adequately tested for health effects and may in fact themselves be hazardous. For example, the search for a nonflammable cleaning solvent led to the use of carbon tetrachloride, which was later found to cause hepatotoxicity and other problems.

In general, these preventive measures tend to be more effective than the following four methods that primarily impact the worker. The four measures that follow potentially reduce the damage that may result from workplace hazards without actually removing the source of the problem:

Education and advice concerning specific work hazards is essential. Workers should always be given full information about workplace hazards and means of reducing their risk (Fig. 4-2). Many safety measures necessitate changed behavior by workers, which also requires education or training. Workers who are not aware of job hazards will not take the health and safety precautions necessary for protecting themselves and their coworkers. (See box on pp. 47–48 on education of workers and information on Hazard Communication Standard in Chapter 10.)

Use of personal protective equipment such as

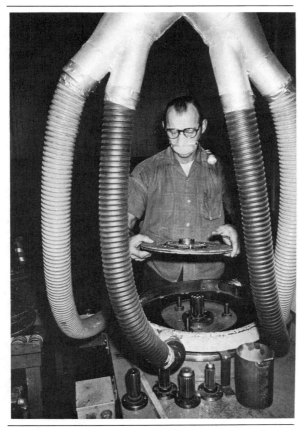

Fig. 4-1. Local exhaust ventilation used to protect a worker from asbestos dust generated in working with clutch plates.
(Photograph by Earl Dotter.)

Administrative measures, taken by the employer, may offer some protection. For example, rotation of workers, such that each worker has less average exposure than one worker performing a hazardous job, may be useful, although it is often impractical. In addition, depending on the dose-response curve of the hazardous effect of a workplace exposure, more aggregate harm may be done by exposing more workers to a hazard, although for a shorter time for each worker. Another preventive administrative measure is a preplacement examination to avoid placing into a job individuals who may be at high risk for specific disease(s) or injury from that job.

Screening for early detection of disease may lead to control measures that prevent further hazardous exposure to workers (see Chap. 6). Unlike the methods described above, which are designed to prevent occurrence of occupational disease by *primary* prevention, screening is part of *secondary* prevention, designed to identify and control disease shortly after it has begun. Screening, however, can lead to primary prevention measures: early detection of disease can identify inadequate control measures and correct them so that other workers do not become sick or injured.

By recognizing potential or existing work-related disease, health professionals can initiate activities leading to one or more of these methods of prevention. They can play an active role in education by informing workers and employers about potentially hazardous workplace exposures and ways of minimizing them. They can advise appropriate use of respirators or other personal protective equipment. They can also screen the worker and facilitate screening of coworkers who may be at high risk for certain diseases. Consultation with occupational health physicians, industrial hygienists, or safety officers may be necessary to facilitate these activities.

respirators, earplugs, gloves, and protective clothing (Fig. 4-3). This approach often has substantial limitations; for example, workers will often not wear such protection because it is cumbersome or causes other difficulties. Effective personal protective equipment programs are surprisingly costly. Proper fit of the equipment is an important factor, especially with respirators. Some personal protective equipment may not be as effective as claimed by its manufacturer.

EFFECTIVELY EDUCATING WORKERS
—Margaret M. Quinn

A prerequisite to effective health and safety programs is education. Therefore, careful consideration must be given to the methods used to present information to workers. It is not uncommon to go into a workplace where labor and management communication is generally good and yet the employees are not even aware that they have received a particular type of health and safety training. Some guidelines for educational programs include:

1. Develop an educational program in the trainee's literal and technical language. All trainees must be able to understand the language that is used to convey the information.
2. Define specific and clearly stated goals.
3. Begin each program with a concise overview and summarize the most important messages.
4. Build an evaluation mechanism that can be easily adapted to each program.
5. Use participatory teaching methods along with or in place of a traditional lecture approach.

Participatory or learner-centered teaching methods are designed to foster maximum worker participation and interaction. They constitute an approach to labor education based on the understanding that adults learn more effectively by doing rather than listening passively.

Learners' experiences are incorporated into the course material and are used to expand their grasp of new concepts and skills. Instructors offer specialized knowledge; workers have direct experience that will help them understand the importance of specific information that is taught during a course. Basing new knowledge on prior practical experience will help the learner solve problems and develop safe solutions to unforeseen hazards. A learner-centered approach to teaching health and safety ac-

knowledges that the worker is the one most familiar with his or her job and that the worker should be included in the development and implementation of safe work practices.

Participatory learning generally requires more trainer-trainee contact than lecture-style presentations. Large groups should be limited to approximately 20 participants, and these groups may break down into groups of four to six for small group exercises. In addition to a traditional classroom lecture, participatory teaching methods rely on:

1. Group discussions, which draw out the participants' work experiences.
2. Small group exercises, where participants work together to review worksheets or case studies and to solve problems.
3. "Brainstorming," where class participants identify existing or potential health and safety problems and their solutions. The trainer elicits information from the participants rather than presenting it in a didactic manner.
4. Hands-on training, where participants actually perform the techniques presented in class, such as respirator fit testing.
5. Role playing, where participants have the chance to practice the new methods presented in class in a supportive, supervised setting.

Participatory learning techniques are well-established methods practiced in labor education programs, schools of education, labor unions, and Coalitions and Committees for Occupational Safety and Health (COSH groups). One example of this type of educational program exists in the courses developed by the United Automobile Workers–General Motors (UAW-GM) National Joint Committee on Health and Safety*. The committee has recently developed four courses, chosen because they deal with a very widespread health hazard (asbestos), a leading cause of on-the-job fatalities among skilled trades workers (failure to lock out energy sources), manlift accidents, and lethal confined-space environments.

Members of the team developing the course stated: "All too often in the past company health and safety training meant a lot of people sitting in rooms, watching a movie, and falling asleep. The workers in our courses will be wide awake. They'll be in motion. They'll be learning every minute."

The new courses reflect a participatory educational philosophy—much more flexible and stimulating than those found in most U.S. schools today.

"Students demonstrate what they have learned at their own pace, rather than in a formal exam at the end. There are no surprise questions, no attempts to catch students off-guard, as in many conventional classrooms.

"Most courses are mandatory, and they have performance criteria—for example, right and wrong ways of entering a confined space, making sure it is safe to do so, and using the buddy system. If students show they can do something right, they don't need to waste class time studying it. They may move through the course faster than other students, or slower. It doesn't matter.

"Once our students find they'll be using a hands-on approach, demonstrating their new skills rather than competing with one another for test scores or risking 'failure,' they really enjoy the training."*

All of the curriculum developers have had "shop floor" experience and understand the teaching process. The curriculum teams researched the hazards. Then they called in skilled trades people and other safety experts to find out what students needed to know. Drafts of the curricula were submitted to the union and GM health and safety departments, revised, tested, and put into final form.

Bibliography

Clement D. The hazards of work: occupational safety and health training manual. New Market, TN: Highlander Research and Education Center, 1980.

Fighting shipyard hazard training manual for stewards: guidance for instructors. Chester, PA: Boilermakers Local 802, 1981.

Massachusetts Coalition for Occupational Safety and Health (MassCOSH) Women's Committee. Occupational safety and health course for working women. Boston: MassCOSH, 1981.

Wallerstein N, Pillar C, Baker, R. Labor educator's health and safety manual. Berkeley, CA: Labor Occupational Health Program, Center for Labor Research and Education, Institute of Industrial Relations, University of California, Berkeley, 1981.

*United Automobile Workers. Teaching about workplace hazards. *Solidarity,* May 1985, Pp. 11–13.

INITIATING PREVENTIVE ACTION

Once a health professional identifies a probable case of work-related disease, or injury, it is crucial to take preventive action. Failure to do so may lead to recurrence or worsening of the disease in the affected worker and the continuation or new occurrence of similar cases among workers in similar jobs—either at the same workplace or others. A health professional has at least the following five opportunities for preventive action after identifying a case of work-related disease.

Advise the Patient

The health professional should always advise the worker concerning the nature and prognosis of the worker's condition and the possible necessity for better engineering of the workplace to remove hazards, for personal protective equipment at work, or even for changing jobs. The patient may be advised to consult with a lawyer if legal issues, such as a contested workers' compensation claim, are involved, or to register a complaint with an appropriate government agency (as discussed below). It

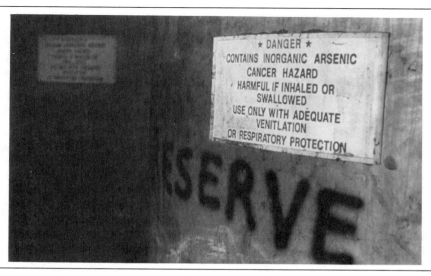

Fig. 4-2. Labels have begun to warn workers of cancer hazards, but many labels still fail to warn about other diseases or their symptoms. (Photograph by Earl Dotter.)

is important to remember that a worker's options may be limited; the worker may not wish to file a claim for workers' compensation or register a complaint with a government agency, fearing job loss or other punitive action. However, it is essential to inform a worker of potential hazards; it is not appropriate to withhold this information because of the possibility of upsetting the patient. A health professional cannot assume that even a large and relatively sophisticated industry will have adequately educated its workers about workplace hazards. (It should be noted that once a patient is informed of the work-relatedness of a disease in writing, this may start the time clock on the notification procedures and statute of limitations for workers' compensation [see Chap. 11]; therefore, one should obtain legal advice.)

Inform the Appropriate Governmental Agency

The health professional may notify the federal Occupational Safety and Health Administration or the appropriate state agency. OSHA establishes and enforces standards for hazardous exposures in the workplace and undertakes inspections, both routinely and in response to complaints from workers, physicians, and others (see Chap. 10). In about half of the states in the United States the program is implemented directly by federal OSHA, which is part of the U.S. Department of Labor; in the other states a state agency—often the state department of labor—implements the program. Both federal OSHA and the state agency may investigate a workplace in response to a complaint. Most state agencies will make recommendations to improve the situation, but only those states with OSHA-delegated authority can order changes to improve health and safety in the workplace and impose fines if these changes are not made. If a case of occupational disease appears to be serious or may be affecting others in the same workplace, it is wise for the health professional or the worker to file a complaint with federal OSHA or the appropriate state governmental agency.

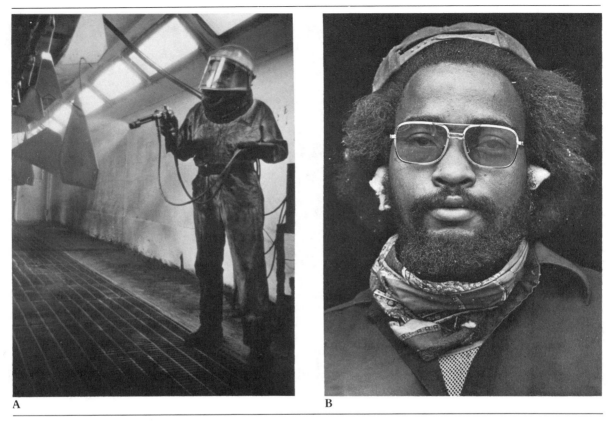

A   **B**

Fig. 4-3. A. Spray painter with respiratory protection. B. Makeshift personal protective equipment. Cotton plugs are not as effective as personal protective equipment. Only adequately fitting earplugs or earmuffs are effective. (Photographs by Earl Dotter.)

The health professional should always inform the patient in advance of notifying federal or state agencies. Although OSHA regulations protect workers who file health and safety complaints against resultant discrimination by the employer (that is, against loss of job, earnings, or benefits), this protection is difficult to enforce, and workers' fears are not unfounded. Health professionals should familiarize themselves with pertinent laws and regulations—for example, if the worker does not file an "11-C" (antidiscrimination) complaint

within 30 days of a discriminatory act, the worker's rights are lost. The health professional and workers (or their union, if one exists) have the right, guaranteed by the Freedom of Information Act, to obtain the results of an OSHA inspection.

The federal Mine Safety and Health Act of 1977 gives miners rights similar to those given other workers by the OSHAct of 1970. Information on this act is contained in a pamphlet entitled "A Guide to Miners' Rights and Responsibilities under the Federal Mine Safety and Health Act of

"1977," which can be obtained from the Mine Safety and Health Administration (MSHA), U.S. Department of Labor. (See box on MSHA in Chap. 10.)

Contact the Patient's Union or Other Labor Organization

If it is agreeable to the affected worker, the health professional should inform the appropriate union or other labor organization of the potential health hazards suspected to exist in the workplace. The provision of this information may help to alert other workers to a potential workplace hazard, facilitate investigation of the problem, possibly identify additional similar cases, and eventually facilitate the implementation of any necessary control measures. (Keep in mind, however, that only about 18 percent of workers in the United States belong to a union.)

Contact the Patient's Employer

The health professional, again only with the patient's consent and without identifying the patient in any way, may choose to report the problem to the employer. This can be effective in initiating preventive action. Many employers do not have the staff to deal with reported problems adequately, but they can obtain assistance from government agencies, academic institutions, or private firms if they are interested in providing a safe workplace. In addition, it may be possible to obtain useful information from an employer concerning exposures and the possibility of similar cases among the other workers.

While the law prohibits employers from firing workers for making complaints to OSHA, it does not prohibit them from firing workers who have a potentially work-related diagnosis. The federal lead and cotton dust standards mandate the removal of workers from jobs that are making them sick. The medical removal protection section of the federal lead standard provides temporary medical removal for workers at risk of health impairment from continued lead exposure, as well as temporary economic protection for workers so removed. It states, "During the period of removal, the employer must maintain the worker's earnings, seniority and other employment rights and benefits as though the worker had not been removed."* The cotton dust standard, however, does not offer such protection.

Contact an Appropriate Research Group

The health professional may choose to report the situation to an agency or other organization con-

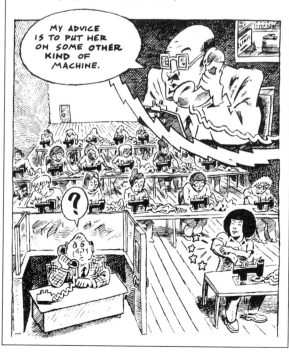

Advice to employees and employers should be practical.
(Drawing by Nick Thorkelson.)

MY ADVICE IS TO PUT HER ON SOME OTHER KIND OF MACHINE.

---

*Occupational exposure to lead: final standard. *Federal Register* 43:52972, 1978.

ducting research on occupational safety and health such as:

The National Institute for Occupational Safety and Health (see Appendix to this chapter entitled "What You Need to Know About NIOSH"). The hazard evaluation group at NIOSH responds to complaints of possibly serious occupational health or safety hazards.

An appropriate state agency, usually within the state departments of labor or public health.

A medical school or school of public health. (Several of these schools have NIOSH-sponsored occupational health and safety Educational Resource Centers; see Appendix B).

Some other group with expertise, experience, and interest in research concerning work-related medical problems.

Occasionally, the health professional who is reporting a work-related medical problem may undertake or assist in a research investigation of this problem. No matter who conducts the research, identifying additional cases and investigating these cases and the workplace will often lead to new information. Publishing epidemiologic studies or even case reports alerts others to newly discovered hazards and ways of controlling them.

THE CONSULTING PHYSICIAN'S ROLE

Health professionals have many other opportunities to be directly involved in the planning and implementation of preventive measures in the workplace. For example, an increasing number of physicians are being asked to advise, consult, or service an industry or a union on a part-time basis. Work for industry often consists primarily of preplacement physical examinations, return-to-work evaluations, and reviews of cases in which there have been workers' compensation claims. A physician consulting on a part-time basis to an employer or a union, however, can and should insist on being permitted to undertake preventive measures; in any such relationship the physician

should have the authority to obtain data, to share data with those who need to have this information, including the workers, and to take preventive and corrective action. The physician's role in the area of prevention may include the following activities:

Visiting the workplace and obtaining sufficient information by direct observation and review of medical and other records to assess more accurately specific health and safety hazards. A workplace visit familiarizes the physician with potentially hazardous processes and substances and also enables the physician to establish rapport with workers and to demonstrate concern about their health (see Chap. 34).

Establishing a surveillance system to monitor the occurrence of diseases among workers, based on reports of cases, baseline and subsequent screening data, and other sources. Such a system may identify clusters of work-related medical problems so that they may be controlled before reaching epidemic proportions.

Monitoring the introduction of new materials or processes to prevent, whenever possible, the addition of new occupational health and safety risks in the workplace.

Presenting educational programs for the employer and workers. This activity may be the difference between success and failure of a prevention program.

Developing cooperative working relationships with occupational health nurses, safety officers, industrial hygienists, personnel managers, union representatives, and workers themselves to ensure that worker health and safety is always the first priority.

Most health professionals are reluctant to go beyond treating or advising their individual patients when they suspect work-related medical problems. Understandably, they do not want to get deeply involved in legal proceedings or other complex situations that may require siding with either employer or employee and for which they feel ill-prepared. Only a few health professionals believe that they have the medical and medicolegal expertise to take on patients with work-related medical problems; preventing such problems, however, requires the active participation of almost *all* health professionals, not only those who have a particular interest or expertise in the field. All health professionals should be willing to take appropriate action as indicated above to ensure that workplace hazards are correctly identified, investigated, and controlled. To do this effectively, health professionals need to develop appropriate methods for advice, consultation, and referral. They also must recognize that persistence—sometimes extraordinary persistence—is necessary to solve complex problems. Nevertheless, there are few other areas of medicine where the health professional has such a vast opportunity to practice prevention and to make such a difference.

APPENDIX
What You Need to Know About NIOSH*

The National Institute for Occupational Safety and Health (NIOSH) was established under the OSHAct. Unlike OSHA, which is in the Department of Labor, NIOSH is in the Department of Health and Human Services; it is part of the Centers for Disease Control of the U.S. Public Health Service.

NIOSH investigates health and safety hazards on request in all kinds of workplaces. After identifying and evaluating the hazards, it recommends procedures for prevention or control. Unlike OSHA, NIOSH does not have the authority to issue citations or fines if employers are violating existing health and safety rules. If NIOSH inves-

tigators discover a hazard, however, NIOSH can and does warn employees and employers and notify the Department of Labor.

Major responsibilities of NIOSH include investigating the cause of workplace illness and accidents and determining the present or potential hazard of a substance, practice, or condition, including on-the-spot evaluation and long-term follow-up; performing research and developing criteria documents that recommend exposure limits to hazardous chemicals, physical agents, and processes; certifying the efficacy of personal protective equipment; providing for the education of industrial hygienists, nurses, physicians, toxicologists, and others in occupational health and safety; and developing sampling and measurement methods to evaluate workplace hazards.

NIOSH publishes a variety of reports and other materials detailing occupational hazards and ways of preventing or controlling them. Many of these publications are for specific industries, types of workers, or specific exposures. If workers want an on-site investigation of actual hazards in their workplace, NIOSH can conduct a health hazard evaluation, which is undertaken not simply to determine compliance with an OSHA or MSHA standard but to explain the cause of a problem. This type of investigation must be requested by an authorized representative of employees, such as a union representative, or by an employer. If the NIOSH investigator finds that any employees may be in imminent danger, the investigator will tell them, the employer, and the Department of Labor immediately.

Through industry-wide studies NIOSH also investigates the effects of long-term exposures to low levels of industrial materials, processes, and stresses that may cause illness, disease, or loss of ability to function. For physicians interested in studying occupational hazards themselves, NIOSH will assist and cooperate in investigations of hazards affecting their patients. Health surveillance conducted by NIOSH is designed to determine the number of workers exposed to specific hazards, what industries they work in, and which

---

*Much of the material for this section was adapted from *A Worker's Guide to NIOSH*, published by the U.S. Department of Health, Education, and Welfare in October, 1978.

jobs they hold. NIOSH also provides a wide variety of training programs in occupational medicine and nursing, industrial hygiene, and occupational safety available through specific courses directly presented by NIOSH and at NIOSH-sponsored Educational Resource Centers (ERCs) (see Appendix B).

In addition, NIOSH develops criteria documents that recommend standards for occupational exposure to hazardous chemicals, physical agents such as noise and heat, and processes. These documents include all available information on hazards, use of materials, and methods for control. The completed document is sent to the Department of Labor for use when OSHA considers setting standards. The purpose of the criteria documentation process is to evaluate thoroughly the problems of the workplace as a first step in protecting the health and well-being of workers. NIOSH recommendations are considered to be objective scientific assessments of hazards; the OSHA standards that are eventually enforced are often compromises among government, industry, and labor.

NIOSH also encourages and responds to phone calls for short-term advice on occupational medical problems, even when a full-fledged investigation is not justified. (See Appendix C for how to contact NIOSH.)

5
Epidemiology

David H. Wegman and Ellen A. Eisen

The relationship between any group of workers and their work environment is dynamic—constantly changing over time due to the aging of the workers, changes in personal habits such as cigarette smoking or diet, and differences in types and levels of exposure (due to job transfers and changes in technology, the production process, and employment status). The epidemiologist uses analytic tools to examine this complex mix of variables in an attempt to develop new understandings of the effects of workplace exposures on disease, disability, or death. The analytic methods used to examine epidemiologic data have become more statistically sophisticated over the past two decades, as the focus of occupational epidemiology has shifted to the detection of early health effects associated with lower-level exposures. Nevertheless, the basic concepts remain fundamentally consistent with intuition and common sense.

The approaches of clinical medicine and epidemiology work together particularly well in addressing occupational health problems. The clinical approach focuses on the individual and is concerned with diagnosis, treatment, and education of the individual regarding risk factors and preventive behavior. The epidemiologic approach, however, focuses on groups and is concerned with identifying subgroups of the population at high risk for a particular disease, providing evidence for new causal associations, estimating dose-response relationships, and determining the effectiveness of exposure control measures. While these two approaches employ different means, they share the same ultimate goal of preventing occupational disease and disability.

All health care providers need to be aware of the importance of epidemiologic concepts in evaluating occupational exposures. A woman may ask her gynecologist if the difficulty she and her husband are having in conceiving a child could be due to work exposure to a chemical. A nurse practitioner may be requested to judge the work-relatedness of a bladder cancer in a 60-year-old patient who has worked for 40 years producing synthetic rubber. A workplace physician may be required to determine if the use of a chemical recently shown to cause cancer in mice has increased the incidence of lung cancer among production workers. A company industrial hygienist may be asked whether the recent introduction of a new chemical is causing acute respiratory irritation in a small group of exposed employees. The director of a state health department may recommend ongoing disease surveillance for various occupational groups. Clearly these decisions require differing levels of epidemiologic expertise—from a familiarity with the literature to the ability to design a health study. The objective of this chapter is to encourage such applications of epidemiologic principles to the prevention of work-related disease.

There are two types of occupational epidemiology: the surveillance of recognized occupational disease (see Chap. 3) and the study of potential health hazards. The most central and distinctive feature of the latter, etiologic epidemiology, is the estimation of exposure-response relationships.

The health "response" may be a discrete endpoint, such as disease diagnosis, or the measurement of a biologic parameter, such as pulmonary function or blood lead. The measure of "exposure" may be as crude as belonging to an occupational group, such as shipbuilders, or as refined as the average daily time-weighted average exposure to a particular substance.

Much greater emphasis has been placed on the measure of response than on the measure of exposure because most epidemiologists have been trained as physicians and, therefore, are more oriented toward measuring health outcomes. Recently, however, epidemiologists have started to collaborate more effectively with toxicologists and environmental scientists to improve the collection of exposure data and to develop models that better estimate cumulative exposure by accounting for uptake, metabolism, and excretion of toxic materials. This collaboration has improved the validity of exposure-response estimation over a broader range of exposure levels allowing more effective prevention strategies.

MEASURING EXPOSURE

In occupational settings, a distinction must be made between *exposure* (what we can measure) and *dose* (what we would like to measure). Exposure is what is measured or measurable in the environment, while dose is what is delivered to the organs or tissues where the effect is manifested. For both, there are two components: intensity and duration. What the epidemiologist wishes to study is the actual dose delivered over a given time period, but what is usually available is only an estimate of exposure. A review of the possible levels of refinement for approximating exposure should place this aspect of the epidemiologic study in perspective.

Potential Exposure

The most common measure of exposure in epidemiologic studies has been a *potential* exposure,

that is, employment in a specific industry or specific job. In either case, the information is in categorical form, such as presence or absence of employment in an industry or job title. It is important to realize that the actual exposure of interest may be greatly diluted by such a surrogate measure. For example, after a recent study of diesel exposure, only 7 percent of railroad workers were found to be exposed to diesel fumes. The title "railroad worker," therefore, was a very crude measure of exposure since 93 percent of railroad workers would be misclassified as exposed. If, however, the association between exposure and response is very strong, the effect of such dilution is not too damaging. For example, asbestos-associated lung cancer excess has been documented with information no more specific than past employment in a shipyard, where less than half of the workers have asbestos exposure [1].

Quantity of Exposure

Ideally, the measure of exposure would reflect both intensity and duration. Because data on duration of employment may be more easily obtained, it is frequently used as a surrogate measure for both. On first inquiry, it is often believed that no data exist on length of employment. Pension plan eligibility, however, may provide at least a dichotomous measure of duration—for example, less than or greater than 10 years of employment. Documentation of the actual number of years employed is preferred. This latter information may be available from payroll records or from union seniority records.

A more refined surrogate for exposure can be created if a complete work history is available for each subject, including documentation of specific jobs, years in those jobs, and potential exposure to specific materials. Information about job-specific potential exposures permits the aggregation of jobs with common exposures [2]. A thorough history would include information on the gaps during time employed, such as time away from work due to prolonged sick leave, periods of layoffs, or military leave.

Estimate of Actual Exposure

Industrial hygiene measurements of work environments permit an estimation of actual exposure. Variation in exposure occurs due to changes in daily work assignments both between days and often within any given day, differences in work habits, seasonal changes in ventilation patterns, and use of personal protective equipment. Current exposure estimates are most relevant for acute effects. Current exposure can only be used to *estimate* past exposure in environments with well-documented stability in the production process.

Estimates of Cumulative Historic Exposure

In occupational studies of chronic disease, the exposure variable of interest is often the total exposure history. Although this has rarely been directly measured, it is generally possible to reconstruct a reasonable approximation. The approach is to estimate job-specific exposures and their variation over time, based on actual measurements along with interviews about estimates of historic change. These estimates are multiplied by the number of years in the job during each exposure era and the products are then summed over all jobs held by each worker. This was done in the Vermont granite industry to estimate a lifetime exposure history. To estimate exposures that occurred prior to the installation of exhaust ventilation, an old granite shed was reopened and operated without environmental controls (operators used personal protective equipment). From measurements collected in these studies, an estimate of the ratio of precontrol to postcontrol exposures was made for each job. This ratio was applied to the number of job-specific years spent in granite sheds before controls.

The assumptions made in the arithmetic cumulation of lifetime exposure should be noted. For example, one year of exposure to a high level (for example, 20 fibers/cc of asbestos) is assumed to be equivalent to 10 years of exposure to a tenth of that level (2 fibers/cc). Second, exposure that occurred 20 years ago is assumed equivalent to the exposure last year. Some investigators have begun to explore the implications of alternatives to these assumptions.

Biological Monitoring

Evaluation of current workers for toxic agents (or their metabolites) in blood, urine, or exhaled air sometimes permits estimation of the actual dose (rather than exposure). The use of urinary hippuric acid levels, for example, is an estimate of the total dose of toluene to an exposed worker via both lung and skin absorption. Such biological monitoring is deservedly receiving much more attention today [3]. Many of the available tests measure, however, only active levels—not total body burden. Also, metabolism of certain materials is so rapid that current levels provide no information on past exposures. Finally, no biological monitoring tests currently exist for a substantial number of hazardous workplace substances.

In summary, there is a wide variety of ways to estimate both current and past exposures. Each has advantages and disadvantages in efficiency and precision. It is important to recognize the range of methods available as well as the assumptions and limitations inherent in each method. An accurate measure of exposure is equally as important as the measurement of response in arriving at an unbiased and precise estimate of an exposure-response relationship.

COMMON MEASURES OF DISEASE FREQUENCY

The number of individuals with a diagnosed disease or with an abnormal test result, in general, cannot be interpreted without some additional information. An exception to this rule is the occurrence of a disease that is so rare that any case is unusual. Three cases of angiosarcoma diagnosed among about 270 workers during a three-year period were sufficient to make a plant physician suspect that the vinyl chloride they were exposed to was a carcinogen [4]. Note, however, the unstated comparison made between three observed cases versus none expected. The more common problem in case counts is illustrated by the example of a study of workers in a coated fabrics plant where 68 individuals were found to have a peripheral neuropathy [5]. This number has little or no meaning without some reference point. There are several different ways to transpose a simple case count into a measure that can be interpreted. Such measures are called rates.

Rates

A rate is the frequency of a disease per unit size of the group (or population) being studied. The simplest rate, known as the *point prevalence rate,* is based on the number of cases present at one point in time.

$$\text{Prevalence rate} = \frac{\text{The number of cases present at a given point in time}}{\text{The total population at risk at that given point in time}}$$

To improve our understanding of the 68 cases of peripheral neuropathy in the coated fabrics plant, we need a denominator. The total plant population was 1157, which results in a plant prevalence rate of 68/1157 = 5.9 percent. This rate can be compared with a general population rate or rate from an appropriate control group to determine if it is excessive. A limitation of a prevalence rate alone, however, is that it counts all cases of the disease, without differentiating between old and new cases.

A rate that removes the background cases and focuses more clearly on new or recent events is the *incidence rate,* which is based on the number of new cases occurring over a specified period of time.

$$\text{Incidence rate} = \frac{\text{The number of new cases of disease during time}}{\text{The total population at risk during time}}$$

In the coated fabrics plant, the number of new cases occurring in the past year was 50. Since 18 cases had onset prior to this year, the population at risk during the study year of developing a new case was 1139. Using these numbers we arrive at a plant-wide incidence rate of 50/1139 = 4.4 percent.

This rate can be better understood if it is subdivided so that an expected rate can be estimated. The population of employees not in the print department was 970, among whom there were 16 new cases for an annual incidence rate of 16/970 = 1.6 percent. In contrast, in the print department 34 of the 169 employees had onset of peripheral neuropathy in the past year for an annual incidence rate of 34/169 = 20 percent. These two rates, when compared, show a striking difference. Contrast this with comparing the numerators alone (34 versus 16) and the additional information expressed in a rate is evident.

Person-Years

When the incidence rate is intended to measure disease onset occurring in the group at risk over more than one year (in contrast to the example above) the appropriate denominator is person-years. This value simultaneously takes into consideration the number of individuals and the time period over which they were observed and considered to be at risk of developing the disease. It therefore permits the inclusion of individuals who were not at risk for the whole time period. This is particularly important when new hires or terminations are counted or when risk in a specific time period is evaluated. In the latter case (Fig. 5-1) [6], some people entered the time period and others left it during the observation period. Only the time spent in the time period (for example, 1955–1960) is appropriate for calculating a rate.

Thus far, the rates discussed are known as crude rates: rates calculated without consideration of factors such as age, race, or sex. If two populations being considered differ, for example, in the proportion of elderly individuals, difference in their crude disease rates may reflect nothing more

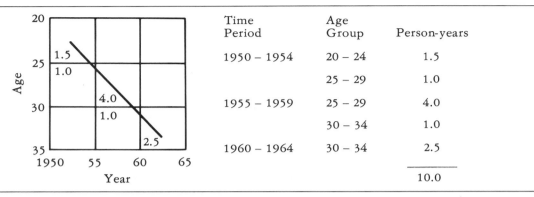

Fig. 5-1. Person-years experienced by a person entering a follow-up at age 23½ in mid-1952 and leaving in mid-1962. (Adapted from RR Monson. Occupational epidemiology. Boca Raton, FL: CRC Press, 1980.)

than differences in age. Therefore it can be desirable to calculate and compare age-specific (or race-specific or sex-specific) rates.

Specific Rates
In some instances, a crude or adjusted rate (see below) for the entire population may obscure an important association. When opposite trends exist in different parts of the age spectrum, these trends may offset each other and be masked by a summary rate. In such cases, it is necessary to examine the data according to homogeneous groups defined by specific levels of each characteristic. For example, in the first published report of the relationship between lung cancer and exposure to bis-chloromethyl ether (BCME), the average age of death for the affected men was 46 years and none was over 55 [7]. The majority of males dying from lung cancer, however, are 55 or older. If these cases of BCME cancer had been collected as part of a sample of lung cancer cases in the general population, no excess rate would have been noted since they would form a very small proportion of all lung cancer. However, if rates were presented on an age-specific basis, the rates for lung cancer in males 35 to 50 years of age would probably have

shown a significant elevation due to the BCME-related lung cancer deaths.

Standardization (Adjustment) of Rates
Although the specific rate can provide invaluable information, it is cumbersome to compare many specific rates. Summary rates, known as adjusted or standardized rates, are therefore helpful in analyzing disease distribution between different populations. To determine such rates, an adjustment or standardization procedure is performed. Two types of adjustment are used:

Direct. The rates of disease in the categories (age groups, for example) of the two groups to be compared are applied to a standard set of age groups forming summary rates that are directly comparable.

Indirect. The category-specific rates of disease in a general population are applied to the appropriate categories of a study group to produce an expected number. This expected number is compared with the observed number in the form of a standardized ratio of observed:expected outcomes. Indirectly standardized rates in two distinct popula-

Table 5-1. Age effect on incidence of asbestosis[a]

Location	Workers < 45 years old			Workers ≥ 45 years old			All workers			
	Cases	Population at risk	Age-specific incidence rate per 1,000	Cases	Population at risk	Age-specific incidence rate per 1,000	Cases	Population at risk	Crude incidence rate per 1,000	Age-adjusted incidence rate per 1,000[b]
Factory 1	4	400	10.0	18	600	30.0	22	1,000	22.0	18.0
Factory 2	10	800	12.5	10	200	50.0	20	1,000	20.0	27.5

[a]The incidence rate is expressed as new cases of asbestosis diagnosed in a 10-year period of observation per 1,000 population.
[b]Based on age distribution summed for Factory 1 and Factory 2.

tions cannot be compared unless the distributions of the categories, such as age groups, are approximately the same in the two study groups.

Table 5-1 gives an example of the use of adjusted rates. For a more detailed description of these types of adjustment, see the appendix at the end of the chapter.

COMPARISONS OF RATES
Independent of whether rates are presented by homogeneous subgroups or adjusted for appropriate variables in the entire group, the rates must be translated into risks to evaluate the effects of exposure. The two major types of risk estimates based on comparisons of rates are the ratio of rates (relative risk) and the difference between rates (attributable risk).

Relative Risk
The relative risk, or rate ratio, is designed to communicate the relative importance of an exposure by comparing rates from an exposed population to an unexposed or normal population. In its simplest form, it is the ratio of two rates (Table 5-2). When evaluating the effect of cigarette smoking on disease outcome, as seen in Table 5-3, the relative risk of lung cancer in smokers compared to nonsmokers is very large (32.4), while that for cardiovascular disease is small (1.4).

Table 5-2. Derivation of relative and attributable risk

Disease	Exposure		
	Present	Absent	Total
Present	a	c	a + c
Absent	b	d	b + d
Total population	a + b	c + d	a + b + c + d

$$\text{Exposed disease rate} = a/(a + b)$$
$$\text{Unexposed disease rate} = c/(c + d)$$
$$\text{Relative risk} = \frac{a/(a + b)}{c/(c + d)}$$
$$\text{Attributable risk} = a/(a + b) - c/(c + d)$$

Attributable Risk
The attributable risk, or risk difference, is designed to communicate the amount of disease that can be attributed to the exposure under study. This concept is particularly useful and necessary in occupational disease studies because few diseases can be attributed solely to an occupational exposure. The attributable risk is calculated by subtracting the rate of the particular disease in the normal or unexposed population from that in the exposed population (see Table 5-2). The risk difference is attributed to the exposure. In contrast to the relative risk, Table 5-3 shows that the smoking-attributable risk for lung cancer (2.20) is smaller than

**Table 5-3. Relative and attributable risks of death from selected causes
associated with heavy cigarette smoking by British male physicians, 1951–1961**

Cause of death	Death rate[a] among nonsmokers	Death rate[a] among heavy smokers[b]	Relative risk	Attributable risk[a]
Lung cancer	0.07	2.27	32.4	2.20
Other cancers	1.91	2.59	1.4	0.68
Chronic bronchitis	0.05	1.06	21.2	1.01
Cardiovascular disease	7.32	9.93	1.4	2.61
All causes	12.06	19.67	1.6	7.61

[a]Annual death rates per 1000.
[b]Heavy smokers are defined as smokers of 25 or more cigarettes per day.
Source: R Doll, AB Hill. Mortality in relation to smoking: ten years' observations of British doctors. Br Med J 1964; 1:1399.

the smoking-attributable risk for cardiovascular disease (2.61). The attributable risk can be viewed as a measure of the impact of a control program. Table 5-3 also shows that the death rate in smokers from cardiovascular disease is over four times higher than that for lung cancer and that elimination of smoking would have a much larger impact on cardiovascular disease than on lung cancer.

TYPES OF EPIDEMIOLOGIC STUDY DESIGNS

Epidemiologic studies can be categorized into two types: cohort and case-control. Cohort studies, in general, are either cross-sectional (characterized by collection of both exposure and effect information at one point in time), or longitudinal (characterized by identification of exposure at a point(s) in time and disease or outcome at a later point(s) in time). In the case-control design, a group with disease is compared to a selected group of nondiseased (control) individuals with respect to current or past exposure. Cohort studies select the study group based on exposure and look ahead to disease outcome, whereas case-control studies select the study group based on disease status and look backward to identify prior exposures.

Cohort Studies (Cross-Sectional or Prevalence Type)

The cross-sectional study is a common approach used in field investigations when an immediate response to a perceived hazard is necessary. In this type of study design, two groups defined by current exposure status are compared for measures of certain disease frequencies. The exposure categories can be defined as exposed versus nonexposed, or high exposure versus low exposure.

Many descriptive epidemiologic studies are cross-sectional in nature and present the age, sex, location, and time-of-onset patterns. In such studies, the distribution of the particular disease may be described in a given work population before an etiologic study. Though these studies usually are designed for health administration purposes, the unusual distribution of a disease may alert the investigator to seek an explanation, work-related or otherwise, in the study group. For example, an unusual prevalence of headaches in a foundry may be cause for concern. The distribution of the reports may lead to the identification of a particular work location (such as an area with excess carbon monoxide exposure). However, a systematic consideration of other potential causes of headaches (such as stress) is necessary before a work association

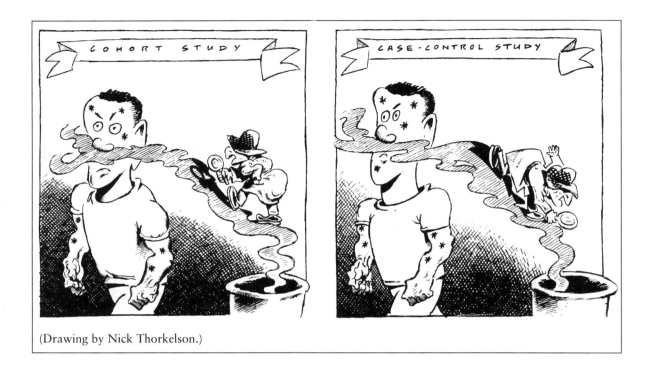

(Drawing by Nick Thorkelson.)

can be concluded. The initial descriptive study assists the investigator in focusing on and planning for a formal etiologic study.

Example (Cross-Sectional Morbidity Study). A pathology resident died of an acute heart attack at the age of 28. In discussing this incident, a number of the other pathology residents noted they had been experiencing abnormal heart rhythms (palpitations). It was discovered that those with palpitations appeared to have worked with fluorocarbon propellants. This led to a study of all employees in the pathology department (the exposed group) where these propellants were used to prepare frozen sections of pathology tissue and to clean instruments or specimen slides. A radiology department (the unexposed group) of similar size and distribution of staff and physicians was selected as an unexposed comparison group. Each

individual was asked about the occurrence of palpitations and the current use of fluorocarbon propellants. Those exposed had twice the rate of palpitations as those unexposed [8].

Cohort Studies (Longitudinal Type)
The most common type of study in work settings is probably the retrospective cohort study. In this study design, a group known to be exposed in the past is selected and followed to disease or death at some point also in the past (Fig. 5-2). In contrast, the prospective cohort study, although conceptually similar, identifies exposure in the past or present, but the outcome (disease or death) is followed into the future. In either type, the study group experience of mortality or morbidity is compared to that of an unexposed group.

It is possible to carry out cohort studies, particularly for mortality, in an exposed and an unex-

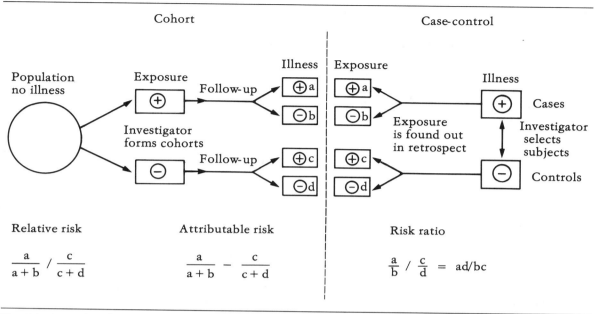

Fig. 5-2. General outline of cohort and case-control studies.

posed cohort so that a relative risk can be directly computed. When a documented unexposed cohort is not available for direct study (because of cost or availability), the cause-specific mortality of the exposed cohort can be compared to that of the general population (assumed to be unexposed). This results in an approximation of a relative risk, known as the *standardized mortality ratio* (SMR). If the number of deaths observed in the exposed cohort is greater than those expected in the standard population, the ratio is greater than one, which denotes an increase in risk. If it is less than one, it suggests a decreased risk. The healthy worker effect (see below) may complicate this latter interpretation.

To construct an SMR, the cause-specific death rates of the general population are applied to the exposed cohort's age distribution, resulting in an indirectly standardized measure (see appendix). Therefore, SMRs for different exposed cohorts should not be compared because the age distributions of each may differ.

To conduct an SMR study, the following information should be obtained for each member of the cohort: date of birth, date of entry into cohort, date of leaving cohort, vital status, and cause of death for those who died. With these data, person-years of risk can be determined that take into consideration workers entering or leaving the exposed group during the study period. This permits a calculation of years at risk, adjusting for different lengths of time since entry into the study. This type of study, however, requires personnel records with accurate employment data. When such data on the total population at risk are lacking, as is often the case, the mortality experience can be evaluated by proportional mortality analysis.

Cause-specific *proportional mortality ratios* (PMRs) are calculated as the proportion of all deaths represented by each specific cause of death.

These ratios in the study population are compared to the cause-specific ratios from the general population and are adjusted for age, sex, race, and year of death (again, indirect standardization).

In contrast to the SMR, however, an excess or deficit of deaths in causes other than the one under scrutiny can affect the *proportional* distributions. Therefore, the PMR results are less reliable than SMR results. For example, an excess of accidental deaths will lead to a reduced proportion of all other causes. When these values are compared to the general population proportions, the deaths from a specific nonaccidental cause may appear to be lower than expected, although they are actually equal or higher. An alternative to the PMR, the Standardized Mortality Odds Ratio (SMOR), has been proposed to address this problem [9]. Despite the greater difficulty in interpreting PMR results, they have often provided the first clue that an occupational factor is associated with a specific cause of death.

Example (Retrospective Cohort Mortality Study, SMR). A study of mortality in steelworkers was planned in 1962. The workers were selected for study if they were employed in 1953 and were followed to the end of 1962 for vital status. Over 59,000 workers were followed and 4,716 deaths recorded. When the number of deaths from specific causes were compared to the number expected, based on deaths in the study county, there appeared to be no excess (SMR for all cancer = 92). The study population was large enough, however, to examine a subgroup and to compare the observed deaths to those expected if the mortality experience of the rest of the workers (documented as unexposed) prevailed. This in-depth evaluation led to the discovery that workers employed on the top of coke ovens had an unusually high risk of lung cancer (Table 5-4) [10]. The large size of the study population permitted detailed examination of a number of subgroups. As a result, the very high risk of lung cancer in coke oven workers was extracted from the overall "normal" results.

Example (Retrospective Cohort Mortality Study, PMR). In 1949, British researchers determined that nickel was an occupational carcinogen. This finding was based primarily on case reports, and an investigation was undertaken to examine the magnitude and duration of risk. Over 15,000 deaths in four districts were grouped according to occupation on the death record and examined for the proportional distribution of lung cancer [11]. Occupations were divided into those using nickel, other occupations with suspected cancer risks, and those with no known suspected cancer risks ("all others"). This permitted use of the last category as

Table 5-4. Standardized mortality ratios for lung cancer among nonwhite males according to employment in coke ovens for five years or more by 1953

Work area	1953–1961			1962–1975		
	Observed	Expected	SMR	Observed	Expected	SMR
Total coke oven	22	5.1	423	29	13.9	209
Side oven	4	3.0	133	15	6.5	231
Part-time topside	4	0.8	500	5	1.5	333
Full-time topside	14	1.3	1077	9	0.6	1500

Source: Adapted from CK Redmond, HS Wieand, HE Rockelle, et al. Long term mortality experience of steelworkers. Department of Health and Human Services (NIOSH) Publication No. 81-120, 1981.

a locally generated comparison group. Based on the age distribution of the nickel workers, almost 10 lung cancers would have been expected if the "all other" occupation proportions applied. However, a total of 48 lung cancer deaths were observed, resulting in a PMR value of 4.86 (or 486 percent). Three explanations of these findings were possible: (1) the "all other" occupations might have had an unusually low number of lung cancer deaths; (2) the nickel workers may have had an unusually low number of "other causes" of death; or (3) the lung cancer excess could be real. The first explanation was excluded since the proportion of lung cancer in the "all other" occupations was very close to that for the country as a whole. The second explanation was considered inappropriate because it would have required deaths from all other causes in nickel workers to be one-fifth of the national experience, a highly unlikely finding. Thus, even though this was a PMR study, the nature of the evidence was convincing. Subsequently, an SMR study confirmed these findings.

Example (Retrospective Cohort Morbidity Study). A local union initiated a survey to assess the possibility of asbestosis in workers in a wallboard manufacturing operation [12]. Fifty-seven workers were examined for current respiratory health by questionnaire, pulmonary function tests, and a limited physical examination. As years employed increased, there was increased prevalence of wheezing, increased prevalence of abnormal chest examination findings (rales), and a decrease in predicted lung function (Table 5-5). Smoking habits were examined and did not explain these findings. Note that in the table a comparison group was created by subdividing the whole study population according to exposure duration.

Example (Prospective Cohort Morbidity Study). Exposure to toluene diisocyanate (TDI) is known to cause asthma. A study was designed to examine whether those without asthma might also suffer adverse respiratory effects. All workers on the first shift of a polyurethane-foam manufacturing firm were examined with pulmonary function tests on a Monday morning. They were divided into three exposure groups and retested at the end of the workday (a one-day prospective study). Generally, lung function does not change in the course of a day, but these workers were shown to lose lung function (presumably due to acute bronchospasm) and the loss was exposure-related (Table 5-6). A person with an acute work-related change in FEV_1 commonly recovers when removed from exposure. Therefore, the question remained whether the acute changes reflected a chronic effect that might persist. As a result, those still employed were retested four years later at the start of the work week before any acute bronchospasm could occur. The same three exposure groups were examined for accelerated decrement in lung function [13]. Again, an exposure-related effect was seen (see Table 5-5). Although all adults lose some

Table 5-5. Asbestos-exposed cohort of workers: Respiratory findings by duration of exposure

Duration of exposure (years)	Percent reporting wheezing	Percent with rales present	Percent predicted forced vital capacity (ml)
0–9	25	4	104
10–19	13	25	97
20–29	27	36	80
30 +	70	60	75

Source: Adapted from DH Wegman, GP Theriault, JM Peters. Worker sponsored survey for asbestosis. Arch Environ Health 1973; 27:105–109.

Table 5-6. Acute and chronic change in FEV$_1$ by exposure group in polyurethane foam manufacturing workers

Exposure group	FEV$_1$ differences from beginning to end of study period	
	Acute (one-day) change	Chronic (four-year) change
Low	78 ml	− 2 ml
Medium	108 ml	133 ml
High	180 ml	242 ml

Source: Adapted from DH Wegman, AW Musk, DM Main, et al. Accelerated loss of FEV-1 in polyurethane production workers: a four year prospective study. Am J Indust Med 1982; 3:209–215.

lung function each year, the high exposure group was losing it at a more rapid rate than the normal (25–30 ml/year). Cigarette smoking habits did not explain the effects noted in either the one-day or the four-year prospective study.

Case-Control Studies
An equally appropriate epidemiologic study for occupational settings is the case-control, or case-referent, study. In this type of study, the investigator selects a particular disease and compares it to another disease (or the absence of disease) for frequency of exposure (see Fig. 5-2). A case-control study is generally performed because the disease of interest is "rare"; therefore, a cohort study would have to be prohibitively large to generate enough cases. Case-control studies can be performed retrospectively or prospectively, but the terms have a different meaning in this context. In both instances, the exposure history is determined *after* the disease occurs. In the retrospective case-control study, people who already have the disease are evaluated for a prior history of exposure(s). In the prospective case-control study, as new cases occur, the past history of exposure(s) is documented.

Unless the case-control study is population-based (which is uncommon), there are no appropriate denominators of people at risk. As a result, actual rates in the exposed and unexposed groups (number with disease divided by population at risk) cannot be calculated, and a relative risk cannot be directly derived. Nevertheless, it can be approximated if three reasonable assumptions are made: (1) the controls are representative of the general population, (2) the cases represent all cases, and (3) the disease frequency is small. If these assumptions apply, the control group has the same distribution of exposure as the general population and can be considered representative. Although this would still not permit calculation of an absolute rate, it does allow calculation of a relative risk approximation, known as the *risk ratio* or *odds ratio*. From Table 5-2, it can be seen that a/a + b is representative of the rate of disease in the exposed population and c/c + d, that of disease in the unexposed population. Since we also assume that "a" is a small portion of "a + b" and "c" a small portion of "c + d," then the relative odds becomes a/b divided by c/d, or ad/bc.

Example (Case-Control Mortality Study). A team of investigators wanted to examine whether excess mortality from lung and blood cancers, heart disease, and cirrhosis of the liver were associated with arsenic exposures [14]. A parish in Sweden surrounding a copper smelter was selected. Deaths from the above four causes were classified into four case groups. Controls included deaths from all other well defined causes. The results for lung cancer alone are presented in Table 5-7. It was assumed that the control group was representative of the general population, that the cases represented all cases, and that lung cancer was relatively infrequent. Thus, the calculation of a relative odds as an approximation of a relative risk was possible.

Example (Case-Control Morbidity Study). Recall the example presented under cohort (cross-sectional or prevalence type) concerning exposure to fluorocarbon propellants among radiology and pathology department staff. In exploring the ex-

Table 5-7. Arsenic exposure and lung cancer mortality

Lung cancer	Arsenic exposure		Total
	Present	Absent	
Cases	18	11	29
Controls	18	56	74
Total	36	67	103

$$\text{Relative odds} = \frac{18 \times 56}{18 \times 11} = 5.1$$

Source: Adapted from O Axelson, E Dahlgran, CD Jarsson, et al. Arsenic exposure and mortality, a case referent study from a Swedish copper smelter. Br J Ind Med 1978; 35:8–15.

perience of the pathology department further, the investigators wanted to examine their impression that fluorocarbon propellants were associated with the palpitations noted. For this purpose, they had to focus on the pathology department, where the propellants were in use. (The frequency of propellant use in the radiology department was already known to be zero.) The group was divided into those with palpitations and those without palpitations. Among those with palpitations 40 percent had exposure, while among those without palpitations only 20 percent had exposure. Furthermore, among those with palpitations, 9 percent had high exposure compared to 3 percent among those without palpitations, resulting in a threefold risk [8].

SELECTION OF TYPE OF STUDY

The study designs described above have relative strengths and weaknesses. The selection of which design to use is based on the variety of factors.

Cohort Studies (Cross-Sectional or Prevalence Type)

Studies of disease prevalence have the advantage of collecting all information at one point in time concerning both exposure and effect. They are, therefore, the simplest and the quickest studies, but they also have significant limitations. Primarily, these studies are based on the not-always-correct assumption that estimates of current exposures are reflective of past exposures and that prevalent cases are the same as incident cases. It is not possible to establish causal relationships based solely on prevalence studies.

Cohort Studies (Longitudinal Type)

These studies focus on exposure and look ahead to outcome or disease. As such, the number of exposures that can be examined is generally small, but the number of outcomes is limited by the investigator's choice of which ones to measure. Such studies can occur completely in the past (retrospective) or in both the past and future (prospective). Retrospective studies have the distinct advantage of permitting quicker results since both exposure and outcome have already occurred. They are, therefore, also cheaper than prospective studies. On the other hand, data collected on exposure retrospectively is dependent on the quality of past records, in contrast to data collected prospectively according to a specific study plan. If questionnaires or interviews about past exposures are used, selective recall is inevitable. Furthermore, since outcome measures in retrospective studies were recorded for purposes other than the study, the endpoint must be fairly concrete, such as death.

Prospective studies have four advantages because the study design is within the investigators' control: (1) exposure data can be collected according to a prearranged plan; (2) several outcomes or diseases can be measured because the subjects can be specifically followed; (3) repeat measures of both exposure and outcome are possible; and (4) the methodology can be standardized and validated. The disadvantages, however, are that such studies take much more time and are usually quite costly. Both types of cohort studies suffer from the common problem that long-term follow-up can be difficult since participants die, move, or drop out of the study.

Case-Control Studies

In contrast to cohort studies, the case-control study starts by identifying disease and seeks information about exposures. It is necessary when the disease is rare because a cohort study is unlikely to produce a sufficient number of cases. It is also preferable when multiple possible exposures are being explored in the etiology of a specific disease. For example, if the investigator wishes to examine diseases associated with an exposure (lead), a cohort study is desirable; but if the interest is in studying the causes of a disease (bladder cancer), the case-control study is more appropriate.

The major advantages of the case-control study are the relative simplicity and the low cost. On the other hand, the exposure information is susceptible to potential bias due to incomplete recall, and there is always the problem of identifying an appropriate control group.

PROBLEMS RELATED TO VALIDITY

No matter what the selected design is, an epidemiologic study will always suffer from not being a planned experiment. The epidemiologist is faced with exposures that have not been assigned to subjects at random. A study's validity (the degree to which the inferences drawn from a study are warranted when account is taken of study methods, sample representativeness, and nature of the source population) needs, therefore, to be carefully considered. The investigator has to identify the potential sources of bias and the methods available for their prevention or control. In this context, bias is defined as a distortion of the measure of association between exposure and health outcome. There are three sources of bias: selection, misclassification, and confounding.

Selection Bias

Selection bias results from inappropriate admission of subjects into either the exposed or the nonexposed group in a cohort study, or into either the diseased or the nondiseased group in a case-control study. Selection bias cannot be corrected or controlled for; it can only be prevented. The basic means for preventing selection bias in cohort studies is masking outcome status when selecting subjects for exposed and nonexposed groups. In fact, it is best to collect outcome information after the groups are formed. Similarly, in case-control studies, the exposure status should be masked while assigning the subjects to diseased or nondiseased categories.

The healthy worker effect is a special case of selection bias. The bias results from subjects' self-selecting out of the study groups rather than as a result of any investigator error. Selection occurs, in general, because employed people are healthier than unemployed. The overall population, therefore, is not strictly comparable since it contains the aged, the infirm, the mentally retarded, and the chronically ill or disabled, most of whom would not be employed. Furthermore, some employers provide health examinations to preplace individuals. For example, preplacement screening will reduce the likelihood of an individual with poor lungs being employed in coke oven work.

As a result, studies of illness or death patterns of employed populations reveal lower rates of chronic disease and death when compared to the general population. That occupational cohorts are so often compared with the general population is of particular concern. For example, in the steelworkers mortality study example, the overall SMR was 82 percent for steelworkers compared to that for the surrounding county. The actual disease risk is underestimated because the comparison group is expected to have *higher* disease rates than the employed steelworkers. However, the healthy worker effect is not great enough to make comparisons with the general population useless.

It is beyond the scope of this chapter to examine ways that the healthy worker effect can be reduced or eliminated. Suffice it to say that studies of work populations, when the general population is the comparison group, must be examined carefully or an exposure-disease relationship may go unnoticed.

Misclassification

Misclassification refers to the investigator's inappropriate placement of an individual into a specific exposure or specific disease category or group. Misclassification can be either differential or nondifferential. *Differential misclassification,* also called information bias, occurs when information is collected in a differential manner in the groups under study. In cohort studies, differential misclassification is commonly prevented by keeping the investigator "blind" about exposure status when collecting outcome information. In this manner, any errors in collection should be randomly distributed over both exposed and nonexposed groups. In case-control studies, controlling such bias is much more complicated; it is difficult for the investigator and generally impossible for the subject to be unaware of the disease status when exposure information is being obtained. Prevention of differential misclassification depends on trying to collect data in as objective a way as possible.

Nondifferential misclassification is more common and results when there is little information on subjects' exposure, and subjects are poorly classified into exposure categories. This error reduces the difference in disease rates between exposed and nonexposed groups.

Confounding

Confounding is the most complex of the three types of bias and is always present to some extent. This kind of bias results when there is a characteristic associated with both the exposure and the disease. For example, coal dust exposure might be epidemiologically examined for its association with stomach cancer. However, chewing tobacco may also be associated with stomach cancer and may be more prevalent in coal miners because lighted tobacco is prohibited in a coal mine. The tobacco chewing, associated with both coal dust exposure and stomach cancer, is a potential confounder. A confounder should be differentiated from an effect modifier, which may dilute or accentuate an effect but not confound it. For example, cigarette smoking in asbestos workers modifies the effect, lung cancer. Cigarette smoking, like asbestos, is associated with lung cancer, but it is not associated with the exposure (asbestos workers are not more likely to smoke than nonasbestos workers); therefore, it is not a confounder.

Confounding can be controlled both in design and in analysis of epidemiologic data. Matching is usually the method employed to control it in the design phase. The cases and controls, or exposed and unexposed individuals, are matched for anticipated confounding factors. In the example above, if stomach cancer were being studied in Appalachia, the cases and controls could be matched on tobacco-chewing habits to eliminate differential distribution of this factor as an explanation of excess cancer. Care must be taken not to "overmatch"—that is, match on some intermediate step in the causal sequence of interest since this will create a negative bias.

Stratification is the major means of controlling confounding in the analysis phase. Here a confounder, such as age, is used to define strata, based, for example, on 10-year age groups. The independent effect of the primary exposure of interest can be examined in each stratum. Stratification, however, presents problems in that the more potential confounders considered, and the more refined the strata (for example, 5-year rather than 10-year age groups), the larger the study group necessary to compute stable estimates of risk.

As the number of strata increases, there are likely to be some strata that contain few or no subjects at all. For example, if age, smoking, and sex must be controlled for simultaneously, there may be no nonsmoking 40-to-45-year-old females in the study population. In this case, stratification becomes an inadequate method of controlling confounding, and one must turn to multivariable models to describe the data.

Multivariate models impose particular mathematical forms on the dose-response relationships, such as a linear form. By restricting the data to a specific structure, one can interpolate between sparse strata. This means of "smoothing" the data can provide more stable adjusted risk estimates.

INTERPRETATION OF EPIDEMIOLOGIC STUDIES

The interpretation of epidemiologic studies depends, in large part, on judgment. This judgment, in turn, is based primarily on the strength of the association, the validity of the observed association, and supporting evidence for causality. The strength of an association is measured by the size of the relative risk estimate for the exposed compared to that for the unexposed. Further evidence of an effect can be provided if the relative risk estimates increase over strata defined by increasing exposure. Although spurious risk estimates can occur, it is much less likely they will occur in an exposure-related manner.

Statistical tests of significance or confidence intervals are generally presented along with the relative risk. Statistical tests, however, do not measure the strength of the association or provide evidence of causality. Statistical tests evaluate the likelihood that the observed association could have occurred by chance alone. For example, "p (probability) < 0.05" indicates that the likelihood of observing an effect at least as large as the one observed is less than one in 20, given that no dose-response effect actually exists (that is, the event can be expected to occur by chance in only one of 20 trials). Some investigators will not interpret an effect as significant unless p is less than 0.01; others will require only that p be less than 0.10. The significance level is a guide to stability, particularly when the available number of subjects is small, and can be used as supporting evidence in the establishment of exposure-related associations.

The power of a study to detect a true effect depends on the background prevalence of the disease or exposure, the size of the cohort, the length of follow-up, and the level of statistical significance required. A small cohort followed for a brief time can result in a falsely negative result. For this reason, it is important, when interpreting a negative study, to examine whether the design itself precluded a positive finding. For example, in a recent retrospective cohort study of formaldehyde exposure, despite having 600,000 person-years of observation, the study had only 80 percent power to detect a fourfold risk in nasal cancer mortality [15]. That is, because nasal cancer has such a low background prevalence, even if the true relative risk were 3.5, the p value associated with such an estimate would have been greater than 0.05, and the finding would have been considered not statistically significant. Formulas for calculating the statistical power associated with a given sample size as well as the converse are available both for case-control and cohort studies.

When an association appears to be present, based on exposure-related relative risk estimates that are significant, the validity of the association still must be evaluated. This evaluation can be done in studies that provide sufficient detail on design and results. The internal validity should be evaluated by examining for selection bias, observation bias, and particularly confounding. All studies will suffer to some degree from problems with validity, so a judgment must be made concerning the importance of the biases. Any systematic errors should be evaluated for the direction and magnitude of their effect.

Finally, the consistency of the association—that is, the repeated demonstration of a particular association in different populations and by different investigations—is valuable supporting evidence of an association. Animal data and reasonable consistency with biology are also important as corroborating evidence of an observed association. A plausible biologic mechanism is particularly helpful, but the absence of one does not necessarily negate the results of a study, since epidemiologic studies may lead to identification of new mechanisms.

Two other considerations should not be overlooked. First, temporal consistency should be demonstrable. The exposure must precede the effect.

Second, the effect of removing a population from exposure should be determined if possible. This should result in a predictable change in disease incidence (unless the disease progresses after removal, as is the case with silicosis). The interpretation of epidemiologic studies and their use to support a causal association depends on the reader's careful evaluation of all aspects of the study and determined application of scientific judgment.

REFERENCES

1. Blot WJ, Harrington JM, Toledo A, et al. Lung cancer after employment in shipyards during World War II. N Engl J Med 1978; 299:620–624.
2. Smith AH, Waxweiler RJ, Tyroler HA. Epidemiologic investigations of occupational carcinogenicity using a serially additive expected dose model. Am J Epidemiol 1980; 112:787–797.
3. Lauwerys RR. Industrial chemical exposure: guidelines for biological monitoring. Davis, CA: Biomedical Publications, 1983.
4. Creech JL, Johnson MN. Angiosarcoma of liver in the manufacture of polyvinyl chloride. J Occup Med 1974; 16:150–51.
5. Billmaier D, Yee HT, Allen N, et al. Peripheral neuropathy in a coated fabrics plant. J Occup Med 1974; 16:665–671.
6. Figueroa WG, Raszkowski R, Weiss W. Lung cancer in chloromethyl methyl ether workers. N Engl J Med 1973; 288:1096–1097.
7. Monson RR. Occupational epidemiology. Boca Raton, FL: CRC Press, 1980:84.
8. Speizer FE, Wegman DH, Ramirez A. Palpitation rates associated with fluorocarbon exposure in a hospital setting. N Engl J Med 1975; 292:624.
9. Miettinen OS, Wang J-D. An alternative to the proportionate mortality ratio. Am J Epidemiol 1981; 114:144–148.
10. Redmond CK, Wieand HS, Rockelle HE, et al. Long term mortality experience of steelworkers. Department of Health and Human Services (NIOSH) Publications No. 81-120, 1981.
11. Doll R. Cancer of the lung and nose in nickel workers. Br J Ind Med 1958; 15:217–223.
12. Wegman DH, Theriault GP, Peters JM. Worker sponsored survey for asbestosis. Arch Environ Health 1973; 27:105–109.
13. Wegman DH, Musk AW, Main DM, et al. Accelerated loss of FEV-1 in polyurethane production workers: a four year prospective study. Am J Ind Med 1982; 3:209–215.
14. Axelson O, Dahlgran E, Jarsson CD, et al. Arsenic exposure and mortality, a case referent study from a Swedish copper smelter. Br J Ind Med 1978; 35:8–15.
15. Blair A, Stewart P, O'Berg M, et al. Mortality among industrial workers exposed to formaldehyde. J Nat Cancer Institute 1986; 76:1071–1084.

BIBLIOGRAPHY

Ahlbom A, Norell S. Introduction to modern epidemiology. Chestnut Hill, MA: Epidemiology Resources, Inc., 1984.
Brief primer on the core ideas underlying epidemiologic research and useful starting point for more advanced reading.
Colton T. Statistics in medicine. Boston: Little, Brown, 1974.
Basic statistics text written in a reasonable fashion with a functional index. Good general reference for statistics.
Kleinbaum DG, Kupper LL, Morgenstern H. Epidemiologic research: principles and quantitative methods. Belmont, CA: Lifetime Learning Publications, 1982.
The basic text in epidemiology that provides principles of epidemiology in substantial detail as well as the quantitative basis for the research methods. Particularly useful as a reference.
Monson RR. Occupational epidemiology. Boca Raton, FL: CRC Press, 1980.
A systematic review of methods as applied specifically to occupational settings. A practical textbook for those doing occupational studies.
Rothman KJ. Modern epidemiology. Boston: Little, Brown, 1986.
Probably the best general text on epidemiologic methods designed both for the novice and the expert. Organized in a way that makes it useful to read through or to use as a general reference.

APPENDIX
Adjustment of Rates

For the purposes of illustration, adjusting for the differences in age will be examined in detail. Table 5-1 presents a hypothetical problem involving the asbestosis experience in two factories. To compare the incidence of asbestosis in Factory 1 and Factory 2, a summary rate is calculated in each factory. If crude rates are calculated, it would appear that workers in Factory 2 have a slightly greater risk. A comparison of these rates, however, ignores the rather striking difference in age distribution of the populations in the two factories. These can be taken into account by adjusting for the differences by either the direct method or the indirect method.

DIRECT ADJUSTMENT

The principle of direct adjustment is to apply the age-specific rates determined in the study groups to a set of common age weights, such as a standard age distribution. The selection of the standard is somewhat arbitrary but often is chosen as the sum of the specific age groups for the two or more study groups. Thus, in Table 5-1, the standard population would be: less than 45 years = 1200, 45 years or older = 800. The specific rates are applied to this set of weights and then added to create an adjusted rate.

Factory 1 $\dfrac{0.010 \times 1200 + 0.030 \times 800}{2000}$

$= \dfrac{12 + 24}{2000} = 0.018$

Factory 2 $\dfrac{0.0125 \times 1200 + 0.050 \times 800}{2000}$

$= \dfrac{15 + 40}{2000} = 0.0275$

Not only is the magnitude of asbestosis affected by the adjustment of the rates, but also the rank order is reversed. Note that if another age distribution had been selected as the standard (for example, < 45 = 1500, ≥ 45 = 500), the standardized rates would change and the rate for Factory 1 would become 0.015 while that for Factory 2 would become 0.022. Thus, the magnitude of the two adjusted rates has no inherent meaning. They can, however, be compared, and although the size of the ratio will change slightly it will be closely

duplicated regardless of the weights; in these two examples of weighting, the ratios of the adjusted rates are 1.52 and 1.46.

INDIRECT ADJUSTMENT

In indirect adjustment standard rates are applied to the observed weights or the distribution of specific characteristics (for example, age, sex, or race) in the study populations. This provides a value for the number of cases (events) that would be expected if the standard rates were operating. These expected cases can be compared to those actually observed for each study group in the form of a ratio. In Table 5-1, assume a national standard rate for asbestosis of 1/1000 (0.001) for those under 45 and 2/1000 (0.002) for those 45 years or older. The expected cases in the two factories would be

Factory 1 = 0.001 × 400 + 0.002 × 600
        = 0.4 + 1.2 = 1.6

Factory 2 = 0.001 × 800 + 0.002 × 200
        = 0.8 + 0.4 = 1.2

These expected values are, in turn, compared to the observed values to calculate a standardized morbidity ratio.

Factory 1 SMR = 22/1.6 = 13.8

Factory 2 SMR = 20/1.2 = 16.7

It is tempting to compare the two SMRs and calculate a ratio similar to that calculated for the directly standardized rates. However, this is one of the drawbacks of indirect standardization. Since the age distributions and age-specific rates are significantly different for the two factories, the resulting comparison of the two SMRs would not distinguish differences due to disease incidence rate from differences due to a different age distribution.

It is reasonable then to ask why indirectly standardized rates are used. One reason is that often only one population is being studied, so comparison to the general population experience is convenient and possibly the only reasonable comparison available. Probably of greater importance is the instability of observed rates. In the example given, if five rather than two age groups were used and it was also necessary to adjust for both race and sex, then the total number of subdivisions necessary would be $5 \times 2 \times 2 = 20$. With a maximum of 22 cases in either factory, several of the subdivisions would contain no cases and therefore have no reliable rate estimate. Even in the illustration provided, one case more or less in Factory 1 workers under 45 years would have changed the age-specific incidence rate to 12.5 or 7.5 respectively, obviously a very large difference.

6
Screening for Occupational Disease

Barry S. Levy and William E. Halperin

Screening for occupational disease is the search for *previously unrecognized* diseases or physiologic conditions that are caused or influenced by work-associated factors. It may be part of an individual physician's evaluation of a patient's health or of a large-scale prevention effort by an employer, union, or some other organization. Screening methods can include questionnaires seeking suggestive symptoms or exposures, examinations and laboratory tests, or other procedures. To be widely used, the methods should be simple, non-invasive, safe, rapid, and usually relatively inexpensive. Screening is one technique in a continuum for the prevention of occupational disease. Other techniques include eliminating hazards from the workplace; containing hazards with engineering controls; protecting workers with personal protective devices such as gloves and respirators; measuring intoxicants in the environment (environmental monitoring) or in biological samples (biological monitoring); and detecting, screening, and treating occupational disease at early stages when it is reversible or more easily treatable [1]. As with screening for nonoccupational diseases, screening for work-related diseases only *presumptively* identifies those individuals who are likely (and those who are unlikely) to have a particular disease. Further diagnostic tests are almost always necessary to confirm the diagnosis and assess the severity of the individual's condition.

Although screening data may eventually lead to more effective primary prevention measures, the purpose of screening is the identification of conditions already in existence at a stage when their progression can be slowed, halted, or even reversed. Screening is therefore a secondary prevention measure. Primary prevention measures that reduce workers' exposure to occupational hazards are, in general, more likely to improve health and prevent disease (see Chaps. 4 and 7).

While the main goal of screening is the early detection and treatment of disease, other goals include the evaluation of the adequacy of exposure control and other means of primary prevention, the detection of previously unrecognized health effects suspected on the basis of toxicologic and other studies, and suitable job placement. Clearly screening data, in addition to their clinical use for the protection of the individual screened, may be useful in a surveillance system to be analyzed epidemiologically for the protection of the community of similarly exposed workers [2].

The employees at a particular workplace are a logical target for screening for occupational disease because they have some risk factors in common (their workplace exposures) and a clear opportunity for prevention in common (reduction or elimination of those exposures). In addition, a workplace may provide excellent opportunities for screening for treatable nonoccupational diseases such as hypertension (see Chap. 34).

To be effective, screening programs for occupational disease must meet the following five criteria:

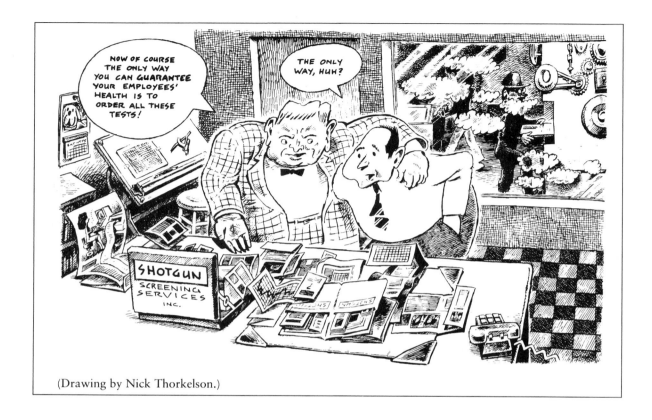

(Drawing by Nick Thorkelson.)

1. *Screening must be selective*—applying only the appropriate tests to the population at risk of developing specific diseases, given its exposures, demographic features, and other factors. A "shotgun" approach, which involves a battery of tests (such as a "chemistry profile") applied indiscriminately without regard to the diseases for which the population is at risk, is generally not effective. The natural history of the exposure-disease relationship should be considered in application of screening tests. For example, screening workers exposed to asbestos in the first few years after the start of exposure may lead to a false sense of security, since the disease process will not have had time to be manifest on screening examination.

2. *Identifying the disease in its latent stage as opposed to identifying it when symptoms appear must lead to treatment that impedes the progres-sion of the disease* in a given individual or to measures that prevent additional cases (Fig. 6-1).

3. *Adequate follow-up is critical, and further diagnostic tests and effective management of the disease must be available, accessible, and acceptable* both to examiner and worker. Lack of follow-up is a frequent deficiency in screening programs for occupational disease. Workers who have been screened should receive test reports along with interpretation of test results and summary data for the entire group tested.* Follow-up also entails that action will be taken to reduce or totally eliminate the hazard. Some follow-up actions are job

*OSHA requires that records of medical surveillance be made available to the affected employee. They can be transmitted to third parties only with the written consent of the worker.

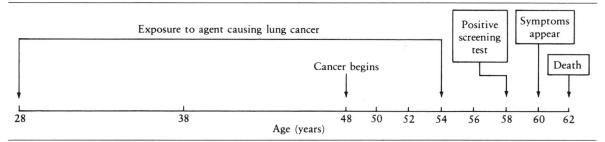

Fig. 6-1. Phases of cancer development. If the course of the disease cannot be positively influenced by early detection and effective treatment, there is no advantage to screening an individual for early detection of the disease. Current screening tests for lung cancer have yet to be proved effective. Screening may detect cancer earlier than would occur without screening, but the eventual time of death is not significantly changed.

transfer for the ill worker and improving the ventilation systems of the plant; job transfer without controlling the underlying problem may mean that another worker will be exposed to the same hazard. The major justification for screening for disease for which there is no therapy is to allow an opportunity to control exposure and prevent disease in others similarly exposed.

4. *The screening test must have good reliability and validity.* Reliability reflects the reproducibility of the test. Validity reflects the ability of the test to identify correctly which individuals have the disease and which do not. Validity is evaluated by examining sensitivity and specificity. *Sensitivity* is the proportion of those with the disease that the test identifies correctly; *specificity* is the proportion of those without the disease that the test identifies correctly. Another measure of a screening test is *predictive value positive,* which is often more useful clinically than sensitivity or specificity; it indicates the proportion of those found with a positive screening test who actually have the disease (Table 6-1).

5. *The benefits of the screening program should outweigh the costs.* Benefits consist primarily of improved quality and length of life—that is, reduced morbidity and mortality. Costs include economic costs (the expenses of performing the screening tests and further diagnostic tests and of managing those with the disease) and human costs

(the risks, inconvenience, discomfort, and anxiety of screening and the diagnostic work-ups of "false positives"). Screening tests in the community must be inexpensive since they compete with other public health resources such as immunization. It should not be assumed that effective screening tests for occupational disease must be inexpensive as they do not compete for the same resources. The cost-benefit equation is often difficult to determine and relies on tenuous assumptions. Therefore, such analysis should not be allowed to obscure the primary objective of screening: early identification

Table 6-1. Hypothetical data: Screening of 100,000 workers for colon cancer*

	Colon cancer present		
Test outcome	Yes	No	Total
Positive	150	300	450
Negative	50	99,500	99,550
Total	200	99,800	100,000

Sensitivity = 150/200 = 75%. The test was (correctly) positive for 75% of actual cancer cases, but 25% of the actual cases were not detected.
Specificity = 99,500/99,800 = 99%. The test was (correctly) negative for 99% of those who actually did not have colon cancer.
Predictive value positive = 150/450 = 33%. Of those with a positive test, 33% actually had colon cancer.

of work-related disease. Advocates of screening should be cautious that increased survival in those detected with disease, as compared with individuals detected when their symptoms occur, is not a result of lead-time bias or length bias. In lead-time bias, the added survival of individuals with detected disease results from adding part of the preclinical detection period to post-diagnosis survival—not from altering the actual time individuals die. In length bias, an apparent increased survival results from the greater probability of detecting indolent, more benign disease, rather than quickly developing disease that is less likely to be detected because it is present for a shorter period of time.

There must be mutual trust among the individuals who have requested or authorized the screening program, the health professionals who are administering it, and the workers being screened. Without such trust, workers may be reluctant to be screened. This trust is developed, in part, by management personnel and health professionals assuring workers that screening data will be kept strictly confidential, will be used only for the stated purpose of the screening program, and will not adversely affect the worker's salary or other benefits. In addition, for any screening program to be effective, it cannot be used as a tool to discriminate—sexually, racially, or otherwise—against a specific group of workers.

SCREENING APPROACHES
Reviewed below are current screening approaches to five major categories of work-related disease: nonmalignant respiratory disease, hearing impairment, toxic effects, cancer, and back problems. As we review these categories, you will note that few current screening approaches for occupational disease meet all five criteria for effective screening.

Nonmalignant Respiratory Disease
Screening for acute work-related respiratory diseases such as irritant pneumonitis is generally not possible. Pathologic changes due to exposure to ir-

ritant or toxic gases and fumes develop so quickly that there is no opportunity to screen for these disorders during a latent stage.

Many chronic work-related respiratory diseases, however, are amenable to screening. These diseases usually have very long periods from initial exposure to first appearance of symptoms—often years. Early identification of workers with asymptomatic pulmonary disease and reduction or elimination of their hazardous exposure may reverse the disease process or at least halt or slow its progression. Once well established, however, most of these diseases are not reversible by currently available treatment, and they account for much morbidity and mortality (see Chap. 21).

Screening approaches for occupational respiratory diseases range from simple questions to sophisticated tests of pulmonary function. The four basic approaches are history of respiratory symptoms, physical examination, chest x-rays, and pulmonary function tests. Usually two or more of these approaches are used in combination. Each approach, of course, has its strengths and weaknesses.

History. By means of direct questioning or use of a standardized questionnaire,* one can elicit information on the presence of respiratory symptoms, including cough, sputum production, wheezing, and dyspnea. The worker is questioned about the presence of these symptoms, their time course, and their relationship to airborne substance exposure, exertion, and work habits. The worker is also questioned about work history and in detail about cigarette smoking history. Although this approach is simple, inexpensive, without risk, usually acceptable to the worker, and capable of being performed by paramedical personnel or the worker, it suffers from major weaknesses. With some dis-

*An excellent questionnaire, developed by the American Thoracic Society, was published in BG Ferris. Epidemiology standardization project. Am. Rev. Respir. Dis. 1978; 118 (2):7–54. It is also available from the National Heart, Lung, and Blood Institute, Bethesda, MD 20892.

eases such as asbestosis, cough, dyspnea on exertion, and other symptoms often do not appear until the disease is moderately advanced. The worker with lung disease may fail to report certain symptoms such as "smoker's cough" that may be considered acceptable or unimportant to smokers. The worker may choose not to report certain symptoms for fear or losing a job or being labelled an unhealthy person. Finally, respiratory symptoms are often due to causes other than chronic lung disease. (The first three of these weaknesses have to do with low sensitivity, the last with low specificity.)

Physical Examination. Performing a physical examination is generally a less helpful screening approach than obtaining a history of previously unrecognized respiratory symptoms. It, too, is simple, inexpensive, without risk, acceptable to the worker, and capable of being done by paramedical personnel; but it, too, has low sensitivity and specificity and is rarely helpful in screening for work-related pulmonary disease. For example, by the time basilar rales are heard in an individual with asbestosis, significant fibrosis has already occurred, and such physical signs as clubbing and cyanosis are usually associated with far-advanced disease.

Chest X-Rays. Chest x-rays also have significant limitations in the early detection of chronic respiratory disease. This screening approach is more expensive and requires special equipment. In addition, with periodic x-rays a given worker may face some cumulative radiation hazard. Moreover, chest films are usually not very sensitive or very specific: the presence or absence of abnormalities does not always correlate with the intensity of symptoms, early physiologic abnormalities, and actual pathology. Chest films also fail to reveal early changes of chronic obstructive pulmonary disease, and they are subject to much variation in technique and interpretation. Despite these limitations, chest films can play an important role in the early diagnosis and assessment of work-related

restrictive diseases, especially if chest x-ray abnormalities begin to appear relatively early in the course of chronic disease. Chest x-rays will be discussed again later in this chapter in the context of lung cancer screening.

Pulmonary Function Testing. Although it requires special equipment and therefore is more costly than performing histories or physical examinations, pulmonary function testing is a reasonably sensitive screening approach for work-related respiratory diseases, and it generally provides more useful screening information than the other approaches (Fig. 6-2). Pulmonary function tests used for screening are relatively easy to perform, and, if properly done, the results are reproducible.

Pulmonary function testing suffers from two general limitations: the range of normal is wide, and if the worker being tested does not cooperate fully, artifacts can appear, especially in tests requiring maximal effort. The first limitation can be countered by periodic testing of the same individual; test results in a given worker can be followed over time and abnormalities identified when greater than expected decreases in function occur. The second limitation can be addressed by applying standardized rules for acceptable tests (see Chap. 21).

The two most frequently used screening tests of pulmonary function are forced vital capacity (FVC) and forced expiratory volume in the first second of expiration (FEV$_1$). FVC is the maximal volume of air that can be exhaled forcefully after maximal inspiration. For most people it closely approximates the vital capacity without a forced effort. FVC is reduced relatively early in restrictive diseases such as asbestosis. FEV$_1$ is the volume of air that can be forcefully expelled during the first second of expiration with a maximal effort after the lungs have been filled completely. It is reduced in both restrictive and obstructive disease but relatively more so than FVC in the latter. In the early course of asthma it returns toward normal when the attack ends spontaneously or with bronchodilators. Advances in assessing pulmonary dysfunc-

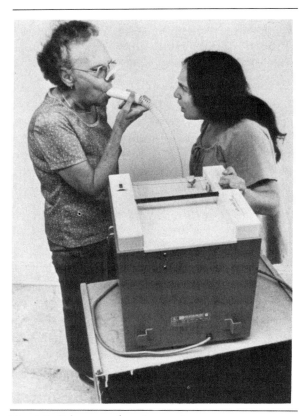

Fig. 6-2. Pulmonary function testing. (Photograph by Earl Dotter.)

tion are occurring but generally require validation before they are ready for routine use [3]. For further discussion, see Chapter 21.

Evaluation of workers for nonoccupational risk factors that may predispose them to occupational pulmonary disease is another, although controversial, approach. This is actually a method of primary prevention rather than screening. For example, some employers identify smokers, who may be at increased risk of acquiring a variety of occupational pulmonary diseases, and restrict them from certain jobs. This approach is sometimes opposed by workers who feel that it is unfair discrimination. One large asbestos company has prohibited workers from smoking in the workplace—even at its corporate offices—and has refused to hire new workers who smoke. This approach is controversial also because it can encourage employers to avoid eliminating hazardous conditions and instead find workers with "iron constitutions" who can withstand these conditions. Decisions on this subject obviously involve both scientific assessments and public policy considerations of equity.

Screening for alpha$_1$-antitrypsin deficiency is an example of a similar approach to risk factor identification. Individuals with a severe deficiency of this protein (1 in 5,000 of the general population) are at very high risk of developing emphysema and chronic bronchitis and should not work in a dusty workplace. But it has not been established if those individuals with lesser degrees of this deficiency are at increased risk of developing respiratory diseases.

Although there are many opportunities to screen for occupational respiratory disease, it is difficult to detect before significant loss of lung function has occurred. Therefore, more reliance should be placed on methods of primary prevention such as ventilation systems, changed work practices, and substitution of hazardous substances with nonhazardous ones.

Hearing Impairment

Several million Americans suffer chronic work-related hearing impairment, and several million American workers are exposed to loud noise at work that poses a threat to hearing (see Chap. 17). Even at the current OSHA standard of 90 dBA (decibels of sound pressure) for eight hours of workplace noise exposure, it is estimated that 10 percent of those exposed for a lifetime will have significant hearing impairment. By the time a worker notices hearing impairment, irreversible sensorineural damage affecting the sound frequencies of human conversation has usually occurred. However, long before a worker notices any hearing impairment, significant changes can be seen in the audiogram. Screening for hearing impairment is therefore important in workers exposed to loud noise.

The first sign of hearing impairment is a dip in the audiogram, usually at 3000 to 6000 hertz (cycles per second). If hearing impairment progresses, the audiologic abnormality becomes more severe and covers a broader range of frequencies. Discovery of an abnormal audiogram can point to the need to prevent hearing impairment by reduction of noise at the source, modification of the work procedures creating the noise, use of personal protective equipment (earmuffs or earplugs), or removal of the worker from a noisy work environment.

Audiograms should be performed as part of the preplacement examination of workers who will be exposed to loud noise at work so that a baseline will be available for comparison with later audiograms. They should be repeated on exposed workers every year. Audiograms should not be performed within 14 hours of any significant noise exposure; if done sooner, a temporary threshold shift may be mistakenly identified as a permanent one. As with other screening tests, it is usually best to compare test results repeated on an individual over time rather than with "normal limits." It is particularly important to note that deterioration of hearing due to loud noise exposure is fairly rapid for the first years of exposure. Therefore, the effectiveness of a screening program is maximal during this initial work period.*

Audiometry is generally accepted as a useful screening approach and is widely performed in industry in the United States. However, its value can be undermined by poor technique such as inadequate calibration of equipment, excess noise in the testing room, headphone position variations,

headset pressure against the external ears, examiner and tester biases, improved performance of the subject after familiarization with the testing procedure, obstruction of the ear canal, tinnitus, simulation or malingering, and fluctuation of the subject's criterion for threshold identification of the test tone. A NIOSH study several years ago indicated that 80 percent of industries surveyed used inadequate audiometric equipment. However, most of these problems can be minimized with appropriately trained technicians and adequate equipment.

Toxic Effects

Three components are involved in the prevention of the toxic effects of workplace chemicals: evaluating the toxicity of the chemical itself (preferably before it is introduced, as the Toxic Substances Control Act now mandates) by animal studies and short-term in vitro assays; environmental monitoring of levels of the chemical in workplace air to determine if it is controlled in accordance with recommended or mandated standards; and biologic monitoring (see also Chap. 14).

Biologic monitoring is the testing of blood, urine, or exhaled air of individuals to determine either the body's level of a hazardous chemical and metabolites or reasonably specific biochemical changes that are associated with cellular damage. The first of these actually provides evidence of exposure; the second is considered screening in the strict sense. For the latter approach to be effective, it must detect early ("sentinel") biologic effects before serious health effects occur. As with other evaluation approaches, once biologic monitoring of any kind indicates that workers have excessive exposure or early toxic effects, measures must be taken to reduce their exposure to the responsible agents. Following are three examples of biologic screening:

Several volatile organic compounds, including benzene and toluene, if inhaled or absorbed

---

*It is useful to remember as a rule of thumb that the maximum temporary threshold shift (i.e., the asymptotic level of threshold shift) determined by several measurements taken consecutively over 8 to 24 hours is considered a possible indicator of future permanent hearing impairment due to continued work in the same noise environment. (Personal communication from R. Hamernik to B. Levy.)

through the skin, produce metabolites that can be measured in urine.

Organophosphate pesticides, before exerting any known health effects, begin to inhibit both plasma and red blood cell cholinesterase. The amount of plasma cholinesterase (pseudocholinesterase) reflects absorption of the organophosphate, and the activity of the red cell cholinesterase correlates well with the degree of adverse effect.

Various tests have been used to evaluate lead exposure or body burden and the biologic effects of lead (Table 6-2). Biologic monitoring for lead is particularly useful because the early effects of lead poisoning are reversible and because symptoms of early toxicity are nonspecific, such as headache and fatigue, or the patient is asymptomatic (see Chaps. 14, 25, 26, and 28).

Biologic monitoring has a different use from environmental monitoring because it takes into consideration host differences in, for example, susceptibility to toxic effects and absorption, distribution, and biotransformation of the substance. It also considers possible multiple exposures (both

Table 6-2. Evaluation of the various tests that have been used to monitor workers with lead exposure

Exposure monitoring tests (evaluation of lead exposure or lead body burden)	Screening tests (evaluation of biologic action of lead)

Lead in blood
  Evaluates amount of lead absorption, therefore reflects intensity of lead exposure
  As absorption increases it reaches a plateau, so it is not an accurate measure of body burden
  Laboratory technique must be very good
Lead in urine
  Ease of obtaining specimens
  Disadvantages of fluctuating kidney function and fluid intake affecting test results
Lead in urine after administration of a chelating agent
  Reflects fraction of lead in body that can be mobilized, therefore probably indicates amount that is metabolically active
  Too complex and dangerous for screening test
Lead in hair
  Indicates past exposure, so of limited use in occupational disease
	Hemoglobin/hematocrit
	  Easy to obtain
	  Do not correlate with blood lead below 70 µg/dl
	Coproporphyrins in urine
	  Low specificity
	  Do not increase until the blood level is about 50 µg/dl
	Free erythrocyte protoporphyrins (including measurement of zinc protoporphyrin [ZPP])
	  Useful, but reflect bone marrow lead 3 months before
	  Some false positives, including iron deficiency
	Porphobilinogen in urine
	  Not useful because increase occurs after toxic symptoms present
	Delta-aminolevulinic acid (ALA) in urine
	  Very useful, reflects amount of metabolically active lead in body
	  Very sensitive, very specific but returns slowly toward normal after exposure ceases
	Activity of delta-aminolevulinic acid dehydratase (ALA-D) in erythrocytes
	  This enzyme inhibited by lead
	  Very sensitive and specific
	  But must keep specimen at 0°C

Source: R Lauwerys. Biological criteria for selected industrial toxic chemicals: a review. Scand J Work Environ Health 1975; 1:139.

occupational and nonoccupational) and multiple routes of absorption. A crucial issue is the relationship of environmental monitoring and biologic monitoring. Since environmental monitoring leads to control of exposure prior to absorption of the hazardous chemical, it is preferable. Biologic monitoring, however, should not be considered a substitute for environmental monitoring. Given the potential for multiple routes of exposure not well assessed by environmental monitoring (for example, percutaneous absorption), biological monitoring should be used as a valuable adjunctive fail-safe technique.

Biologic monitoring—at present—is still in its infancy and has several limitations. There is no health effect parameter for many substances; as each new parameter is developed, its relation must be established, on the one hand, to the amount of exposure and, on the other, to the disease. The biologic half-lives of many toxins are not known, and screening may be done at the wrong time to identify acute intoxication or transient effects. For many known biologic parameters, the range of normal is wide, so it is necessary to base the interpretation of testing on a series of tests on the same individual over time. This demonstrates the importance of performing baseline biologic screening specific to known or anticipated hazards during the preplacement examination. Quality control in laboratories varies; it is essential that the laboratories performing the biological monitoring can ensure accurate results.

These potential problems make it crucial to plan biologic screening carefully. Workers who may be exposed must be identified. The appropriate parameter to monitor them must be chosen. Baseline measurements made before exposure and measurements after exposure must be appropriately timed. There is also much room for error in the choice of specimen, the storage and handling of specimens, and the interpretation of results. However, biologic screening holds much promise, and with the increase of toxic substances in the workplace and greater recognition of toxic hazards, it can play an important preventive role.

Cancer

Screening has a limited role in occupational cancer control. National Cancer Institute data support the concept that early detection of cancer followed by appropriate treatment can increase survival of some patients with certain cancers. Approaches that have been used to screen for different cancers include examination of exfoliated cells by the Papanicolaou technique (Pap smear); x-rays; proctosigmoidoscopy; identification of a substance in the blood or other body fluid that may be a specific marker for a given malignancy; breast self-examination; measures of organ function; and tests to detect colon cancer by identifying occult blood in the stool. These approaches are of widely varying degrees of effectiveness (see Chap. 15).

Few screening approaches of any kind, however, have been proved to reduce mortality from cancer. As with screening for most chronic diseases, discussion of the effectiveness of cancer screening has been greatly confused by studies that do not differentiate between true mortality reduction and merely earlier identification.

A dramatic increase in lung cancer mortality has taken place in the past fifty years. Attempts to detect lung cancer early have recently focused on periodic chest x-rays and cytologic examinations of sputum, which tend to complement one another: chest x-rays are more useful for detecting peripherally situated cancers while sputum cytology can identify early squamous cell carcinoma involving major airways. Relatively few cases of lung cancer give a positive result on both tests at the same time. Although these tests are often used to screen for lung cancer, neither has been convincingly shown to be effective. Usually, by the time either of these tests presumptively identifies a lung cancer, it has metastasized and is incurable. Well-controlled studies have demonstrated that addition of sputum cytology to chest x-ray screening does not significantly reduce mortality from all types of lung cancer but suggests that mortality from squamous cell carcinoma is reduced [4]. A report of three randomized trials of screening for early lung cancer suggests that sputum cytology detects 15 to

20 percent of all lung cancer, mostly squamous cell carcinoma, with a relatively good prognosis, and that chest x-ray alone may be a more effective test for early-stage lung cancer than previous reports have suggested. However, a randomized clinical trial at the Mayo Clinic has shown that both procedures offered every 4 months had no advantage in survival over standard medical practices [5].

The status of attempts to screen for bladder cancer is much the same as that for lung cancer. The approaches used most frequently in recent years have been a search for occult blood and cytologic examination of exfoliated cells in urine. These approaches have been successfully used to identify asymptomatic individuals with early bladder cancer in a population at high risk of bladder cancer because of exposure to aromatic amines [6]. However, whether screening in this or similar high-risk groups will lead to prolongation of life or decreased morbidity has not been evaluated in a controlled clinical trial.

Given the continued high incidence of cancer (and the substantial incidence of occupational cancer), its severity, and frequent lack of effective treatment, attempts will no doubt continue to develop better screening tests. In the meantime, health professionals should not raise false hopes of workers with most currently available screening tests of unproved effectiveness and should concentrate on measures of primary prevention. These measures include testing workplace substances for carcinogenicity, limiting exposure to proved or suspected carcinogens, and encouraging smoking cessation, since smoking is associated with lung, bladder, and other cancers.

Back Problems

When the term *screening* is used to refer to back problems in the workplace, it usually refers to preplacement identification of preexisting back problems, both work-related and not, or of a predilection to back problems. Three methods have been traditionally used to try to identify workers at high risk of work-related back problems: history, physical examination, and x-rays of the lumbosacral spine. None of these methods has been effective in controlling low back injuries. X-rays have been used on the basis of a hypothesis, now shown to be false, that developmental abnormalities of the spine predispose to low back injury. The persistent use of back x-rays to detect such abnormalities not only is without benefit but also discriminates unnecessarily against prospective workers with x-ray abnormalities. X-rays do not necessarily predict future back injury risk and create unnecessary x-ray exposure. Although the only effective control for back problems today seems to be the ergonomic approach of designing the job to fit the worker, some evidence indicates that measurements of strength and fitness prior to start of work can predict back injuries (see Chaps. 8 and 22). In addition, strength measurements can be used to match a worker's strength to job requirements.

POSSIBILITIES FOR IMPROVED SCREENING

Opportunities for effective screening for occupational diseases at present are relatively limited, and most available screening approaches do not meet the criteria outlined earlier in this chapter. Unless screening approaches are improved, much time, effort, and limited resources may be wasted; workers may face unnecessary risks and experience unnecessary anxiety and inconvenience; and workers and employers may become disillusioned with preventive approaches in general.

The general industry standards for specific hazardous exposures, published by OSHA, specify requirements for medical surveillance of exposed workers [8]. They may include preplacement and periodic screening histories, examinations, and tests. Table 6-3 illustrates some of the specific screening tests required by OSHA. OSHA also requires employers to keep records of this surveillance and to make these records available to affected employees. The records can also be made available to physicians or other third parties on specific written request.

Suggested principles for screening and biologic

Table 6-3. Selected OSHA standards for medical surveillance

Exposure	History	Physical examination	Other tests/procedures
Airborne asbestos	Especially respiratory symptoms	Especially chest examination	Chest x-ray FVC and FEV_1
Vinyl chloride	Especially alcohol use, history of hepatitis, transfusions	Especially liver, spleen, and kidneys	Liver function tests
Inorganic arsenic	Yes	Especially nasal and skin examinations	Chest x-ray Sputum cytology
Benzene	Including alcohol use and medications	Yes	Complete blood count Reticulocyte count Serum bilirubin
Dibromochloropropane (DBCP)	Including reproductive history	Especially genitourinary system	FSH, LH Males: also sperm count Females: also total estrogen

Source: Occupational Safety and Health Administration, U.S. Department of Labor. General Industry: OSHA Safety and Health Standards (29 CFR 1910). Washington, D.C.: U.S. Government Printing Office, 1984.

monitoring of the effects of exposure in the workplace and many related articles were the subject of an intensive national conference held in Cincinnati in July 1984 and published as the August and October 1986 issues of the *Journal of Occupational Medicine*. Extensive discussions of various aspects of screening are included in these issues. A central theme expressed in these discussions is the following: "Screening and monitoring, in and of themselves, prevent nothing; only the appropriate intervention, in response to results of these tests, can prevent" [7].

REFERENCES

1. Halperin, WE, Frazier, TM. Surveillance for the effects of workplace exposure. Annu Rev Public Health 1985; 6:419–432.
2. Halperin, WE, et al. Medical screening in the workplace: proposed principles. J Occup Med 1986; 28:547–552.
3. Kreiss, K. Approaches to assessing pulmonary dysfunction and susceptibility in workers. J Occup Med 1986; 28:664–669.
4. Frost, JK, et al. Sputum cytopathology: use and potential in monitoring the workplace environment by

screening for biological effects of exposure. J Occup Med 1986; 28:692–703.
5. Fontana, RS. Lung cancer screening: the Mayo program. J Occup Med 1986; 28:746–750.
6. Schulte, P, Ringen, K, Hemstreet, G. Optimal management of asymptomatic workers at high risk of bladder cancer. J Occup Med 1986; 28:13–17.
7. Millar, JD. Screening and monitoring: tools for prevention. J Occup Med 1986; 28:544–546.
8. OSHA, U.S. Department of Labor. General industry: OSHA safety and health standards (29 CFR 1910). Washington, D.C.: U.S. Government Printing Office, 1978.

BIBLIOGRAPHY

Halperin WE, Schulte PA, Greathouse DG (eds. Part I) and Mason TJ, Prorok PC, Costlow RD (eds. Part II). Conference on medical screening and biological monitoring for the effects of exposure in the workplace. J Occup Med 1986; 28:543–788, 901–1126.
An in-depth, up-to-date, comprehensive review on screening in the workplace.
World Health Organization. Early detection of occupational diseases. Geneva: WHO, 1986.
An excellent guide on the principles of early detection and approaches to early detection and control of various occupational diseases.

Baselt RC. Biologic monitoring methods for industrial chemicals. Davis, CA: Biomedical Publishers, 1980.
A good compendium of monitoring methods.

Halperin WE, et al. Medical screening in the workplace: proposed principles. J Occup Med 1986; 28:547–552.
Questions the adequacy of current recommendations on screening in the workplace and proposes a revised set of principles for such screening.

Lauwerys RR. Industrial chemical exposure: guidelines for biological monitoring. Davis CA: Biomedical Publications, 1983.
Presents concepts of biological monitoring and reviews current knowledge on numerous specific agents.

Morrison AS. Screening in chronic disease. Monographs in epidemiology and biostatistics, volume 7. New York and Oxford: Oxford University Press, 1985.
An excellent text on the epidemiology of screening.

Proctor NH, Hughes JP. Chemical hazards in the workplace. Philadelphia: Lippincott, 1978.
Includes recommended screening exams and tests for workers exposed to any of almost 400 substances.

Rothstein MA. Medical screening of workers. Washington, DC: Bureau of National Affairs, 1984.
A presentation of the legal issues involved in screening.

Zielhuis RL. Biologic monitoring. Scand J Work Environ Health 1978; 4:1.
A good review article.

7
Industrial Hygiene

Thomas J. Smith

Industrial hygiene is the environmental science of identifying and evaluating physical, chemical, and biologic hazards in the workplace and devising ways to control or eliminate them. It encompasses the study of toxicology, industrial processes, the chemical and physical behavior of air contaminants, environmental sampling techniques and statistics, the design and evaluation of ventilation systems and noise control and radiation protection programs, and the health effects of occupational hazards. Typically an industrial hygienist would be asked to determine the composition and concentrations of air contaminants in a workplace where there have been complaints of eye, nose, and throat irritation. The hygienist in this situation would also determine if the contaminant exposures exceeded the permissible exposure limits required by the Occupational Safety and Health Administration (OSHA). If the problem was the result of airborne materials (a conclusion that might be reached in consultation with a physician or epidemiologist), then the hygienist would be responsible for selecting the techniques used to reduce or eliminate the exposure such as installing exhaust ventilation around the source of the air contaminants and isolating it from the general work area, and follow-up sampling to verify that the controls were effective. Most industrial hygienists have earned either a bachelor's degree in science or engineering or a master of science degree in industrial hygiene.

Industrial hygienists must work with physicians to develop comprehensive occupational health programs and with epidemiologists to perform research on health effects. It has been traditional to separate industrial hygiene and safety, but the present trend is to broaden the training for each to include the other. This trend will probably lead to the formation of a single specialty for identifying, evaluating, and controlling all types of environmental hazards in the workplace. At present industrial hygienists generally do not deal with mechanical hazards or job activities that can cause physical injuries; these are the responsibility of the safety specialists (see Chap. 8). However, it is not uncommon for private companies to have a single individual responsible for both industrial hygiene and safety who has no formal training in either area.

Most industrial hygienists work for large companies or governmental agencies. A small but growing number work for labor unions. For whomever they work, industrial hygienists unfortunately are often located in organizational units where they have little organizational power to force necessary changes. Hygienists who work for labor unions may be restricted in their access to the workplace for sampling and exposure measurements, which can limit their ability to assess and control hazards.

The closeness of working relationships between industrial hygienists and occupational physicians varies. Some have close collaborative activities with an extensive exchange of information, while others operate with nearly complete independence and have little more than formal contact. A physician who is familiar with the workplace, job activities, and health status of workers in all parts of the process may be very helpful in guiding the industrial hygienist in assessing environmental hazards and vice versa. The same is true of industrial hygienists and safety specialists. Where contact among these groups is minimal, many opportunities are lost for improving the effectiveness of health hazard control and the prevention of adverse effects.

IDENTIFICATION, EVALUATION, AND CONTROL OF HAZARDS

Industrial facilities are usually complex collections of simpler units organized to manufacture a product or to perform a service. The occupational hazards present in an industrial plant may be most easily evaluated if the plant is subdivided into its component unit processes. In this stepwise fashion the processes with hazards can be identified, the worker exposures evaluated, and the exposures in nearby areas assessed. Examples of some common unit processes and their hazards are given in Table 7-1. This general approach, and the hazards of a wide range of common industrial processes, are discussed in more detail in Burgess' *Recognition of Health Hazards in Industry: A Review of Materials and Processes* (see Bibliography).

This approach to hazard identification can be illustrated by considering a small company that manufactures tool boxes from sheets of steel by a six-step process: (1) sheets of steel are cut into the specified shape; (2) sharp edges and burrs are removed by grinding; (3) sheets are formed into boxes with a sheet metal bender; (4) box joints are spot welded; (5) boxes are cleaned in a vapor degreaser in preparation for painting; and (6) boxes are painted in a spray booth. Production steps 2, 4, 5, and 6 use unit processes with known hazards given in Table 7-1 and should be evaluated. It may also be necessary to evaluate the exposures of workers involved with steps 1 and 3 because they may be located near enough to the operations with hazards to have significant exposure.

The design of job tasks by management and an individual's work habits can both have an important influence on exposures. For example, a furnace tender's exposure to metal fumes will depend on the length of tools provided to scrape slag away from the tapping hole in the furnace and on the instructions for performing the task. If management does not provide adequate tools or give sufficient operating instructions, the worker may be exposed excessively. Similarly, the furnace tender who is positioned close to the slag as it runs out of the furnace may receive a much higher exposure than a coworker who stands farther away from the slag. Therefore, an important part of an evaluation is the observation of work practices used in hazardous unit processes.

When assessing the problems in a new or unfamiliar workplace, the industrial hygienist engages in the following activities:

Collection of background information on processes and associated hazards.

Visits to the workplace to become familiar with unit processes and their hazards, observe work practices, collect samples to determine the range of exposure, and, if necessary, develop a plan for a full-scale survey. These visits are crucial for detecting unique aspects of the workplace that may strongly affect exposures, such as the placement of work stations near windows, which may sharply reduce exposures when the wind blows in the windows. Sampling may show that sensory impressions under- or overestimate exposures; for example, the odor threshold for most solvents is well below the level at which they present a toxic exposure hazard.

Evaluation of operations and exposures by sampling and environmental measurements and observation of process activities in a full-scale survey. The full-scale survey will examine all phases of workplace activities—both normal activities and abnormal or infrequent ones such as maintenance, reactor cleaning, or simulation of malfunctions. The survey activities

Table 7-1. Common unit processes and associated hazards by route of entry*

Unit process	Route of entry and hazard
Abrasive blasting (surface treatment with high velocity sand, steel shot, pecan shells, glass, aluminum oxide, etc.)	Inhalation: silica, metal, and paint dust Noise
Acid/alkali treatments (dipping metal parts in open baths to remove oxides, grease, oil, and dirt)	
Acid pickling (with HCl, HNO_3, H_2SO_4, H_2CrO_4, HNO_3/HF)	Inhalation: acid mist Skin contact: burns and corrosion
Acid bright dips (with HNO_3/H_2SO_4)	Inhalation: NO_2, acid mists
Molten caustic descaling	Inhalation: smoke and vapors
Bath (high temperature)	Skin contact: burns
Blending and mixing (powders and/or liquid are mixed to form products, undergo reactions, etc.)	Inhalation: dusts and mists of toxic materials Skin contact: toxic materials
Crushing and sizing (mechanically reducing the particle size of solids and sorting larger from smaller with screens or cyclones)	Inhalation: dust, free silica Noise
Degreasing (removing grease, oil, and dirt from metal and plastic with solvents and cleaners)	
Cold solvent washing (clean parts with ketones, cellosolves, and aliphatic, aromatic, and stoddard solvents)	Inhalation: vapors Skin contact: dermatitis and absorption Fire and explosion (if flammable) Metabolic: carbon monoxide formed from methylene chloride
Vapor degreasers (with trichloroethylene, methyl chloroform, ethylene dichloride, and certain fluorocarbon compounds)	Inhalation: vapors; thermal degradation may form phosgene, hydrogen chloride, and chlorine gases Skin contact: dermatitis and absorption
Electroplating (coating metals, plastics and rubber with thin layers of metals) Copper Chromium Cadmium Gold Silver	Inhalation: acid mists, HCN, alkali mists, chromium mists Skin contact: acids, alkalis Ingestion: cyanide compounds
Forging (deforming hot or cold metal by presses or hammering)	Inhalation: hydrocarbons in smokes (hot processes), including polyaromatic hydrocarbons, SO_2, CO, NO_x, and other metals sprayed on dies (for example, lead and molybdenum) Heat stress Noise

Table 7-1 (**continued**)

Unit process	Route of entry and hazard
Furnace operations (melting and refining metals; boilers for steam generation)	Inhalation: metal fumes, combustion gases, for example, SO_2 and CO Noise from burners Heat stress Infrared radiation, cataracts in eyes
Grinding, polishing, and buffing (an abrasive is used to remove or shape metal or other material)	Inhalation: toxic dusts from both metals and abrasives Noise
Industrial radiography (x-ray or gamma ray sources used to examine parts of equipment)	Radiation exposure
Machining (metals, plastics, or wood are worked or shaped with lathes, drills, planers, or milling machines)	Inhalation: airborne particles, cutting oil mists, toxic metals, nitrosamines formed in some water-based cutting oils Skin contact: cutting oils, solvents, sharp chips Noise
Materials handling and storage (conveyors, forklift trucks are used to move materials to/from storage)	Inhalation: CO, exhaust particulate, dusts from conveyors, emissions from spills or broken containers
Mining (drilling, blasting, mucking to remove loose material and material transport)	Inhalation: silica dust, NO_2 from blasting, gases from the mine Heat stress Noise
Painting and spraying (applications of liquids to surfaces, for example, paints, pesticides, coatings)	Inhalation: solvents as mists and vapors, toxic materials Skin contact: solvents, toxic materials
Soldering (joining metals with molten alloys of lead or silver)	Inhalation: lead and cadmium particulate ("fumes") and flux fumes

Welding and metal cutting
(joining or cutting metals by heating them to molten or semi-molten state)
  Arc welding
  Resistance welding
  Flame cutting and welding
  Brazing
	Inhalation: metal fumes, toxic gases and materials, flux particulate, etc.
	Noise: from burner
	Eye and skin damage from infrared and ultraviolet radiation

*The health hazards may also depend on the toxicity and physical form(s) (gas, liquid, solid, powder, etc.) of the materials used. For further information see WA Burgess. Recognition of health hazards in industry: a review of materials and processes. New York: Wiley, 1981.

may take several weeks or months in a complex manufacturing or chemical plant.

The evaluation techniques used by the hygienist are based on the nature of the hazards and the routes of environmental contact with the worker. For example, *air sampling* can show the concentration of toxic particulates, gases, and vapors that workers may inhale; *skin wipes* can be used to measure the degree of skin contact with toxic materials that may penetrate the skin; and *noise dosimeters* record and electronically integrate workplace noise levels to determine total daily exposure. Both acute and chronic exposures should be considered in the evaluation because they may be associated with different types of adverse health effects. The workplace is not a static environment: Exposures may change by orders of magnitude over short distances from exposure sources, such as welding, and over short time intervals because of intermittent source output or incomplete mixing of air contaminants. It is also common that operations and materials used or produced may change, as do job titles and definitions. The nature of these changes and their possible effects must be recognized and taken into consideration by the industrial hygienist. The effects of environmental controls such as ventilation and personal protective equipment must also be considered.

The hygienist's decision on whether a hazard is present is based on three sources of information: (1) scientific literature and various exposure limit guides such as the Threshold Limit Values (TLVs) of the American Conference of Governmental Industrial Hygienists* (ACGIH), a set of consensus standards developed by industrial hygienists, toxicologists, and physicians from governmental agencies and academic institutions; (2) the legal requirements of OSHA (in some cases these are less stringent than the TLVs because the TLVs have been updated); and (3) interactions with other health professionals who have examined the ex-

posed workers and evaluated their health status. In cases where health effects are present but exposures do not exceed either the TLVs or OSHA requirements, the prudent hygienist will assume a relationship if it is consistent with the facts. Exposure limits of either type are designed to prevent adverse effects in most exposed workers but are not absolute levels below which effects could not occur. The supporting data for many of these exposure limits are sometimes viewed as insufficient, out-of-date, or based too much on evidence of toxic effects and not enough on recent evidence of carcinogenicity, mutagenicity, or teratogenicity.

Once a hazard is identified and the extent of the problem evaluated, the hygienist's next step is to design a control strategy or plan to reduce exposure to an acceptable level. Such controls may include (1) changing the industrial process or the materials used; (2) isolating the source and installing engineering controls such as ventilation systems; and (3) using administrative directives to limit the amount of exposure a worker receives, or, as a final resort, requiring the use of personal protective equipment. The approaches in (3) are less reliable because they depend on enforcement by management and conscientious application by the workers, both of which can fail. Usually the control strategy will include a combination of these approaches, particularly where there may be delays in installing engineering controls. Education of both workers and supervisors is an important part of any control strategy; both must understand the nature of the hazards and support the efforts taken to control or eliminate them.

After hazards are controlled, the hygienist may recommend a routine environmental surveillance program to ensure that controls remain adequate. This type of surveillance is most effective when done in close association with a medical surveillance program designed to detect subtle effects that may occur at low levels of exposure.

The following sections indicate how assessment and control techniques are utilized in connection with several major categories of environmental hazards: toxic materials, noise, and radiation and

---

*Can be obtained from: ACGIH, 6500 Glenway Ave., Bldg. D-5, Cincinnati, Ohio 45211.

radioactivity. The industrial hygienist may also be involved with the evaluation and control of other hazards such as heat, poor lighting, or infectious agents.

Toxic Materials
The hazard of a given exposure to a toxic material depends on the toxicity of the substance and on the duration and intensity of contact with the substance. Thus, adverse effects can result from chronic low-level exposure to a substance or from a short-term exposure to a dangerously high concentration of it. However, the pharmacologic mechanisms by which effects are caused differ for acute and chronic effects. Industrial hygienists are concerned with both long-term, low-level exposures and brief acute exposures and strive to characterize both.

In assessing a given hazardous material, the hygienist determines the route of exposure by which workers contact it and by which it may enter their bodies. There are four major routes of exposure: (1) direct contact with skin or eyes; (2) inhalation with deposition in the respiratory tract; (3) inhalation with deposition in the upper respiratory tract and subsequent transport to the throat and ingestion; and (4) direct ingestion of contaminated food or drink. In the workplace, several routes of exposure may occur for a single toxic substance.

Inhalation of airborne particulates, vapors, or gases is by far the most common route of exposure and therefore occupies much of a hygienist's efforts at assessment and control. Skin absorption may be important if the substance is lipid soluble or the skin's barrier is damaged or otherwise compromised. Ingestion of contaminated food and drink is a problem, especially for particulate and liquid materials, whose degree of risk may depend on the worker's awareness of the hazard and personal hygiene habits and on the availability of adequate facilities for washing and eating at the workplace. Contamination of cigarettes with toxic materials and their subsequent inhalation is also a problem for some substances.

For example, workers handling lead ingots are exposed to a low-level hazard from ingesting small amounts of lead by eating contaminated food or by inhaling small amounts of lead fumes from contaminated cigarettes. However, workers refining lead at temperatures above 800°F are exposed to a serious hazard from inhaling large amounts of lead fume if they work too close to unventilated refining kettles for several hours daily. Workers handling liquid nitric acid are exposed to the hazard of direct contact with the liquid on their skin, but they may also be exposed to a respiratory hazard from inhaling acid mist generated by an electroplating process using the nitric acid. In these examples the toxic materials cause different types and magnitudes of hazards because their physical forms vary: solid material versus small-diameter airborne particulates, and liquid material versus airborne droplets.

Identification. The first problem the hygienist faces in evaluating an unfamiliar workplace for toxic hazards is the identification of toxic materials. In many cases, such as at a lead smelter or pesticide manufacturing facility, they are clearly evident. But even in these examples some hazards may not be evident without a careful examination of an inventory of the chemicals used in the facility, including raw materials, by-products, products, wastes, solvents, cleaners, and special-use materials. Lead smelter workers are also exposed to carbon monoxide and sometimes to arsenic and cadmium; pesticide workers are subject to solvent exposures. Relatively nontoxic chemicals may be contaminated with highly toxic ones; for example, low-toxicity chlorinated hydrocarbons used in weed killers (2,4-T) may contain dioxin, which is highly toxic, and technical grade toluene may contain significant amounts of highly toxic benzene.

Material safety data sheets, which list the composition of commercial products, are available from manufacturers and can be useful, but they are sometimes too general or out-of-date. Toxicity data on specific substances can be obtained by literature searches—either manually or by computer—or by searches of toxic data indices (see appendix to Chap. 3).

As noted earlier, exposure to toxic substances can also occur by contamination of food, drink, or cigarettes. Therefore, the hygienist determines if facilities physically separated from the work area are available for eating and drinking, if facilities for washing are close to eating areas, and if sufficient time is permitted workers to use both of these facilities. Protective clothing and facilities for showering after a work shift should also be provided. Workers' understanding of hazards from toxic materials they are using must also be assessed. Finally, the hygienist determines the existence and enforcement of rules prohibiting eating, drinking, and smoking in areas with toxic substances.

Measurement Techniques. Once the toxic substances and routes of exposure have been identified, the hygienist decides which exposures are likely to be hazards and need to be quantified with environmental samples. Two types of techniques are available to make these measurements.

Direct reading instruments have sensors that detect the instantaneous air concentration and may produce a reading on a dial; some are expensive and require careful calibration and maintenance to obtain accurate data. The detector tube is another type of direct reading instrument of considerable use in determining approximate concentrations of air contaminants. This simple device uses a small hand pump to draw air through a bed of reagent in a glass tube that changes color or develops a length of stain that is proportional to the concentration of a given gaseous air contaminant. In spite of its popularity and wide use, it has important limitations: It takes only a short sample, which can misrepresent long-term average exposures; it is relatively inaccurate and imprecise; and it is prone to interference from a variety of materials.

Sample collectors that remove substances from the air for analysis in a laboratory are a less expensive alternative to direct reading instruments. *Personal sampling* is a common approach used by the industrial hygienist to obtain accurate and precise measurements of workers' exposures to particulate and gaseous air contaminants: the worker wears the sampler like a radiation dosimeter. Particulate contaminants are collected with filters, and gases and vapors are collected by solid adsorbents or liquid bubblers. The sampling apparatus is generally quite simple, consisting of a small air pump usually worn on a worker's belt, connected by tubing to the collector, and attached to the worker's lapel. (Some gas and vapor collectors are passive—they use diffusion instead of an air pump to move the contaminant into the sampler.) With the appropriate selection of a gas or particulate collector, it is possible to measure the average concentration of an air contaminant in the worker's breathing zone during an eight-hour work shift.

Collection devices for toxic particulates may capture either total dust—that is, all particle sizes that can enter the collector—or only the respirable dust—that is, only particles that can penetrate the terminal airways and alveolar spaces (less than 5 µ). Total particulate samples are collected if the toxic substance causes systemic health problems, as lead and pesticides do. Respirable dust samples are collected if the particulate causes chronic pulmonary disease such as pneumoconiosis. There is some controversy about the size of particles that cause chronic bronchitis and, therefore, which type of sample to collect.

Charcoal tubes are the most common adsorption collectors for gases and vapors; a small amount of charcoal inside a small glass tube acts as an activated surface that will retain nonpolar materials such as benzene. These collectors are commonly used to measure inhalation exposures to solvents such as vapor exposures of printers. Collectors such as impingers or bubblers will collect gases and vapors into liquid from air drawn through them. Bubblers are less convenient to use than charcoal tubes but may be required for some compounds such as sulfur dioxide. The specific methods are discussed in detail in the NIOSH *Manual of Analytical Methods* (see Bibliography).

The passive or badge type samplers are much more convenient to use for gas and vapor sampling than the collectors requiring air pumps, and they have better worker acceptance because many workers do not like the weight of the pumps. After the sampling period is completed, the cover is replaced on the badge and it is sent to a laboratory for analysis. Although they are convenient and relatively inexpensive, the accuracy of the passive samplers is not proved.

Sampling Strategy. When the airborne toxic exposures have been identified and the appropriate measurement techniques selected, then the hygienist must design a sampling strategy that takes into account the types of hazards, variations in exposure, and routes of exposure. The use of personal measurement in the strategy is designed to reflect the accumulation of exposure from a variety of sources that a worker may encounter in the course of a workshift. In some cases exposure may only occur during certain operations, and it may be decided that sampling will only be done during the period of exposure. It is frequently found that workers in adjacent areas, not directly involved with the air contaminant of interest, may also have significant exposures because the air contaminant drifts into their work areas.

The personal sampling plan must take into account the considerable day-to-day variation in air concentrations at a given operation and between samples on different workers at the same job, either because of personal work habits or variations in the process itself. Therefore, it is usually important to collect several samples from each worker in a given work area over several days to be fully informed about the nature of air exposures. Single samples are generally avoided wherever possible because it is difficult to know whether the sample value is representative.

In addition to personal sampling, the industrial hygienist also uses fixed location sampling in the sampling strategy. In this approach the sampler is set at a given location that has some useful relationship to the source of exposure. This type of sampling is advantageous because it can allow determination of features of the exposure that would be difficult with personal samples. For example, a large sampler can be used to determine the particle size distribution of airborne dust in a work area or to collect a large quantity of airborne material for detailed chemical analysis if the composition of the contaminants is not known. As with personal sampling, to get the most out of the effort, it is very important to select carefully the sampling location and strategy for fixed location sampling. In some cases a combination of personal and fixed location samples is used to describe a given problem completely; for example, personal samples are used to describe the highly variable exposures of steel workers tending a blast furnace while stationary samples measure exposures to the uniform, well-mixed air levels they experience while waiting in the lunchroom for their next job assignment (2 to 4 hours per work shift).

In general, the principal applications of fixed location sampling are to identify and characterize sources within a work area and to evaluate the effectiveness of emission control systems such as local exhaust ventilation. In some cases, such as cotton dust exposures, only fixed location sampling techniques are available.

In some occupational settings the most important route of exposure is skin contact. Skin contact is difficult to evaluate with environmental sampling because even if the amount of skin contamination can be determined, it is not possible to know how much of the contaminant has already penetrated into the body or would penetrate given sufficient time. Two principal sampling approaches are employed. First, cloth patches can be used to cover given locations of skin, such as the forehead, back of the neck, back of the hands, and forearms, to measure the amount of contamination per unit area that resulted during a period of exposure. The second approach is to use wipe sampling in which an area of skin is washed with an appropriate solvent to determine the quantity of contamination. Both of these techniques have been used to estimate pesticide exposures of agricultural workers. Additionally, wipe sampling can also be used to measure contamination on surfaces in the workplace with which workers may come in contact. While this type of sampling may be useful in estimating the risk of one person relative to another or of one area relative to another, it is difficult to know in absolute terms the quantity of contaminant that may actually penetrate the worker and become a health problem. Biologic monitoring is probably the best method for determining the intensity of skin exposures to a substance for which such a monitoring test is available (see Chap. 6).

Some nonpolar substances such as pesticides and solvents may enter the body both via the respiratory tract and through skin contact. In these cases both skin contact and air exposure must be evaluated to completely assess the risk. Biologic sampling that integrates these two routes of intake may be a practical necessity. However, two important theoretical problems are associated with biologic monitoring. Some types of tests may represent detection of adverse effects, such as monitoring red blood cell cholinesterase in pesticide-exposed workers. As a result they detect excessive exposures only after the effects have occurred. Tissue levels of environmental contaminants represent a dynamic interaction because the exposure is rarely constant. As a result, there is a complex relationship between exposures and levels of compounds and metabolites in blood, urine, exhaled breath, and other biologic media. This relationship is controlled by toxicokinetics of the particular agents [1]. Consequently, proper interpretation of findings from biologic monitoring for a given worker requires some knowledge of the temporal variations in the worker's exposure. In many situations, biologic monitoring should only be used to verify that exposures have been controlled. Its use in detecting high exposures should be limited (for example, when absorption is primarily through the skin).

It is almost never possible to evaluate ingestion as a route of exposure with sampling. Occasionally, samples of food and drink may be collected to assess the level of contamination; however, this sort of exposure is likely to be extremely variable and episodic in nature, so that environmental sampling is usually an ineffective way of assessing exposure. Again, biologic monitoring is the method of choice to monitor this route of exposure.

Controls. The three basic approaches to controlling exposures to toxic materials are (1) substitution of less toxic or nontoxic materials for a toxic substance; (2) limitation of release or prevention of buildup of environmental contamination by isolation of the source and using engineering controls; and (3) limitation of contact between worker and toxic materials by personal protective equipment and administrative methods. The method of choice, whenever possible, is substitution: to change the process or materials used in a process so that toxic substances are not used. For example, less-toxic toluene may be an adequate replacement for benzene.

If substitution is not possible, then the next step is to attempt to control or limit releases and prevent the buildup of toxic materials in the worker's environment (Fig. 7-1). Local exhaust ventilation combined with source isolation will control process emissions. General room ventilation is used to prevent the buildup of emissions in the work area and may be the only control used if the amount and toxicity of the emissions are low. An example of these two ventilation approaches is shown in Figure 7-2.

Local exhaust systems surround the point of emission with a partial or complete enclosure and attempt to capture and remove the emissions before they are released into the worker's breathing zone. Figures 7-3 through 7-5 show several examples of local ventilation systems; a wide variety of types is available with differing degrees of effectiveness. Unfortunately, it is not possible before installation to determine precisely the effectiveness of a particular system. As a result it is important to measure exposures and evaluate how much con-

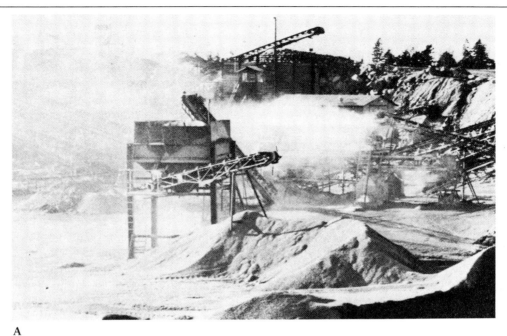

A

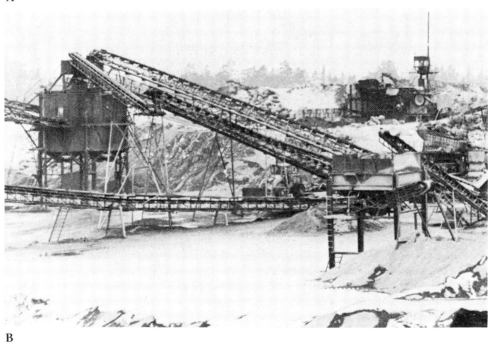

B

Fig. 7-1. Rock crushing. A. Before dust control. B. After dust control.
(From L. W. Holm. Limit values in Sweden—targets and means. *Newsletter*, National Swedish Board of Occupational Safety and Health, January, 1981, p. 5.)

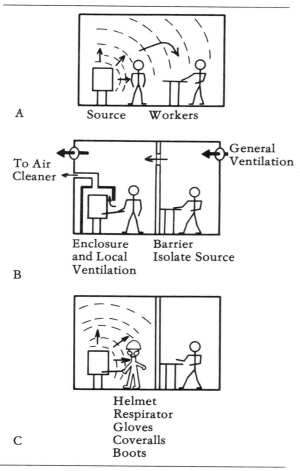

Fig. 7-2. Examples of controls for airborne exposures. A. Workers with primary and secondary exposure to source emissions. B. Ventilation and source isolation to control exposures. C. Personal protection and source isolation to control exposures.
(From Harvard Occupational Health Program.)

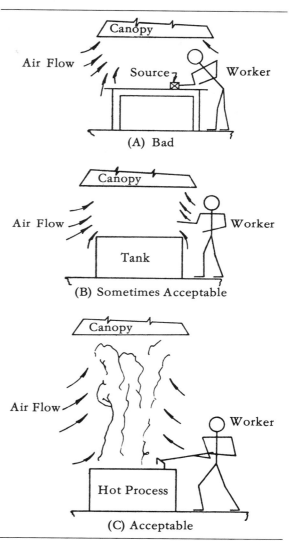

Fig. 7-3. The proper use of a canopy hood, which will not draw the air contaminants through the worker's breathing zone. The worker's location is crucial. (From National Institute for Occupational Safety and Health. *The Industrial Environment—Its Evaluation and Control.* Washington, D.C.: NIOSH, 1973, p. 599.)

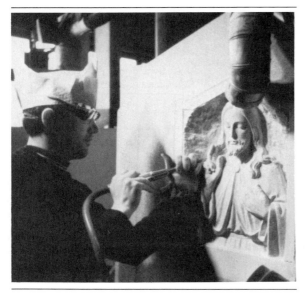

Fig. 7-4. Local exhaust ventilation successfully captures dust produced by stone cutting.
(From Harvard Occupational Health Program.)

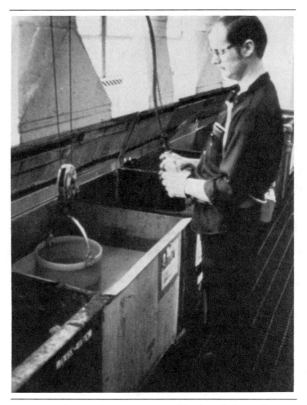

Fig. 7-5. Electroplating protected by local slot exhaust ventilation.
(From Harvard Occupational Health Program.)

trol has been achieved after a system is installed. Unless contaminant sources are totally enclosed, collection will only capture a percentage of the total emission: A good system may collect 80 to 99 percent, but a poor system may capture only 50 percent or less. Careful maintenance must be performed on the system to maintain efficiency. Poor maintenance is probably most responsible for system failures.

Most industrial settings have general ventilation in work areas to dilute and remove those emissions that are not collected by the local exhaust system and to prevent buildup of toxic materials in the workplace. If the air contaminants are of a low order of toxicity, a workplace may have only general ventilation without local exhaust systems. The increasing cost of energy has made the practice of ventilating work areas with outside fresh air an increasingly expensive process; considerable effort is being directed to the design of systems that can

recirculate decontaminated air so the heat value is not lost.

The third important approach to controlling exposures to toxic materials is to limit worker contact either by isolating processes using toxic materials from the remainder of the work area so that the potential for contact with these materials is limited (Fig. 7-6), or by furnishing workers with personal protective equipment such as dust or gas masks (respirators) or hoods or suits with externally supplied air for controlling inhalation of toxic materials (Fig. 7-7). Many people mistakenly think that the use of respirators is a simple and

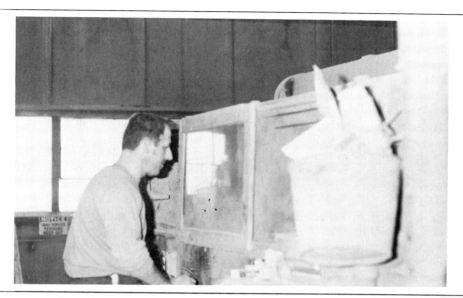

Fig. 7-6. Sandblaster protected from dust exposure by enclosed blasting booth. (From Harvard Occupational Health Program.)

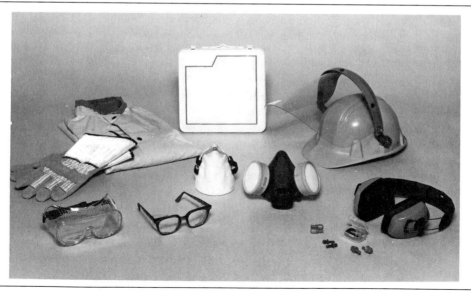

Fig. 7-7. Several types of personal protective equipment. (Courtesy of James Schaepe, M.D.)

inexpensive way to control exposure to toxic airborne materials. However, there is discomfort in wearing these masks, poor worker acceptance, and variable levels of protection achieved. There are extensive OSHA requirements for an adequate respirator program to ensure that the quality of the devices is maintained and that workers are receiving adequate protection. It should be noted that the cost of a good respirator program for lead dust exposures is reported to be as much as $1,000 per worker per year. The fitting of respirators is an extremely important aspect that is commonly neglected; a poorly fitting respirator provides substantially less protection than expected because, even if the filters are highly efficient, air leaks around the edges of the face mask.

The use of rubber gloves and protective clothing does not automatically ensure that workers are protected adequately. Toluene and other aromatic solvents readily penetrate rubber gloves; thus, glove composition must be matched to the chemical nature of the substance. Similarly, long-sleeved shirts or coveralls may not prevent skin contact with toxic dusts because small dust particles can sift through the openings between threads in woven cloth. A study of orchard workers showed the effects of pesticide exposures even though they had been wearing dust masks to prevent inhalation of the dust and long-sleeved shirts to prevent skin exposure. Special testing indicated that, despite their wearing the shirts, their arms were covered with dust that contained pesticide.

An important part of limiting contact with hazardous substances is the requirement that protective clothing be changed each day and not worn outside the work area. This effort is also facilitated by the requirement for showers after the work shift.

Some reduction in exposure can be obtained by administrative controls such as schedules where workers spend limited amounts of time in areas with potential exposure, with the overall result that the exposure is at or below recommended guidelines. While this approach may be effective in certain situations, it requires good exposure data

to demonstrate its effectiveness and the careful attention of supervisory personnel, may be an inefficient use of workers, and may be inappropriate for controlling exposures to carcinogens.

Ideally, all the control approaches described should be used together to develop an overall control strategy that will deal with all aspects of toxic material exposure in a particular workplace. Short-term measures such as extensive use of personal protective equipment may be adopted immediately after a problem is recognized to allow time for developing engineering controls or process modifications that will provide more long-term control. In spite of their undesirable aspects (OSHA's previous policy was to use them only as a last resort), respirators may be the only effective control device for some exposures such as those faced by maintenance or clean-up workers.

Noise Problems

Occupational exposure to excessive noise is an important problem that is evaluated and controlled in part by industrial hygienists (see also Chap. 17). An industrial hygienist is trained to measure the intensity and quality of noise, assess its potential for producing damage, and devise means to control noise exposures. Two principal types of workplace noise have somewhat different techniques of evaluation and control:

> *Continuous noise* is produced by high-velocity air flow in compressors, fans, gas burners, and motors. Crushing, drilling, and grinding are important sources of continuous noise because a large amount of energy is used in a small space.
>
> *Impact noise* results from sharp or explosive inputs of energy into some object or process such as hammering or pounding on metal or stone, dropping heavy objects, or materials handling.

During the evaluation of a workplace an industrial hygienist looks for sources of excessive noise, determines which workers are exposed, and then selects an evaluation strategy to clarify the nature and extent of the exposures. If the noise is continuous or almost continuous, an industrial hygienist will use a hand-held noise survey meter to determine the noise levels at the worker's location. If the exposure involves impact noises, an electronic instrument that records and averages the high-intensity but short-duration pulses is used to characterize the source and exposures.

Typically, workers spend variable amounts of time exposed to noise sources, and they may work at different distances from the sources, which will alter their exposures. Exposures may also vary because the output of noise sources may change over time. Therefore, the average (time-weighted) exposure may not be easy to estimate, even though the sources may present clear potential for overexposure. This problem has been solved by the use of small noise dosimeters worn by the workers that electronically record sound levels and indicate average noise levels during the work shifts. Dosimeters are very useful for describing average exposures, but they give relatively little data on sources. Therefore, a typical noise evaluation will include both source noise level and dosimeter measurements.

OSHA requirements and TLV guidelines are used by the hygienist to evaluate noise data and decide if a hazard is present. In addition to the hazard to hearing, noise also affects verbal communication, which may create a hazard by interfering with warnings and worker detection of safety hazards such as moving equipment. The current OSHA standard for continuous noise for 8 hours is 90 dBA.* Higher levels are permitted for shorter periods of time [2]. The OSHA standard allows levels of noise exposure that will protect some but not all workers from the adverse effects of workplace noise. The TLV for noise (1980) is 85 dBA, lower than the 90 dBA OSHA standard for (continuous) noise.

Although techniques exist to obtain an overall time-weighted average of noise exposures received in several different work settings, no techniques exist for assessing the hearing risks of combined exposure to both continuous and impulse noise. Workers exposed to both continuous and impulse noise are numerous; they include brass foundry workers who are exposed to continuous noise from gas burners and to impulse noise from brass ingots dropping into a metal bin from a conveyor.

The strategies for controlling noise are similar to those used for toxic material control:

Substitution. Use another process or piece of equipment: electrically heated pots for melting metal can be used instead of gas heated pots to eliminate burner noise.

Prevent or reduce release of noise. Modify the source to reduce its output, enclose and soundproof the operation, or install mufflers or baffles: noisy air compressors can be fitted with mufflers and placed in soundproofed rooms to control their noise.

Prevent excessive worker contact. Provide personal protective equipment such as earplugs or earmuffs.

As with toxic materials, the overall strategy to control exposures usually involves approaches for various aspects of the problem. It may be necessary to consult an acoustical engineer with advanced evaluation and engineering expertise for dealing with complex noise problems. If engineering controls are not completely effective or are impractical, ear protectors may be required; however, the effectiveness of these devices is limited because sound may also reach the ear by bone conduction. A full shift exposure above 120 dBA cannot be controlled adequately using earplugs or muffs (see Chap. 17).

Radiation Problems

Radiation hazards are commonly first identified by industrial hygienists, but the responsibility for their evaluation and control overlaps among the industrial hygienist, the health physicist, and the

---

*dBA means decibels on the "A" scale, which is related to the human ear's response to sound.

radiation protection officer (see Chaps. 16 and 18).

Exposure to ionizing radiation can be external (from x-ray machines or radioactive materials) or internal (from radioactive substances in the body). External exposures can be monitored instrumentally by several methods; the type of detector system chosen for a given problem depends on the nature of the ionizing radiation. Personal monitoring is commonly performed with badges of photographic emulsions, thermal luminescent materials, or induced radiation materials that will indicate the cumulative dose during the period worn. Data from these measurement systems can be used to construct relatively accurate estimates of tissue exposure.

Nonionizing radiation is also an external exposure problem. This type of radiation includes a variety of electromagnetic waves ranging from short wavelength ultraviolet, through visible and infrared, to long wavelength microwaves and radiowaves. Exposures to ultraviolet, visible, and infrared radiation are measured with photometers of various types. Microwaves and radiowaves can also be measured by several nonstandardized techniques, but there is some controversy over the exposure intensities required to produce adverse effects. No personal monitoring systems have yet been developed for nonionizing radiation exposures.

Exposures to radioactive materials can be evaluated with similar methodology to that used for toxic substances. Personal air sampling, surface sampling, and skin contamination measurements can be used to quantify exposures by their route of contact or entry into the body. For example, personal air sampling in uranium mines can measure the miners' exposure to respirable radioactive particles that will be deposited in their respiratory tracts. Internal levels of some radionuclides can be detected outside the body and measured directly if they emit sufficient penetrating radiation, such as gamma rays emitted from radioactive cobalt. However, most cannot be detected externally; the quantities of radioactive substances reaching sensitive tissues usually must be estimated by determining the worker's external exposures and making assumptions about the amount entering the body and being transported to the site(s) of adverse effects.

The Nuclear Regulatory Commission has set standards for allowable ionizing radiation exposures for both external and internal sources. These exposure limits, based on the work of an earlier governmental agency, the National Council on Radiation Protection and Measurements, can be used, like TLVs, to decide if a given exposure presents a health risk. They also have many of the same problems associated with TLVs: They were based on limited data obtained at high-dose levels and include many assumptions and extrapolations that have not been verified. They are especially controversial because they contain an inherent assumption of a threshold below which there is no cancer risk. Radiation protection programs have strict requirements about techniques for handling radioactive materials and working with radiation sources and also require extensive routine exposure monitoring and medical monitoring.

Exposure limits for nonionizing radiation have been set by OSHA based on published scientific data, the TLVs developed by the ACGIH, and standards developed by the American National Standards Institute. The eyes and the skin are the critical organs to be protected, and the standards are set for the most susceptible areas. Standards also have been developed for lasers based on ophthalmoscopic data and irreversible functional changes in visual responses. As with other types of standards, the numerical limits cannot be treated as absolute, and the margin of safety for many is uncertain.

Control of external ionizing and nonionizing radiation exposures is achieved by minimizing the amounts of radiation used, isolating the processes, shielding the sources, using warning devices and interlocking door and trigger mechanisms to prevent accidental exposures, educating workers and supervisors about the hazards, and, if necessary, requiring use of personal protective equipment.

For example, an industrial x-ray machine used to check castings for flaws is placed in a separate room with extensive lead shielding, and the x-ray machine cannot be triggered when the door is open. The room also has signs warning of the hazard. A red warning light inside the room is lit for 30 seconds before the x-rays are released so that a worker inside the room when the door is closed could activate an emergency override switch to prevent operation of the x-ray machine. All personnel working around the x-ray operation are required to wear film badges to monitor their accumulated x-ray exposure.

Control of internal radiation exposures from radioactive materials is very similar to controls for toxic materials. The objectives are to use minimal amounts of radioactive materials; isolate the work areas; enclose any operations likely to produce airborne emissions; use work procedures that prevent or minimize worker contact with contaminated air or materials; have workers wear personal protective equipment to prevent skin contact, eye exposure, or inhalation of materials; monitor environmental contamination levels; and educate workers about the hazards. Some or all of these measures will be used in a typical radiation control problem. Careful supervision of work activities and monitoring of program implementation are required to provide adequate protection.

REFERENCES

1. Fiserova-Bergerova V. Modeling of inhalation exposure to vapors: uptake, distribution, and elimination. Boca Raton, FL: CRC Press, 1983.
2. Occupational Safety and Health Administration, U.S. Department of Labor. General Industry: OSHA Safety and Health Standards (29 CFR 1910). Washington, D.C.: U.S. Government Printing Office, 1984.

BIBLIOGRAPHY

Cralley LV, Cralley LJ, eds. Patty's industrial hygiene and toxicology. New York: Wiley, 1978 (Vol. I), 1979 (Vols. IIA and IIB), 1981 (Vol. III), and 1982 (Vol. IIC).

National Institute for Occupational Safety and Health. The industrial environment—its evaluation and control. Washington, D.C.: NIOSH, 1973.
Two useful and comprehensive general references on industrial hygiene. The Cralley volumes, although somewhat unwieldy, are the professional's reference work. The NIOSH volume has the advantage of being reasonably priced, but can be difficult to use for specific problems because of the poor quality of its index.

American Conference of Governmental Industrial Hygienists. Industrial ventilation, 19th ed. Cincinnati: ACGIH, 1986.
Manual containing the latest recommendations for the design and operation of ventilation systems to control air contaminants.

American Conference of Governmental Industrial Hygienists. Air sampling instruments, 6th ed. Cincinnati: ACGIH, 1983.
A useful reference containing detailed discussions of instrument operating principles, usage, and limitations that can be helpful in interpreting the quality of industrial hygiene data.

Burgess WA. Recognition of health hazards in industry: a review of materials and processes. New York: Wiley, 1981.
The source of much of the data in Table 7–1 and a highly recommended reference.

Considine DM. Chemical and process technology encyclopedia. New York: McGraw-Hill, 1974.
A technical source for gathering background information.

Leidel NA, Busch KA, Lynch JR. Occupational exposure sampling strategy manual. Washington, D.C.: NIOSH, 1977.
While this manual contains much useful information, it is difficult to follow in places and requires a strong background in statistics. It is important because it lays out the rationale for sampling strategies to determine compliance with OSHA's permissable exposure limits.

National Institute for Occupational Safety and Health. Manual of analytical methods, 3rd ed. Washington, D.C.: NIOSH, 1984.
Designed for the laboratory chemist and industrial hygienist.

The way things work (Vols. I and II). New York: Simon & Schuster, 1967 and 1971.
A practical encyclopedia on industrial processes and other technological items that can be used to obtain basic background information to guide a hazard evaluation.

8
Occupational Safety: Preventing Accidents and Overt Trauma

W. Monroe Keyserling

An *accident* is an unanticipated, sudden event that results in an undesired outcome such as property damage, bodily injury, or death. *Injury* is physical damage to body tissues caused by an accident or by exposure to environmental stressors. Many work injuries are directly associated with accidents, such as a heavy object falling and crushing bones in the feet. Some work injuries, however, are not associated with accidents but result from normal, "everyday" exposures, such as tendinitis from a highly repetitive assembly-line job. The occupational basis of these nonacute injuries may not always be recognized because of the lack of a well-defined causative event.

Each year, occupational accidents result in staggering costs in terms of loss of life, pain and suffering, lost wages for the injured worker, damage to production facilities and equipment, and lost production opportunity. In 1984, workplace accidents in the United States caused 11,500 deaths, 1,900,000 disabling injuries, and over 40 million lost workdays. The estimated cost, including lost wages, medical and rehabilitation payments, insurance administrative costs, property losses, production losses, and other indirect costs was approximately $33 billion [1]. These figures underestimate the true count and cost of all work injuries, however, because of underreporting of nonacute injuries by many industrial recordkeeping systems.

As a result of the aggressive implementation of industrial safety programs following World War II and the passage of the Occupational Safety and Health Act in 1970, the annual rate of accidental industrial fatalities in the United States declined from about 33 per 100,000 workers in 1945 to 11 per 100,000 in 1984. Certain industries, such as mining, agriculture, and construction, however, have continued to experience high rates of fatal accidents. Death rates for these industries ranged between 39 and 60 per 100,000 workers in 1984 [1]. Considering only fatalities, the safest U.S. industries in 1984 were retail trade (such as apparel and furniture stores) and service (e.g., insurance, real estate, and education) where death rates ranged between 5 and 7 per 100,000 workers [1]. While nonfatal accidents have also declined dramatically during the last four decades, the construction, agriculture, manufacturing, transportation, and mining sectors continue to experience high rates of disabling injuries. For these reasons, the prevention of industrial accidents and injuries continues to be a high priority in occupational health.

The principal responsibility of the safety professional is to minimize the risk of occupational injuries by preventing accidents and controlling exposures to hazardous stressors in the work environment. Common examples of these injuries are listed in Table 8-1. Traditionally, safety professionals have concentrated their efforts on the prevention of *acute trauma* injuries such as lacerations, burns, and electrocution. These injuries typically are immediately apparent to the victim and can be directly linked to a well-defined accident or event. In recent years, safety professionals have also become concerned with the prevention of *cumulative trauma* such as chronic back pain,

Table 8-1. Selected examples of overt and cumulative trauma and commonly affected occupational groups

	Overt trauma	
Cause	Injury or disorder	Affected occupations
Mechanical energy	Lacerations	Sheet metal workers, butchers, press operators, sawyers, fabric cutters
	Fractures	Materials handlers, miners, construction workers
	Contusions	Materials handlers, any worker exposed to low energy impacts
	Amputations	Press operators, butchers, machine operators
	Crushing injuries	Materials handlers, press operators, construction workers, rubber workers
	Eye injuries (struck by foreign objects)	Miners, grinders, saw mill operators, machine shop employees
	Strains or sprains (overt)	Materials handlers, miners, baggage handlers, mail handlers, construction workers
Thermal energy	Burns	Foundry workers, smelter workers, welders, glass workers, laundry workers
	Heat strain	Firefighters, steelworkers, smelter workers
	Cold strain	Utility workers, lumberjacks, butchers
Chemical energy (including acute toxicity)	Burns	Masons, process workers, hazardous waste workers
	Asphyxiation, acute toxicity	Firefighters, confined space workers, hazardous waste workers
Electrical energy	Electrocution, shocks, burns	Utility workers, construction workers, electricians, users of electric hand tools or machines
Nuclear energy	Radiation burns, illness	Hospital workers, industrial radiographers, nuclear workers
	Cumulative trauma	
Cause	Injury or disorder	Affected occupations
Heavy lifting, prolonged sitting, awkward posture	Back pain	Materials handlers, nurses, truck drivers, sewing machine operators
Frequent or repetitive forceful hand motions with awkward posture	Upper extremity cumulative trauma disorders (tendinitis, carpal tunnel syndrome, epicondylitis, degenerative joint disease)	Assembly line workers; garment workers; poultry, meat, or fish processors; clerical workers; press operators; fruit pickers; musicians
Vibration	Raynaud's syndrome	Lumberjacks, grinding machine operators, jackhammer operators

tendinitis, and carpal tunnel syndrome. These problems are rarely associated with a specific accident or event but with repeated low-level insults to a localized body region. Furthermore, because of differences in individual tolerance to the stresses that cause cumulative trauma injuries, only a small fraction of workers on a particular job may actually be affected.

This chapter focuses on topics related to the prevention of acute trauma. (For discussions of cumulative trauma disorders and injuries, see Chap. 22.)

SAFETY HAZARDS IN THE INDUSTRIAL ENVIRONMENT

Safety hazards and the injuries they cause can be classified and categorized in many different ways. The American National Standards Institute (ANSI, see Appendix C) has developed a system for clas-

Table 8-2. Major causes of work injury classified by accident type

Struck by
Caught in, under, or between (CIUB)
Fall from elevation
Fall on same level
Overexertion
Motor vehicle accident
Contact with electric current
Struck against
Contact with temperature extremes (see Chap. 18)
Rubbed or abraded
Bodily reaction
Contact with radiation, caustics, toxic and noxious substances (see Chapters 14, 16, and 18)
Public transportation accident
Other
Unknown

Source: This material is reproduced with permission from American National Standard Method of Recording Basic Facts Relating to the Nature and Occurrence of Work Injuries, ANSI Z16.2, copyright 1962 by the American National Standards Institute. Copies of this standard may be purchased from the American National Standards Institute at 1430 Broadway, New York, N.Y. 10018.

sifying the cause of work injuries according to accident type. This approach, summarized in Table 8-2, considers the conditions and events that caused the accident and has been adopted by workers' compensation boards in many states. ANSI classifications for major accident types are discussed below.

Struck By

The classification "struck by" applies to a broad variety of cases in which the worker is hit by a moving object or particle. Typical accident scenarios include: a construction worker suffers a concussion when hit by a hammer accidentally kicked off a scaffold, a warehouse worker fractures a leg when hit by a moving forklift, and a grinding machine operator is permanently blinded when struck in the eyes and face by the fragments of an exploding grinding wheel.

Approximately one-third of these accidents are caused by falling objects. Items accidentally dropped from overhead (such as hand tools, construction materials, and equipment being hoisted to an upper floor of a building) can cause severe head, neck, and shoulder injuries, such as fractures, concussions, and lacerations. In some instances, these injuries are fatal. Effective methods for preventing these events include:

1. Installing covers or side rails to enclose or contain materials carried on overhead conveyor systems (Fig. 8-1)
2. Placing toeboards on all overhead work platforms
3. Installing nets or gratings above workers assigned to hazardous areas
4. Providing and requiring the use of safety helmets
5. Training workers to follow safe rigging practices when hoisting materials overhead
6. Painting safety warnings on floors to indicate work zones where overhead hazards are present

Objects that are dropped during materials handling tasks, such as lifting and carrying, can cause

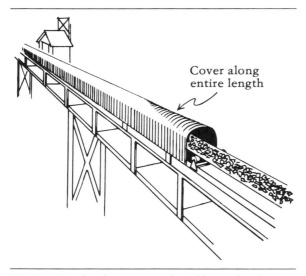

Fig. 8-1. Overhead conveyors should be enclosed to prevent loose materials from falling on people walking or working below.
(Reprinted with permission. National Safety Council. Accident prevention manual for industrial operations: engineering and technology, [9th ed.]. Chicago: National Safety Council, 1988, p. 118.)

severe "struck by" injuries to the feet and toes; crush injuries, fractures, and contusions are quite common. Heavy objects that are manually carried should be equipped with handles that allow workers to maintain a firm grasp and should weigh no more than workers' strength capabilities. (See discussion of manual materials handling in Chap. 9.) Finally, it is essential that foot protection (safety shoes and metatarsal guards) be provided and worn whenever these hazards exist.

Flying objects are another cause of "struck by" injuries. Small airborne particles released during operations such as grinding, chipping, and machining can cause severe eye injuries and blindness. These operations should be fully enclosed whenever possible. The use of compressed air for cleaning dust and chips may also be hazardous because small particles can rapidly accelerate to very high velocities. OSHA regulations require that the pressure of cleaning air be limited to 30 pounds per square inch (PSI) to minimize this hazard. Eye and face protection is a critical factor in the prevention of eye injuries. All workers exposed to operations that can release flying particles and fragments must be provided with and *constantly* wear the appropriate personal protective equipment, such as safety glasses, safety goggles, and face shields (see Chap. 24).

The remainder of "struck by" injuries are caused by a variety of factors. In-plant vehicles, such as forklifts and other industrial trucks, can strike workers and cause injuries such as fractures and severe trauma to internal organs. Machines with moving parts that can strike a worker, such as the rotating blades of a lawnmower, are common hazards. All rotating and reciprocating parts of machines and power transmission systems that can either strike or ensnare a person should be fully enclosed within a barrier guard (Fig. 8-2). Programmable robots, which are becoming common in many industries, can create special hazards. Many robots do not have the sensory capabilities, such as vision, hearing, and touch, to detect the presence of a worker. A person entering the work zone of a "live" robot without taking the necessary

Fig. 8-2. The belt drive in this power transmission system is completely enclosed by a barrier guard.
(From Occupational Safety and Health Administration. Concepts and techniques of machine guarding. OSHA Pub. No. 3067. Washington, D.C.: Occupational Safety and Health Administration, 1980: 13.)

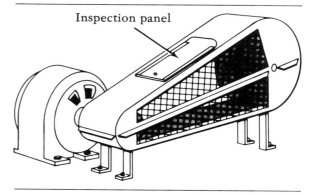

precautions to deactivate all sources of machine power may be struck during subsequent movements of the system. Research is being conducted to improve the sensory abilities of robots to avoid this type of accident. In the meantime, however, all workers assigned to robot installations should receive special training in robot safety. (For a case study of a robot-related fatality, see box.)

Caught In, Under, or Between

Accidents classified as "caught in, under, or between" (frequently abbreviated as CIUB) include

---

A ROBOT-RELATED FATALITY

A 34-year-old male operator of an automated die-cast system went into cardiorespiratory arrest and died after being pinned between the back-end of an industrial robot and a steel safety pole (Fig. 8-8.) The robot had been installed in an existing production line to remove parts from a die-cast machine and transfer these parts to a trimmer. The victim had 15 years' experience in die-casting and had completed a one-week course in robotics three weeks before the fatal incident.

The victim entered the work zone of the operating robot prior to the accident, presumably to clean up scrap metal that had accumulated on the floor. Despite training and warnings to avoid this practice, the victim apparently climbed over, through, or around the safety rail that surrounded two sides of the robot's work envelope. The entry gate in the safety rail was interlocked. (Had the worker used the gate, power to the robot should have been shut off.) No other presence-sensing devices (for example, electric eyes, pressure-sensitive floor mats) were operative in the system.

This preventable fatality demonstrates the growing problem of the failure of workers to recognize all of the hazards associated with robots and the weaknesses in the design of some robotic systems. While workers may readily recognize hazards associated with movement of the robotic arm, they may not recognize dangers associated with the movement of other parts of the assembly. In this case, the victim was trapped between a fixed object (a steel pole) and the active back-end of the robot. Because the worker was not standing in the movement envelope of the robot's working arm, he apparently presumed that he was in a nondangerous zone. Furthermore, the existing enclosure system for isolating the robot (a safety rail and interlock gate) failed to accomplish its intended purpose of preventing access to the robot's work zone during powered phases of the operation.

To prevent recurrences of this type of accident, several actions must be taken. First, the design of robotic systems must be enhanced to ensure that enclosure barriers cannot be bypassed simply by walking around a fence or passing through or under a rail. Furthermore, the design must ensure that hardware is placed in a nonpowered, safe condition whenever a safety barrier is opened or crossed. Inside the barrier, floors should be painted to indicate zones of movement for all parts of the robot system. Second, workers must be trained to recognize all hazards associated with a specific robot installation. This training must be enhanced periodically with refresher courses to prevent complacency and overconfidence when working near robots. Finally, supervisors must ensure that no worker is ever permitted to enter the operational area of a robot without first putting the system into safe condition.

Adapted from NIOSH Publication No. 85-103. Request for assistance in preventing the injury of workers by robots. Cincinnati: National Institute of Occupational Safety and Health, December 1984.

those in which the injury is caused by the crushing, squeezing, or pinching of a body part between a moving object and a stationary object, or between two moving objects. Frequently, these accidents are associated with operations that involve the use of mechanized equipment, such as power presses and calenders. A power press is a machine used to produce contoured sheet metal products, such as automobile body parts and metal furniture. When operating a power press, unprocessed stock material (typically a flat piece of sheet metal) is loaded to the machine and placed on the lower die. The machine is then activated, which causes the upper die to slam down on the sheet metal with tremendous force (up to several tons), to form the desired shape. If a worker's hand is between the dies during this action, it may be severely crushed or amputated (Fig. 8-3). Calenders are large heavy rolls used to compress raw materials, such as slabs of steel or rubber, into sheets of precise thickness. It is possible for a limb to become caught in the "in-running pinch point" between these rollers and to be crushed or amputated (Fig. 8-4). Occasionally, the entire body may be drawn into the rollers, killing the worker.

When power presses and calenders are used, the most hazardous operations involve the feeding and removal of stock, since these tasks place workers' hands near moving machine parts. Effective systems for preventing accidents during these activities include *barrier guards,* devices that enclose the dangerous zone before the machine can be activated; *two-handed "safety" buttons,* devices that are positioned in a safe location and require simultaneous activation to start the machine (Fig. 8-5); and *presence-sensing systems,* devices such as electric eyes that prevent the operation of a machine while the hands are in a danger zone. In addition, all machines that can catch clothing or body parts in a "pinch point" should be equipped with emergency stop buttons that can be easily reached by the operator with either hand. Because all of the above systems are quite sophisticated, it is essential that they be designed and installed only by qualified personnel.

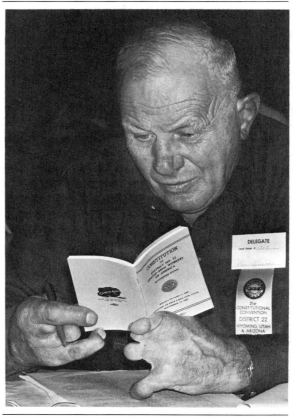

Fig. 8-3. Although not necessarily totally disabling, finger amputations are disfiguring and may reduce job opportunities.
(Photograph by Earl Dotter.)

Maintenance activities, such as set-up, clean-up, unjamming parts, and repair, are also associated with CIUB accidents. These operations are particularly hazardous because of the necessity to remove or bypass guards to reach locations that require maintenance. (Such was the case in a robot-related fatality described in the box.) Maintenance workers require special training in safe procedures for working with powered machines and equipment that are temporarily unguarded.

Maintenance activities should be performed only when the machine has been put into a non-

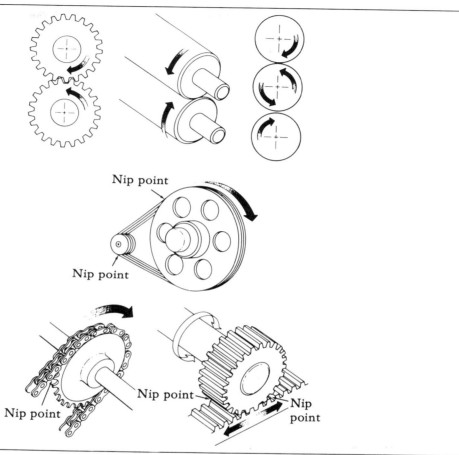

Fig. 8-4. Common examples of in-running pinch points.
(From Occupational Safety and Health Administration. Concepts and techniques of machine guarding. OSHA Pub. No. 3067. Washington, D.C.: Occupational Safety and Health Administration, 1980: 3–4.)

powered state, which can be done using "lock-out" procedures that prevent the machine from being started during servicing (Fig. 8-6). Lock-out is a relatively simple but highly reliable procedure for protecting maintenance workers. Prior to performing any servicing to a piece of equipment, the power switch is placed in the "off" position. The switch is then secured in the "off" position using the personal padlocks of each maintenance worker assigned to the job. Because each worker carries the key to his or her padlock, it is virtually impossible to restart the machine until all workers have left the danger zone and removed their locks.

Fall from Elevation
The "fall from elevation" category covers incidents in which a worker falls to a lower level and is injured on impact against an object or the ground.

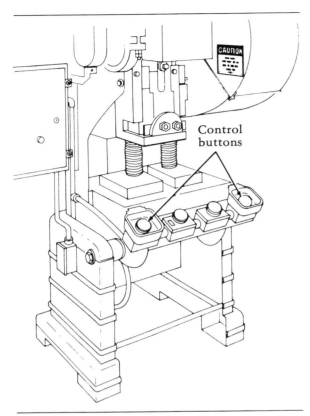

Control buttons

Fig. 8-5. Two-handed safety buttons assure that both hands are out of the danger zone before the machine cycle starts.
(From Occupational Safety and Health Administration. Concepts and techniques of machine guarding. OSHA Pub. No. 3067. Washington, D.C.: Occupational Safety and Health Administration, 1980: 38.)

Typical injuries include fractures, sprains, strains, contusions, damage to internal organs, and death. The nature and severity of the injury is primarily determined by the velocity and orientation of the body at the time of impact. Over 40 percent of these falls occur in the construction industry, in which work activities are frequently performed on temporary, elevated structures that are exposed to rain, snow, and ice (Fig. 8-7). Maintenance work-

ers in manufacturing plants frequently fall while performing repairs from ladders and other temporary work surfaces. Falls from elevated scaffolds, walkways, and work platforms are usually due to insufficient or nonexistent guardrails. The American National Standards Institute (ANSI, see Appendix C) has developed standards for the design and safe use of scaffolds and elevated work platforms. Many of these standards have been adopted by OSHA.

Falls from ladders account for over 20 percent of work injuries in the "fall from elevation" category. In a common fall scenario, the accident is initiated by a slippage of the worker's shoe on a ladder rung, which is followed by a loss of hand grip. Prevention of this type of accident is difficult, particularly in outdoor locations where the ladder is slippery. Other falls are caused by slippage or breakage of the ladder itself, which can be prevented in many cases by close compliance with safety standards developed by OSHA and ANSI.

Personal protective devices have been developed to reduce the risk of severe injuries and fatalities that result from falls from elevations. These devices include safety belts, harnesses, lanyards, and lifelines. It is recommended that these devices be equipped with a deceleration control system—that is, a shock absorber—to minimize injuries caused by the jerk that occurs when the fall is suddenly stopped. In spite of the protection offered by these devices, contusions, fractures, strains, and deceleration injuries to internal organs may occur when fall protection devices are used.

Fall on the Same Level
Although rarely fatal, serious injuries such as fractures, sprains, strains, and contusions can occur when workers lose their footing or balance and fall to the surface supporting them. Slipping, a loss of traction between the shoes and the floor, accounts for about half of all "same level" falls in industry. Most slips are caused by an unanticipated reduction in shoe-floor friction, such as when walking from a dry surface to a wet or oily

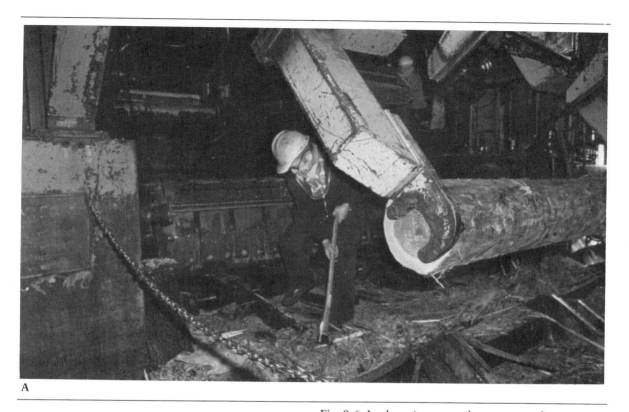

A

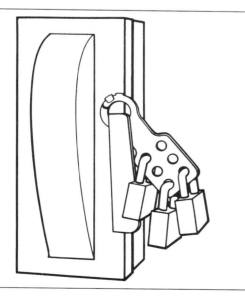

B

Fig. 8-6. Lockout is a control measure used to prevent premature accidental activation of a power switch. A. Maintenance worker has locked operating switch in the "off" position with a personal key. Without lockout, he could be caught in this machine when the operator restarts it.
(Photograph by Earl Dotter.)
B. In this diagram, three workers' locks are in place, preventing accidental activation of the power switch.
(From Occupational Safety and Health Administration. Concepts and techniques of machine guarding. OSHA Pub. No. 3067. Washington, D.C.: Occupational Safety and Health Administration, 1980: 60.)

surface, or from a nonskid surface to a highly polished one. These accidents can be controlled by using similar floor surfaces throughout a work area and by preventing liquid spills. Many slips occur on floor surfaces where friction is relatively uniform but low, such as in slaughterhouses and food processing plants and on floors where oil spills are common. In these environments, shoe soles and tread designs must be carefully selected to provide maximum friction. Due to the unpredictable interactions among sole materials, floor materials and surface treatments, and floor contaminants, it is recommended that in-house friction experiments be performed to select the best shoe or floor surface treatment.

Trips and missteps, which usually occur because of unseen objects on a floor or unexpected changes in floor elevation, are common causes of "same level" falls. These accidents can frequently be prevented through good housekeeping (keeping floors and aisles clear), good maintenance (repairing cracks and uneven surfaces) and good lighting. Finally, warning devices, such as caution signs, may be useful in situations where a hazardous floor condition is temporary (such as during mopping and other maintenance).

Overexertion and Repetitive Trauma

Overexertion and repetitive trauma injuries, such as low back pain, strains, sprains, and tendinitis, are caused by jobs that involve excessive physical effort or highly repetitive patterns of localized muscle and joint usage. Awkward work posture is frequently a confounding or aggravating factor in these injuries. In recent years, overexertion and repetitive trauma injuries have accounted for over one-fourth of workers' compensation costs in the United States. These injuries frequently occur on jobs that involve manual materials handling (where human power is used to lift, push, pull, or carry an object) or highly repetitive hand motions, such as working on an assembly line or operating a sewing machine. Despite many efforts in recent years to develop effective control programs, over-

exertion and repetitive trauma injuries continue to plague many industries as the principal causes of lost workdays and work restrictions. Many cases of these injuries are not associated with a specific event or accident but result from the cumulative effects of repeated physical exertions. (For a detailed discussion of the recognition and prevention of these injuries, see Chap. 22.)

Motor Vehicle Accidents

Motor vehicle accidents are frequently overlooked as occupational hazards. While motor vehicle accidents account for less than 10 percent of workers' compensation payments, they are responsible for almost one-third of work-related deaths. Controlling injuries and deaths due to vehicle accidents is a complex problem. Driver selection and training may help reduce the frequency and seriousness of accidents. Vehicle inspection programs, routine preventive maintenance, and regular use of seat belts also reduce accident frequency. Detailed investigations to determine the causes of motor vehicle accidents can lead to measures that prevent recurrences. Details on these and other loss control programs for motor vehicles are available from the National Safety Council, the Insurance Institute for Highway Safety, and the National Highway Traffic Safety Administration (see Appendix C).

Other Causes of Physical Trauma

About one-fourth of work accidents do not fall into any of the categories discussed above. "Contact with electrical current" results in shocks and electrical burns, which are sometimes fatal. The critical factor in the effect of electric shock is the amount of current that flows through the victim, particularly through the chest cavity. Studies have shown that an alternating current of only 100 milliamps at the commercial frequency of 60 hertz (standard in the United States) may cause ventricular fibrillation or cardiac arrest if the current passes through the chest cavity. Power supplies commonly found at construction sites, in manufacturing facilities, and even in households are suf-

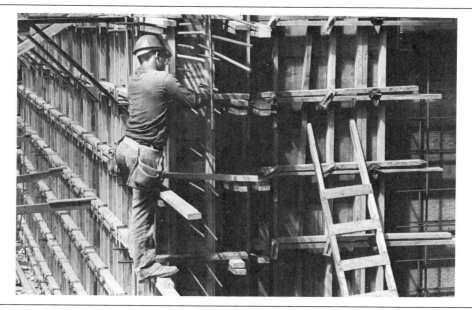

Fig. 8-7. Construction workers have high rates of occupational injuries, many of which are caused by falls.
(Photograph by Ken Light.)

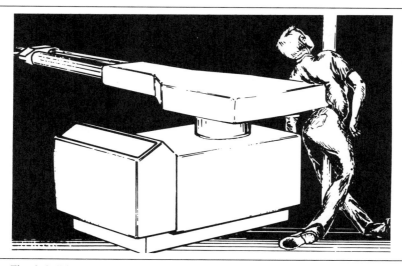

Fig. 8-8. Die-cast operator crushed between "back-end" of robot and post.
(From National Institute for Occupational Safety and Health. Request for assistance in preventing the injury of workers by robots. Pub. No. 85-103. Cincinnati: National Institute for Occupational Safety and Health, 1984.)

ficiently high to drive fatal currents through the body.

Construction workers are frequently the victims of electrical accidents because they use electrically-powered tools and equipment in outdoor locations that are unprotected from climatic elements. Control programs for construction sites should include effective grounding of all electrical equipment, double insulation of all electrical hand tools, or ground fault circuit interrupters. In addition, regular inspections of all equipment and power cords should be performed to ensure that insulation is intact. Personal protective devices, such as insulated gloves, boots, and clothing, should be worn. Metal ladders and heavy equipment, such as cranes and "cherry pickers," present a special problem at construction sites since they can accidentally become energized on contact with "live" overhead wires. Special precautions must be taken when working below or near overhead lines, such as substituting wood ladders and de-energizing power sources.

The classification "struck against" is used to describe cases in which a worker collides with a stationary object. Typical injuries include contusions, abrasions, lacerations, and fractures. Head injuries are common and are associated with low ceilings and confined spaces. Hand and finger injuries are also common and are frequently caused by forceful exertions with poorly designed tools. The severity of "struck against" injuries can sometimes be controlled by using personal protective equipment, such as safety helmets and gloves, and through improved design of work stations and tools.

"Contact with temperature extremes" refers to incidents in which tissue damage (burning or freezing) results from exposure to hot or cold solids, liquids, or gases. Control measures include insulating thermal hazards, using robots in extreme thermal environments, or using personal protection equipment such as heat-resistant clothing and gloves. (For additional information on thermal extremes, see Chap. 18.)

The category "rubbed or abraded" refers to relatively minor tissue damage resulting from prolonged contact with rough or sharp objects. Common sites of these injuries are the hands (using abrasives for cleaning or polishing) and the knees (prolonged kneeling on a rough surface). In most instances, these incidents can be controlled by covering the objects with padded materials or handholds or by wearing protective clothing.

COMPONENTS OF AN OCCUPATIONAL SAFETY PROGRAM
Organization and Responsibilities

An effective safety program results from a multi-disciplinary effort involving inputs from and interactions among many groups within an organization. To institute a successful program, it is necessary to establish a plant-level safety committee with overall responsibility for administering the program. This "steering" committee should include upper-level "line" managers (typically the plant manager or designate and heads of production departments), the plant physician or nurse, the safety manager, plant-level staff managers (from the engineering, purchasing, maintenance, and industrial relations departments), and labor representatives (the president or safety steward in plants with union representation, employee representative(s) in plants without unions). This committee should oversee the activities of departmental safety committees, which run the day-to-day safety program and solve problems on the plant floor. For the safety program to be effective, it is essential that the departmental committees be organized to encourage active participation by supervisors and hourly workers.

Upper-level managers must establish a safety policy, develop the policy into a program, and ensure that the program is effectively executed. Although safety policies vary from one organization to another, most safety policies will include the following items:

1. A commitment to provide the greatest possible safety to all employees and to ensure that all facilities and processes will be designed with this objective. Similarly, purchasing policies must provide that all equipment, machines, and tools meet the highest safety standards.
2. A requirement that all occupational injuries and accidents be reported and corrective action taken to ensure that similar incidents do not occur.
3. Clear explanations to all employees of the safety and health hazards to which they are exposed and the establishment of training programs to inform employees of how to minimize their risk of being affected.
4. Regularly scheduled systems safety analyses of all processes and work stations to identify potential safety hazards so that corrective actions can be taken before accidents occur. (Systems safety is discussed later in this chapter.)
5. Disciplinary procedures for employees who engage in unsafe behavior and for supervisors who encourage or permit unsafe activities.

While the chief executive officer is ultimately responsible for the safety of all employees, this responsibility should be delegated throughout all levels of management.

Line and floor supervisors play a key role in the execution of safety programs because of their direct contact with employees. Supervisors must ensure that all pieces of equipment comply with applicable safety standards and regulations and that employees use safe work practices. In addition, the supervisor must make certain that all injuries are promptly reported and treated. Some organizations use "safety competitions," in which supervisors compete to achieve the best safety record. These contests yield beneficial results when supervisors are encouraged to bring their departments into compliance with applicable safety standards and regulations. Unfortunately, however, such competitions sometimes discourage the accurate reporting of accidents or appropriate medical care for injuries. For this reason, safety competitions may lead to unintended and counterproductive results and should be undertaken with caution. Care should also be taken to avoid giving supervisors incompatible goals, such as unreasonably high production standards, when lower rates are necessary to guarantee safety.

Larger worksites usually have a full-time safety director, a manager responsible for the day-to-day administration of the safety program. Typical responsibilities include developing and presenting safety training, inspecting facilities and operations for unsafe conditions and practices, conducting accident investigations, maintaining accident records and performing analyses to identify causal factors, and developing programs for hazard control. The safety director must work with the engineering and purchasing departments to ensure that equipment and facilities are designed and purchased in compliance with all applicable safety standards. The safety director also works closely with the plant's medical staff to ensure that all injuries and illnesses are properly recorded and investigated. A full-time safety director should be certified by the Board of Certified Safety Professionals (BCSP). For smaller worksites that do not employ a full-time safety director, the duties described above should be assigned to managerial personnel on a parttime basis or to a qualified safety consultant.

Regardless of the size and structure of the plant's medical services, physicians and nurses play an essential role in the plant safety program through primary treatment of injured workers and by helping to identify workplace hazards. While the causes of overt trauma injuries are usually obvious, causes of cumulative trauma are often subtle and difficult to identify. By evaluating patterns of employee injuries, disorders, and complaints, the physician or nurse can provide early detection of potentially hazardous operations and processes. Whenever disorders or complaints are suspected of being work-related, this information should be reported to the plant safety director and the responsible supervisor. The physician or nurse should participate in the subsequent worksite investigations to identify specific hazards or stresses potentially causing the observed injuries and in planning the subsequent hazard control programs. Finally, physicians and nurses must work closely and cooperatively with supervisors to ensure the prompt reporting and treatment of all work-related health and safety problems.

The maintenance department and skilled trades (for example, electricians and millwrights) play a critical role in the success of the safety program by routinely inspecting facilities, equipment, and tools, and servicing them when necessary. Individuals in these groups should receive special training to enhance their knowledge of safety hazards and control technology.

Finally, workers play an essential role in the successful execution of a safety program. Prior to a new assignment, a worker must be educated regarding specific hazards associated with the new job. Training should include both hazard recognition and control techniques. If personal protective equipment is required to ensure safety, training must cover how to inspect, maintain, and wear such equipment. Training must emphasize the responsibility of each worker to maintain a safe work station and to comply with safe work practices. Part of this responsibility includes reporting unsafe conditions to supervisors and employee safety representatives so that corrective action can be taken.

Employee participation is an important component of the total safety program. Each worker is an expert in his or her job and should be actively involved in inspections and systems safety analyses. If modifications are deemed necessary to reduce hazards, worker acceptance of new equipment, tools, and work methods is an essential ingredient in the successful implementation of change. For this reason, workers should actively participate in the design of equipment and process safety features and the selection of personal protective equipment.

Hazard Discovery and Identification

A totally successful safety program would identify and eliminate all hazards before any accidents occur. Systems safety analysis is a subdiscipline of safety engineering concerned with the discovery and evaluation of previously unrecognized hazards. Over 30 different systems safety methodologies have been developed for specific applications, such as aircraft design and consumer product safety. One of these methodologies, *Job Safety Analysis* (JSA), has been found to be particularly useful for identifying hazards in the work environment.

JSA is performed by an interdisciplinary team composed of the worker, supervisor, safety specialist, and medical specialist. If the analyzed job or process is technically complex, the responsible engineers and skilled trades workers should also participate. The first step in JSA is to break the job down into a sequence of work elements. The next step is to scrutinize each element to identify existing or potential hazards. To do this effectively, the worker must simulate or "walk through" each element, explaining the details of the element to the team and describing previous accidents or "near misses" and the associated hazards. Team members rely on experience and expertise in their specialty areas to identify any additional hazards. The results of this analysis are used to recommend changes to the work station, process, or methods to eliminate or effectively control all identified hazards.

JSA is widely regarded as a useful technique for the identification and control of hazards *prior* to accidents, injuries, or illnesses. To maximize its effectiveness, JSA must be formally incorporated into the safety program and practiced on a regular basis.

REFERENCES

1. National Safety Council. Accident facts. Chicago: National Safety Council, 1985.
2. National Institute for Occupational Safety and

Health. Request for assistance in preventing the injury of workers by robots. Publication No. 85-103. Cincinnati: National Institute for Occupational Safety and Health, 1984.

BIBLIOGRAPHY

Clemens PL. A compendium of hazard identification and evaluation techniques for systems safety application. Hazard Prevention, March 1982.
Provides a brief summary of 25 frequently-used systems safety techniques. An excellent bibliography directs the reader to detailed descriptions of each approach.

Ferry TS. Modern accident investigation and analysis. New York: Wiley-Interscience, 1981.
Presents thorough coverage of accident investigation methods. Emphasizes importance of accident investigation as a method of preventing recurrences.

Fullman JB. Construction safety, security, and loss prevention. New York: Wiley-Interscience, 1984.
Discusses management and engineering aspects of construction safety. Covers hazards unique to the construction environment such as scaffolding and excavations.

Greenberg L, Chaffin DB. Workers and their tools. Midland, MI: Pendell Publishing, 1977.
A comprehensive discussion of safety considerations in the design and use of industrial hand tools. Well illustrated, with many examples.

Hammer W. Occupational safety management and engineering. Englewood Cliffs, NJ: Prentice-Hall, 1985.
A useful reference text that covers both engineering and management aspects of occupational safety. Engineering chapters are organized by generic hazard types; management chapters provide topical coverage of training, workers' compensation, and safety legislation.

Heinrich HW, Peterson D, Roos N. Industrial accident prevention. New York: McGraw-Hill, 1980.
Discusses theoretical models of accident causation and approaches to accident prevention with emphasis on theory of unsafe behavior. Special appendix covers principles of machine guarding.

McElroy FE, ed. Accident prevention manual for industrial operations: engineering and technology. 8th ed. Chicago: National Safety Council, 1980.
Reference manual for identification and control of generic safety hazards. Well-illustrated, topical chapters summarize relevant safety standards and established control technology.

9
Occupational Ergonomics: Designing the Job to Match the Worker

W. Monroe Keyserling

Ergonomics is the study of humans at work to understand the complex relationships among people, physical and psychological aspects of the work environment (such as facilities, equipment, and tools), job demands, and work methods. A fundamental principle of ergonomics is that all work activities cause the worker to experience some level of physical and mental stress. As long as these stresses are kept within reasonable limits, work performance should be satisfactory and the worker's health and well-being should be maintained. If stresses are excessive, however, undesirable outcomes may occur in the form of errors, accidents, injuries, or a decrement in physical or mental health.*

Ergonomists are concerned with evaluating stressors that occur in the work environment and the corresponding abilities of people to cope with these stressors. The goal of an occupational ergonomics program is to establish a safe work environment by designing facilities, furniture, machines, tools, and job demands to be compatible with workers' attributes (such as size, strength, aerobic capacity, and information processing capacity) and expectations. A successful ergonomics program should simultaneously improve health and enhance productivity.

The following examples call attention to ergonomic activities that are relevant to the prevention and control of a broad range of health and safety problems in the contemporary workplace. These examples illustrate applications of ergonomics in the prevention of accidents, job-induced fatigue, and work-related musculoskeletal disorders.

Prevention of Accidents

Designing a machine guard that will allow a worker to operate a piece of equipment with smooth, nonawkward, time-efficient motions. (This minimizes any inconvenience introduced by the guard and decreases the likelihood that it will be bypassed or removed.)

Studying the biomechanics of human gait to determine forces and torques acting at the interface between the floor and the sole of the shoe. (This information can be used to improve the friction characteristics of floor surfaces and shoe soles to reduce the risk of a slip or fall.)

Prevention of Fatigue

Designing a computer work station (equipment and furniture) so that an operator can use a video display terminal (VDT) for an extended period of time without experiencing visual or postural fatigue.

Evaluating the metabolic demands of a job performed in a hot, humid environment to recommend a work-rest regimen that will prevent heat stress.

---

*An *accident* is defined as an unanticipated, sudden event that results in an undesired outcome such as property damage, injuries, or death. An *injury* is defined as physical damage to body tissues. Injuries can be associated with accidents but can also result from normal stressors in the environment.

Prevention of Musculoskeletal Disorders

Evaluating lifting tasks to determine biomechanical stresses acting at the lower back and designing lifting tasks to ensure that these stresses will not cause back injuries.

Evaluating work station layout to discover potential causes of postural stress and recommending changes to eliminate or reduce nonneutral work postures that could cause cumulative trauma disorders. (Eliminating awkward posture can also reduce fatigue.)

Evaluating highly repetitive manual assembly operations and developing alternative hand tools and work methods to reduce the risk of cumulative trauma disorders such as tendinitis, epicondylitis, tenosynovitis, and carpal tunnel syndrome.

The remainder of this chapter describes several subdisciplines of ergonomics concerned with safety and health in the workplace.

HUMAN FACTORS ENGINEERING

Human factors engineering, sometimes called engineering psychology, is the subdiscipline of ergonomics concerned with the information processing aspects of work. The objective of human factors engineering in the context of occupational safety and health is to design procedures, equipment, and work environments to minimize the likelihood of an accident caused by human error. Common causes of work accidents caused by human error include:

1. *Failure to perceive or recognize a hazardous condition or situation.* To react to a dangerous situation, it is necessary to perceive that the danger exists. Many workplace hazards are not easily perceived through human sensory channels, such as excessive pressure inside a boiler that could cause an explosion, a forktruck approaching from behind in a noisy factory, unguarded machinery in a poorly lit room, or the sudden release of an odorless, colorless toxic gas. In these situations, it is necessary to supplement the sensory functions with special informational displays, such as a pressure gauge with "redline" marks to indicate a dangerous condition inside the boiler, a horn or beeper on the forktruck that sounds automatically while it is in motion, a well-lit warning sign at the entrance to the poorly lit equipment room, or an emergency alarm system that indicates the release of toxic gases.

2. *Failures in the information processing or decision-making processes.* Decision making involves combining new information with existing knowledge to provide a basis for action. Errors can occur at this stage if the information processing load is excessive; for example, in the accident at the Three Mile Island nuclear power plant, operators were required to react to multiple simultaneous alarms. Errors can also occur if previous training was incorrect or inappropriate for handling a specific situation.

3. *Failures in motor actions following correct decisions.* Following a decision, it is frequently necessary for a worker to perform some motor action by using a control to implement the desired change, such as flipping a switch or adjusting a knob. Failures can occur if these controls are not designed to be consistent with human motor abilities (for example, the force required to adjust a control valve in a chemical plant should not exceed human strength ability), or if manipulation of the control causes an unexpected response. Controls that start potentially dangerous machinery or equipment should be guarded to prevent accidental activation, usually by covering the control or placing it in a location where it cannot be accidentally touched.

Effective human factors engineering is essential for workplace safety, even when the simplest equipment and machines are involved.

WORK PHYSIOLOGY

Work physiology is the subdiscipline of ergonomics concerned with stresses that occur during the metabolic conversion of biochemical energy sources such as glucose to mechanical work. If these stresses are excessive, the worker will experience fatigue. Fatigue may be localized to a relatively small number of muscles or may affect the entire body.

Static Work and Local Muscle Fatigue
Static work occurs when a muscle or muscle group remains in a contracted state for an extended period of time without relaxation. High levels of static work can be caused by sustained awkward posture, such as that of a mechanic who must continuously flex the trunk to perform repairs to an automobile engine, or by high strength demands associated with a specific task, such as using a tire iron to unfreeze a badly-rusted wheelnut when changing a tire.

When a muscle contracts, the blood vessels that supply nutrients and remove metabolic wastes are compressed by the adjacent contractile tissue. As a result, vascular resistance increases with the level of muscle tension and the blood supply to the working muscle decreases. If the muscle is not allowed to relax periodically, the demand for metabolic nutrients may exceed the supply. Furthermore, metabolic wastes can accumulate. The short-term effects of this condition include ischemic pain, tremor, or a reduced capacity to produce tension. Any of these effects can severely inhibit work performance [1].

The temporal relationship between the intensity of a static exertion and loss of contractile capability is presented in Figure 9-1. A contraction of maximum intensity can be held for only about 6 seconds. At a 50 percent effort, the duration of a static contraction is limited to approximately 1 minute. To sustain a static contraction indefinitely, muscle tension must be kept at or below 15 percent of maximum strength. It is evident from the graph in Figure 9-1 that prolonged static exertions

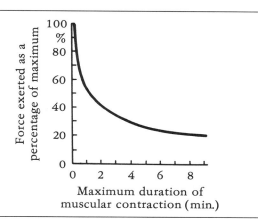

Fig. 9-1. Maximum duration of a static muscle contraction for various levels of muscular contraction. (From WM Keyserling, TJ Armstrong. Ergonomics. In: JM Last, ed. Maxcy-Rosenau public health and preventive medicine. 12th ed. Norwalk, CT: Appleton-Century-Crofts, 1986.)

should be avoided, particularly when high muscle forces are involved [1].

In addition to discomfort and decreased performance capacity of the affected muscle, static work causes a temporary increase in the peripheral resistance of the cardiovascular system. Significant increases in heart rate and mean arterial blood pressure have been observed in conjunction with short-duration static contractions [2]. Caution should be exercised to avoid placing a person with a history of cardiovascular disease on a job that requires moderate to heavy static exertions.

In most situations, dynamic activities involving cyclical contraction and relaxation of working muscle are preferable to static work. If, however, the job requires highly repetitive or forceful exertions, a variety of localized cumulative trauma injuries may occur to musculoskeletal tissue or peripheral nerves. (These injuries are discussed below and in Chap. 22.)

Dynamic Work and Whole-Body Fatigue
Dynamic, whole-body work occurs when multiple groups of large skeletal muscles repeatedly contract and relax in conjunction with the performance of a task. Common examples of dynamic work activities include walking on a level surface, pedaling a bicycle, climbing stairs, and moving a load (by carrying, pushing, pulling, or shoveling) from one location to another.

The intensity of whole-body, dynamic work is primarily limited by the capacity of the pulmonary and cardiovascular systems to deliver sufficient oxygen and glucose to working muscles and to remove products of metabolism. Whole-body fatigue occurs when the collective metabolic demands of working muscles throughout the body exceed this capacity. Common symptoms of whole-body fatigue include shortness of breath, weakness in working muscles, and a general feeling of tiredness. These symptoms will continue and may increase until the work activity is stopped or decreased in intensity.

For extremely short durations of whole-body dynamic activity (typically 4 minutes or less), a person can work at an intensity equal to his or her aerobic capacity. As the duration of the work period increases, the work intensity must be adjusted downward. If a task is to be performed continuously for 1 hour, the average energy expenditure for this period should not exceed 50 percent of the worker's aerobic capacity. For a job that is performed for an 8-hour shift, the average energy expenditure should not exceed 33 percent of the worker's aerobic capacity.

Aerobic capacity varies considerably within the population. Individual factors that determine aerobic capacity include age, sex, weight, heredity, and the current level of physical fitness. Table 9-1 presents average values of aerobic capacity for males and females of various ages. It is important to note that these are average values for each age-sex stratum and do not reflect the full range of variability in aerobic capacities among the adult population. This variability is an important consideration in evaluating ergonomic stress; a job

Table 9-1. Average aerobic capacities of males and females for various ages*

Age	Males	Females
10	9.8	8.8
20	17.1	12.8
30	15.1	10.8
40	14.2	10.3
50	12.7	9.8
60	11.7	9.1

*Values in kcal/min.
Source: WM Keyserling, TJ Armstrong. Ergonomics. In: JM Last, ed. Maxcy-Rosenau public health and preventive medicine. Norwalk, CT: Appleton-Century-Crofts, 1986.

that is relatively easy for a person with high aerobic capacity can be extremely fatiguing for a person with low capacity.

The prevention of whole-body fatigue is best accomplished through good job design. The energy expenditure requirements of a job should be sufficiently low to accommodate the adult working population, including those individuals with limited aerobic capacity. These requirements can be met by designing the workplace to minimize unnecessary body movements (excessive walking or climbing) and providing mechanical assists (such as hoists or conveyors) for handling heavy materials. If these approaches are not feasible, it may be necessary to provide additional rest allowances to prevent excessive fatigue, particularly in hot, humid work environments because of the metabolic contribution to heat stress (see Chap. 18).

In establishing metabolic criteria for jobs that involve repetitive manual lifting. NIOSH [3] has recommended that the average energy expenditure rate for an eight-hour work shift should not exceed 3.5 kcal/min. Applying the "33 percent" rule to the values in Table 9-1, the NIOSH rate would be acceptable to the majority of the adult working population. Individuals with aerobic capacities less than 10.5 kcal/min could have trouble, however, maintaining a 3.5 kcal/min work pace. Caution should be practiced when placing persons with low levels of physical fitness on metabolically strenuous jobs.*

To assess the potential for whole-body fatigue, it is necessary to measure or estimate the energy expenditure rate for a specific job, which is usually done in one of three ways:

1. *Table reference.* Extensive tables of the energy costs of various work activities have been developed (see Bibliography for references).
2. *Indirect calorimetry.* Energy expenditure can be estimated for a specific job by measuring a worker's oxygen uptake while performing the job.
3. *Modeling.* The job is analyzed and broken down into fundamental tasks such as walking, carrying, and lifting. Parameters describing each task are measured and substituted into equations to predict energy expenditure.

There is no "best" method for determining energy expenditure. The selection of a specific method is often a trade-off between the availability of published tables or prediction equations and the inconvenience associated with taking the measurements required for indirect calorimetry.

BIOMECHANICS

Biomechanics is the subdiscipline of ergonomics concerned with the mechanical properties of human tissue, particularly the resistance of tissue to mechanical stresses. Some of the injury-causing mechanical stresses in the work environment are associated with overt accidents, such as crushed bones in the feet resulting from the impact of a dropped object. The hazards that cause these injuries can usually be controlled through safety engineering techniques (see Chap. 8). Other injurious mechanical stresses are more subtle and can

cause cumulative trauma injuries. These stresses can be external, such as a vibrating chain saw that causes Raynaud's syndrome, or internal, such as compression on spinal discs during strenuous lifting. These stresses are most effectively controlled through ergonomics—that is, designing job demands so that resulting mechanical stresses can be tolerated without injury.

According to a 1985 NIOSH report [4], occupationally caused or aggravated musculoskeletal disorders (MSDs) are ranked as one of the most serious health problems affecting U.S. workers. Specifically:

1. MSDs rank first among health problems in the frequency with which they affect quality of life (as indicated by activity limitation).
2. MSDs are the leading cause of disability of people during the working years. MSDs affect nearly one-half of the nation's workforce at some time, resulting in time lost from work.
3. Based on lost earnings, workers' compensation payments, and medical payments, MSDs are more costly than any other single health disorder.

Although musculoskeletal disorders can occur in all parts of the body, the back and upper extremities are the most commonly affected areas.

Ergonomic approaches to preventing back and upper extremity problems are discussed below.

Low Back Pain and Manual Lifting

Manual lifting of heavy objects is the most commonly cited risk factor in the development of low back pain. In an effort to reduce the frequency and severity of lifting-related injuries, NIOSH has developed and issued a technical report, *Work Practices Guide for Manual Lifting* (see box). This document discusses the various risk factors associated with lifting and describes procedures for evaluating lifting tasks and reducing lifting hazards. To use the NIOSH Guide, it is first necessary to measure the following six task variables:

---

*Aerobic capacity can be determined by measuring oxygen uptake and carbon dioxide production during a graded stress test. For additional information on measuring or estimating aerobic capacity, see Astrand and Rodahl.

USING THE NIOSH WORK PRACTICES
GUIDE FOR MANUAL LIFTING

The magnitude of the acceptable lift (AL) (in lbs) is determined algebraically using the formula:

$$AL = 90\ lb \times HF \times VF \times DF \times FF \quad \text{(Equation 1)}$$

where:

HF is a discounting factor based on horizontal location,

VF is a discounting factor based on the vertical location of the object at the origin of the lift,

DF is a discounting factor based on the lift distance, and

FF is a discounting factor on the lift frequency.

All of the discounting factors in Equation No. 1 range between 0 and 1 and can be estimated using the graphs in Figure 9-3. Because the discounting factors are multiplicative, the maximum value of the AL is 90 lbs—that is, when all factors are equal to 1. This situation occurs when a lift is ergonomically ideal (close to the body, comfortable initial height, short travel distance, and low frequency). As conditions deviate from the ideal, the corresponding values of the discounting factors decrease, thus reducing the magnitude of the AL. The computed value of the AL is particularly sensitive to the horizontal distance. (Increasing the horizontal distance from 6 to 12 inches reduces the horizontal discount factor from 1.0 to 0.5.) Highly frequent lifting also substantially reduces the value of the AL.

Once the AL has been determined, it is easy to compute the maximum permissible lift (MPL) using the following formula:

$$MPL = 3 \times AL \quad \text{(Equation 2)}$$

For additional details on using and interpreting Equations 1 and 2, refer to the NIOSH *Work Practices Guide for Manual Lifting.*

---

1. *Object weight (L)*—measured in kilograms or pounds.
2. *Horizontal distance (H)*—the location of the object's center of gravity measured in the sagittal plane from a point midway between the ankles. (The sagittal plane bisects the body, dividing it into symmetric left and right sections.) This measurement should be made for the origin and the destination of the lift, in inches or centimeters (Fig. 9-2).
3. *Vertical location (V)*—the location of the hands at the origin of the lift, measured vertically from the floor or working surface in inches or centimeters (see Fig. 9-2).
4. *Lift distance (D)*—the vertical displacement of the object (origin to destination), measured in inches or centimeters.
5. *Lifting frequency (F)*—the number of lifts per minute, averaged over the time that manual lifting is performed.
6. *Duration of lifting*—classified as *occasional* if lifting activities can be performed in less than one hour or *continuous* if lifting activities are performed for more than one hour.

Variables 2 through 5 are used to determine two limits, an acceptable lift (AL) and a maximum permissible lift (MPL). Procedures for determining the AL and MPL are discussed in the above box.

After the AL and MPL have been determined, the job can be classified into one of three risk categories:

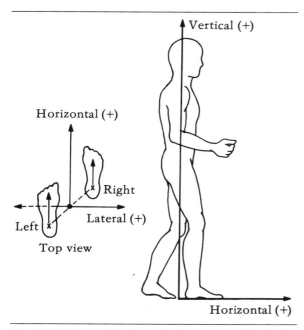

Fig. 9-2. Horizontal and vertical locations of the hands when using the NIOSH *Work Practices Guide for Manual Lifting*.
(From National Institute for Occupational Safety and Health. Work practices guide for manual lifting. NIOSH Pub. No. 81-122. Cincinnati: National Institute for Occupational Safety and Health, 1981.)

1. *Acceptable.* If the weight of the lifted object is less than the AL, the job is considered acceptable, which implies that most individuals in the workforce could perform the job with only a minimal risk of injury.
2. *Administrative controls required.* If the weight of the object falls between the AL and the MPL, the job is assigned to this category, implying that some individuals in the workforce would have difficulty in performing the job (because of limited strength) or would be at increased risk of injury. Action should be taken to protect these individuals, such as redesigning the job so that it would fall into the acceptable cate-

gory or implementing administrative procedures such as employee selection or training.
3. *Hazardous.* If the lifted object weighs more than the MPL, the job is considered hazardous. This category implies that most individuals in the workforce would be at substantial risk of injury when performing the job. The only acceptable approach to resolving this situation is redesigning the job to eliminate lifting stresses or reducing these stresses to acceptable levels.

The most effective method to control low-back injuries associated with lifting is to design task requirements to match the capabilities of the worker, which typically requires re-engineering the job to reduce stress. Common examples of effective engineering changes include reducing the weight of the load such as by placing fewer parts in a package; modifying the work station layout to improve horizontal or vertical reach requirements; reducing the frequency of lifting tasks such as by rotating or enriching jobs; and providing mechanical assists such as lift tables, hoists, conveyors, and robots (Fig. 9-4).

In limited instances, the capital expenditures required to redesign a job may prove to be prohibitively expensive. In such situations, performance-based employee selection procedures may be an appropriate method for matching the worker to the job. Isometric strength testing has been demonstrated to be an effective method for accomplishing this match, and its application has led to the reduction of injuries [5]. To establish a strength testing program, it is first necessary to perform an intensive job analysis to identify critical strength-demanding elements. Isometric tests are developed to simulate the strength demands of these critical tasks. The results of the strength tests are used by the plant physician or personnel officer when making placement decisions.

Low Back Pain and Awkward Trunk Posture

Awkward trunk posture during work activities can be caused by the interaction of several factors, in-

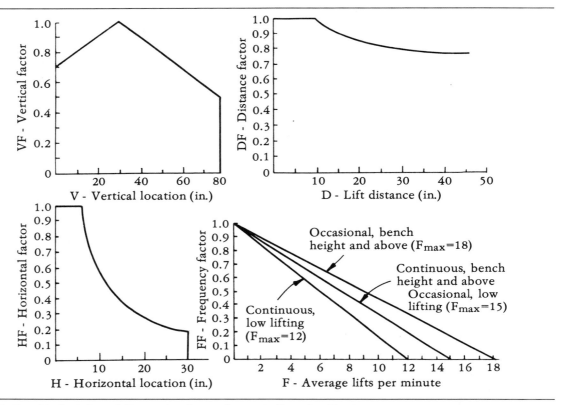

Fig. 9-3. Graphic depiction of discounting factors for use in Equation No. 1.
(From National Institute for Occupational Safety and Health. Work practices guide for manual lifting. NIOSH Pub. No. 81-122. Cincinnati: National Institute for Occupational Safety and Health, 1981.)

cluding poor work station layout (such as low reaches that require stooping), incorrect work methods, or the anthropometric characteristics (body size and reach capabilities) of the worker. Laboratory studies of trunk posture have demonstrated that forward flexion, lateral bending, or axial twisting increase the level of localized muscle fatigue (particularly when the nonneutral posture is maintained for prolonged periods) and intradiscal pressures. Refer to Figure 9-5 for an illustration of nonneutral trunk postures [6].

The posture classification system in Figure 9-5 was recently used in a case-control study of auto-

mobile assembly workers to evaluate the relationship between nonneutral trunk posture and complaints of back pain [7]. Cases consisted of all workers who reported to the plant medical department with an injury to the trunk, and on interview met criteria for persistent pain. Controls were workers randomly selected from the same departments of the plant who had not reported a trunk injury and who on interview did not report persistent pain. The use of each nonneutral trunk posture was compared among cases and controls by computing odds ratios. Workers classified as cases were approximately five times more likely

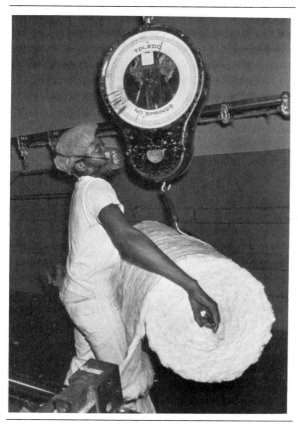

Fig. 9-4. Lift assists are necessary to prevent the risk of back injury on this job. (Photograph by Earl Dotter.)

with significant postural demands should be redesigned where feasible to eliminate postural stress. Trunk flexion (forward bending) can usually be attributed to one of two causes: (1) reaching down to grasp an object that is lower than the level of the hands when standing with the arms hanging in a relaxed, vertical position, or (2) reaching forward to grasp an object that is too far in front of the body. Trunk bending or twisting is usually associated with reaching for objects that are located either to the side or behind the worker's body.

Prevention of awkward posture can usually be accomplished through improved work station layout. Recommendations to avoid trunk flexion and twisting include designing the work station and task so that

1. The hands do not have to reach below a height of 28 in. (measured from the floor) to obtain an object, handle a tool, or manipulate a control. (This height is the lowest that a large male can reach without excessive trunk flexion.)
2. Forward reach distances are minimized. All reaches should be easily accomplished using only the arms and should require no trunk flexion.
3. All reaches are performed in front of the body— that is, in or near the sagittal plane. If this goal cannot be achieved through better layout, workers should be instructed to rotate their bodies by moving the feet instead of twisting the trunk.

Because working posture is a function of an individual's anthropometry (body size), a work station layout that is good for one operator may not be appropriate for workers who are considerably larger or smaller. For this reason, adjustability should be incorporated into the work station wherever possible.

Cumulative Trauma Disorders of the
Upper Extremities
Cumulative trauma disorders (CTDs) are a major cause of lost time and workers' compensation pay-

than controls to work with the trunk in mild flexion for at least part of the normal work cycle and were approximately six times more likely to work with the trunk in severe flexion, or bent and twisted sideways. Furthermore, the magnitude of the odds ratios increased with the length of exposure to each nonneutral posture. For both mild and severe trunk flexion, there was substantial increase in risk if the posture had to be maintained for more than 10 percent of the work cycle.

The results reported above suggest that nonneutral posture is a contributing factor to the development of injuries and disorders of the trunk. Jobs

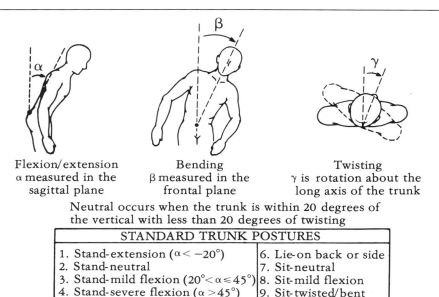

Flexion/extension
α measured in the
sagittal plane

Bending
β measured in the
frontal plane

Twisting
γ is rotation about the
long axis of the trunk

Neutral occurs when the trunk is within 20 degrees of
the vertical with less than 20 degrees of twisting

STANDARD TRUNK POSTURES	
1. Stand-extension ($\alpha < -20°$)	6. Lie-on back or side
2. Stand-neutral	7. Sit-neutral
3. Stand-mild flexion ($20° < \alpha \leq 45°$)	8. Sit-mild flexion
4. Stand-severe flexion ($\alpha > 45°$)	9. Sit-twisted/bent
5. Stand-twisted/bent (β or $\gamma > 20°$)	

Fig. 9-5. A method for classifying nonneutral trunk postures.
(From WM Keyserling. Postural analysis of the trunk and shoulders in simulated real time. Ergonomics 1986; 29:569–583.)

ments in many hand-intensive jobs. These disorders affect the musculoskeletal system or the peripheral nervous system at the fingers, hand, and wrist (including tenosynovitis, DeQuervain's disease,* trigger finger, digital neuritis, carpal tunnel syndrome, Guyon tunnel syndrome,† degenerative joint disease of the fingers); elbow and forearm (including epicondylitis, cubital tunnel syndrome, pronator teres syndrome); and shoulder (such as rotator cuff tendinitis, bicipital tenosynovitis, and thoracic outlet syndrome). (For additional information on these disorders, see Chap. 22.)

While the etiology of any CTD is quite complex,

occupational exposures such as highly repetitive hand exertions, forceful hand exertions, awkward posture of the upper extremities, vibration, and localized mechanical pressure are considered contributing factors. In many hand-intensive jobs, more than one of these risk factors may be present (Fig. 9-6).

Highly repetitive work has been defined as jobs in which the length of the fundamental work cycle is less than 30 seconds or in which more than 50 percent of the work cycle is spent performing the same basic hand actions [8]. Where possible, repetitive work should be avoided, sometimes accomplished through job enrichment (adding more tasks to an individual's job description to increase the length of the basic work cycle) or through job rotation (alternating a worker between a hand-intensive job and a less strenuous job to reduce cu-

*DeQuervain's disease is a stenosing tenosynovitis of the extensor or abductor tendons of the thumb.
†Guyon tunnel syndrome is an entrapment of the ulnar nerve as it passes through the base of the palm.

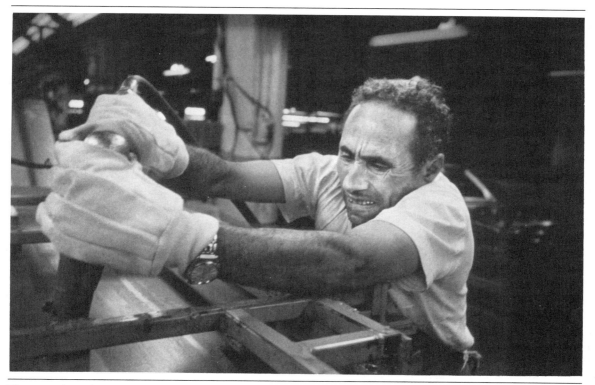

Fig. 9-6. This job involves exposure to several risk factors associated with the development of upper extremity cumulative trauma disorders.
(Photograph by Earl Dotter.)

mulative exposure to upper extremity stresses). In implementing either job enrichment or job rotation as a control technique, it is necessary to perform job analyses to determine that the new tasks do not involve the same types of upper extremity stresses found on the original job.

Forces on the tendons and nerves are related to hand posture and to the magnitude of forces exerted by the hand. While critical force levels are not known, there is general agreement that force is an important factor in the development of many CTDs [8]. Where feasible, forceful exertions should be eliminated or reduced in magnitude,

sometimes accomplished by reducing the effective weight of an object or tool, such as by suspending a heavy tool using a counter-weight or balancing device, or by using both hands to lift a heavy object. The force required to lift and hold a heavy object can also be reduced if the object is gripped near its center of gravity. Internal muscle forces are lowest when an object or tool can be held in a power grip (the grip used when holding a suitcase handle or tennis racket). Four to five times as much force must be exerted to hold objects with a pinch grip than with a power grip.

Nonneutral wrist posture, such as flexion or ex-

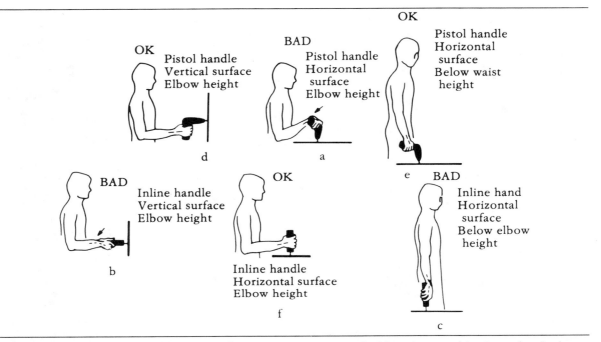

Fig. 9-7. Examples of neutral and nonneutral wrist postures associated with various combinations of tool selection and work station layout.
(From T Armstrong. An ergonomics guide to carpal tunnel syndrome. Akron: American Industrial Hygiene Association, 1983. Reprinted with permission by American Industrial Hygiene Association.)

treme extension, has been associated with tenosynovitis of the flexor and extensor tendons and with carpal tunnel syndrome. Ulnar and radial deviations have been associated with tenosynovitis at the base of the thumb (DeQuervain's disease). These nonneutral postures can usually be controlled through proper location and orientation of the work surface and through proper design of handles. Figure 9-7 illustrates these relationships for two common handle configurations found on a powered screwdriver. To drive a screw into a vertical surface at elbow height, a pistol-shaped tool is preferred because it can be used with a nondeviated wrist. The use of an in-line (straight-handled) tool in this situation causes an ulnar deviation. To drive a screw into a horizontal surface at

elbow height, the in-line tool is preferred. A pistol-shaped tool for this task results in substantial wrist flexion. The pistol-shaped tool is preferred again, however, when driving a screw into a horizontal surface below waist height. The use of an in-line tool in this situation causes flexion or ulnar deviation. As these examples illustrate, *there is no such thing as an ergonomic tool.* Instead, it is necessary to consider work station layout and the functional demands of the task to select the proper tool.

Other risk factors associated with the development of upper extremity CTDs include mechanical pressure on musculoskeletal tissue or nerves (such as when exerting high forces on the handles of a pair of pliers), vibration, low temperature, and the use of gloves (see Chaps. 18 and 22).

REFERENCES

1. Astrand P, Rodahl K. Textbook of work physiology. New York: McGraw-Hill, 1970.
2. Armstrong TJ, Chaffin DB, Faulkner JA, et al. Static work elements and selected circulatory responses. Am Ind Hyg Assoc J 1980; 41:254–260.
3. National Institute for Occupational Safety and Health. Work practices guide for manual lifting (NIOSH Pub. No. 81-122). Cincinnati: National Institute for Occupational Safety and Health, 1981.
4. National Institute for Occupational Safety and Health. Prevention of musculoskeletal injuries: a proposed synoptic strategy. Cincinnati: National Institute for Occupational Safety and Health, 1985.
5. Keyserling WM, Herrin GD, Chaffin DB. Isometric strength testing as a means of controlling medical incidents on strenuous jobs. J Occup Med 1980; 22:332–336.
6. Keyserling WM. Postural analysis of the trunk and shoulders in simulated real time. Ergonomics 1986; 4:569–583.
7. Keyserling WM, Punnett L, Fine LJ. Trunk posture and back pain: Identification and control of occupational risk factors. App Ind Hyg 1988; 3:87–92.
8. Silverstein BA. The prevalence of upper extremity cumulative trauma disorders in industry (Ph.D. dissertation, The University of Michigan). Ann Arbor, MI: University Microfilms International, 1985.

BIBLIOGRAPHY

Armstrong T. An ergonomics guide to carpal tunnel syndrome. Akron, OH: American Industrial Hygiene Association, 1983.
Discusses etiology and prevention of upper extremity cumulative trauma disorders. Covers design and selection of hand tools useful in controlling biomechanical stresses on musculoskeletal tissue and peripheral nerves.
Chaffin DB, Andersson GBJ. Occupational ergonomics. New York: Wiley-Interscience, 1984.
This text discusses in detail the biomechanical basis of many occupational injuries and disorders. Quantitative methods of job analysis are presented with numerous examples of ergonomic approaches to equipment, tool, and work station design.
Durnin JVGA, Passmore R. Energy, work, and leisure. London: Heineman Educational Books, 1967.
Presents numerous tables of the metabolic cost of common occupational, household, and recreational activities. A useful reference text.

Garg A, Chaffin DB, Herrin GD. Prediction of metabolic rates for manual materials handling jobs. Am Ind Hyg Assoc J 1978; 39:661–674.
Describes the development and validation of a modeling approach to estimate energy expenditure rates associated with common materials handling tasks. Equations for predicting energy expenditure are included in an appendix to this paper.
Grandjean E. Fitting the task to the man—an ergonomic approach. London: Taylor and Francis, 1980.
A well-written survey text that covers all aspects of ergonomics. Chapters on fatigue and work physiology provide an excellent introduction to these topics.
Keyserling WM, Herrin GD, Chaffin DB. Isometric strength testing as a means of controlling medical incidents on strenuous jobs. J Occup Med, 1980; 22:332–336.
Describes the development and implementation of isometric strength tests used in the selection of workers for 20 strenuous jobs in a tire and rubber plant. Medical incidents of workers selected using the strength tests and those selected using traditional screening techniques are compared.
Keyserling WM, Armstrong TJ. Ergonomics. In: Last JM, ed. Maxcy-Rosenau Public Health and Preventive Medicine. 12th ed. Norwalk, CT: Appleton-Century-Crofts, 1986; 734–750.
A general review of occupational ergonomics with emphasis on human factors engineering, anthropometry, work physiology, and biomechanics. References include many recent journal articles on ergonomic topics.
McCormick EJ, Sanders MS. Human factors in engineering and design. New York: McGraw-Hill, 1987.
A useful reference text for many topics in human factors engineering including: lighting, displays, controls, and information processing. Well illustrated with numerous examples.
National Institute for Occupational Safety and Health. Work practices guide for manual lifting (NIOSH Pub. No. 81-122). Cincinnati: National Institute for Occupational Safety and Health, 1981.
Provides a comprehensive literature review of recent research on manual lifting and presents standardized procedures for evaluating lifting hazards. Excellent bibliography and illustrations.
Tichauer ER. The biomechanical basis of ergonomics. New York: Wiley Interscience, 1978.
This monograph discusses the biomechanical causes of occupational accidents and diseases with emphasis on the back and upper extremities. Principles of ergonomic design for equipment, tools, and work methods are presented.

10
Federal Regulation of Occupational Health and Safety in the Workplace

Nicholas A. Ashford

The use of chemicals, materials, tools, machinery, and equipment in industrial, mining, and agricultural workplaces is often accompanied by health and safety hazards or risks (Fig. 10-1). These hazards cause occupational disease and injury that place heavy economic and social burdens on both workers and employers. Because voluntary efforts in the free market have not succeeded historically in reducing the incidence of these diseases and injuries, government intervention into the activities of the private sector has been demanded by workers. This intervention takes the form of the regulation of health and safety hazards through standard-setting, enforcement, and the transfer of information.

In the United States, toxic substances in the workplace are regulated primarily through three federal laws: the Mine Safety and Health Act of 1969 (see box on page 137), the Occupational Safety and Health Act (OSHAct) of 1970, and the Toxic Substances Control Act (TSCA) of 1976. The OSHAct established the Occupational Safety and Health Administration (OSHA) in the Department of Labor to enforce compliance with the act, and the National Institute for Occupational Safety and Health (NIOSH) in the Department of Health and Human Services (under the Centers for Disease Control) to perform research and conduct health hazard evaluations. The Office of Toxic Substances in the Environmental Protection Agency (EPA) administers TSCA.

The evolution of regulatory law under the OSHAct has profoundly influenced other environmental legislation and will probably similarly af-

fect the evolution of TSCA. This chapter addresses federal regulation, focusing on standard-setting, enforcement mechanisms, and Right-to-Know provisions.

The OSHAct requires OSHA to (1) encourage employers and employees to reduce hazards in the workplace and to implement new or improved safety and health programs; (2) develop mandatory job safety and health standards and enforce them effectively; (3) establish "separate but dependent responsibilities and rights" for employers and employees for the achievement of better safety and health conditions; (4) establish reporting and recordkeeping procedures to monitor job-related injuries and illnesses; and (5) encourage states to assume the fullest responsibility for establishing and administering their own occupational safety and health programs, which must be at least as effective as the federal program.

As a result of these responsibilities, OSHA inspects workplaces for violations of existing health and safety standards; establishes advisory committees; holds hearings; sets new or revised standards for control of specific substances, conditions, or use of equipment; enforces standards by assessing fines or by other legal means; and provides for consultative services for management and for employer and employee training and education. In all of its procedures, from the development of standards through their implementation and enforcement, OSHA guarantees employers and employees the right to be fully informed, to participate actively, and to appeal its decisions.

The coverage of the OSHAct initially extended

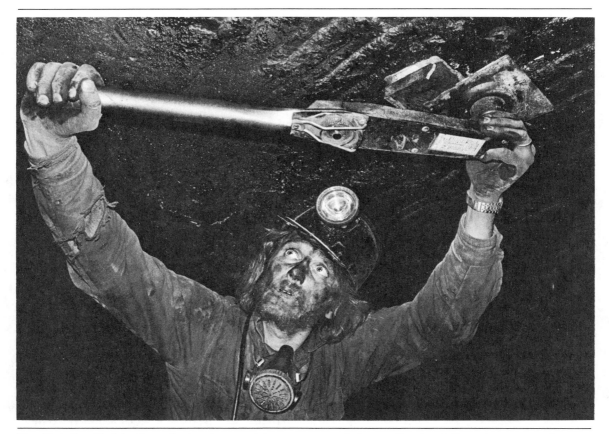

Fig. 10-1. Roof bolting in coal mines is essential to prevent roofs from collapsing. Miners face many other injury risks as well.
(Photograph by Earl Dotter.)

to all employers and their employees, except self-employed people, family-owned and -operated farms, and workplaces already protected by other federal agencies or other federal statutes. In 1979, however, Congress exempted from routine OSHA safety inspections approximately 1.5 million businesses with 10 or fewer employees. (Exceptions to this are allowed if workers claim there are safety violations.) Since federal agencies, such as the U.S. Postal Service, are not subject to OSHA regulations and enforcement provisions, each agency is required to establish and maintain its own effec-

tive and comprehensive job safety and health program. OSHA provisions do not apply to state and local governments in their role as employers. OSHA requires, however, that any state desiring to gain OSHA support or funding for its own occupational safety and health program must provide a program to cover its state and local government workers that is at least as effective as the OSHA program for private employees.

OSHA can begin standard-setting procedures either on its own or on petitions from other parties, including the Secretary of Health and Human

WHAT YOU NEED TO KNOW ABOUT THE MINE SAFETY AND HEALTH ADMINISTRATION
—James L. Weeks

The Mine Safety and Health Act is similar in structure and function to the Occupational Safety and Health Act, although there are some important differences. It is designed to protect the approximately 350,000 miners engaged in the most dangerous industrial occupation in the United States. Historically, federal government intervention in mine safety and health was the responsibility of the U.S. Bureau of Mines in the Department of the Interior. The bureau was organized in 1910 for the purpose of conducting research into mine disasters and thereafter acquired increasing authority and responsibility to promote mine safety. This role culminated in the federal Coal Mine Health and Safety Act of 1969, which created the Mining Enforcement Safety Administration (MESA). This act was amended in 1977, at which time MESA's name was changed to the Mine Safety and Health Administration (MSHA), it was moved to the Department of Labor, and all mines (not only coal mines) were included under its jurisdiction.

MSHA has functions similar to those of OSHA. In general, it is required to write and enforce regulations and employs a corps of inspectors to inspect mines. Citations carry penalties that mine operators may appeal in court, including the U.S. Supreme Court. Mine operators may request variances from standards and may receive technical assistance from MSHA or the Bureau of Mines. Miners have the right to request inspections and to participate in most aspects of rule-making and enforcement. They are promised protection from discrimination for engaging in activities protected by the act.

MSHA, however, differs from OSHA in some important ways. All mines are covered by the act, without exception. Inspections of mines on a regular basis is mandatory (quarterly for underground mines, semiannually for surface mines), and penalties are mandatory. Inspectors have the authority to close all or parts of mines in the event of imminent danger and have done so. OSHA inspectors do not have the authority to close workplaces, even in the event of imminent danger; they must request a court order. Unlike OSHA, MSHA has no "general duty" clause. Finally, under the Mine Safety and Health Act, miners are required to undergo extensive training, both before working full-time and annually thereafter.

The act also created measures to control respiratory disease in miners, commonly called "black lung," by requiring mine operators to provide chest x-rays at regular intervals and by setting a statutory limit for exposure to coal mine dust. Miners who have a positive chest x-ray for pneumoconiosis have the opportunity to transfer to less dusty areas of a mine without loss of pay or seniority. Exposure to dust, including free silica, must be monitored on a regular basis in both surface and underground coal mines.

The 1969 act created a novel federal government program to compensate miners who were totally disabled by pneumoconiosis. Largely because of difficulty in establishing a precise etiology for miners' respiratory disease, the black lung program is complex and controversial. By the mid-1980s, approximately $1.6 billion in payments was being sent annually to recipients and their families. Initially, payments were made out of the general treasury and the program was administered by the Social Security Administration. Several amendments to the act moved the program to the Department of Labor and payments are currently made by the miner's last mining employer or, if that employer cannot be found, out of a disability trust fund (see Chap. 11).

Services, NIOSH, state and local governments, any nationally recognized standards-producing organization, employer or labor representatives, or any other interested person. The standard-setting process involves input from advisory committees and from NIOSH. When OSHA develops plans to propose, amend, or delete a standard, it publishes these intentions in the *Federal Register*. Subsequently, interested parties have opportunities to present arguments and pertinent evidence in writing or at public hearings. Under certain conditions OSHA is authorized to set emergency temporary standards, which take effect immediately but expire within six months. OSHA must first determine that workers are in grave danger from exposure to toxic substances or new hazards and are not adequately protected by existing standards. Standards can be appealed through the federal courts, but filing an appeals petition will not delay the enforcement of the standard unless a court of appeals specifically orders it. Employers may make application to OSHA for a variance from a standard or regulation if they lack the means to comply readily with it or if they can prove that their facilities or methods of operation provide employee protection that is at least as effective as that required by OSHA.

OSHA requires employers of more than 10 employees to maintain records of occupational injuries and illnesses as they occur. All occupational injuries and diseases must be recorded if they result in death, one or more lost work days, restriction of work or motion, loss of consciousness, transfer to another job, or medical treatment (other than first aid).

STANDARD-SETTING AND OBLIGATIONS OF THE EMPLOYER AND THE MANUFACTURER OR USER OF TOXIC SUBSTANCES
Legal Background for OSHA Obligations
The OSHAct provides two general means of protection for workers: (1) a statutory general duty to provide a safe and healthful workplace, and (2) adherence to specific standards by employers. The act imposes on virtually every employer in the private sector a general duty "to furnish to each of his employees employment and a place of employment which are free from *recognized hazards* that are causing or are likely to cause death or serious physical harm. . . ." A recognized hazard may be a substance for which the likelihood of harm has been the subject of research, giving rise to reasonable suspicion, or a substance for which an OSHA standard may or may not have yet been promulgated. The burden of proving that a particular substance is a recognized hazard and that industrial exposure to it results in a significant degree of exposure is placed on OSHA. Since standard-setting is a slow process, protection of workers through the employer's general duty obligation is especially important, but it is crucially dependent on the existence of reliable health effects data.

The OSHAct addresses specifically the subject of toxic materials. It states, under Section 6(b)(5) of the act, that the Secretary of Labor (through OSHA), in promulgating standards dealing with toxic materials or harmful physical agents, shall set the standard that "most adequately assures, to the extent *feasible*, on the basis of the *best available evidence* that *no* employee will suffer material impairment of health or functional capacity, even if such employee has a regular exposure to the hazard dealt with by such standard for the period of his working life." By these words, one can see that the issue of exposure to toxic chemicals or carcinogens that have long latency periods, as well as to reproductive hazards, is covered by the act in specific terms.

Under Section 6(a) of the act, without critical review, OSHA initially adopted as standards the 450 Threshold Limit Values (TLVs) recommended as guidelines from protection against the toxic effects of these materials. In the 1970s, under Section 6(b), OSHA set formal standards for asbestos, vinyl chloride, arsenic, dibromochloropropane (DBCP), coke oven emissions, acrylonitrile, lead, cotton dust, and a group of 14 carcinogens. More recently, OSHA has regulated benzene, ethylene oxide, and formaldehyde as carcinogens and asbestos more rigidly as a carcinogen at 0.2 fibers per cubic centimeter.

The burden of proving the hazardous nature of a substance is placed on OSHA, as is the requirement that the proposed controls are technologically feasible. The necessarily slow and arduous task of setting standards substance by substance makes it impossible to realistically deal with 13,000 toxic substances or 2,000 suspect carcinogens on NIOSH lists. Efforts have been made to streamline the process by proposing generic standards for carcinogens.

The inadequacy of the 450 TLVs adopted under Section 6(a) of the act is widely known. The TLVs originated as guidelines recommended by the American Conference of Governmental Industrial Hygienists (ACGIH) to protect the *average* worker from either recognized acute effects or easily recognized chronic effects. The standards are based on animal toxicity data or the limited epidemiologic evidence available at the time of the establishment of the TLVs. They do not address the sensitive populations within the workforce or those with prior exposure or existing disease, nor do they address the issues of carcinogenicity, mutagenicity, and teratogenicity. These standards were adopted en masse in 1971 as a part of the consensus standards that OSHA adopted along with those dealing primarily with safety.

As an example of the inadequacy of protection offered by the TLVs, the 1971 TLV for vinyl chloride was set at 250 ppm, whereas the later protective standard (see below) recommended no greater exposure than 1 ppm—a level still recognized as unsafe but the limit that the technology could detect. Another example is the TLV for lead, which was established at 200 μg per cubic meter, whereas the later lead standard required a level no greater than 50 μg per cubic meter, also recognizing that that level was not safe for all populations, such as pregnant women or those with prior lead

exposure. The ACGIH is considering adding a list of carcinogens to its TLV list. While useful, this list will have little legal significance unless formally adopted by OSHA.

Under Section 6(b) of the OSHAct, new health standards dealing with toxic substances were to be established utilizing the mechanism of an open hearing and subject to review by the U.S. Circuit Courts of Appeals. The evolution of case law associated with the handful of standards that OSHA promulgated through this section is worth considering in detail. The courts addressed the difficult issue of what is adequate scientific information necessary to sustain the requirement that the standards be supported by "substantial evidence on the record as a whole." The cases also addressed the extent to which economic factors were permitted or required to be considered in the setting of the standards, the meaning of "feasibility," the question of whether a cost-benefit analysis was required or permitted, and, finally, the extent of the jurisdiction of OSHAct in addressing different degrees of risk.

The Carcinogens Standard

In an early case challenging OSHA's authority to regulate 14 carcinogens, the District of Columbia Circuit Court of Appeals first addressed the issue of substantial evidence. For eight of the 14 carcinogens, there were no human (epidemiologic) data. Industry challenged OSHA's ability to impose controls on employers in the absence of human data. Here the court expressed its view that some facts, such as the establishment of human carcinogenic risk from animal data, were on the "frontiers of scientific knowledge" and that the requirement for standards to be supported by substantial evidence in these kinds of social policy decisions could not be subjected to the rigors of other kinds of factual determinations. Thus, OSHA was permitted to require protective action against substances known to produce cancer in animals but with no evidence of producing cancer in humans. It was not until 1980 that the U.S. Supreme Court in the benzene case (see below) placed limits on the extent of OSHA's policy determinations on carcinogenic risk.

The Asbestos Standard

In the challenge to OSHA's original asbestos standard—in which asbestos was regulated as a classic lung toxin and not as a carcinogen—the Industrial Union Department of AFL-CIO unsuccessfully challenged the laxity of the standard, claiming that OSHA improperly weighed economic considerations in its determination of feasibility. OSHA indeed was permitted to consider economic factors in establishing feasibility. The District of Columbia Circuit Court of Appeals went on to state, however, that a standard might be feasible even if some employers were forced out of business, as long as the entire asbestos-using industry was not disrupted. In 1986, OSHA revised the standard from 2 fibers per cubic centimeter to 0.2 fibers per cubic centimeter, thus finally acknowledging it as a carcinogen.

The Vinyl Chloride Standard

In the industry challenge to OSHA's regulation of vinyl chloride at 1 ppm, the Second Circuit Court of Appeals reiterated OSHA's ability to make policy judgments with regard to matters "on the frontiers of scientific knowledge" when it declared that there could be no safe level for a carcinogen. In addition, the court said that since 1 ppm was the lowest feasible level, OSHA was permitted to force employers to comply even though it had performed no formal risk assessment or knew how many tumors would be prevented by the adoption of this protective level. Another noteworthy aspect of the case was the recognition that OSHA could act as a "technology forcer" and require controls not yet fully developed at the time of the setting of the standard.

The Lead Standard

Protection from lead exposure had been provided through the TLV of 200 μg per cubic meter. This level was long recognized as inadequate for workers who accumulated lead in their body tissues and for women (and possibly men) who intended to have children. As a result, based on the limits of technological feasibility, OSHA promulgated a new standard that permitted no exposure greater than 50 μg per cubic meter, averaged over an 8-hour period. In addition, because this was still unsafe for many workers, OSHA also provided that workers be removed with pay and employment security if their blood lead levels exceeded 50 μg per deciliter of blood *or* if there were grounds to remove them based on risks to their reproductive system. The legality and necessity of this additional provision, known as Medical Removal Protection (MRP), was unsuccessfully challenged by the Lead Industries Association. (MRP has since been required in a limited way in the cotton dust and benzene standards.) OSHA specifically provided that workers in workplaces with air-lead levels over an "action level" of 30 μg per cubic meter have the benefit of a continuing medical surveillance program, including periodic sampling of blood-lead levels and removal from exposure above the action level after finding of blood-levels in an individual worker above 50 μg per deciliter, with job return when the worker's level fell below 40 μg per deciliter.

Removal could also be triggered by other medical conditions deemed to create an unusual risk for lead exposure (for example, pregnancy). OSHA provided that workers' pay and seniority be maintained by the employer during any periods of medical removal (up to 18 months), even if such removal entailed sending the worker home. In actual practice, many employers have reduced the ambient air-lead level well below 50 μg per cubic meter, which results in the removal of fewer workers.

The Benzene Standard

Following the first serious successful industry challenge of an OSHA benzene standard in the Fifth Circuit Court of Appeals, the U.S. Supreme

Court, in a controversial and divided majority opinion, chided OSHA for not attempting to evaluate the benefits of changing the permissible exposure level for benzene from 10 ppm (the former TLV) to 1 ppm. The Court argued that OSHA is obligated to regulate only "significant risks" and that without a risk assessment of some kind OSHA could not know whether the proposed control addressed a significant risk. The Court was careful to state that it was not attempting to "statistically straitjacket" the agency, but that at a minimum the benefits of regulation needed to be addressed to meet the substantial evidence test. The Court did not give useful guidance concerning what constituted a significant risk. It stated that a risk of death of 1 in 1,000 was clearly unacceptable, while a risk of 1 in 1,000,000 might be tolerated. This three-orders-of-magnitude range, of course, represents the area on which the arguments have always been centered.

The implications of the benzene decision for future standards will depend on the nature of the particular OSHA administration. There is little question that had OSHA performed a risk assessment for benzene at the time, it could have argued that the risk it was attempting to address was actually significant. The precise requirement and nature of a risk assessment sufficient to meet the substantial evidence test remains quite unclear. In late 1985, OSHA again proposed to lower the permissible exposure limit from 10 ppm to 1 ppm, and in 1987, the standard was set at that level. OSHA, however, after intervention by the Office of Management and Budget (OMB), declined to establish a short-term exposure limit.

The petroleum industry argued in the benzene case that not only must a risk assessment be performed, but a cost-benefit analysis must also be done in which the risks of exposure must be balanced against the benefits of the chemical. The question, however, was not decided in the benzene case but was addressed in a later case challenging OSHA's cotton dust standard. The Supreme Court not only acknowledged that cotton dust did represent a significant risk but also indicated that a cost-benefit balancing was neither required nor permitted by the OSHAct since Congress had already struck the balance heavily in favor of worker health and safety.

The Generic Carcinogen Standard

In 1980, OSHA promulgated a generic carcinogen standard by which questions of science policy, already settled as law in cases dealing with other standards, were codified in a set of principles. During the process of developing the generic carcinogen standard, OSHA and NIOSH developed lists of chemical substances that would probably be classified as suspect carcinogens. Each agency composed a list of approximately 250 substances. Thus far, OSHA has declined to formally list any substance under the carcinogen standard.

In setting or revising standards for formaldehyde, ethylene oxide, asbestos, and benzene, the agency has proceeded to act as if the generic carcinogen standard did not exist, thus following the historically arduous and slow path to standard-setting.

The Consumer Product Safety Act

The implementation of the OSHAct, with burden of proof placed on the government, cannot keep pace with the proliferation of chemicals in the work environment, and it is certainly no safeguard against general environmental contamination or consumer product hazards. The burden of proving "unreasonable risk" in consumer products is placed on the Consumer Product Safety Commission, which has taken action on only a few chemical problems, including fluorocarbons, vinyl chloride, and formaldehyde in foam insulation.

The Toxic Substances Control Act (TSCA)

TSCA enables the Environmental Protection Agency (EPA) to require data *from industry* on the production, use, and health and environmental effects of chemicals. EPA may regulate by requiring labeling, setting tolerances, or banning completely and requiring repurchase or recall. EPA may also order a specific change in chemical process technology. In addition, TSCA gives aggrieved parties, including consumers and workers, specific rights to sue for damages under the act, with the possibility of awards for attorneys' fees. (This feature was missing in the OSHAct.)

Under TSCA, EPA must regulate "unreasonable risks." EPA has issued a regulation for worker protection from asbestos at the new OSHA limit of 0.2 fibers per cubic centimeter, which applies to state and local government asbestos abatement workers not covered by OSHA. EPA has declared formaldehyde a "probable carcinogen" and will proceed to regulate it to supplement OSHA's actions.

The strength of TSCA is in its ability to shift onto the producer the requirement to prove that a substance is safe to the extent that exposure to it does not present an "unreasonable risk of injury to human health or the environment." Used together, the OSHAct and TSCA provide potentially comprehensive and effective information-generation and standard-setting authority to protect workers. In particular, the information-generation activities under TSCA can provide the necessary data to have a substance qualify as a "recognized hazard," which, even in the absence of specific OSHA standards, must be controlled in some way by the employer to meet the general duty obligation under the OSHAct to provide a safe and healthful workplace.

ENFORCEMENT ACTIVITIES

Standard-setting, of course, is only the beginning of the regulatory process. For a regulatory system to be effective, there must be a clear commitment to the enforcement of standards. Under OSHA, a worker can request workplace inspection if the request is in writing and signed. Anonymity is preserved on request. When an inspector visits a workplace, a representative of the workers can accompany the inspector on the "walkaround."

If specific requests for inspections are not made, OSHA makes random inspections of those workplaces with worse-than-average safety records. However, the inspection frequency is low. Furthermore, firms with significant exposures to chemicals may not be routinely inspected, simply because their record for *injuries* (which dominate the reported statistics) is good.

Inspections are usually conducted without advance notice, but an employer may insist that OSHA inspectors obtain a court order before entering the workplace. In 1987, federal OSHA had fewer than 1,100 inspectors (compared to 1,300 in 1980) and state agencies fewer than 2,000. Clearly not all 5 million workplaces covered by the act could be inspected.

OSHA can fine employers up to $1,000 for each violation of the act that is discovered during workplace inspection and up to $10,000 if the violation is willful or repeated. Management can appeal violations, amounts of fines, methods of correcting hazards, and deadlines for correcting hazards (abatement dates). Workers can appeal only deadlines. All appeals are processed through the Occupational Safety and Health Review Commission, which also was established by the OSHAct.

The act requires OSHA to encourage states to develop and operate their own job safety and health programs. State programs, when "at least as effective" as the federal program, can take over enforcement activities. Once a state plan is approved, OSHA funds half of its operating costs. About 20 state plans, which OSHA monitors, are in effect (see Appendix C). State safety and health standards under such approved plans must keep pace with OSHA standards, and state plans must guarantee employer and employee rights as does OSHA.

During the 1980s OSHA inspection policy has seen directives given to the field staff to deemphasize general duty violations. In addition, inspectors are actually evaluated by the managers of the establishments they inspect. Follow-up inspections after violations are often restricted to checks by telephone. Thus, incentives for aggressive inspection activity are not great under the present Administration.

THE RIGHT TO KNOW

The transfer of information regarding workplace exposure to toxic substances has received considerable public attention. It is clear that workers need an accurate picture of the nature and extent of probable chemical exposures to decide whether to enter or remain in a particular workplace. Workers also need to have knowledge regarding past or current exposures to be alert to the onset of occupational disease. Regulatory agencies must have timely access to such information if they are to devise effective strategies to reduce disease and death from occupational exposures to toxic substances. Accordingly, laws designed to facilitate this flow of information have recently been promulgated at the federal, state, and local levels. Indeed, the Right to Know has become a political battleground in many states and communities and has been the subject of intensive organizing efforts by business, labor, and citizen-action groups.

In essence, the Right to Know embodies a democratization of the workplace. It is the mandatory sharing of information between management and labor. Through a variety of laws, manufacturers and employers are directed to disclose information regarding toxic substance exposure to workers, to unions in their capacity as worker representatives, and to governmental agencies charged with the protection of public health. The underlying rationale for these directives is the assumption that this transfer of information will prompt activity that will improve worker health.

Although the phrase *Right to Know* is a useful generic designation, it is an inadequate description of the legal rights and obligations that govern the transfer of workplace information on toxic substances. One cannot have a meaningful *right* to information unless someone else has a corresponding *duty* to provide that information. Thus, a worker's Right to Know will be secured by requiring a manufacturer or employer to disclose. The disclosure requirement can take a variety of forms, and the practical scope of that requirement may depend on the nature of the form chosen. In particular, a duty to disclose only such information as has been requested may provide a narrower flow of information than a duty to disclose all information, regardless of whether it has been requested. The various rights and obligations in the area of toxics information transfer may be grouped into three categories. Though they share a number of similarities, each category is conceptually distinct.

1. *The duty to generate or retain information* refers to the obligation to compile a record of certain workplace events or activities or to maintain such a record for a specified period of time if it has been compiled. An employer may, for example, be required to monitor its workers regularly for evidence of toxic exposures (biologic monitoring) and to keep written records of the results of such monitoring.
2. *The right of access* (and the corresponding duty to disclose on request) refers to the right of a worker, a union, or an agency to request and secure access to information held by a manufacturer or employer. Such a right of access would provide workers with a means of obtaining copies of biologic monitoring records pertaining to their own exposure to toxic substances.
3. Finally, *the duty to inform* refers to an employer's or manufacturer's obligation to disclose, without request, information pertaining to toxic substance exposures in the workplace. An employer may, for example, have a duty—independent of any worker's exercise of a right to access—to inform workers whenever biologic monitoring reveals that their exposure to a toxic substance has produced bodily concentrations of that substance above a specified level.

Rights and duties governing toxic information transfer in the workplace can originate from a variety of sources. Some will be grounded in state common law, while others will arise out of specific state statutes or local ordinances. Although the states have been increasingly active in this field, the primary source of regulation is federal law. Most federal regulation in this area emanates from three statutes: the OSHAct, TSCA, and the National Labor Relations Act (NLRA), administered by the National Labor Relations Board (NLRB).

The scope of a particular right or duty will depend on many factors. The first, and perhaps most important, is the nature of the information required to be transferred.

Scientific information refers to data concerning the nature and consequences of toxic substance exposures. These data, in turn, can be divided into three subcategories:

1. *Ingredients information* provides the worker with the identity of the substances to which he or she is exposed. Depending on the circumstances, this information may involve only the generic classifications of the various chemicals involved or may include the specific chemical identities of all chemical exposures and the specific contents of all chemical mixtures.
2. *Exposure information* encompasses all data regarding the amount, frequency, duration, and route of workplace exposures. This information may be of a general nature, such as the results of ambient air monitoring at a central workplace location, or may take individualized form, such as the results of personal environmental or biological monitoring of a specific worker.
3. *Health effects information* indicates known or potential health effects of workplace exposures. This information may be general data regarding the effects of chemical exposure, usually found in a material safety data sheet (MSDS) or a published or unpublished workplace epidemiologic study, or it may be individualized data, such as worker medical records compiled as a result of medical surveillance.

In general, the broadest coverage is found in rights and duties emanating from the OSHAct. By its terms, that act is applicable to all *private* employers and thus covers the bulk of workplace exposures to toxic substances. Most private industrial workplaces are also subject to the NLRA. Farmworkers and workers subject to the Railway Labor Act, however, are exempt from NLRA coverage. TSCA provides a generally narrower scope. While many of the act's provisions apply broadly to both chemical manufacture and use, its information transfer requirements extend only to chemical manufacturers, processors, and importers. On the state level, the relevant coverage of the various rights and duties will depend on the specifics of the particular state and local law defining them. In general, common law rights and duties will evidence much less variation than will those created by state statute or local ordinance.

Under OSHA's Hazard Communication Standard, employers have a duty to inform workers in the manufacturing sector of the identity of substances with which they work through labeling the product container and disclosing to the purchaser (the employer) using MSDSs.

Employers are under no obligation to amend inadequate, insufficient, or incorrect information provided by the manufacturer. Employers must, however, transmit certain information to their employees: (1) information on the standard and its requirements; (2) operations in their work areas where hazardous chemicals are present; and (3) the location and availability of the company's hazard communication program. The standard also requires that workers must be trained in (1) methods to detect the presence or release of the hazardous chemicals; (2) the physical and health hazards of the chemicals; (3) protective measures, such as appropriate work practices, emergency procedures, and personal protective equipment; and (4) the details of the hazard communication program developed by the employer, including an explanation of the labeling system and the MSDSs, and how employees can obtain and use hazard information.

OSHA is now under court order to extend the standard to nonmanufacturing sectors. The federal standard preempts state Right-to-Know laws in the worker notification area in a minority of jurisdictions; it would appear to be coexistent with state requirements in most jurisdictions, although its stated intent is to preempt all state efforts.

Under OSHA's Medical Access Rule, an employer may not limit or deny an employee access to his or her own medical or exposure records. The current OSHA regulation, promulgated in 1980, grants employees a general right of access to medical and exposure records kept by their employer. Furthermore, it requires the employer to preserve and maintain these records for 30 years. There appears to be some overlap in the definitions of *medical* and *exposure* records, because both may include the results of biological monitoring. Medical records, however, are generally defined as those pertaining to "the health status of an employee," while the exposure records are defined as those pertaining to "employee exposure to toxic substances or harmful physical agents."

The employer's duty to make these records available is a broad one. The regulations provide that upon any employee request for access to a medical or exposure record, "the employer *shall* assure that access is provided in a reasonable time, place, and manner, but in no event later than 15 days after the request for access is made."

An employee's right of access to medical records is limited to records pertaining specifically to that employee. The regulations allow physicians some discretion as well in limiting employee access. The physician is permitted to "recommend" to the employee requesting access that the employee (1) review and discuss the records with the physician; (2) accept a summary rather than the records themselves; or (3) allow the records to be released instead to another physician. Furthermore, where information in a record pertains to a "specific diagnosis of a terminal illness or a psychiatric condition," the physician is authorized to direct that such information be provided only to the employee's designated representative. Although these pro-

visions were apparently intended to respect the physician-patient relationship and do not limit the employee's ultimate right of access, they could be abused. In situations in which the physician feels loyalty to the employer rather than the employee, the physician could use these provisions to discourage the employee from seeking access to his or her records.

Similar constraints do not apply to employee access to exposure records. Not only is the employee assured access to records of his or her own exposure to toxic substances, but the employee is also assured access to the exposure records of other employees "with past or present job duties or working conditions related to or similar to those of the employee." In addition, the employee has access to all general exposure information pertaining to the employee's workplace or working conditions and to any workplace or working condition to which he or she is to be transferred. All information in exposure records that cannot be correlated with a particular employee's exposure is accessible.

One criticism of the OSHA regulation is that it does not require the employer to compile medical or exposure information but merely requires employee access to such information if it is compiled. The scope of the regulation, however, should not be underestimated. The term *record* is meant to be "all-encompassing," and the access requirement appears to extend to all information gathered on employee health or exposure, no matter how it is measured or recorded. Thus, if an employer embarks on any program of human monitoring, no matter how conducted, he or she must provide the subjects access to the results. This access requirement may serve as a disincentive for employers to monitor employee exposure or health, if it is not clearly in the employer's interest to do so.

The regulations permit the employer to deny access to "trade secret data which discloses manufacturing processes . . . or . . . the percentage of a chemical substance in a mixture," provided that the employer: (1) notifies the party requesting access of the denial; (2) if relevant, provides alternative information sufficient to permit identification of when and where exposure occurred; and (3) provides access to all "chemical or physical agent identities including chemical names, levels of exposure, and employee health status data contained in the requested records."

The key feature of this provision is that it ensures employee access to the precise identities of chemicals and physical agents. This access is especially critical for chemical exposures. Within each "generic" class of chemicals, there are a variety of specific chemical compounds, each of which may have its own particular effect on human health. The health effects can vary widely within a particular family of chemicals. Accordingly, the medical and scientific literature on chemical properties and toxicity is indexed by specific chemical name, not by generic chemical class. To discern any meaningful correlation between a chemical exposure and a known or potential health effect, an employee must know the precise chemical identity of that exposure. Furthermore, in the case of biological monitoring, the identity of the toxic substance or its metabolite is itself the information monitored.

Particularly in light of the public health emphasis inherent in the OSHAct, disclosure of such information does not constitute an unreasonable infringement on the trade secret interests of the employer. In general, chemical health and safety data are the least valuable to an employer of all the "proprietary" information relevant to a particular manufacturing process.

TSCA imposes substantial requirements on chemical manufacturers and processors to develop health effects data. TSCA requires testing, premarket manufacturing notification, and reporting and retention of information. TSCA imposes no specific medical surveillance or biological monitoring requirements. However, to the extent that human monitoring is used to meet more general requirements of assessing occupational health or exposure to toxic substances, the data resulting from such monitoring are subject to an employer's recording and retention obligations.

The EPA has promulgated regulations requiring general reporting on approximately 300 chemicals, including information related to occupational exposure. The EPA administrator may require the reporting and maintenance of those data "insofar as known" or "insofar as reasonably ascertainable." Thus, if monitoring is undertaken, it must be reported. The EPA appears to be authorized to require monitoring as a way of securing information that is "reasonably ascertainable."

In addition to the general reports required for specific chemicals listed in the regulations, the EPA has promulgated rules for the submission of health and safety studies required for 169 substances. A health and safety study includes "[a]ny data that bear on the effects of chemical substance on health." Examples are "[m]onitoring data, when they have been aggregated and analyzed to measure the exposure of humans . . . to a chemical substance or mixture." Only data that are "known" or "reasonably ascertainable" need be reported.

Records of "significant adverse reactions to [employee] health" must be retained for 30 years under Section 8(c). A recently promulgated rule implementing this section defines significant adverse reactions as those "that may indicate a substantial impairment of normal activities, or long-lasting or irreversible damage to health or the environment." Under the rule, human monitoring data, especially if derived from a succession of tests, would seem especially reportable. Genetic monitoring of employees, if some basis links the results with increased risk of cancer, also seems to fall within the rule.

Section 8(e) imposes a statutory duty to report "immediately . . . information which supports the conclusion that [a] substance or mixture presents a substantial risk of injury to health." In a policy statement issued in 1978, the EPA interpreted "immediately" in this context to require receipt by the agency within 15 working days after the reporter obtains the information. Substantial risk is defined exclusive of economic considerations. Evidence can be provided by either designed, controlled studies or undesigned, uncontrolled studies, including "medical and health surveys" or evidence of effects in workers. In the EPA's rule for Section 8(c), Section 8(e) is distinguished from Section 8(c) in that "[a] report of substantial risk of injury, unlike an allegation of a significant adverse reaction, is accompanied by information which reasonably supports the seriousness of the effect or the probability of its occurrence." Human monitoring results indicating a substantial risk of injury would thus seem reportable to the EPA. Either medical surveillance or biological monitoring data would seem to qualify.

Section 14(b) of TSCA gives the EPA authority to disclose from health and safety studies the data pertaining to chemical identities, except for the proportion of chemicals in a mixture. In addition, the EPA may disclose information, otherwise classified as a trade secret, "if the Administration determines it necessary to protect . . . against an unreasonable risk of injury to health." Monitoring data thus seem subject to full disclosure.

In addition to the access provided by OSHA regulations, individual employees may have a limited right of access to medical and exposure records under federal labor law. Logically, the right to refuse hazardous work (see below), inherent in Section 7 of the NLRA and Section 502 of the Labor Management Relations Act, carries with it the right of access to the information necessary to determine whether or not a particular condition is hazardous. In the case of toxic substance exposure, this right of access may mean access to all information relevant to the health effects of the exposure and may include access to both medical and exposure records. These federal labor law provisions are clearly not adequate substitutes for OSHA access regulations, however, as there is presently no systematic mechanism for enforcing this right.

Collective employee access, however, is available to unionized employees through the collective bargaining process. In four recent cases, the NLRB has held that unions have a right of access to exposure and medical records so that they may bargain effectively with the employer regarding conditions of employment. Citing the general proposition that employers are required to bargain on health and safety conditions when requested to do so, the NLRB adopted a broad policy favoring union access: "Few matters can be of greater legitimate concern to individuals in the workplace, and thus to the bargaining agent representing them, than exposure to conditions potentially threatening their health, well-being, or their very lives."

The NLRB, however, did not grant an unlimited right of access. The union's right of access is constrained by the individual employee's right of personal privacy. Furthermore, the NLRB acknowledged an employer's interest in protecting trade secrets. While ordering the employer in each of the four cases to disclose the chemical identities of substances to which the employer did not assert a trade secret defense, the NLRB indicated that employers are entitled to take reasonable steps to safeguard "legitimate" trade secret information. The NLRB did not delineate a specific mechanism for achieving the balance between union access and trade secret disclosure. Instead, it ordered the parties to attempt to resolve the issue through collective bargaining. Given the complexity of this issue and the potential for abuse in the name of "trade secret protection," the NLRB may find it necessary to provide further specificity before a workable industrywide mechanism can be achieved.

The legal avenues for worker and agency access to information relevant to workplace exposures to toxic substances have been expanded substantially. Despite certain inadequacies in the current laws and despite current attempts by OSHA to narrow the scope of some of these even further, access to toxics data remains broader than it has ever been. By itself, however, this fact is of little significance. The mere existence of information-transfer laws will mean little unless those laws are employed aggressively to further the objective of the Right to Know: the protection of workers' health. Currently, the various rights and duties governing toxics information transfer in the workplace present workers, unions, and agencies with a magnificent opportunity. The extent to which they seize this opportunity over the next few years will be a true measure of their resolve to bring about meaningful improvement in the health of the American worker.

THE RIGHT TO REFUSE HAZARDOUS WORK

The NLRA and the OSHAct provide many employees a limited right to refuse to perform hazardous work. When properly exercised, this right protects an employee from retaliatory discharge or other discriminatory action for refusing hazardous work and incorporates a remedy providing both reinstatement and back pay. The nature of this right under the NLRA depends on the relevant collective bargaining agreement, if there is one. Nonunion employees and union employees whose collective bargaining agreements specifically exclude health and safety from a no-strike clause have the *collective* right to stage a safety walkout under Section 7 of the NLRA. If they choose to walk out based on a good faith belief that working conditions are unsafe, they will be protected from any employer retaliation. Union employees who are subject to a comprehensive collective bargaining agreement may avail themselves of the provisions of Section 502 of the NLRA. Under this section, an employee who is faced with "abnormally dangerous conditions" has an *individual* right to leave the job site. The right may be exercised, however, only where the existence of abnormally dangerous conditions can be objectively verified. Both exposure and medical information are crucial here.

Under a 1973 OSHA regulation, the right to refuse hazardous work extends to all employees, *individually*, of private employers, regardless of the existence or nature of a collective bargaining agreement. Section 11(c) of the OSHAct protects an employee from discharge or other retaliatory action arising out of his or her "exercise" of "any right" afforded by the act. The Secretary of Labor has promulgated regulations under this section defining a right to refuse hazardous work in certain circumstances: where an employee reasonably believes there is a "real danger of death or serious injury," there is insufficient time to eliminate that danger through normal administrative channels, and the employer has failed to comply with an employee request to correct the situation.

Under the federal Mine Safety and Health Act, miners also have rights to transfer from unhealthy work areas if there is exposure to toxic substances or harmful physical agents or if there is medical evidence of pneumoconiosis.

BIBLIOGRAPHY

Ashford A. Crisis in the workplace: occupational disease and injury, a report to the Ford Foundation. Cambridge: MIT Press, 1976.
A policy-focused overview of science, law, economics and public policy dealing with occupational disease and injury.

Caldart C. Promises and pitfalls of workplace right-to-know. Sem Occup Med. 1986; 1:81–90.
Legal and ethical considerations concerning the transfer of toxic substances information in the workplace.

La Dou J, ed. Occupational health law. New York: Marcel Dekker Publications, 1981.
A collection of articles written by attorneys on various aspects of occupational health law.

US Congress, Office of Technology Assessment. Preventing illness and injury in the workplace. Washington, DC: U.S. Government Printing Office, 1985.
An update and comprehensive assessment of the political problems faced in preventing occupational disease and injury.

US Department of Labor. Protecting people at work, a reader in occupational safety and health. Washington, DC: U.S. Government Printing Office, 1980.
A collection of short articles on various aspects of occupational health and safety written by authors in government, industry, labor, and academia.

11
Workers' Compensation
Leslie I. Boden

Workers' compensation is a legal system designed to shift some of the costs of occupational injuries and illness from workers to employers. Workers' compensation laws generally require employers or their insurance companies to reimburse part of injured workers' lost wages and all of their medical and rehabilitation expenses. This chapter describes workers' compensation systems in the United States, discusses the role of the physician, and analyzes the very difficult problems of compensating victims of chronic occupational disease.

HISTORICAL BACKGROUND
Prior to the passage of the first workers' compensation act in 1911, workers generally bore the costs of their work-related injuries. Injured workers and their families were forced to cope with lost wages and medical care and rehabilitation costs. Under the common law* workers had to prove in a court of law that their injuries were caused by employer negligence to recover these costs.

For several reasons it was extremely difficult for workers to win such negligence suits. The injured worker had the burden of proof and had to show that the employer was negligent, that there was a work-related injury, and that the negligence caused the injury. To sustain this burden of proof, the worker had to hire a lawyer (which was costly) and often had to rely on the testimony of fellow

workers (who, along with the suing worker, might be fired for their part in the suit). All of this was enough to deter most workers from bringing suit.

In addition, employers had three very strong defenses that usually protected them from losing negligence suits when they were brought:

Doctrine of contributory negligence: If employees were found by judges to have contributed in any way to their injuries, they were barred from winning.
Fellow-servant rule: If fellow employees' actions were found by judges to have caused the injuries, employers were not considered responsible.
Assumption of risk: If injuries were found to be caused by common hazards or unusual hazards of which workers were aware, they could not recover damages.

In the late nineteenth century these defenses were widely used, and less than one-third of all employees who brought such negligence suits won any award. In one case a New York woman lost her arm when it was caught between the unguarded gears of the machine she had been cleaning. Unguarded gears were in violation of the laws of New York State at that time, and prior to the accident she had complained to her employer about this hazard. Still, her employer refused to guard the machine. After the accident the worker sued her employer, but the court held that she could not be compensated; she had obviously known about the hazard and of her own free will had continued to

---

*The common law is a body of legal principles developed by judicial decisions rather than by legislation. Legislation (statutory law) can override these judge-made laws.

work. This evidence showed that she had "assumed the risk" and that her employer was not responsible for the consequences.

The inability to hold employers responsible for their negligent actions persisted in the face of the high and increasing toll of occupational death and disability at the beginning of this century. After a disabling injury workers and their families were left largely to their own resources and to assistance from relatives, friends, and charities.

By 1920 some efforts had been made to provide better means of compensation to injured workers and their families. Some of the larger corporations had established private compensation schemes, and several states and the federal government had enacted employers' liability acts. These laws retained the basic common law liability scheme but reduced the role of the three common law defenses.

Most injured workers, however, were not able to take advantage of these changes. They were not employed by companies with private programs and were still not able to win negligence suits. There was growing support for a major change in the law, not only from the social reformers of the Progressive Era but also from major corporations. It is not entirely clear why the major corporations were promoting legislative reform. Some observers believe that industrial leaders realized that the burden of workplace injuries could spur independent, radical political action by workers. Others believe that employer defenses were already being weakened by legislation and that corporate leaders feared a rapid rise in the costs of employer liability suits. Still others argue that the basic motives to support new laws were humanitarian in nature.

These pressures gave rise to the passage of the first workers' compensation law in New York State in 1911. Many other states rapidly followed suit, and by 1920 all but eight states had passed similar laws, although most did not cover occupational disease. Mississippi, in 1948, was the last state to establish a workers' compensation system.

DESCRIPTION OF WORKERS' COMPENSATION

Workers' compensation provides income benefits, medical payments, and rehabilitation payments to workers injured on the job as well as benefits to survivors of fatally injured workers. There are 50 state and three federal workers' compensation jurisdictions, each with its own statute and regulations.

While state and federal systems are different in numerous ways, they have several characteristics in common. Benefit formulas are prescribed by law. Generally, medical care and rehabilitation expenses are fully covered, but lost wages are only partially reimbursed. Employers are legally responsible for paying benefits to injured workers. Some large employers pay these benefits themselves, but most pay yearly premiums to insurance companies, which process all claims and pay compensation to injured workers. Workers' compensation is a no-fault system. Injured workers do not need to prove that their injuries were caused by employer negligence. In fact, employers are generally required to pay benefits even if the injury is entirely the worker's fault.

The change to a no-fault system was established to minimize litigation. For a worker to qualify for workers' compensation benefits only three conditions must be met: There must be an injury or illness; the injury or illness must "arise out of and in the course of employment"; and there must be medical costs, rehabilitation costs, lost wages, or disfigurement. Clearly, these conditions are much easier for the injured worker to demonstrate than is employer negligence. For example, if a worker falls at work and breaks a leg, all three conditions are easily demonstrated. Unusual cases sometimes arise in which the question of the relationship of an injury to employment is difficult to resolve, and there may be questions about when a worker is ready to return to work. Such issues may result in litigation, but they are the exception not the rule. In most cases a worker files a claim for compensation with the employer, and the claim is accepted and paid either directly by the employer or by the workers' compensation insurance carrier of the employer.

The following case is typical of the events that follow many minor claims for workers' compensation:

Mr. Fisher had a painful muscle strain while lifting a heavy object at work on Monday afternoon. He went to the plant nurse and described the injury. He was sent home and was unable to return to work until the following Friday morning. On Tuesday the nurse sent an industrial accident report to the workers' compensation carrier and a copy to the state workers' compensation agency. Two weeks after he returned to work Mr. Fisher received a check from the insurance company covering part of his lost wages—as mandated by state statute—and all of his out-of-pocket medical expenses related to the muscle strain.

Workers' compensation has wider coverage than did the common law system. Under workers' compensation workplace injuries and illnesses are compensable even if they are only in part work-related. Suppose, for example, a worker with preexisting chronic low back pain becomes permanently disabled as a result of lifting a heavy object at work. In this case the worker's preexisting condition may just as easily have been aggravated by carrying out the garbage at home, but the fact that the disabling event occurred at work is generally sufficient for compensation to be awarded.

Cases in which an occupational injury or illness becomes disabling as a result of non-work exposures are more complicated. A worker with non-disabling silicosis may leave a granite quarry job for warehouse work. Without further exposure the silicosis will probably never become disabling. However, the worker begins to smoke cigarettes and loses lung function until partial disability results. In most states this worker should receive compensation from the owner of the granite quarry if the work relationship can be demonstrated.

Generally, diseases are considered eligible for

Table 11-1. Likelihood of compensation, by source of preexisting condition and source of ultimate disability

Source of ultimate disability	Source of preexisting condition	
	Work-related	Non-work-related
Work-related	Compensable	Generally compensable
Non-work-related	Generally compensable	Not compensable

Source: Adapted from PS Barth, HA Hunt. Workers' compensation and work-related illnesses. Cambridge: MIT Press, 1980.

compensation if occupational exposure is the *sole cause* of the disease, is *one of several causes* of the disease, was *aggravated* by or aggravates a nonoccupational exposure, or *hastens* the onset of disability (Table 11-1). Several states, including California and Florida, allow disability to be apportioned between occupational and nonoccupational causes. While at first this may seem like a sensible approach, apportionment creates some difficult decisions for workers' compensation administrators. Many disabilities are not additively caused by two separable exposures. With silica exposure or cigarette exposure alone, the worker in the above example would not have become disabled. Often, as in the case of lung cancer caused by asbestos exposure and smoking, the contribution to disability or death of two factors is many times greater than that of one alone. Such issues make the apportionment of disability very difficult if not impossible.

When workers' compensation was introduced, workers gained a swifter, more certain, and less litigious system than existed before. In return, however, covered workers waived their right to sue employers through common law. They also accepted lower awards than those given by juries in negligence suits: Workers' compensation provides no payments for "pain and suffering" as there might be in a common law settlement. In addition, disability payments under workers' compensation are often much less than lost income, especially for more severe injuries.

The United States does not have a unified workers' compensation law. Each state has its own system with its own standards and idiosyncracies. In addition, federal systems cover federal employees, longshoremen and harbor workers, and workers employed in the District of Columbia. Almost all states require employers either to purchase insurance or to demonstrate that they are able to pay any claims that might be made by their employees. In most states private insurers underwrite workers' compensation insurance paid for by premiums from individual employers. In some states a non-profit state workers' compensation fund has been established; the state government therefore acts as an insurance carrier, collecting premiums and disbursing benefits. State funds seem to be very effective in delivering benefits: They disburse a higher percentage of premiums in the form of benefits than do private insurance carriers.

COMMON LAW SUITS

While workers' compensation coverage bars workers from suing their employers at common law, it generally does not bar suits against a third party whose negligence caused a worker's injury or illness. If workers are injured by faulty machinery, workers' compensation coverage does not bar them from suing the manufacturer(s) of the equipment. Similarly, workers whose asbestosis is work-related may sue the asbestos manufacturer. In both circumstances, of course, negligence must be demonstrated. In a case decided in the U.S. Eighth Circuit Court of Appeals it was ruled that the manufacturer of an "unreasonably dangerous" product, asbestos, was negligent because it did not warn exposed workers of the hazards of being exposed to this product.

THE ROLE OF THE PHYSICIAN IN WORKERS' COMPENSATION

Workers' compensation is basically a legal system, not a medical system. The decision points for claims in this complex system are shown in Fig. 11-1. If a claim is rejected by the workers' compensation carrier or self-insured employer, it will generally be necessary for the injured worker to hire a lawyer. The worker's lawyer may then bargain with the lawyers for the insurance carrier in an attempt to settle the dispute informally. If this bargaining does not result in agreement, the claim must either be dropped or taken before an administrative board—a quasi-judicial body established by state statute—for a hearing. To the worker or to a physician who may be called to testify in such a hearing, such a proceeding may be indistinguish-

Fig. 11-1. Decision points for workers' compensation claims.

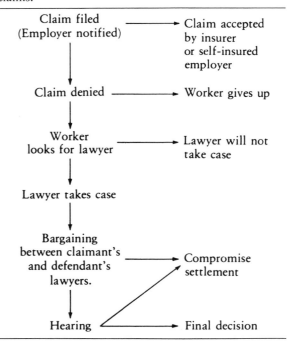

able from a formal trial: Witnesses are sworn, rules of evidence are followed, and testimony is recorded.

As a part of this legal proceeding medical questions are often raised. There may be disagreement about the degree of disability of a worker, when an injured worker is ready to return to work, or whether a particular injury or illness is work-related. To settle these disputes physicians may be called on to give their medical opinions about employees' disabilities. Many physicians do not like to testify in such hearings, and most are not prepared by their training or experience to assume this role. Their expertise may be challenged; moreover, they may be confused by the different meanings of legal and medical terminology.

In workers' compensation, decisions are based on legal definitions, and the legal distinction between disability and impairment is often unclear to physicians (see Chap. 12). A physician called in to testify about whether or not a worker is permanently and totally disabled may understand total disability as a state of physical helplessness and may therefore testify that the injured worker is not totally helpless. However, this standard is not what a workers' compensation board would apply; the term *disability* as used in workers' compensation proceedings means that wages have been lost, while *total disability* means that the injured worker loses wages as a result of not being able to perform gainful employment. This definition is in contrast to total *impairment,* which might imply that the injured worker could, in addition, not feed him- or herself or get out of bed. For example, a worker who has been exposed to silica at work may have substantially reduced pulmonary function and therefore impairment. However, if the worker continues to work at the same job, no wages have been lost and therefore no disability payment is made. Many states, however, offer specified payments for disfigurement or losses of sight, hearing, or limbs, with compensation based on impairment and not on disability (Table 11-2).

Table 11-2. Income benefits for scheduled injuries in selected jurisdictions (as of January 1, 1986)*

Jurisdiction	Arm at shoulder	Hand	Thumb	First finger	Foot
Alabama	$ 48,840	$ 37,400	$13,640	$ 9,460	$ 30,580
Alaska	59,000	45,400	14,000	8,700	39,700
California	58,975	53,540	7,595	3,360	33,740
Connecticut	123,864	100,044	37,715	21,438	74,636
Delaware	58,923	51,852	17,677	11,785	37,710
Georgia	34,875	24,800	9,300	6,200	20,925
Illinois	120,275	97,244	35,827	20,472	79,331
Mississippi	26,600	19,950	7,980	4,655	16,625
New York	46,800	36,600	11,250	6,900	30,750
Washington	36,000	32,400	12,960	8,100	25,200
Wisconsin	50,000	44,800	17,920	6,270	28,000
Federal employees	305,729	239,096	73,493	45,075	200,880
U.S. longshoremen	185,715	145,239	44,643	27,381	122,024

*Amounts in table reflect maximum potential entitlement.
Source: Reprinted with the permission of the Chamber of Commerce of the United States of America from *Analysis of Workers' Compensation 1986* © 1986 Chamber of Commerce of the United States of America.

While physicians may feel that they have not been trained adequately for their role in workers' compensation, workers do need their support in this area. A lack of assistance may mean unnecessary financial hardship for the victim of an occupational injury or disease. The best way a physician can help identify a work-related disease or injury is by taking an occupational history (see Chap. 3). If the physician suspects a work-related disease or injury, the patient should be informed of the right to receive workers' compensation and the time limits on such claims. (The period for filing a claim generally begins when the patient is informed that the disease is work-related.) Physicians should also suggest the possibility of seeking legal counsel, and they can provide direct help by completing any required reports, including descriptions of the illness or injury and why it is believed to be work-related. The extent of probable disability should also be noted (see Chap. 12). None of these steps requires testimony before a workers' compensation board; most workers' compensation claims are either paid without contest or settled without a hearing.

The National Institute for Occupational Safety and Health has published *A Guide to the Work-Relatedness of Disease* (rev. ed., 1979) (edited by S. Kusnetz and M. K. Hutchison). It proposes that such a determination be made on the basis of evidence of disease, epidemiologic data, evidence of exposure, and validity of testimony. A primary care physician may be the only person willing and able to provide documentation for an employee wishing to file a workers' compensation claim. Support for valid compensation claims not only assists injured workers but also helps to ensure that employers and their insurance carriers will shoulder the costs that result from workplace hazards. If these costs are not paid under workers' compensation, they will be borne by workers and their families or by all of us through our share of the costs of third-party medical payments, welfare, Social Security, and other public support programs.

THE ADEQUACY OF WORKERS' COMPENSATION FOR OCCUPATIONAL INJURIES

The fundamental problems of the common law scheme were that litigation was a necessary element of compensation and that it was very difficult for workers to win suits against their employers. Even when workers won negligence suits, payments were made long after they were injured, and a large amount of each settlement was diverted for legal fees. Today workers with minor injuries covered by workers' compensation generally can expect to receive payments promptly and without a contest. In fact, less than 10 percent of all claims for occupational injuries—as opposed to occupational diseases—are contested.

Under workers' compensation, insurance carriers or self-insured employers have the right to contest a claim. A claim may be contested because the injury is not considered work-related, for example, or because the claim is for a larger settlement than the insurer is willing to pay. However, in most injury cases the employer or insurance carrier has little incentive to contest because proof of eligibility is easy, and the potential gain to the insurer of postponing or eliminating small payments is not enough to offset the legal costs of pursuing a claim. For expensive injury claims such as permanent total disability and death claims, insurance companies are much more likely to contest. Even if they do not win, a contest enables them to keep the settlement money temporarily, invest it, and receive investment income until the case is closed and the claimant paid. Since a contest delays the date of payment, this investment income is an incentive to contest even those cases that the insurer is very likely to lose. The higher the potential settlement, the stronger the incentive to contest. This analysis is supported by the fact that claims for permanent disability and death are contested five times more frequently than are claims for temporary disability.

Aside from the incentives to contest major claims, several other important problems can be cited in the more than 50 workers' compensation systems in the United States. In theory, workers' compensation should cover all employees; however, many states exempt agricultural employees, household workers, or state and municipal employees. Another problem is that, while compensation systems generally provide replacement for close to two-thirds of lost wages for temporary disability, benefits for victims of permanent disability are characterized by low maximum weekly ceilings and low statutory limits on total benefits, with the worker generally receiving the smaller of two-thirds of lost wages or the state maximum benefit. The maximum weekly benefit provided varies widely among the states: the highest on Jan-

uary 1, 1986, was in Alaska ($1114) and the lowest in Mississippi ($133) (Table 11-3). Many jurisdictions do not provide for cost-of-living adjustments, so that a person injured 20 years ago but still disabled may receive total disability payments of only $10 to $20 a week. They also do not account for the increased wages that would have been earned if the employee had continued to work.

MEDICOLEGAL ROADBLOCKS TO COMPENSATION FOR OCCUPATIONAL DISEASES

The burden of proving that occupational injuries arose "out of and in the course of employment" is

Table 11-3. Maximum weekly benefits for total disability provided by workers' compensation statutes of selected states (as of January 1, 1986)

Jurisdiction	Fraction of worker's wage	Maximum weekly benefit (to nearest dollar)
Alabama	$2/3$	303 (SAWW)
Alaska	$4/5$ of worker's spendable earnings	1114
California	$2/3$ up to $4/5$ of worker's spendable earnings	224
District of Columbia	$2/3$	432 (SAWW)
Florida	$2/3$	315 (SAWW)
Iowa	$4/5$ of worker's spendable earnings	598 (200% of SAWW)
Massachusetts	$2/3$	360 (SAWW)
Michigan	$4/5$ of worker's spendable earnings	375 (90% of SAWW)
Mississippi	$2/3$	133
New Hampshire	$2/3$	462 (150% of SAWW)
New York	$2/3$	300
North Carolina	$2/3$	294 (SAWW)
Ohio	72% first 12 weeks, then $2/3$	365 (SAWW)
Pennsylvania	$2/3$	347 (SAWW)
Texas	$2/3$	217
West Virginia	$7/10$	333 (SAWW)
Federal employees	$2/3$ to $3/4$*	871 to 890
U.S. longshoremen	$2/3$	595 (twice NAWW)

*Maximum is $3/4$ if one dependent or more.
Key: SAWW = State's average weekly wage; NAWW = national average weekly wage.
Source: Reprinted with the permission of the Chamber of Commerce of the United States of America from *Analysis of Workers' Compensation 1986* © 1986 Chamber of Commerce of the United States of America.

Table 11-4. Roadblocks to compensation for occupational disease

Limitations of medical science	Statutory limitations	Other limitations
Difficulty of differential diagnosis	Time limits	Lack of exposure records (duration and intensity)
Lack of epidemiologic and toxicologic studies	Burden of proof	
Multiple causal pathways	Restrictive definitions of disease	
Limitations of physician training		

usually straightforward. However, workers with occupational illnesses face a different situation (Table 11-4). The workers' compensation system expects a physician to say whether or not a worker's illness was caused by or aggravated by work. Physicians are asked, "Was this illness caused by workplace conditions?" This is a question for which medical science often does not have a simple answer.

Many aspects of occupational diseases make the disabled worker's burden of proof difficult to sustain. Physicians may not realize that their patients may have become ill as a result of workplace exposures. Many physicians are not able to identify occupational diseases because their medical training in this has been inadequate; many have not even been trained in taking occupational histories. Furthermore, the signs and symptoms of most occupational diseases are not uniquely related to an occupational exposure. Medical and epidemiologic knowledge may be insufficient to distinguish clearly a disease of occupational origin from one of nonoccupational origin. For example, shortness of breath, an important symptom of occupational lung disease, is also associated with other chronic lung diseases.

Another complicating factor is that a disease may have multiple causes only one of which is occupational exposure. A worker who smokes and is exposed to ionizing radiation at work may develop lung cancer. Since both cigarette smoke and ionizing radiation are well-established risk factors

for lung cancer, it may be impossible to say which of these two factors "caused" the disease. In many cases occupational disease may develop many years after exposure began, and perhaps many years after exposure ceased. Consequently, memories of events and exposures may be unclear, and records of employment may not be available.

Some occupational injuries occur as a result of extended exposure to a hazard. These are "cumulative trauma" injuries, such as carpal tunnel syndrome, noise-induced hearing loss, and chronic low back pain. As with chronic occupational diseases, it may be difficult to prove the work-relatedness of these injuries. Moreover, records of exposure to occupational hazards are not often kept, so that even when a worker knows the type, level, and duration of exposure, no written evidence of this can be presented.

These aspects of occupational disease mean that many victims do not even suspect that their disease is job-related. For those who do and wish to make a claim, the causal relationship between disease and workplace exposures may be very difficult to establish. These are major reasons why so few claims for compensation for occupational disease are filed. A study of occupational disease in Washington and California revealed that, of the 51 probable cases of occupational respiratory conditions, only one was reported as a workers' compensation claim.

When claims for chronic occupational disease are filed, many are contested by the insurance car-

Table 11-5. Percent of alleged occupational disease cases controverted (contested) by category of disease

Category	Percent
Dust disease	88
Disorders due to repeated trauma	86
Respiratory conditions due to toxic agents	79
Cancers and tumors	46
Poisoning	37
Skin diseases	14
Disorders due to physical agents	10
Other	54
All diseases	63*

*In contrast, the percentage for all injuries is 10 percent.
Source: Adapted from PS Barth, HA Hunt. Workers' compensation and work-related illnesses. Cambridge: MIT Press, 1980.

Table 11-6. Delays in compensation for occupational disease by category of disease

Category	Mean number of days from notice to insurer to first payment
Skin diseases	59
Dust diseases	390
Respiratory conditions due to toxic agents	389
Poisoning	111
Disorders due to physical agents	79
Disorders due to repeated trauma	362
Cancers and tumors	260
Other illnesses	180*

*In contrast, the mean delay for all injuries is 43 days.
Source: Adapted from PS Barth, HA Hunt. Workers' compensation and work-related illnesses. Cambridge: MIT Press, 1980.

rier or self-insured employer (Table 11-5). Therefore, payments to disabled workers are delayed and uncertain (Table 11-6). Workers with chronic occupational diseases wait an average of more than a year to receive compensation payments. In addition, administrative and legal costs absorb many of the resources devoted to compensating occupational diseases.

ESTABLISHING WORK-RELATEDNESS FOR COMPENSATION

The burden of proving that disease is occupational in origin lies with workers. They must find physicians who are convinced that their illnesses are occupational in origin or that their illnesses were aggravated or hastened by occupational exposures. Physicians must then be able to convince referees who hear the cases that the diseases are indeed work-related.

The burden of proof might at first seem to be impossible for those diseases that are not uniquely occupational in origin. For example, lung cancer may be caused by smoking, air pollution (although not definitely established), occupational or non-occupational radiation exposure, or all of these factors.

Suppose that a worker with lung cancer has smoked cigarettes, has had diagnostic x-rays, and has also been occupationally exposed to ionizing radiation in a uranium mine. Since occupational lung cancer does not have distinctive clinical features, an expert medical witness, using clinical judgment, cannot say that the disease is without question occupational in origin. The expert witness cannot even say with certainty that occupational exposure to ionizing radiation was one of several causes or if it hastened the onset of the cancer. At best all that can be determined is that the worker has an increased risk of lung cancer as a result of the job. In this case the legal standard is that there must be a "preponderence of evidence" that the disease is occupational in origin, or the case is unlikely to be settled in favor of the disabled worker. A "preponderence of evidence" means that it is more likely than not (probability greater than 50 percent) that the illness in question was caused by, aggravated by, or hastened by workplace exposure.

In some cases workers' compensation laws have been written so that payment of a claim may be denied even though convincing evidence is presented that the illness was caused by or aggravated by the worker's employment. Some states require that a disease not be "an ordinary disease of life." In other words, diseases such as emphysema and hearing loss may not be compensable because they often occur among people with no occupational exposure. More than 20 states have a related requirement that diseases are only compensable if they are "peculiar to" or "characteristic of" a worker's occupation.

All jurisdictions have a statute of limitations (often one or two years) on claims for workers' compensation. A two-year statute of limitation means that the claim must be filed by the worker within two years of a given event. A time limit of two years after the worker has learned that a disease is work-related imposes no particular hardship on occupational disease victims. In some states, however, the time period begins when the disease becomes symptomatic, even if this takes place before the disease is diagnosed or determined to be work-related. The latter policy for starting the statute of limitation may be a special problem if the worker's physician is not familiar with the occupational disease. The most burdensome statutes require that a claim be filed one or two years after exposure. Since chronic occupational diseases commonly do not manifest themselves until five, ten, twenty, or more years after exposure, such rules effectively eliminate the possibility of compensation for workers with these illnesses. In a recent study, occupational disease compensation among a group of asbestos insulators was only half as great in states with these restrictive statutes of limitation as in other states. Time limits for filing workers' compensation claims are described in Table 11-7.

THE PROBLEM OF COMPROMISE SETTLEMENTS

A workers' compensation claim that is denied by the employer or insurer does not automatically go to a hearing. The injured worker must first find a lawyer who will take the case (see Fig. 11-1). The lawyer's fee is often based on the portion of the award attributed to lost wages, which means that the lawyer's fee will be small in a small award and that the lawyer will receive nothing if the claim is denied. Thus, it is hard for injured or ill workers to find lawyers to represent them when claims are small or success is unlikely.

Lawyers generally prefer to bargain informally with the defendant's lawyers rather than go to trial. If a compromise settlement can be reached prior to trial, no preparation for a hearing is necessary, and the lawyer will therefore have more time to work on other cases and earn additional income. A settlement reached outside the courtroom is called a compromise settlement because the amount paid to the claimant generally is a compromise between the maximum amount that the claimant could receive in a court decision and the amount (if any) of the settlement if the claimant lost.

In the face of protracted litigation with uncertain results, a compromise settlement may seem very attractive to an injured worker who may have no wage income for a considerable period and may be facing large medical bills. The injured worker may therefore prefer a small settlement paid immediately to a much larger but uncertain settlement that would not be available for one or two years. Especially where the worker does not foresee a quick return to work, a settlement may be accepted that might seem quite small to an outside observer. Insurers may use their knowledge of the financial pressures on the claimant to obtain a small settlement; they will thus contest, delaying the time when the case is closed in the hope of obtaining a small compromise settlement.

The compromise settlement will usually be paid in a lump sum to the injured worker and the attorney. This lump sum settlement will take the place of future payments for lost earnings and medical and rehabilitation costs. Many compromise settlements also release the insurer from future liability: If the claimant's condition should change at a later date or if future medical needs

Table 11-7. Time limits on filing occupational disease claims in selected jurisdictions (as of January 1, 1986)

Jurisdiction	Time limit on claim filing
Alabama	Within 2 years after injury, death, or last payment; radiation—within 2 years after disability or death and claimant knows or should know relation to employment.
California	Disability—within 1 year from injury or last payment; death—within 1 year after death and in no case more than 240 weeks after injury, except for asbestos-related disease claims. Date of injury is defined as when claimant is disabled and knows or should know of relation to employment.
Colorado	Within 3 years after commencement of disability or death; within 5 years in case of ionizing radiation, asbestosis, silicosis, or anthracosis.
Massachusetts	Within 1 year after injury or death; delay excusable.
Michigan	Within 2 years after claimant knows or should know of relation to employment.
New York	Within 2 years after disability or death, or 2 years after claimant knows or should know of relation to employment.
North Carolina	Within 2 years after disablement, death, or last payment; radiation—within 2 years after incapacity and claimant knows or should know relation to employment.
Oregon	Within 5 years after last exposure and within 180 days after disablement or physician informs claimant of disablement. 10 years after last exposure for radiation disease.
Utah	Within 1 year after claimant knows or should know relation to employment, but no later than 3 years after death; permanent partial disability—within 2 years.
Virginia	Within 2 years after diagnosis is first communicated to worker or within 5 years after exposure, whichever is first; within 3 years after death, occurring within limit for disability.
Federal employees	Within three years after injury, death, or disability and claimant knows or should know relation to employment; delay excusable.
U.S. longshoremen	Within 1 year after injury, death, last payment, or knowledge of relation to employment.

Source: Reprinted with the permission of the Chamber of Commerce of the United States of America from *Analysis of Workers' Compensation 1986* © 1986 Chamber of Commerce of the United States of America.

were inadequately estimated, the insurer would not incur the costs of any increased disability or medical or rehabilitation expenses. The injured worker who has accepted a "compromise and release" settlement may later need additional medical care but not have the resources to pay for that care.

For example, a worker with a back injury was denied compensation by his employer, who claimed that the injury was not work-related. He then took action that led to his being offered a lump sum settlement:

I went to my union representative and filled out the forms for the industrial accident board, and about three weeks later they sent me an award which was about $600 . . . and I wouldn't take it.

But then I applied for an attorney and talked to my attorney, and then filed suit. They turned around and told my attorney that they would consider [the injury] an industrial accident. So, I never did go to court. All they did was talk to my lawyer. They settled out of court. My lawyer told me while I was in the hospital that they wanted to settle it for $7,500. The fee for him [would be] $2,500.*

*Adapted from Subcommittee on Labor, Committee on Labor, and Public Welfare, U.S. Senate. Hearings on the National Workers' Compensation Standards Act, 1974. Statement of Lawrence Barefield.

If the settlement of $7,500 was the result of a compromise and release agreement, the insurer or employer will not be liable for any future disability or medical costs resulting from this injury.

RECOMMENDATIONS OF THE NATIONAL COMMISSION

As part of the Occupational Safety and Health Act of 1970 Congress established the National Commission on State Workmen's Compensation Laws to "undertake a comprehensive study and evaluation of State workmen's compensation laws in order to determine if such laws provide an adequate, prompt, and equitable system of compensation." In 1972 the Commission released its report, which described many problems of workers' compensation and made many recommendations for improving state workers' compensation systems including these seven "essential" recommendations:

1. Compulsory coverage. Employees could not lose coverage by agreeing to waive their rights to benefits.
2. No occupational or numerical exemptions to coverage. All workers, including agricultural and domestic workers, should be covered. All employers, even if they have only one employee, should be covered.
3. Full coverage of work-related diseases—the elimination of arbitrary barriers to coverage such as highly restrictive time limits, occupational disease schedules, and exclusion of "ordinary diseases of life."
4. Full medical and physical rehabilitation services without arbitrary limits.
5. Employees' choice of jurisdiction for filing interstate claims.
6. Adequate weekly cash benefits for temporary total disability, permanent total disability, and fatal cases.
7. No arbitrary limits on duration or sum of benefits.

Since this report was issued, many states have changed their statutes to follow the recommendations of the National Commission. By increasing coverage and raising benefits, they have substantially improved the value of workers' compensation to injured employees. However, general changes in coverage have done little to discourage the litigation of occupational disease claims and costly occupational injury claims.

THE FUTURE OF WORKERS' COMPENSATION

The common law system in effect during the nineteenth century was time-consuming, inefficient (because of litigation costs), and uncertain. Workers' compensation was designed to minimize litigation, but in spite of the change to a no-fault system more than 80 percent of all compensation claims for chronic occupational diseases are contested (see Table 11-5), and almost half of all injury claims for permanent total disability or death are also contested. This process of contests leads to delays of a year or more in settling workers' compensation claims (see Table 11-6). The settlements may be compromised and may thereby leave claimants seriously undercompensated. Also, legal fees, commonly 15 to 20 percent of the compensation award for lost wages, must be paid by the claimant. For cases of permanent total disability from occupational disease for which the average award for lost wages was about $9,700 in 1975, the average worker received only about $8,000 after legal costs were paid.

Two essential elements of workers' compensation that lead to so many contested cases are (1) the necessity of proving that a disease is work-related, and (2) the fact that large medical and wage replacement payments to compensated workers come directly from their employers or employers' insurance carriers. The first element leaves room for much legal argument; the second gives considerable incentive for employers or their insurance carriers to pursue such arguments. If contesting claims were less rewarding, more difficult, and less likely to be successful, employers might instead find it cheaper to pay them, thereby reducing the amount of litigation in the system.

In one proposed reform aimed at eliminating incentives for litigation, benefits would be paid from industry-wide funds rather than by individual employers or their insurance carriers. This plan would mean that individual employers or carriers would not gain financially by contesting an award and would thereby have little incentive to do so. A concern about such an arrangement, however, is that if workers submit claims for nonoccupational injuries and illnesses, insurers would have little incentive to screen out such claims.

A second proposed reform would establish expert medical boards to make decisions about the compensability of each contested case of alleged occupational disease as soon as a claim was denied by the employer's insurance carrier. If the medical board ruled that a disease was occupational in origin, the burden of proof would be lifted from the worker. The employer or insurer would be able to contest the decision of the medical board, but there would remain a strong presumption that the claim was valid.

Another way of reducing the burden of proof of causation would be to establish presumptive standards. A presumptive standard defines a level of evidence sufficient to demonstrate legally a causal relationship between occupation and disease. For example, a history of ten years of work in a coal mine, combined with specific medical test results consistent with coal workers' pneumoconiosis ("black lung"), could be defined as legally sufficient evidence to presume that a specific disease is work-related. An employer or insurance company would then have the burden of proving that the disease was not work-related to avoid paying the claim.

The compensation of victims of occupational disease may also be improved through publicly funded programs such as Social Security Disability Insurance (SSDI). Currently, SSDI offers disability payments to people suffering from total disability, whether or not that disability is work-related. If SSDI were broadened to cover partial disability, those unable to receive workers' compensation disability payments would still receive income support. Similarly, a mandatory medical insurance program would assure medical benefits for treatment of injuries and illnesses regardless of cause.

Other countries have workers' compensation systems with considerably less controversy surrounding compensation for occupational diseases. Part of the reason for this is these countries have social programs that provide medical benefits and disability benefits that are substantially greater than those provided to many American workers; thus, a worker who does not receive workers' compensation still can pay for needed medical care and continue to help support the family through disability payments. Countries with national health systems such as Great Britain and Sweden provide free medical care whether or not illnesses are occupational; Belgium and Denmark have excellent social insurance and disability programs, which provide a significant amount of wage replacement for disabled workers whether or not their disability is work-related.

BIBLIOGRAPHY

Ashford NA. Economic issues. II. Workmen's compensation. In Crisis in the workplace. Cambridge: MIT Press, 1976.
Provides a good summary of the goals of workers' compensation, the problems in meeting these goals, and how well they are actually met. The shortest overview among the references cited here.

Barth PS, Hunt HA. Workers' compensation and work-related illnesses. Cambridge: MIT Press, 1980.
The most complete description available of how workers' compensation programs handle occupational diseases. Describes how different states compensate occupational diseases and gives an overview of litigation and settlement of workers' compensation disease claims in the United States. Also reviews workers' compensation in other countries.

Chamber of Commerce of the United States. Analysis of

workers' compensation laws. Washington DC, 1986.
An annual review of workers' compensation laws in the United States and Canada. Compensation statutes are continually changing, and reading this review is one way of keeping up-to-date on the coverage, payment levels, and administrative arrangements of different laws.

Kusnetz S, Hutchison MK, eds. A guide to the work-relatedness of disease. revised ed. Washington DC: NIOSH, 1979.
Designed primarily as an aid to state agencies and others concerned with occupational disease compensation, this presents one method for assembling and evaluating evidence that may be relevant in determining the work-relatedness of a disease in an individual. Information on 14 disease-producing agents is presented to illustrate the decision-making process.

National Commission on State Workmen's Compensation Laws. Report and compendium on workmen's compensation. Washington DC: US Government Printing Office, 1972 and 1973.
The National Commission was created by the OSHA Act of 1970 to evaluate the status of workers' compensation. It undertook a 2-year study. The Compendium is a descriptive report on workers' compensation in 1973, while the Report makes recommendations to upgrade workers' compensation programs.

Selikoff IJ, ed. Disability compensation for asbestos-associated disease in the United States. New York: Mt. Sinai School of Medicine, 1983.
Reviews the asbestos occupational health problem in detail and discusses the workers' compensation and tort litigation experience of asbestos-exposed workers.

Somers HM, Somers AR. Workmen's compensation. New York: Wiley, 1954.
A general description of workers' compensation, written from a policy perspective, which was so well done that it is still worth reading decades later.

US Department of Labor, Assistant Secretary for Policy, Evaluation and Research. An interim report to congress on occupational diseases. Washington DC, 1980.
Report of a task force in the U.S. Department of Labor that conducted a study of the compensation of occupational respiratory diseases. Discusses the problems of compensating occupational diseases and suggests ways of improving that compensation.

12
Work Incapacity, Impairment, and Disability Evaluation

Jay Himmelstein and Glenn S. Pransky

Basic knowledge needed by clinicians for treating work incapacity and performing effective impairment and disability evaluations includes an awareness of the distinction between impairment and disability, the regulations of specific disability systems, familiarity with the impairment rating process, and a sensitivity to the social and legal contexts of disability. The health care provider willing to become more informed about the process of impairment and disability determinations can provide an important service to patients.

Patients frequently present to clinicians with a chief complaint (or symptom) of inability to work. Such visits may be triggered by (1) the patient's need for medical treatment to return to work, or (2) a requirement for medical evaluation or certification of "disability" by employers, insurance companies, or government agencies. The medical evaluation and treatment of work incapacity is surprisingly complicated, both medically and sociologically, and provides unique challenges to the clinician.

The purpose of this chapter is to increase clinicians' effectiveness in dealing with work incapacity by describing (1) key definitions related to the disability evaluation process, (2) common features of disability insurance plans, (3) the clinician's role in the disability evaluation process, and (4) the unresolved controversies and potential role conflicts for the clinician.

In reviewing the variety of compensation plans and the associated roles for the health care provider, it is important to recognize a few key concepts. Most important is the distinction between *impairment* and *disability*.

Impairment is defined as the loss of function of an organ or part of the body compared to what previously existed. Ideally, impairment can be defined and described in purely medical terms and quantified in such a way that a reproducible measurement is developed (for example, severe restrictive lung disease with a total lung capacity of 1.6 liters).

Disability, on the other hand, is usually defined in terms of the impact of an impairment on societal or work functions. A disability evaluation would therefore take into account the loss of function (impairment) *and* the patient's work requirements and home situation. Certain agencies use a more restrictive definition of disability; for example, the Social Security Administration defines disability as "inability to perform any substantial gainful work." Often, private disability insurance defines disability as an "inability to perform the essential tasks of the usual employment." In all cases, the determination of disability is predicated on an assessment of impairment, followed by a determination of the loss in occupational or societal functioning that results from the impairment. In general, the determination of impairment is performed by a health care professional (usually a physician), whereas the determination of disability and extent of disability may be done by a person who is not a physician using physician-generated information on impairment.

A worker who is injured and cannot do any

work because of the injury is *totally disabled.* If this person can work but has some limitations and cannot do his or her customary work, a *partial disability* exists. Either type of disability is *temporary* as long as a complete resolution of the impairment is expected. When no significant functional improvement is expected, it is inferred that a *medical end-result* (sometimes called maximal medical improvement) has been achieved. Often, disability compensation systems assume that if a condition has not changed over a one-year period, then a medical end-result has occurred, and a temporary (partial or total) disability would then be legally regarded as a *permanent disability.*

A *work-related* injury or disease has resulted from some exposure (physical, chemical, biological, or psychological) in the workplace. In acute traumatic injuries, the relationship of the injury to the workplace is usually clear (Fig. 12-1). In chronic conditions, however, it may be difficult to be medically certain of the relationship between work and disease. It is recommended that the physician's determination of work-relatedness should be based on the evidence of disease, the exposure history, and the epidemiologic evidence linking exposure and disease [1].

Health professionals must be aware, however, that the legal definition of cause may be less exacting than the medical definition and that most disability systems are based on the legal standard. A legal definition of a work-related condition is one ". . . arising out of or in the course of employment" or "caused or exacerbated by . . . employment" [2]. Thus, a preexisting condition, unrelated to work, that becomes substantially worse because of work may legally be work-related. The legal standard of proof is that a condition is work-related if it is "more likely than not" that the condition would not have been present had the work exposure not occurred. (See Chapters 3 and 11 for more discussion of work-relatedness.)

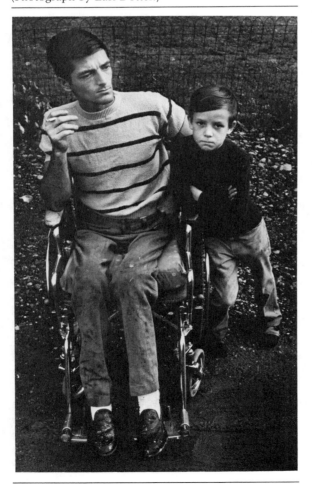

Fig. 12-1. Coal miner disabled from mine roof fall and his son.
(Photograph by Earl Dotter.)

DISABILITY COMPENSATION SYSTEMS

Some of the confusion regarding disability assessment stems from the multitude of disability plans, since each has its own definition of disability and criteria for impairment. The majority of compensation systems, however, fall into one of three major categories (Table 12-1).

Table 12-1. Compensation systems

Program	Eligibility	Source of benefits	Basis for claim	Clinician's role
1. WORKERS' COMPENSATION (WC) SYSTEMS—"CAUSE" OF DISABILITY IS DETERMINANT.				
State Federal Railroad workers	Private employees Federal employees Railroad employees	Employer insurance Taxes Employer	Work-related illness or injury	Evaluate work-relatedness, impairment, and disability
Black lung benefits	Coal miners	Tax on coal	Lung disease	Report chest x-ray, pulmonary and function tests and examination results only
2. PROGRAMS FOR SEVERELY DISABLED—INABILITY TO PERFORM GAINFUL ACTIVITIES IS DETERMINANT.				
Social Security Disability Insurance (SSDI)	Contributing workers	Workers' contributions Taxes	Severe disability	Evaluate and report impairment
Supplemental Security Income (SSI)	The aged, blind, and severely disabled			
3. PRIVATE DISABILITY PLANS—REGARDLESS OF CAUSE, PROTECT INCOME IF UNABLE TO PERFORM REGULAR JOB.				
Short-Term Disability (STD) Long-Term Disability (LTD)	Enrolled workers	Payments by employee, employer, or union	Any illness preventing usual employment	Evaluate impairment and disability

Occupational physicians are most familiar with workers' compensation insurance, which is offered to federal, state, and private employees. All of these plans are designed to provide compensation for medical expenses and lost wages due to work-related injuries and illnesses.

The federal government sponsors the major compensation programs for the severely disabled. These programs pay a limited amount of compensation to those who are unable to achieve gainful employment regardless of the cause of disability.

Private disability insurance is often purchased by individuals or provided as an employer or union benefit and is designed to provide compensation for those who are unable to work at their regular jobs regardless of the cause of disability.

So, a patient who can no longer work because of injury or illness might receive support from his or her employer's insurer, a federal or state agency, or a private insurance policy that has been purchased.

Although each plan has different eligibility criteria and payment schedules, all share a few common features:

1. In every plan, many people or employers at risk of financial losses contribute to a pool, from which a few individuals are reimbursed. This uses the concept of *shared risk*. The cost of entering the pool for an individual is partially determined by the actuarial risk of future events for that person. Thus, private disability insur-

ance (often purchased to supplement benefits available through Social Security for non-work-related disability) is much more expensive per year for a 55-year-old than for a 20-year-old, since the older worker has a higher risk of disabling medical illness. Workers' compensation insurance is more expensive per employee for a construction company (higher risk of injury to employees) than for a stock brokerage firm.

2. Because payments into the pool are predictable, *finite resources* are available to the potential recipients in each plan. Therefore, eligibility criteria are structured so that the limited resources go to those in greatest need. Workers' compensation plans often do not replace lost wages for fewer than 6 days of absence from work, since doing so might greatly increase the cost of the program. Many private disability insurance plans do not begin coverage until 30 days to 6 months of illness absence has occurred. The Social Security Disability Income (SSDI) plan does not begin payments until a year of sickness absence has occurred.

3. Before medical evaluation of impairment, a potential recipient of benefits must first demonstrate *legal eligibility*. The basis for eligibility is different in each plan. For example, to be eligible for SSDI, one must have worked for 5 of the past 10 years. Workers' compensation covers only regular employees—not consultants or subcontractors. Private disability insurance often does not cover illness occurring during the first 60 to 90 days of enrollment.

4. *Medical information* on impairment is requested once a legal basis for a claim has been established. In every system, a medical diagnosis is necessary; in the workers' compensation system, physicians are also asked their opinions on the *work-relatedness* of employees' conditions, the prognosis for eventual return to work, and the restrictions or job accommodations that might be necessary to return the worker to employment.

5. The information from the physician, however, does not determine whether benefits are award-

ed or how much is paid; all of these systems are under *administrative control*. In the SSDI system, an administrator-physician team reviews the medical information from the evaluating physician and compares it with specific criteria for eligibility. In the workers' compensation systems, if there is a significant discrepancy between the employer's report of an injury and the physician's report, benefits may be withheld pending an investigation by the insurance company.

6. *Benefits are limited* and are intended to provide only a proportion of lost wages, medical expenses related to the specific impairment, and vocational rehabilitation. Only in rare circumstances are workers' compensation benefits intended to punish gross negligence by an employer in causing the injury.

7. Any applicant has a *right of appeal* of an administrative or medical decision, with review by a third party. In the SSDI system, applicants who are initially denied benefits can appeal to a second administrator-physician team, then to a Social Security benefits coordinator, then to an administrative law judge, and finally to the federal courts, if desired. In most workers' compensation plans, the claimant can request an administrative hearing and be represented by an attorney. The agencies providing benefits also conduct periodic reviews of cases to verify that continued eligibility (disability) exists.

Workers' compensation insurance is reviewed in Chapter 11. To summarize, the United States does not have a unified workers' compensation law, and each state has developed its own system. In addition, there are a number of workers' compensation programs that are occupation-specific; these programs often have developed their own definitions of disability and related eligibility criteria. The Black Lung Program, for example, provides payments to coal miners with a documented work history and respiratory insufficiency meeting certain criteria. All disabling respiratory insufficiency is assumed to be related to mining if the miner meets a standard of number of years worked in the mines. Other examples of occupations with workers' compensation-type programs include railroad workers, longshoremen, military veterans, and municipal workers such as police and firefighters.

The purpose of each plan is to reimburse workers for medical expenses, rehabilitation expenses, and lost wages that result from a work-related injury or illness. Plans are designed to be nonadversarial so that, in most cases, limited benefits are paid to injured workers without the necessity of a formal hearing. In most cases of acute traumatic injuries (for example, fractures or lacerations occurring at work), the relationship to work is unquestionable and the system works reasonably well at compensating the injured worker. In many cases, however, the relationship to work is less clear, and the demand on the physician more complicated, as the following case illustrates.

A 50-year-old truck driver followed by his physician for 6 years because of chronic low back pain came to the physician stating "I cannot take it anymore." Although he could not recall a specific injury, he found that the requirements of driving a long-haul tractor trailer caused him severe discomfort that was no longer relieved by rest or analgesics. His back discomfort generally improved while he was on vacation but was clearly aggravated after more than 2 hours of driving or after any heavy lifting (at home or at work). He had been out of work for one week because of his discomfort and required a note from the physician before returning to work. Physical examination revealed a mild decrease in anterior flexion. X-rays were consistent with osteoarthritis of the spine. The patient wanted to know the physician's opinion on whether his back problems were due to his work as a truck driver, whether he should change his vocation because of his discomfort, and whether he should file a workers' compensation claim for work-related injuries.

This case illustrates some of the difficulties in evaluating and treating the patient with work incapacity. The patient went to the physician because his back discomfort was interfering with his

ability to do his job. Like most patients with chronic low back pain, his symptoms and examination findings were nonspecific. The standard recommendations of rest and avoidance of exacerbating activities met with transient success, but his symptoms reappeared with his return to work. It is logical at this point to explore with the patient any opportunity for altering the nature of the job demands at work, and, if no alternatives are available, for him to seek employment that would not exacerbate the symptoms. The patient, for a variety of reasons, however, may be reluctant to consider changing to another line of work, despite the discomfort associated with the current job.

With regard to causality, the high prevalence of nonspecific low back pain in the general population and the multifactorial etiology of this common condition make it impossible to say with medical certainty that this patient's back discomfort was caused in its entirety by his work. Several epidemiologic studies, however, have linked truck driving with a higher incidence of chronic disabling low back pain and have attributed this increase to excessive vibration, sitting, and heavy lifting [3]. Despite medical uncertainty, it is likely that most compensation systems would recognize this patient's low back pain as a condition that is aggravated by work and that the patient's medical bills and lost wages related to his back pain would be covered by workers' compensation insurance.

The Social Security Administration, in the U.S. Department of Health and Human Services, administers two plans that provide benefits to those unable to work regardless of the cause for the disability.

Social Security Disability Insurance (SSDI) is a true insurance plan in that all nongovernmental employees in the United States contribute to the plan through mandatory deductions from wages. Eligibility requires 5 years of contributions to the plan over the previous 10 years and is determined by the federal Social Security Administration. State rehabilitation commissions are given the responsibility of determining whether the applicant's impairment qualifies for benefits. To qualify, an impairment must be the result of a documented medical illness and must be expected to result in at least one year of inability to work, or death, but does not have to be a consequence of work. Once a claim is accepted, there is a 6-month waiting period until benefits begin. Claims are reevaluated periodically to determine that a severe impairment continues to exist, and updated medical information is requested. The condition must be as severe as the standard description listed in the Social Security Administration's publication *Disability Evaluation Under Social Security.* If a condition is not listed in the regulations, it must be medically equivalent to one that is listed. A sufficient impairment must result in inability to perform *any* gainful employment, not only the person's usual job. In cases where the impairment does not meet the established criteria, the examiner will take into account age, education, and prior work history in determining the likelihood that an applicant would be able to find any future employment. The following case illustrates the basic medical considerations involved in the Social Security disability determination process.

A 60-year-old male was referred for Social Security disability for evaluation related to chronic lung disease. The patient had worked as a maintenance worker since age 25 and had moderate exposure to asbestos when he worked as a "fireman" on a Navy ship during World War II. He smoked one to two packs of cigarettes a day for the past 42 years until quitting 6 months prior to this evaluation. He had been short of breath for 7 years. He became exhausted by merely dressing himself in the morning. Physical examination revealed him to be thin, with a respiratory rate of 18 at rest. His breath sounds were distant posteriorly, and there was no clubbing or cyanosis. Chest x-ray showed flattened diaphragms, emphysematous changes, and bilateral pleural plaques. His pulmonary function tests showed severe obstructive lung disease with an FEV_1 of 1.1 liters (35 percent of predicted), an FVC of 3.1 liters (68 percent of predicted), a TLV of 5.4 liters (80 percent of predicted), and an FEV_1/FVC ratio of 35 percent.

In this case, a patient with severe chronic lung disease was being evaluated for disability under Social Security. His exposure history was significant for occupational exposure to asbestos and nonoccupational exposure to cigarette smoke. His physical examination, chest x-ray, and pulmonary function tests were consistent with diagnoses of (1) severe obstructive lung disease and possible restrictive lung disease, and (2) asbestos-related pleural plaques.

A number of systems have been developed for the evaluation of severe pulmonary impairment. These systems are not identical in the level of impairment that is considered severe. For 20- and 60-year-old males who are each 70 inches tall, the FEV_1 values for "severe impairment" are different for each system (Table 12-2). Comparison of this

Table 12-2. Comparison of levels of FEV_1 required for severe impairment for 40- and 60-year-old males, 70 in. (178 cm) tall, in five different sets of criteria

Criteria	Actual FEV_1 (liters) and percent predicted*	
	Age	
	40	60
Social Security Administration (1979)	1.40 (35%)	1.40 (41%)
American Medical Association (1977)	2.19 (55%)	1.89 (55%)
Wilson, et al. (1964)	1.60 (40%)	1.23 (36%)
Gaensler, et al. (1966)	1.59 (40%)	1.37 (40%)
Department of Labor Proposed Black Lung Benefits (1978)	2.38 (60%)	2.06 (60%)

*Percent predicted is based on RJ Knudson, et al. The maximal expiratory flow volume curve. Am Rev Resp Dis 1976; 113:587.

patient's pulmonary function tests with the guidelines for SSDI demonstrate that people of this height who have an FEV_1 of less than 1.4 liters are considered disabled under Social Security.

The patient's occupational exposure to asbestos might have played a small etiologic role in the development of pulmonary insufficiency. It is worth noting however that this would have *no* effect on the patient's application for SSDI.

Supplemental Security Income (SSI) is a program, funded through federal taxes (not by employee contributions), for blind, disabled, or elderly people who do not qualify for SSDI. Although criteria for disability are identical to those for SSDI, benefits are generally lower and do not begin until the claimant's assets and benefits from all other sources are exhausted.

Private disability insurance is available from over 25 different insurers in the United States. These programs provide benefits supplementing SSDI and have much less stringent criteria for acceptance of claims. Usually, the claimant need only have his or her physician state that an impairment exists that prevents working at the usual job. Most plans provide a fixed income level for the first 2 years of disability, if one is unable to work at his or her usual job because of illness. Afterwards, full benefits are paid only if the claimant is totally disabled from (any type of) work; if the claimant can do work with lower wages than previously, the difference between current potential wages and prior wages determines the reimbursement level. Programs usually provide for maintenance of health insurance and certain other employee benefits, and benefits usually end at retirement age. Many variations and supplements exist that can be purchased by an employee. The next case illustrates a typical situation that would be covered through private disability insurance.

A 60-year-old male maintenance worker, who formerly smoked cigarettes, was referred by his employer for a return-to-work evaluation. The patient had been out of work for 3 months following hospitalization for an inferior myocardial infarction (MI). Despite a good medical regimen, the patient continued to have fatigue after minimal exertion but no chest pain. His home activities were limited to 20 minutes of walking twice a day. On physical examination he was in no acute distress, with a resting heart rate of 80 beats per minute. His lungs were clear to auscultation, and his heart sounds showed a normal rate and rhythm without murmur or gallop. The ECG showed evidence of his MI. A recent exercise test had been discontinued after 4 minutes because of fatigue, but there were no signs of active ischemia or arrhythmia. His job as a maintenance worker involved walking long distances in the plant, pushing a 45-kg (100-lb) maintenance cart, and performing scheduled and unscheduled machinery repair.

In summary, this patient showed evidence of cardiopulmonary deconditioning after a myocardial infarction. The patient demonstrated decreased exercise capability by his symptoms and exercise tolerance test performance. This deconditioning would probably prevent him from performing his normal job tasks. He had probably not achieved a medical end-result by the time of his evaluation. It would, therefore be appropriate to refer this patient to a cardiac rehabilitation program in an attempt to increase his exercise tolerance before making any judgment about permanent impairment. He would be supervised in a progressive exercise program, which might restore much of his exercise capacity. Until fit enough to return to work, this patient would be eligible for continued short-term disability compensation from his company-sponsored plan. This patient would *not* be eligible under Social Security because the disability was not expected to last more than one year and did not meet the relevant guidelines. Since outcome of rehabilitation efforts may be difficult to predict at the outset, the treating physician would want to monitor the patient's progress and reevaluate his disability once a plateau in reconditioning has been reached.

STEPS IN THE DISABILITY EVALUATION PROCESS

The following questions are involved in disability evaluation:

1. What is the patient's medical diagnosis?
2. Does the individual have any impairment related to this diagnosis? If an impairment is present, is it temporary or permanent?
3. What is the extent of any impairment? (see box on pages 171–173.)
4. Is the patient's impairment or disease caused or aggravated by work?
5. What is the impact of this impairment on the individual's ability to obtain employment in specific occupations and to perform specific jobs?
6. In consideration of the answers to the above questions, to what, if any, economic benefit is the individual entitled?

Physicians generally play a major role in answering the first four questions but not the last two. The answer to the fifth question often depends on the specialized skills of a vocational evaluation unit and is based on legal-administrative criteria. The last question is usually resolved by administrators using legal guidelines.

Physical examination findings that support the degree of impairment and the stated diagnosis are important. For example, SSDI claims without positive objective physical findings (symptoms without physical or laboratory findings) are rejected. Evaluations often include measurement of strength and endurance, length of scar, degree of visual impairment, and other relevant items (see box, pp. 171–173.) Serial measurement of these findings over time provides an objective basis for deciding whether a medical end-result has been achieved. Since the physician's office usually has meager resources to fully evaluate functional capacity, referral to an occupational therapist or vocational evaluation specialist for work capacity evaluation may be appropriate. A series of standardized tasks can be performed to document functional impairment [3].

The physician is often asked to determine whether the impairment is permanent or whether a medical end-result has been achieved. For example, in the first case, it is likely that the patient would feel better once he had been away from work for a few weeks. However, his physician's experience has shown that this patient consistently develops back pain soon after returning to this type of work. Although some improvement of symptoms is likely, the patient probably will not improve enough medically to allow him to continue working as a truck driver. Therefore, in terms of functional ability, a medical end-result has been achieved; although his discomfort is not likely to be permanent, the medical limitations to his working as a truck driver probably will not change.

At times, insurance companies or lawyers ask for a determination of permanency that seems to require a crystal ball. In many cases, the prognosis for functional improvement is uncertain. Pressures from a lawyer or insurer may be present to declare a medical end-result so that a case can be settled. However, it is important to communicate uncertainty, both to the patient and to others involved with the case; patients do not benefit from a premature medical determination of permanent disability.

In workers' compensation and in private-insurance disability cases, the physician is often asked whether the impairment is disabling—in what way it impedes the person's usual work. A clear job description is the basis for evaluating whether the employee can perform all the essential functions of the job. Often, this cannot be determined without knowing what accommodations at work might be available. So, in the second case, it cannot be determined whether the patient is totally disabled until it is known whether any alternate work is available. The same considerations apply to determining disability for private insurance. A visit to the workplace usually will resolve the lack of clarity that frequently is present in standard job de-

STANDARDIZED MEASURES OF IMPAIRMENT

Most systems providing disability benefits require objective evidence of functional loss. However, clinicians' assessments tend to integrate subjective impressions with objective data in their evaluations, since this integrative model has proved useful in treating patients. Therefore, impairment measurements may differ considerably among evaluators. A number of systems to standardize impairment measurement have been developed, such as the American Medical Association (AMA) *Guidelines to the Evaluation of Permanent Impairment,* to limit these differences. Any system that attempts to evaluate disability in the absence of detailed information on job requirements, however, will be seriously flawed. Although the AMA *Guidelines* were developed primarily to aid in legal determinations, they are arbitrary and their use is not widely accepted.

Why bother to develop standardized measures of impairment? First, since most reimbursement systems rely on objective medical data (physical examination findings and laboratory test results) to verify impairment, standardization might allow for a common method of describing impairment. Second, consistent examination methods and reliance on objective findings rather than on subjective descriptions would eliminate much of the conflict over degree of functional loss and resulting compensation benefits. Third, quantifiable measurements of residual function in various organ systems should be linked with data on functional ability required by various jobs; this linkage might be helpful in designing individualized rehabilitation programs. Finally, objective measurements of function have been shown to aid in measuring progress in a rehabilitation program, or lack of progress when a medical end-result has been reached.

For over 30 years, the AMA and the Social Security Administration (SSA) have worked to develop guides for objective impairment quantification. Both organizations' guides divide evaluations by organ systems, specifying the medical information required for the evaluation. The SSA guide provides threshold criteria for impairments sufficient for eligibility; the AMA guides express impairment as a percentage of total body function that has been lost. For example, the AMA guides provide reproducible information for impairment from hand injuries, allowing documentation of functional changes over time. The validity of these so-called standardized measures of impairment in predicting actual functional losses in other organ systems has not been established.

A number of problems frustrate attempts to develop measures of impairment that are reproducible, valid, and standardized. The absence of a "pre-injury" baseline evaluation usually forces the examiner to use population-derived norms to predict degrees of functional loss. For example, the results of simple lung function tests are often compared to the distribution of test results in a population, standardized by age, sex, height, and race, to determine what percentage of a predicted value is present in an individual. An individual who originally had large lung volumes and lost a significant percentage of function because of disease might have a substantial respiratory impairment but may still have "normal" lung volumes by testing. Conversely, another person may have always had lung volumes below the population-derived norm, and a slight decrease on lung function tests may result in a misleading label of "abnormal lung function." Exercise testing with oxygen uptake monitoring provides a much better measure of how well the lungs perform in their essential function of oxygen transport; these tests can reveal critical limitations of gas exchange not revealed by simple spirometric testing [4]. Therefore, a static test of lung volume might be quick and inexpensive but would not reveal information about actual ability that a test of function, such as exercise testing, shows. Inaccuracies caused by poor cardiovascular conditioning, lack of understanding, fear of test procedures, or poor motivation can confound even the best test in providing estimates of actual functional ability. A determination of medical end-result may be frustrated by an illness with a variable course or presentation, where signs and symptoms wax and wane.

Several devices have been developed to quantify musculoskeletal function. These devices measure ability to exert a rotational or linear force against a mobile or stationary object. Output of the device, which is usually reproducible, usually indicates the degree or distance of motion and the maximum force applied. Many programs have used these devices in assessment and rehabilitation of extremity injuries. These devices have not been shown to accurately predict ability to perform occupational tasks, since the actions required to operate them are usually unrelated to job tasks. Musculoskeletal function measurement is an area of intensive research, and new devices for assessment are frequently introduced. When considering purchase, the physician should carefully review the scientific data supporting any advantages over existing forms of assessment and rehabilitation.

The following case is an example of an impairment and disability evaluation, where standardized measurement of impairment had been attempted:

A physician had been treating a 58-year-old clerk for apparently non-work-related carpal tunnel syndrome of both hands, mainly the right (dominant) hand. Her job required filing, answering phones, and occasional typing. Six months after successful carpal tunnel surgery, her pain and numbness largely resolved, although she still complained of considerable weakness of the right hand. Physical examination showed a well-healed scar and considerable loss of sensation of the right hand in a median nerve distribution. Grip strength by dynamometer was 5.4 kg (12 lb) with the left hand, and 4.5 kg (10 lb) with the right. She had been out of work for 6 months, and the physician believed her condition had stabilized. She was concerned that "no one will hire me because I have hand problems" and wanted the physician to examine her for Social Security Disability Insurance (SSDI) eligibility.

1. What was the patient's medical diagnosis?

   Carpal tunnel syndrome: status—post-carpal tunnel release, with residual median nerve damage.

2. Was impairment present?

   Yes. There was loss of normal function of the right hand, and the information suggested that no further return of function was likely to occur.

3. What was the level of impairment?

   One could first quantify the impairment using the AMA guides. History and examination revealed that the left hand was normal; however, there was evidence of considerable sensory loss of the right hand. She stated that she could do most of the activities of self-care but had difficulty with digital dexterity: physical examination revealed considerable loss of two-point discrimination, pain sensation, and sensation to fine touch over the affected area; and decreased oppositional strength between the thumb and other fingers. According to the charts in the AMA guides, she had a 7 percent loss of motor function in the upper extremity caused by median nerve motor injury (20 percent loss of strength in the hand, multiplied by 35 percent loss of upper extremity strength). Similar calculations revealed a 22 percent loss of function in the upper extremity from sensory deficit. These values were combined for a 16 percent impairment of the whole person. This calculation has limited medical significance, although the structured examination could be repeated in the future to aid in determining whether any medical progress has been made.

For the SSDI application, the physician must provide a description of the patient's functional status by history and examination; it would be helpful to describe her attempts to move objects in the office. The evaluation report should also include a copy of the nerve conduction studies and the statement that a medical end-result had been reached.

4. Was the patient's impairment caused or aggravated by work?

No report of forceful or repetitive movements required at work was indicated. A careful review of the job tasks with the patient might have uncovered a history of unusual activities that might have exacerbated or even caused the carpal tunnel syndrome, such as folding large quantities of paper, typing on a manual typewriter, or using scissors extensively. Work-relatedness is not an issue in SSDI.

5. What was the impact of the impairment on the individual's ability to obtain employment or perform specific jobs?

The amount of impairment here may have interfered with typing and filing but may not have interfered with other duties. If these activities were required in the job, then the physician might have had to ask the patient to demonstrate her ability to perform these skills;

the exercise in the AMA guides would not have been helpful in determining disability. The actual abilities of the patient over an 8-hour workday are difficult to determine by a cursory office examination and are best determined by a vocational evaluation specialist with a thorough understanding of a patient's functional ability and job demands. The history of current household activities may also aid in assessment of functional ability.

6. To what, if any, economic benefits was this patient entitled?

It is unlikely that she would have initially received SSDI, since the criteria in *Disability Evaluation Under Social Security* require that both upper extremities be substantially affected by a process that "results in sustained disturbance of gross and dexterous movements in two extremities." If on case review she demonstrated limited education and work experience and impairment preventing performance of practically any job, her claim might have been accepted. The physician's input in this regard is not considered; Social Security disability determination services often employ vocational assessors to perform this function. However, if the patient were applying for private disability insurance, the physician may have to determine whether the essential job tasks could be performed by the patient.

scriptions and may have an important role in encouraging an employer to provide accommodations for an injured employee.

Most insurance systems theoretically reimburse individuals for loss of earning capacity caused by objective impairment. It is often difficult to determine whether sufficient impairment exists for one to qualify for benefits under a given plan. Physicians usually lack the experience, technical facilities, and ability to accurately estimate vocational

potential; in these situations, early involvement with a qualified vocational rehabilitation specialist is worthwhile. Specialized skills and a broad data base are required to predict residual earning capacity when an employee is no longer able to return to previous work. For example, factors related to worker autonomy, such as the availability of self-paced work, educational and experience levels, and self-employment, have been shown to be more important in determining disability status in patients with rheumatoid arthritis than the extent of medical findings [5]. In workers' compensation plans and in most private disability plans, the treating or reviewing physician is required only to determine that the impairment is sufficient to prevent work. However, in the Social Security, Veteran's Administration, and Black Lung programs, there are often specific criteria for impairment that determine whether one is eligible for benefits, which vary from plan to plan. For example, the Black Lung and Social Security programs have threshold pulmonary function values; if an applicant's lung function is better than the threshold, then he or she does not qualify for disability. In the Veteran's Administration system, the degree of lost function is expressed as a percentage of total lung function. Benefits are assigned based on the percentage of function lost; in contrast, the Social Security and Black Lung programs usually provide a fixed amount of benefits only if a worker is totally disabled according to the threshold criteria. Physicians are often frustrated with the arbitrary nature of the determination process. Under these criteria, some individuals with truly disabling impairments will be refused compensation, while others capable of gainful employment will receive benefits.

THE CLINICIAN'S ROLE

Within the disability evaluation process, three different and potentially conflicting roles for the clinician become clear: patient advocate, provider of information, and medical adjudicator. It is important to understand the requirements of each of these roles so that the patient can best be served.

Clinicians must not neglect their role as patient advocate in treating patients with work incapacity and, when appropriate, assisting them in obtaining benefits to the extent entitled by a particular disability system. The clinician should not let personal feelings about a specific disability or impairment rating system interfere with judgment in assisting patients.

As patient advocates, clinicians need to be aware that depression is often a complicating factor in the patient with long-term disability. Patients frequently are limited financially and socially by their work incapacity, and social isolation frequently accompanies isolation from the workplace. Patients may be upset at how they have been handled by the "system," especially if benefits have been delayed or denied. They may be angry at the apparent insensitivity of their employer, insurer, or physician and this anger often complicates their evaluation and treatment. Patients are often afraid of returning to the workplace where a serious injury occurred, or they may be afraid of being dismissed once they have successfully returned to work. Being aware of the complicated social, legal, and psychological state of disabled workers is an essential aspect of assisting their recovery. Appropriate referral for psychological diagnosis and treatment should be considered in every case of prolonged work incapacity. Mindful of the adverse psychological, physical, and economic consequences of disability, the clinician should be careful to avoid removing patients from gainful employment, whenever possible.

Patients may also have significant concerns about the disability evaluation itself. Since patients are aware that the outcome of the evaluation may determine their access to or continuation of benefits, they may feel the need to emphasize the extent of the disability to "prove" their case. They may have residual anger from previous examinations in which clinicians seemed unsympathetic or doubted their "true" disability.

As a patient gradually loses function because of a progressive disease process, the physician should anticipate the possibility that earning capacity may be lost and discuss this potential with the patient. Patients should be made aware of the potential loss of self-esteem and income and the uncertainty of receiving benefits while out of work. Actively assisting patients in vocational rehabilitation and early selection of jobs that will not conflict with physical limitations can avoid unnecessary time out of work. Physicians should learn of possible accommodations in the workplace by

REHABILITATION MANAGEMENT FOR WORK-RELATED INJURIES
—Charles D. DelTatto and
  Edward C. Swanson

The physical restoration and ultimate reorientation of injured workers has become a multifocal process involving a multidisciplinary team of professionals. Members of this team include physicians, physical therapists, occupational therapists, occupational health nurses, and safety personnel. In large corporations, all team members may be within the same health unit. For small employers, the team members may be consultants to the workplace or be professionals practicing in the community. Regardless of the setting, it is essential that the team be clearly identified and utilized.

Historically, occupational injuries have been grouped together with other injury cases and have been expected to respond to similar interventions. However, analysis of case outcomes reveals the need to rethink current management models and to give occupational injuries a more specialized approach.

On the surface, this approach may appear no different from any other acute medical model. However, here the processes of triage, diagnosis, and treatment are predicated on unique information: (1) a clear understanding of the worker's job, especially those physical demands contributing to the injury; and (2) environmental and other physical demands the worker will encounter.

Each member of the team must consider this information when designing an effective rehabilitation program that will result in return to work and avoidance of reinjury. This goal is achieved by early integration of physical restoration and injury prevention measures.

To facilitate this approach an early referral to physical or occupational therapy is desirable. In so doing, critical information required by the team will be gathered in a systematic way.

First, the job description at the time of injury should be requested from the occupational nurse or other appropriate person at the workplace. This description will form the baseline measurement for the physical restoration program and provide the framework for any specific medical release. Initial investigation of the factors that contributed to the injury should also begin. This information can be collected by the workplace safety officer or industrial nurse. A plan to eliminate or minimize factors that contributed to the injury should be implemented prior to the worker's return and should be coordinated with the physical restoration process. The therapist may also be able to assist in task redesign and worker instruction in proper material handling techniques, if deemed appropriate [1, 2].

Because the therapist, in most cases, will spend the greatest amount of time with the injured worker, he or she must act as investigator, mediator, and sounding board for the rest of the team.

Program design must be specific to the nature of the injury and expected physical demands. Simulated work tasks should also be incorporated into any restoration plan [3]. These tasks will serve as an objective measure of the worker's progress and form the basis of specific return-to-work recommendations.

Modification of treatment approach may be necessary and will largely depend on the team's ability to identify both the physical and emotional signs of any delayed recovery [4].

Frequent communication of critical information must be made among team members, allowing for a clear mutual understanding of where the injured worker is in the recovery process and when return-to-work planning should begin.

Any breakdown in communication among team members leads to misunderstanding and often unnecessarily protracts the restoration process. Nowhere is this breakdown more evident than at the time of medical release. Often the employer receives little information at this point, usually in the form of a vague physician's order to "return to light duty" or "do not lift over 15 lb". It is very difficult for the employer to translate this into functional terms, and consequently the employee is often not allowed back to the workplace without a medical release stating he or she is 100 percent fit for duty.

What makes return to work optimal is a medical release that addresses specific alternative jobs or tasks that the worker can safely perform and includes a timetable for progressive reemployment, if the worker is unable initially to sustain a full workday. This kind of specific medical release is only possible if the restoration program is designed to yield this type of information from its start.

The successful rehabilitation of injured workers depends on a team approach. Program design must address expected physical demands while the contributing factors of the original injury are identified and controlled, if not totally eliminated, prior to return to work. Communication among all involved parties is most critical and will ultimately determine the success of the entire process.

References

1. Ayoub MA. Control of manual lifting hazards: training in safe handling. J Occup Med 1982; 24:573–577.

2. Ayoub MA. Control of manual lifting hazards: training in safe handling. J Occup Med 1982; 24:668–676.
3. Matheson L. Work capacity evaluation, 1986, VI pp. 2–26; VII pp. 2–23. Anaheim, CA: Employment Rehabilitation Institute of California.
4. Tullis W, Devebery VJ. Delayed recovery in the patient with a work compensable injury. J Occup Med 1983; 25:829–835.

Bibliography

Cyriax J. Diagnosis of soft tissue lesions. In: Textbook of orthopedic medicine. Vol. 1, 8th ed. London: Balliere-Tindall, 1979.
Manual of techniques for the systematic approach to evaluation and treatment of soft tissue lesions.
Saunders H. Orthopedic physical therapy evaluation and treatment of musculoskeletal disorders. 1982.
Saunders' evaluation and treatment planning of musculoskeletal conditions including indication for, contraindication to, and effects of physical exercise and physical agents.
Alexander D. Palat BM. Industrial ergonomics, a practitioner's guide. Norcross, GA: Industrial Engineering & Management Press, 1985.
This text explains through example and illustration the use of ergonomics in the industrial setting. All articles are original works or adaptations written especially for this book.
Mayer et al. Objective assessment of spine function following industrial injury. JAMA 1987; 258:1763–1767.
This article details comprehensive assessment and treatment of patients with low back pain compared with a control group of chronic patients who did not participate in a treatment program.

contacting the personnel manager or the patient's supervisor. With this information, the physician can often help the employee return to work earlier, thus preserving earning capacity and often providing an additional stimulus to recovery.

In the routine care of patients, clinicians will frequently be asked to provide information relating to their patient's medical condition for the purposes of determining impairment or disability.

Such requests may originate from employers, insurance companies, state agencies, or patients. When such requests are accompanied by the patients' signed requests for release of information, it is appropriate to release information that is relevant to the request. (However, it would not be appropriate, for example, to comment on or release records about a patient's diabetes or epilepsy when the request was for information about impairment from a injury to the lower back.) Since records relating to workplace injuries must be routinely supplied in workers' compensation cases, it may be worthwhile to make and provide office notes that are separate from the notes relating to other, non-work-related problems. Since a worker's reimbursement is frequently tied to the receipt of records from the attending clinician, it is important that clinicians be prompt in responding to such requests to minimize financial difficulties for their patients.

Several sources of information can aid in the provision of relevant information. For example, most private disability plans have a short guide on eligibility requirements for clinicians, state workers' compensation boards often publish free guidebooks on the subject, and the Social Security Administration office will provide a free copy of the disability determination guide.

The greatest potential conflict arises between the primary clinician's traditional role as patient advocate and his or her gatekeeper or adjudicator role, brought about by a request from an employer or insurance company for professional evaluation of impairment. This situation can lead to hostility between patient and clinician because of unrealistic expectations and inexperience with disability systems. Frequently, patients are not aware of the requirements of different systems and will blame their clinicians if benefits are denied. Clinicians will frequently share their patients' frustration with the arbitrary nature of a particular disability system. Clinicians occasionally resent their patients for "trying to take advantage" of an insurance system, and patients may rightly resent the need to "prove" their illness. All of these feelings may interfere with a satisfactory clinician-patient relationship.

When a clinician is acting as an adjudicator, therefore, it is important to clarify the purpose of the evaluation and the limitations of the clinician's situation. It may be appropriate for the clinician to refer the patient to a social worker, lawyer, or union representative for clarification of the social, legal, and financial issues surrounding application for disability. It is often appropriate for a clinician to seek an independent opinion about impairment and disability when there is a potential for conflict with a patient or significant uncertainty about the cause or extent of disability.

REFERENCES

1. Kusnetz S, Hutchinson MK, eds. A guide to the work-relatedness of disease. Revised edition (NIOSH Pub. No. 79-116). Washington DC: U.S. Government Printing Office, 1979.
2. Barth PS, Hunt HA. Workers' compensation and work-related illnesses. Cambridge: MIT Press, 1980.
3. Pope MH, Andersson G, Chaffin, D. "The workplace" In: Pope M. Frymoyer J, Andersson G, eds. Occupational low back pain. New York: Praeger Publishers, 1984.
4. Becklake MR. Organic and functional impairment: Overall perspective. Am Rev Respir Dis 1984; 129: Suppl. S96–S100.
5. Yelin E. et al. Work disability in rheumatoid arthritis: Effects of disease, social and work factors. Ann Intern Med 1980; 95:551–556.

BIBLIOGRAPHY

Committee on Mental and Physical Impairment, American Medical Association. Guidelines to the evaluation of permanent impairment. 2nd ed. Chicago: American Medical Association, 1984.
These guidelines offer a quantitative approach to the measurement of permanent impairment. They are easy to use and well illustrated. There is no documentation concerning the validity of the impairment ratings. However, the guidelines are a useful starting point in impairment evaluations.
Becklake MR. Organic and functional impairment: Overall perspective. Am Rev Respir Dis 1984; 129: Suppl. S96–S100.
Thorough, yet concise, discussion of the problems inherent in development and use of "normal" values for interpretation of lung function tests and methods of cardiopulmonary disability determination.
Carey TS, Hadler NM. The role of the primary physician in disability determination for Social Security and workers' compensation. Ann Intern Med 1986; 104:706–710.

A good overview of the physician's role in these systems.

National Institute for Occupational Safety and Health. Occupational characteristics of disabled workers. Washington DC: U.S. Government Printing Office, 1980.

A study of the relationship between the rates of disability and various occupations.

Social Security Administration. Disability evaluation under Social Security, Social Security Administration Pub. No. 05-10089, Washington, DC: U.S. Department of Health and Human Services, 1986.

A guide to SSA medical criteria for disability.

13
Ethics and Occupational Health

Kathleen M. Rest

Case 1: A respected epidemiologist, having just completed a mortality study of the relationship between chemical X and liver cancer, is asked by OSHA to testify and make recommendations regarding the advisability of regulating chemical X as a carcinogen. The study found a weak association between chemical X and cancer. Previous animal studies showed a strong causal association; one other human study was equivocal. In the interest of protecting worker health, should the epidemiologist recommend regulation of chemical X as a human carcinogen, even though the human scientific evidence is weak?

Case 2: Company Y manufactures chemical X. In the past, the company industrial hygienist expressed strong concern about its safety and recommended an environmental monitoring program and several engineering controls. The company did not implement these recommendations. Does the industrial hygienist have any obligation to take further action, or has he done enough in making recommendations to the company?

Case 3: Company Y has asked its physician to implement a biological monitoring program for its employees. They are especially interested in liver function and have asked the physician to include liver function tests in all future examinations, including those done for employment purposes. What ethical issues should the physician consider before she agrees to undertake the requested screening program?

These cases illustrate the range of issues and types of ethical questions that occupational health specialists, scientists, regulators, epidemiologists, and other health professionals can expect to encounter on a regular basis. Ethics is the study of what constitutes good and bad human conduct [1]. It is more than law, social custom, personal preference, or consensus of opinion. Ethics is a fundamental and internally consistent system that provides a basis for making decisions that can be justified by appeal to commonly accepted principles of conduct and that can withstand close moral scrutiny [2].

Not all difficult decisions are dominated by ethical considerations; some may be simple disagreements about facts, methods, or desired outcomes. Other decisions may have clear ethical dimensions but involve nonmoral elements as well. Then there are moral dilemmas or quandaries—situations in which there are several conflicting avenues of action, each ethically justifiable and desirable in some respects, but none clearly preferable. When confronted with difficult choices, it is important to define exactly where the conflict lies, recognizing that a variety of other nonmoral factors may be problematic as well.

Numerous ethical theories attempt to reduce analysis to one or more moral principles. This chapter provides only a very brief and simplified discussion of the more important principles, while focusing on several occupational health policy and practice issues that present ethical problems.

CURRENT ETHICAL ISSUES IN OCCUPATIONAL HEALTH

Science, technology, public policy, and the practice of the occupational health professions all provide seeds for heated debate on issues with clear relevance to workplace health and safety.

Science and Policy

In occupational health, most discussion about science and public policy focuses on the regulation of health and safety hazards (see Chap. 10). Regulation has been viewed in disparate ways. It has been described as the codification of a shared moral code [3], and as a device developed to compensate for the grave moral defects of society [4]. Health and safety regulation invariably transfers choices about acceptable risk from the individual to the government and, thus, almost by definition, evokes conflict between autonomy and the public good [3].

In regulating health and safety hazards, process *and* outcome have important ethical dimensions. To understand the current state of occupational health and safety in the United States, both must be considered.

Process Issues. While most scientists assert that their research and scientific inquiry is value-free, most individuals will agree that the use of information generated by such inquiry is not [5]. In some senses, one can even question the value-free nature of the inquiry. Some observers argue that individual and social values as well as the values of funding agencies may influence what scientists decide to study, how they frame questions, what data they collect, and, therefore, the science itself [6]. Others feel that such pressures do not usually detract from the quality of the science [7]. The peer review process allegedly weeds out most studies that are biased or fail to acknowledge and address conflicting findings from other research.

Some argue that scientists should and can ignore policy questions in their pursuit of objective scientific data [7]. Others suggest that scientists should participate in policy questions through in-

forming and advising the regulatory process [5]. These views may reflect different understandings of the duties imposed by concerns for nonmaleficence, beneficence, and justice.

The epidemiologist in Case 1 has been asked to make recommendations about regulating the chemical he studied. His actions will involve issues of nonmaleficence and beneficence. Nonmaleficence is the moral principle that proscribes doing harm. Beneficence is a closely related principle that imposes a duty to do or promote good. While there is debate about the extent to which individuals are morally obligated to take positive action to contribute to the welfare of others, most moral philosophers agree that some situations impel positive action to prevent harm and to do good. If the epidemiologist does not recommend regulation, workers may be at increased risk of developing liver cancer. If he recommends regulation, chemical manufacturers may suffer substantial financial loss. Even if he choses not to become directly involved, his study will have significant impact on OSHA's decision-making process. Perhaps he was not aware that his science would be used in this way, but now his methods, results, intentions, and even allegiances may be questioned and criticized.

This case further illustrates the distinction between risk assessment and risk management currently made in occupational and environmental health. The former is alleged to be scientific and value-free, while the latter is considered political and value-laden. But is the division really so clearcut? Will our risk-assessing epidemiologist be willing to call chemical X a human carcinogen? Is his decision a scientific determination or a policy determination? Will policy-makers decide that the level of scientific proof is sufficient to trigger regulatory action? These decisions reflect value judgments about certainty of risk and therefore about one's duty to prevent harm from befalling others. In the face of uncertainty, some will prefer to take the risk of future harm rather than expend resources and impose costly regulation; others will prefer to err on the side of caution and regulate, recognizing that sometimes resources may be needlessly expended. Without stating their values in explicit terms, these individuals make decisions that involve issues of fairness, distributive justice, nonmaleficence, and beneficence. Such value-laden decisions could surely benefit from an ethical analysis in addition to the economic analyses imposed by the federal Office of Management and Budget (OMB). To be meaningful, such ethical considerations should be applied throughout the decision-making process and not simply be appended at the end.

Mention of OMB raises the specter of another important process issue in regulating health and safety hazards—cost-benefit analysis. Following on the heels of President Ford's "economic impact statements" and President Carter's "regulatory impact analyses," President Reagan issued an executive order in 1981 that set an explicit cost-benefit decision rule: "Regulatory action shall not be taken unless the potential benefits for the regulation outweigh the potential costs" [8]. The order further specifies that "regulatory objectives should be chosen to maximize the benefits to society" [8]. It requires that costs and benefits be quantified in monetary terms to the extent possible.

While the appropriateness and technical difficulties of applying cost-benefit analysis to the regulation of health and safety hazards remains a controversial topic, it is important to recognize the ethical dimensions of this economic tool. It places a high priority on maximizing benefits but seldom considers issues of distributive justice. Justice is a complex principle that involves notions of fairness and desert—that is, giving persons what is due to them. In the context of cost-benefit analysis, distributive justice suggests questions that relate to the fair distribution of benefits and burdens of regulating and not regulating. Who actually benefits from regulating or not regulating? Who bears the costs? Who bears the risk? What is the relationship between those who bear the costs and those who receive the benefits? If an ethical analysis accompanied every cost-benefit analysis, decision-makers would be forced to consider such issues of fairness.

Outcome Issues. While controversy has accompanied virtually every piece of occupational health and safety regulation, several recent initiatives aptly illustrate the ethical dimensions of such regulation.

OSHA's lead standard reflects issues of justice, nonmaleficence, and beneficence. The regulatory debate on lead included scientific questions about safe airborne levels and the merits of using blood levels as the primary measure of compliance with the standard. An interesting part of the debate centered on the establishment of medical removal protection with (hourly) rate retention for employees found to have elevated blood lead levels. There was little argument about the wisdom of removing workers with high blood lead levels from exposure. The conflict arose over a proposal that obligated employers to maintain the workers' hourly rates and seniority rights during the period of removal. The Lead Industries Association argued against such medical removal protection on legal grounds, stating that Congress did not intend OSHA to have the power to require such policies and that it violated provisions of the Occupational Safety and Health Act [9]. Workers' representatives focused on issues of autonomy and fairness, noting that workers would chose not to participate in a blood lead screening program that might threaten their livelihoods. Although medical removal was in the best interest of the workers' health, workers' representatives felt it was unfair to penalize them by putting their wages and seniority benefits at risk in an exposure situation over which they had no control.

The courts ruled in favor of the medical removal with rate retention policy, but the ethical issues did not abate. Recognizing the reproductive effects of lead, some employers began to institute "fetal protection policies." Such policies seek to protect actual and potential fetuses of women who are pregnant or of reproductive capacity. These policies reflect consideration of the principles of beneficence and nonmaleficence and may clash with the principles of autonomy and justice. In weighing options, employers who adopt such policies place a higher value on protecting the fetus from harm (and thereby protecting their own future financial interests) than providing autonomous choices to female employees who may take steps to control their fertility. Furthermore, as is the case with lead, some reproductive toxins affect male and female workers prior to conception. In such instances, one can question the fairness of differentially protecting female and male employees. As scientific research provides more information about the effects of toxins on the reproductive system, we can expect to examine more frequent and increasingly complex ethical issues.

More recent regulatory action regarding Right to Know places the ethical concept of autonomy in clear view. Autonomy is the moral principle that concerns respect for persons and an individual's right to self-determination without constraint. Self-governance and noninterference are tightly guarded and highly cherished rights, which frequently clash with the notion of public good. In the context of Right to Know, the following ethical questions emerge: Do workers have an unlimited right to information about the substances with which they work? Do employers have a correlative duty to provide this information to workers at the possible risk of revealing something commercially valuable? Should this information be provided on request or even without a request? The principle of autonomy suggests that individuals have a right to self-determination, the right to control their own behavior without coercion. In the context of work, this principle implies that individuals have a right to decide if they are willing to assume risks to their health and safety on their jobs. To make autonomous decisions, one requires information— in this case, information about the health effects of substances used in the workplace and the risks of acquiring a disease by working with them. On the other hand, management has a property interest in proprietary information. This interest results in an ethical dilemma, one that is resolvable but problematic nonetheless.

Current federal, state, and local legislation grants workers the Right to Know about hazard-

ous exposures to varying degrees. The federal Hazard Communication Standard confers some rights and positive duties on workers and employers in the private sector. Numerous state and local laws provide broader coverage and extend these protections and duties to community residents, thus addressing the issue of fairness in the distribution of health and safety information. Although some have questioned the basic ability of most individuals in this country to make truly autonomous choices about where they work, especially in the absence of full employment [10], workers would be far less able to exercise any control over exposure situations without the type of information provided by Right-to-Know laws.

While the promise of Right-to-Know legislation is great, it is not without dangers. One author suggests that "to contribute to worker autonomy in any real sense, Right-to-Know must facilitate enough of a change in the employer-employee relationship to enable the worker to effect changes in workplace technology (or changes in the way in which workplace technology is employed in the workplace). . . . If all Right-to-Know does is provide a mechanism whereby workers are able to summon the courage to risk occupational disease and reproductive disaster, it will be an empty exercise" [11].

A more subtle and perhaps unexpected result of the Right-to-Know initiatives has been a push for what is being called "worker- or high-risk notification." This effort seeks to provide information about health risks to subjects of epidemiologic studies conducted by NIOSH and other federal agencies and to other worker populations at risk. Proponents of the initiative suggest that these agencies have a duty to inform individuals and worker groups when they have identified a disease-exposure relationship. Such notification would allow these individuals to make informed decisions about their continued employment in the industry, seek medical attention and advice in a timely manner, take action to decrease their exposure, and, thus, perhaps prevent the development of an occupational disease. Such notification seems justified by appeal to the principles of autonomy and justice and to the moral duties of preventing harm and doing good.

Yet the initiative poses real ethical dilemmas for policy makers. How much scientific evidence is needed to trigger notification? Is personal notification required? Will a notification policy make employers more reluctant to give researchers access to worker populations and to exposure data? If so, is a legal requirement to notify workers without a corresponding legal right to access relevant workplace information really in the best interest of worker health? Congress is presently considering these difficult ethical issues along with other scientific, technical, and economic dimensions of enacting legislation to notify workers at risk.

OCCUPATIONAL HEALTH PRACTICE

It is one thing to describe and act on ethical principles in the process of making public policy. It is quite another to use them for decision-making in the everyday practice of occupational health. Occupational physicians, nurses, and industrial hygienists, among others, routinely encounter difficult ethical issues in the performance of their work. And, more than legislators and policy-makers, these individuals suffer the consequences of their decisions in very personal ways. Their actions can enhance their reputation, status, and esteem or can incur the wrath and distrust of their employers, patients, or coworkers. Their actions can affect their income, employability, standing in their professional community, and respectability in the eyes of individuals for and to whom they are responsible.

This section examines the ethical aspects of several situations frequently encountered by occupational health professionals.

Working for Companies

Physicians who work for companies find themselves in a unique position. Although their goals and interests may be similar to those of their colleagues who practice medicine in the community, the goals of their employers and patients are certainly very different. The company's primary purpose and interest is the manufacture of a product or the delivery of a service. The physician's patients, who are also employed by the company, are primarily interested in the benefits and opportunities of continued employment. The relationship between the physician and these individuals is undeniably different from the traditional doctor-patient relationship. While the workers may be the physician's *patients*—one can question the appropriateness of using this term at all in these circumstances—the relationship is complicated by the fact that the physician's *client* is actually the company.

Within this structure, the practice of occupational medicine, nursing, or industrial hygiene is inherently difficult and challenging. These professionals may find themselves in the middle of the competing and the conflicting interests of the parties involved in the workplace. Employers may expect physicians and nurses to function as agents of social control, making determinations about when, where, and if an individual will work. They may limit the ability of their industrial hygienists and safety officers to take action on preventing or controlling workplace hazards. Workers, on the other hand, may expect occupational health professionals to protect their interests and function as their advocates when problems arise. In situations where the client's interests differ from those of the patient, it is not surprising that skepticism and distrust arise on all fronts.

An ethical issue frequently discussed in the context of working for companies relates to confidentiality. How much of the personal and medical information obtained by physicians and nurses is the company entitled to? Should employers be informed that a job applicant has diabetes or has had cancer? Should the employer be told that the executive up for promotion is seeing a psychiatrist because of a family crisis? Physicians and nurses may encounter direct or indirect pressure to release this type of information to help the company protect its legitimate business interests. But such disclosure invades workers' privacy and may threaten their job status. The rights of the client conflict with the rights of the patient.

As difficult as the issue of confidentiality seems, other more subtle pressures may create even larger and more difficult problems. These problems relate to the extent to which occupational health professionals are responsible for taking action on suspected or actual health and safety problems in the workplace. The hygienist in Case 2 had previously expressed his strong concern about the safety of chemical X and had made recommendations for controlling the exposure. The company took no action on his recommendations. Having expressed this concern to the employer, does the hygienist have any further obligation to follow-up on this suspected hazard? Do the moral principles of nonmaleficence and beneficence impose an ethical duty on the hygienist? Should he notify OSHA? Should he alert the workers? How far should the company-employed occupational health professional go to protect worker health and safety?

Organizations of occupational health professions have acknowledged these dilemmas and have sought to provide guidance through the development of codes of ethics. The American Occupational Medical Association, the American Academy of Industrial Hygiene, and the American Association of Occupational Health Nurses have promulgated codes of ethics for occupational health professionals in their respective fields (pp. 185–187). The American Occupational Medical Association (AOMA) code exhorts physicians to give the health and safety of the worker the highest priority and to treat as confidential whatever is learned about individuals unless the law or an overriding public health concern dictates otherwise. Some concerns have been raised about the lack of clarity, directness, strength, and practical usefulness of this code [12, 13]. The code of the American Academy of Industrial Hygiene clearly advises hygienists to hold their responsibilities to the employer or client subservient to their ultimate responsibility of protecting employee health. The American Association of Occupational Health Nurses ethical code clearly makes the worker the primary focus. Certainly, these codes offer some guidance, but one cannot reasonably expect codes to offer solutions to the very real moral dilemmas that arise in the practice of occupational medicine, nursing, and industrial hygiene in the company setting.

In the final analysis, the problems encountered by these company-related occupational health specialists may hinge on the principle of autonomy. Can they exercise professional judgment and make decisions free of undue pressure? Can they take action, even if such action conflicts with the goals and priorities of the company or places the company at risk of future liability? (For a detailed and excellent discussion of these and related issues, see reference 14.)

Participation in Screening Programs
There is probably no other single issue in the practice of occupational medicine that raises as many ethical questions as worker screening (see Chap. 6). Whether employed by a company or delivering health care services in other settings, most physicians will at some time be asked to do some sort of worker screening examination—from preplacement physicals and OSHA-mandated, exposure-specific examinations to the more controversial testing for drug use, AIDS antibody, and genetic imperfections.

Medical screening is usually done for one of two reasons: (1) for job placement purposes—that is, to assess an individual's ability to perform a job, including making recommendations on work restrictions; and (2) to predict an individual's risk of future health problems that would inhibit job performance or result in large economic expenditures for the company [15]. Such predictions are usually based on certain genetic, behavioral, physiologic, or biochemical factors. A variety of technical and descriptive terms are commonly used and frequently confused in discussions of worker screen-

CODE OF ETHICAL CONDUCT
FOR PHYSICIANS PROVIDING
OCCUPATIONAL MEDICAL SERVICES
—Developed by the American Occupational
Medical Association and adopted by its board
of directors, July 23, 1976.

These principles are intended to aid physicians
in maintaining ethical conduct in providing occupational medical service. They are standards
to guide physicians in their relationships with
the individuals they serve, with employers and
workers' representatives, with colleagues in the
health professions, and with the public.

Physicians should:

1. accord highest priority to the health and
   safety of the individual in the workplace;
2. practice on a scientific basis with objectivity
   and integrity;
3. make or endorse only statements which reflect their observations or honest opinion;
4. actively oppose and strive to correct uneth-
   ical conduct in relation to occupational
   health service;
5. avoid allowing their medical judgment to be
   influenced by any conflict of interest;
6. strive conscientiously to become familiar
   with the medical fitness requirements, the
   environment and the hazards of the work
   done by those they serve, and with the
   health and safety aspects of the products
   and operations involved;
7. treat as confidential whatever is learned
   about individuals served, releasing information only when required by law or by
   over-riding public health considerations, or
   to other physicians at the request of the individual according to traditional medical
   ethical practice; and should recognize that
   employers are entitled to counsel about the
   medical fitness of individuals in relation to
   work, but are not entitled to diagnoses or
   details of a specific nature;
8. strive continually to improve medical
   knowledge, and should communicate information about health hazards in timely and
   effective fashion to individuals or groups
   potentially affected, and make appropriate
   reports to the scientific community;
9. communicate understandably to those they
   serve any significant observations about
   their health, recommending further study,
   counsel or treatment when indicated;
10. seek consultation concerning the individual
    or the workplace whenever indicated;
11. cooperate with governmental health per-
    sonnel and agencies, and foster and main-
    tain sound ethical relationships with other
    members of the health professions; and
12. avoid solicitation of the use of their services
    by making claims, offering testimonials,
    or implying results which may not be
    achieved, but they may appropriately advise
    colleagues and others of services available.

ing. These include medical monitoring, surveillance, genetic testing, and biologic monitoring.
Each term has a precise definition. For the purposes of this chapter, they will not be differentiated, but rather considered under the broad rubric of medical screening.

Issues of privacy, confidentiality, fairness, informed consent, and informed refusal pervade almost every form of worker screening. They may
relate to the screening program or to the use of the
results of the screening program.

As in Case 3, many employers require individuals to undergo medical screening prior to and during the course of their employment. Physicians
must be aware that an individual's compliance
with this requirement does not usually reflect an
entirely autonomous decision. Individuals often
consent to these examinations because they need

AMERICAN ACADEMY OF INDUSTRIAL
HYGIENE CODE OF ETHICS
FOR THE PROFESSIONAL PRACTICE
OF INDUSTRIAL HYGIENE

Purpose

This code provides standards of ethical conduct
to be followed by industrial hygienists as they
strive for the goals of protecting employees'
health, improving the work environment, and
advancing the quality of the profession. Industrial hygienists have the responsibility to practice their profession in an objective manner following recognized principles of industrial
hygiene, realizing that the lives, health, and welfare of individuals may be dependent upon their
professional judgment.

Professional Responsibility

1. Maintain the highest level of integrity and
   professional competence.
2. Be objective in the application of recognized
   scientific methods and in the interpretation
   of findings.
3. Promote industrial hygiene as a professional
   discipline.
4. Disseminate scientific knowledge for the benefit of employees, society, and the profession.
5. Protect confidential information.
6. Avoid circumstances where compromise of
   professional judgment or conflict of interest
   may arise.

Responsibility to Employees

1. Recognize that the primary responsibility of
   the industrial hygienist is to protect the
   health of employees.
2. Maintain an objective attitude toward the
   recognition, evaluation, and control of
   health hazards regardless of external influences, realizing that the health and welfare of
   workers and others may depend upon the industrial hygienist's professional judgment.
3. Counsel employees regarding health hazards
   and the necessary precautions to avoid adverse health effects.

Responsibility to Employers and Clients

1. Act responsibly in the application of industrial hygiene principles toward the attainment of healthful working environments.
2. Respect confidences, advise honestly, and report findings and recommendations accurately.
3. Manage and administer professional services
   to ensure maintenance of accurate records to
   provide documentation and accountability in
   support of findings and conclusions.
4. Hold responsibilities to the employer or
   client subservient to the ultimate responsibility to protect the health of employees.

Responsibility to the Public

1. Report factually on industrial hygiene matters of public concern.
2. State professional opinions founded on adequate knowledge and clearly identified as
   such.

Source: Am Ind Hyg Assoc J (40), June 1979.

AMERICAN ASSOCIATION OF
OCCUPATIONAL HEALTH NURSES
CODE OF ETHICS ADOPTED
IN JUNE 1986

This code of ethics has been developed as a guide for registered professional nurses to maintain ethical conduct in providing occupational health services.

Occupational health nurses should:

1. conserve, protect and promote the health and safety of the employee in the workplace.
2. provide health care in the work environment with respect for human dignity, unrestricted by considerations of social or economic status, national origin, race, religion, sex or the nature of health problems.
3. safeguard the employee's right to privacy by protecting confidential information and releasing information only upon written consent of the employee or as required by law.
4. maintain individual competence in occupational health nursing practice, recognizing and accepting responsibility for individual actions and judgments.
5. participate in activities (such as research and case-finding) that contribute to the ongoing development of the profession's body of knowledge when assured that the employee's and the employer's rights are protected.
6. contribute to the ongoing efforts of the profession to define and upgrade standards for occupational health nursing practice and education.
7. incorporate standards of practice into the occupational health nursing service by using them as criteria to assure quality of care.
8. collaborate with other health professions and community health agencies to promote efforts to meet the health needs of America's workers.

to work. They may knowingly divulge highly personal and sensitive information to the physician, or they may reveal such information unknowingly through their consent to laboratory tests. They may not know how or even if the information will be passed on to others. In Case 3, the physician will be gathering information on workers' liver function, a variable that may reflect certain lifestyle factors that workers would rather keep confidential.

The content of the screening program may pose problems for the physician as well. Many screening programs are ill-conceived from both a scientific and ethical point of view. Problems with test validity (sensitivity, specificity) and predictive value may weaken any appeal to beneficence. For example, some employers still insist on using lumbosacral x-rays to screen out individuals with back problems despite the low predictive value of the x-rays to forecast future back injury. The use of such a test provides no real benefit to the company and, in fact, may cause harm to the worker. The use of cardiovascular stress testing in healthy young adults applying for jobs in the hazardous waste industry is another questionable practice. In Case 3, one can reasonably ask if liver function tests are appropriate for screening job applicants for employment at company Y. The physician should also consider how the results of the employee biological monitoring program will be used. How does the occupational health practitioner balance fairness to the employer with protection of the prospective or current employee? Will workers be informed of their test results and counseled about their meaning? Will individuals be removed from their jobs if their liver function tests are elevated? Will such elevations trigger implementation of the hygienist's recommendations? If the institution of a medical screening program is the employer's sole method of reducing risk of workplace illness and injury, physicians should be wary and weigh their involvement very carefully.

These factors place stringent ethical obligations

on physicians and nurses who participate in worker screening programs. They must decide if the content of the proposed screening is medically reasonable and ethically justifiable. In doing so, they must identify and weigh the interests of the employer and the worker.

To respect the autonomy of individual workers, physicians must strive to provide them with enough information to obtain informed consent to any screening examination. Arguably, this information should not only be about medical risks but also about possible risks to employability and job tenure as well. Workers have a right to know what information will be released to their employers so they can decide if they wish to participate in the screening program.

Physicians and nurses also must decide how much information employers need for health and safety purposes and what should be retained in confidence. Concerns for nonmaleficence and beneficence must also be applied to decisions about follow-up action. Such action may adversely affect the employer, the employee, and, possibly, the physician's own standing with the company.

While this chapter cannot examine all the relevant aspects of worker screening programs, it can summarize the thoughts of several authors who have considered the issues carefully. They suggest the following: Screening should not only monitor an individual's exposure but also lead to action that improves conditions in the workplace [16]. Screening should not divert attention and resources from reducing toxic exposures in the workplace [17]. Worker participation in screening programs should be voluntary when possible. Employees should be informed of the purpose of the testing and who has access to the results. Confidentiality should be respected and the employee should be informed of the results [18]. Because there are few legal protections for workers involved in medical screening, occupational health professionals must take care in designing and participating in worker screening programs.

Participation in Compensation

The issue of compensation is an integral part of occupational health and one that causes physicians a lot of discomfort. They are commonly reluctant to get involved with the bureaucratic and administrative requirements of the compensation system (see Chap. 11). Many physicians feel intimidated by the adversarial nature of the legal system. There is also the very real issue of the physician's ability or willingness to diagnose an individual's disease as occupational. Physicians are often uncomfortable with the legal definition of proof and have difficulty bridging the gap between medical and scientific certainty regarding causation and the legal definition of the same. The physician's willingness or unwillingness to accept the legal definition of causation—that is, "more likely than not"—reflects his or her concept of fairness.

Few would deny that individuals who suffer disease and disability related to their work deserve some sort of compensation to help them with medical expenses and income maintenance. Patients with occupational disease often need the physician's help to obtain compensation; without this help, they are unlikely to receive it. Do physicians who see working patients have obligations that extend beyond the preventive and therapeutic realm? What if the patient works for a company that is the physician's client? Is the physician obligated to assist the patient with compensation under these circumstances? It has been argued that when rights to health conflict with rights to property, the former must prevail [19]. To the extent that just compensation contributes to health and quality of life, one can argue that the patient's rights to compensation take precedence over the client's rights to protection of their financial interests. Moreover, if individuals have positive moral duties to do good and physicians are ethically obligated to work in their patient's best interest, then one can contend that physicians have an obligation to assist their patients in this way.

Making Decisions

With all the conflicting demands and expectations, what guidance can we offer conscientious occupational health practitioners? How should they go about making decisions in the face of uncertainty or competing interests?

They can begin by trying to determine the medical and scientific facts. Part of the difficulty may be a simple disagreement about what is known, what a test can do, or how a study is interpreted. A second step is to review and evaluate any relevant legal constraints. In many cases, the law has already considered issues of fairness and justice and has provided legal remedies and guidance. The weight of the law may persuade recalcitrant or inflexible individuals who are attempting to influence the occupational health professional to act in certain ways. A third step demands more careful consideration and introspection. Occupational health specialists should attempt to identify and examine the true goals and intentions of the parties involved. There may be hidden agendas that will shed considerable light on the decision-making process. Examination of these intentions and agendas may help occupational health professionals expose the values of the individuals involved. Physicians, nurses, industrial hygienists, and safety professionals must discover their own values as well, as they are of paramount importance. These values determine how much responsibility they are willing to assume in protecting worker health, how far they are willing to go to assure safe working conditions for their own patients and for others in the particular workplace [18].

In considering the ethical dimensions of a decision, occupational health professionals should try to identify all possible options and ask pointed questions about each. Who will benefit or who will be harmed by each alternative? What is the relationship between those who stand to gain from a decision and those who will bear the cost of it? Who is the least advantaged individual or group in the situation? Are the needs and preferences of this individual or group known? What are the long-term consequences of each action? What will happen if a particular action is *not* taken? What harm or benefit will such inaction cause? What are the occupational health professional's own ethical responsibilities in the situation? Why does he or she feel reluctant to do one thing or another? What does the occupational health practitioner stand to lose or to gain from each possible alternative?

Although these steps may not make the decision easy, especially when alternative actions have merit and ethical justification, they will help clarify the values involved in the process.

In conclusion, the field of occupational health is fraught with ethical problems and dilemmas that are not easy to solve. Ethical analyses that include consideration of the moral principles of autonomy, nonmaleficence, beneficence, and justice can help guide decision-making but may not make hard choices any easier in the practical sense. The rapidly changing health care system presages even more complex ethical problems. The time is ripe for considering structural safeguards for occupational health professionals. Unless these professionals can somehow be insulated from personal and economic reprisals, it will remain difficult for them to make the bold decisions that are needed to ensure worker health and safety. Developing these structural solutions demands creativity and a willingness to question and look beyond the status quo. Until such solutions are found, occupational health professionals will continue to find themselves in the middle of formidable ethical problems.

REFERENCES

1. Barry V. Moral aspects of health care. Belmont, CA: Wadsworth, 1982:4.
2. Beauchamp TL, Childress JF. Principles of biomedical ethics. New York: Oxford University Press, 1983.
3. Hutt PB. Five moral imperatives of government

regulation. The Hastings Center Report. 1980; 10(1):29–30.

4. MacIntyre A. Regulation: a substitution for morality. The Hastings Center Report. 1980; 10(1):31–3.

5. Ashford NA, Gregory KA. Ethical problems in using science in the regulatory process. Natural Resources and the Environment. American Bar Association. 1986; 2(2):13–57.

6. Ashford NA. A framework for examining the effects of industrial funding on academic freedom and the integrity of the university. Science, Technology, and Human Values. 1983; 8(2):16–23.

7. Rothman KJ, Poole C. Science and policy-making. Am J Pub Health 1985; 75(4):340–42.

8. Reagan R. Federal regulation, executive order no. 12291. Federal Register. Feb 17 1981:46(33): 13193.

9. Lead Industry Association. Lead Industry Association Inc. versus Donovan. 1981:453 U.S. 913, 11 OSHC 1264.

10. Kilburn KH. Human values and social responsibility: a response to Mr. Ward. Am J Ind Med 1986; 9:25–7.

11. Caldart CC. Promise and pitfalls of workplace right-to-know. Semin Occup Med 1986; 1(1):81–90.

12. Whorton D, Davis ME. Ethical conduct and the occupational physician. Bull NY Acad Med 1978; 54:733–41.

13. Ilka R. Necessity and adequacy of the American Occupational Medical Association code of ethics. Semin Occup Med 1986; 1(1):59–65.

14. Walsh DC. Corporate physicians: between medicine and management. New Haven: Yale University Press, 1987.

15. Rothstein MA. Medical screening: a tool with broadening use. Bus Health 1986; 3(10):7–9.

16. Atherley G. Biomedical surveillance. Am J Ind Med 1985; 7:269–71.

17. Ashford NA. Medical screening in the workplace: legal and ethical considerations. Semin Occup Med 1986; 1(1):67–79.

18. Rest KM, Patterson WB. Ethics and moral reasoning in occupational health. Semin Occup Med 1986; 1(1):49–57.

19. Gewirth A. Human rights and the workplace. Am J Ind Med 1986; 9:31–40.

BIBLIOGRAPHY

Ashford NA, Gregory K. Ethical problems in using science in the regulatory process. Natural resources and the environment. American Bar Association 1986; 2(2):13–57.
A provocative discussion of the role of values in science and regulation and the ethical dilemmas that confront scientists who participate in the regulatory process.

The environment of the workplace and human values. Am J Ind Med 1986; 9:1–113.
Proceedings of a 1982 conference cosponsored by the Labor Policy Institute and the Marshall-Wythe School of Law at the College of William and Mary. An excellent collection of papers dealing with the role of human rights and values in science, technology, policy, regulation, law, and workplace health and safety.

Lappe M. Ethical issues in testing for differential sensitivity to occupational hazards. J Occup Med 1983; 25(11):797–808.
A detailed and excellent analysis of the ethical aspects of using biochemical indices of worker susceptibility to prevent and control workplace hazards.

Rothstein M. Medical screening of workers. Washington, DC: Bureau of National Affairs, 1984.
This valuable book explores medical screening from the perspectives of law, medicine, economics, epidemiology, and ethics. It covers issues of disability, susceptibility, predictive screening, reproductive hazards, and the use of medical screening in employment decisions. It describes relevant state and federal laws, as well as important court decisions that relate to the screening of workers.

Schulte P, Ringen K. Notification of workers at high risk: an emerging public health problem. Am J Pub Health 1984; 74(5):485–91.
A thoughtful commentary on the scientific, ethical, economic, and institutional aspects of notifying workers at high risk of occupational disease.

Semin Occup Med 1986; 1(1):49–96.
This issue of the journal contains five articles that deal with ethics and occupational health. The papers on medical screening, Right to Know, and the AOMA code of ethics are especially informative and provocative.

Walsh DC. Corporate physicians: between medicine and management. New Haven: Yale University Press, 1987.
An interesting study of "medicine's man in the middle," the company physician. This lively and easy-to-read book reflects a series of interviews with corporate physicians. It traces the historical development of the occupational medicine profession, describes the structure and organization of contemporary occupational medicine practice, examines the roles and functions of corporate physicians, and concludes with inferences for theory and practice.

III
Hazardous Workplace Exposures

14
Toxins and Their Effects

Howard Frumkin

A toxin is generally understood to be a substance that is harmful to biologic systems, but within this simple concept lies a great deal of variability. A substance that is harmful at a high dose may be innocuous or even essential at a lower dose. A toxin may damage a specific body system, or it may exert a general effect on an organism. A substance that is toxic to one species may not be toxic to another because of different metabolic pathways or protective mechanisms. And the biologic damage may be temporary, permanent over the organism's lifetime, or expressed over subsequent generations.

Toxicology is the study of the harmful effects of chemicals on biologic systems. It is a hybrid science built on advances in biochemistry, physiology, pathology, physical chemistry, pharmacology, and public health. Toxicologists describe and quantify the biologic uptake, distribution, effects, metabolism, and excretion of toxic chemicals. A subfield, environmental toxicology, focuses on exposures to toxic substances in the atmosphere, in food and water, and in occupational settings. These exposures have important effects both on humans and on the ecosystem in which we live.

The course of most toxicologic interactions takes the form of uptake → distribution → metabolism → excretion. Storage and biologic effects are other important events that may, but need not, occur. A knowledge of each of these steps is essential for a complete understanding of the effects of a chemical.

CLASSES OF TOXIC SUBSTANCES

Toxic or harmful substances encountered in the workplace may be classified in various ways. A simple and useful classification is given below, along with definitions adopted by the American National Standards Institute (ANSI).

Dusts Solid particles generated by handling, crushing, grinding, rapid impact, and detonation of organic or inorganic materials such as rocks, ore, metal, coal, wood, and grain. Dusts do not tend to flocculate except under electrostatic forces; they do not diffuse in air but settle under the influence of gravity.

Fumes Solid particles generated by condensation from the gaseous state, generally after volatilization from molten metals, and often accompanied by a chemical reaction such as oxidation. Fumes flocculate and sometimes coalesce.

Mists Suspended liquid droplets generated by condensation from the gaseous to the liquid state or by breaking up a liquid into a dispersed state, such as by splashing, foaming, or atomizing.

Vapors The gaseous form of substances that are normally in the solid or liquid state and can be changed to these states by either increasing the pressure or decreasing the temperature. Vapors diffuse.

Gases Normally formless fluids that occupy the space of enclosure and can be changed to

CARBON MONOXIDE EXPOSURE IN AIRCRAFT FUELERS

A 51-year-old fueler was found dead in the cab of his fuel truck at a major airport. Since circumstances suggested the possibility of carbon monoxide (CO) poisoning, investigators examined the fuel trucks. It was noted that the exhaust pipe ran forward under the cab to a muffler mounted behind the front bumper. This configuration, apparently standard at airports, is intended to minimize the proximity of the exhaust system to the jet fuel in the truck and aircraft.

Soon thereafter NIOSH investigated the potential hazard in the airport's fuel trucks. With the windows closed and the heaters turned on to simulate winter operating conditions, 8 of 18 trucks tested had excessive CO concentrations in their cabs. One truck averaged 300 parts per million (ppm), six times the permissible level set by OSHA.

In this case, it was not proved that CO contributed to the death of the fueler, but the investigation indicated the presence of a remediable health hazard. NIOSH recommended that the employer minimize exposure time of the fuelers, maximize fresh air ventilation in the trucks, and improve the maintenance of the vehicles [1].

Carbon monoxide is an occupational hazard for workers involved with internal combustion engines and for those working near any gas- or oil-fueled heating process, such as in potteries, foundries, petroleum refineries, pulp mills, steel mills, and coke ovens. It is a colorless, odorless gas. Following inhalation, CO combines with hemoglobin to form carboxyhemoglobin, compromising the oxygen-carrying capacity of the blood. Moderate levels may cause headache, dizziness, and drowsiness; higher levels lead to nausea, vomiting, collapse, coma, and death. Even very low levels have been shown to reduce exercise tolerance in subjects with angina, and smokers, who generally have carboxyhemoglobin levels in the 5 to 10 percent range, are probably especially susceptible (see Chap. 27).

This case serves to illustrate several principles. First, not every toxic exposure is exotic or mysterious. Second, workers, when exposed to an asphyxiant or intoxicant, become less alert and less able to react briskly to hazards. In a manner analogous to chemical synergy, their risk of accidents is enhanced markedly. Third, in an environment with very high gas concentrations every breath boosts the blood level of the gas, and toxicity can develop remarkably rapidly. Such acute exposures are common in enclosed spaces like reaction tanks; other workers who rush to the victim's aid can be quickly overcome as well. Finally, when a worker is found unconscious or dead following an unknown exposure, a blood sample should always be taken. Carboxyhemoglobin concentration can be determined as can evidence of numerous other toxicities. In this way the cause of death would likely have been verified.

---

the liquid or solid state only by the combined effect of increased pressure and decreased temperature. Gases diffuse.

This classification does not include the obvious categories of solids and liquids that may be harmful, nor does it encompass physical agents that cannot be considered "substances." Living agents such as bacteria and fungi constitute another group of "substances" that would appear in a comprehensive classification of occupational health hazards.

ABSORPTION

In the workplace chemicals are taken up by three main routes: the respiratory system, the skin, and the gastrointestinal tract. Other routes of absorption, generally of less importance, include mucous membranes and open lesions. If these routes of exposure are remembered by a health professional while taking an occupational history, the importance of each can be evaluated with appropriate questions (see Chap. 3).

Respiratory Tract
Inhalation is the major route of entry of the gases, vapors, mists, and airborne particulate matter encountered in the workplace. To analyze this process we need to consider gases, vapors, and mists separately from particles.

Gases, Vapors, and Mists. Gases, vapors, and mists can damage the respiratory tract; they can pass from the lungs to the bloodstream for distribution to other parts of the body; or both may occur.

Irritant gases are an important example of respiratory tract toxins (see Chap. 21). Their effects may be immediate or delayed. Gases that are very water soluble like hydrogen fluoride, ammonia, and sulfuric acid tend to dissolve in the moist lining of the upper respiratory tract, often producing immediate irritation, which forces an exposed worker to flee the area. Less soluble irritant gases, such as nitrogen dioxide, ozone, and phosgene, reach the bronchioles and alveoli where they dissolve slowly and may cause acute pneumonitis and pulmonary edema hours later. Long-term exposure at low concentrations may lead to chronic changes such as emphysema and fibrosis. Whether acute or chronic, the effects of irritant gases are seen mainly in the respiratory tract.

Asphyxiants are inhaled substances that exert toxicity by interrupting the supply or use of oxygen. *Simple asphyxiants* such as methane or nitrogen have relatively little direct physiologic effect, but by displacing oxygen in ambient air, they can cause severe hypoxia. This is a common problem in enclosed spaces such as silos and storage tanks. *Chemical asphyxiants* block the delivery or use of oxygen at the cellular level through one of several mechanisms. One example is carbon monoxide, a product of incomplete combustion found in foundries, coke ovens, furnaces, and similar facilities. It binds tightly to hemoglobin, forming a carboxy-hemoglobin complex (COHb) that is ineffective at oxygen transport. Another example is cyanide, which is used in plastic production, metallurgy, electroplating, and other processes. Cyanide inhibits the cytochrome oxidase enzymes, compromising oxidative metabolism and phosphorylation. A third example, hydrogen sulfide, a gas found in mines, petrochemical plants, and sewers, also inhibits cytochrome oxidase. Unfortunately, occupational fatalities from all these exposures remain common.

Gases, vapors, and mists that are highly fat soluble can cross from the alveoli to the bloodstream and migrate from there to binding sites or fat depots for which they have a special affinity. Substances that are readily absorbed following inhalation and exert their effects elsewhere include carbon disulfide, volatile aliphatic and aromatic hydrocarbons, volatile halogenated hydrocarbons, and aliphatic saturated ketones such as methyl ethyl ketone. Because of the impressive variety of substances involved and the wide spectrum of acute and chronic effects that may result, this is an important pathway of absorption in workplace settings.

The toxic action of some inhaled gases, vapors, and mists may be considerably enhanced when they are adsorbed to respirable particles. Presumably, the particles transport these toxins to deep parts of the respiratory tree, which would otherwise be inaccessible. An example is radon gas: This substance increases lung cancer incidence among uranium miners, but, if it is experimentally inhaled in dust-free air, then almost none is retained by the lung and little or no carcinogenic effect is seen.

Several other variables influence the delivery of gases, vapors, and mists to the lower respiratory tract. With rapid, deep breathing, as occurs during strenuous exertion, the delivered dose increases. When a respirator is incorrectly chosen, poorly fit, or inadequately maintained, significant amounts of airborne toxins can reach workers' lungs (see Chap. 7).

Particles. Inhaled particles, unlike most gases and vapors, are of interest primarily for their pathologic effects on the lungs. Their deposition, retention, and clearance are influenced by several well-defined factors.

One factor is inertia, which tends to maintain moving particles on a straight course. A second is gravity, which tends to move particles earthward, promoting the early settling out of larger and denser particles. A third is Brownian diffusion, the random motion that results from molecular kinetic energy. When these forces cause a particle to strike the airway wall or alveolar surface, deposition occurs.

Three factors influence the location and extent of deposition: anatomy of the respiratory tract, particle size, and breathing pattern. Branching, angling, and narrowing at each point in the airways define the local velocity and flow characteristics of the inspired air, which in turn influence particle deposition. For example, the nasopharynx features sharp bends, nasal hairs, and narrow cross-sections with resulting high linear velocities, which together promote the impaction of inhaled particles.

This principle has some well-known applications. Nasal cancers are rare in the general population, but they occur with an increased incidence in certain occupational groups, probably due to nasal deposition of inhaled dusts that contain carcinogens. Examples include workers in furniture manufacturing who are exposed to wood dust, and workers in leather shoe and boot manufacturing who are exposed to leather, fiberboard, rubber, and cork dusts. A similar phenomenon is thought to occur farther along the airways. Most bronchogenic carcinomas arise at airway branch points, where particle deposition is promoted by locally turbulent air flow.

The effective anatomy of the respiratory tract changes significantly with a simple shift from nose-breathing to mouth-breathing, as occurs normally during physical exertion. This bypasses the more efficient filtration of larger particles by the nasopharynx and results in greater deposition in the tracheobronchial tree. Through such a transition workers performing physical labor may lose the benefit of a major natural defense mechanism.

Since particle density and shape also influence deposition, these parameters are subsumed in a conceptual measure of size, the *effective aerodynamic diameter.* Comparisons among unlike particles, as if they were spherical and of unit density, are thus possible. As Figure 14-1 shows, deposition is very efficient for particles with an effective aerodynamic diameter above several microns (μ), reaches its minimal level at about 1.0 μ, and increases again below 0.5 μ. Particles with an effective aerodynamic diameter of between 0.5 and 5.0 μ (the respirable fraction) can persist in the alveoli and respiratory bronchioles after deposition there, the first step in the development of pneumoconiosis. Smaller particles are cleared by macrophages, lymphatics, and the bloodstream, while larger particles are filtered out in the upper airways. The size of a particle is not always constant; hygroscopic particles such as some salts can expand significantly when hydrated in the upper airways. The result is a higher proportion of upper airway deposition.

As minute volume increases, the deposition of particles in the airways increases, especially of larger particles. In contrast, a change to rapid, shallow breathing diminishes the residence time of airborne particles in the lungs and hence the probability of deposition. Deep breathing, as during strenuous exertion, delivers a larger proportion of inhaled air to the distal airways and promotes alveolar deposition. Thus, with some basic knowledge of the particles in question and the nature of the inhalation exposure, one can evaluate, in general terms, the seriousness of a workplace exposure.

Filtration of particles in the upper airways and clearance of particles that do arrive distally are accomplished mainly by the mucociliary escalator. Particles that impact on ciliated regions of the air-

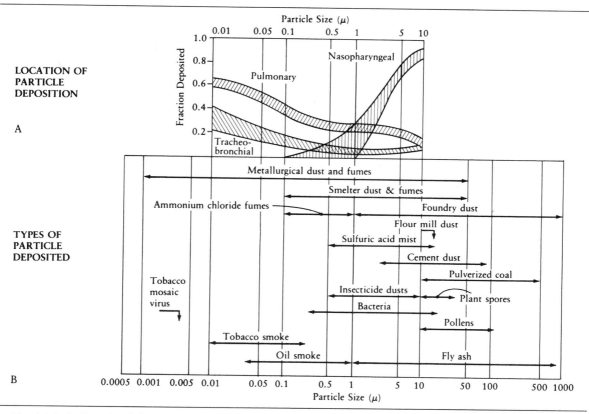

Fig. 14-1. A. Fractional deposition plotted against particle size (effective aerodynamic diameter) for three functional parts of the respiratory tree, based on the model of the International Committee on Radiation Protection. The broad bands reflect large standard deviations. B. Examples of inhaled particles, classified by size. By comparing (A) and (B), one can generate approximate predictions of the deposition pattern of each particle. (Adapted from JD Brain, PA Valberg. Aerosol deposition in the respiratory tract. Am Rev Resp Dis 1979; 120:1325–1373).

ways are carried toward the pharynx within hours and thus have little chance to dissolve or undergo leaching. However, particles deposited in nonciliated regions may be more persistent. If they are removed from surface sites by alveolar macrophages, they reach the mucociliary escalator and are cleared within 24 hours. (Materials that are carried to the pharynx by the mucociliary escalator are then swallowed, resulting in gastrointestinal exposure and possibly explaining the elevated

incidence of gastrointestinal cancer among asbestos workers.)

Alternatively, particles that reach nonciliated regions may penetrate into fixed tissue, such as connective tissue or lymph nodes, where they may reside for years, sometimes eliciting pathologic reactions. This penetration is especially likely when the performance of the mucociliary escalator is somehow compromised, as it is in smokers or in some chronically exposed workers. In general, the mucociliary escalator is an effective defense against the retention of most inhaled particles. But when it is overrun, particles are retained and the stage is set for subsequent pathology.

Skin

Human skin consists of three layers (the epidermis, dermis, and subcutaneous fat) and three kinds of glandular structures (sebaceous glands, apocrine sweat glands—both part of the "pilosebaceous unit"—and eccrine sweat glands) (see Fig. 23-1). The outermost layer of the epidermis, the stratum corneum or horny layer, provides some of the skin's structural stability and much of its chemical resistance. This layer consists mainly of thickened cell envelopes and a combination of sulfur-rich amorphous proteins and sulfur-poor fibrous proteins known as keratin.

There are two forms of percutaneous absorption: *transepidermal* (through the epidermal cells) and *appendageal* (through the hair follicles and sebaceous glands). The appendageal route offers greater permeability and plays an important role early in exposure and in the diffusion of ions and polar nonelectrolytes. However, the transepidermal route is generally more prominent because of its far greater absorbing surface.

Transepidermal transport occurs by passive diffusion, and several mechanisms have been hypothesized. According to one theory, the intracellular keratin matrix of the stratum corneum provides the main resistance to penetration by toxins, with polar and nonpolar molecules appearing to permeate through distinct channels. Alternatively, a two-phase series model postulates a protein-rich "cytoplasm" and a lipoidal "cell wall" to describe the passage of alcohols and steroids through the stratum corneum. A third possibility is that the stratum corneum limits the passage of polar molecules, while aqueous "boundary layers" prevent the diffusion of more lipophilic substances. Even very soluble substances encounter a relative barrier at the skin; in one experiment mustard gas was found fixed in the epidermis and dermis of human skin 24 hours after application. (An interesting possibility is that the skin acts as a reservoir due to in situ fixation. After exposure ceases, toxins could continue to enter the bloodstream from skin stores. This process has been documented with some steroids.)

A tremendous variety of aliphatic and aromatic hydrocarbons, metals, and pesticides can undergo at least some percutaneous absorption. Generally, fat soluble substances show a greater flux than water soluble ones, and substances that are soluble in both fat and water show the greatest flux. For any substance the relative importance of percutaneous absorption must be evaluated in light of other significant routes of entry: Although volatile solvents such as trichloroethylene and toluene are absorbed through the skin, inhalation would be far more significant in most occupational settings; on the other hand, for a substance such as benzidine, which is readily absorbed by the skin but has low volatility, percutaneous absorption may be the major route of entry.

A variety of factors can influence the extent of percutaneous absorption. Some are properties of the skin such as wetness, location on the body, and vascularization. Prior damage, such as abrasion or dermatitis, can dramatically increase absorption. Certain organic solvents, such as dimethyl sulfoxide (DMSO), and mixtures, such as ethanol/ether or chloroform/methanol, are efficient delipidizing agents, which compromise the barrier function of the stratum corneum. Occlusion is often used to promote the absorption of medications, but in the workplace occlusion can have untoward results. For example, if a worker wears rubber gloves that contain a solvent, absorption may be enhanced. Other factors that influence percutaneous absorption reside in the substance being absorbed and include concentration, phase (aqueous or dry), pH, molecular weight, and vehicle. In fact, the best single determinant of the flux of a substance across the skin is its *partition coefficient* between stratum corneum and vehicle, which varies with the vehicle.

Skin absorption, of course, is necessary but not sufficient for the development of percutaneous toxicity. Cutaneous exposure may be followed by local effects (as discussed in Chap. 23), by systemic effects (as discussed later in this chapter), or by no effects at all.

Gastrointestinal Tract

Ingestion of hazardous substances is generally not a major route of workplace exposure, although there are important exceptions. Workers who mouth-breathe or who chew gum or tobacco can absorb appreciable amounts of gaseous materials during a workday. Inhaled particulates swept upward by ciliary action from the airways can be swallowed. And materials on the hands may be brought to the mouth during on-the-job eating, drinking, and smoking.

Several features of the gastrointestinal (GI) tract help to minimize toxicity by this route. Gastric and pancreatic juices can detoxify some substances by hydrolysis and reduction. Absorption into the bloodstream may be inefficient and selective. Food and liquid present in the GI tract can dilute toxins and can form less soluble complexes with them. Finally, the portal circulation carries absorbed materials to the liver, where metabolism can begin promptly. As a result, the most serious GI exposures to consider are those with slowly cumulative action such as mercury, lead, and cadmium.

DISTRIBUTION

Some toxins exert their effects at the site of initial contact. For example, the skin can be "burned" by strongly acidic or basic solutions or delipidized by some solvents, inhalation of phosgene can lead to delayed pulmonary edema, and inhalation of cadmium fume can lead to pneumonitis. But many toxins are taken up by the bloodstream and transported to other parts of the body, where they may exert biologic effects or be stored. The destination of a chemical is largely determined by its ability to cross various membrane barriers and by its affinity for particular body compartments.

Membranes are the main obstacle to the free movement of chemicals among the various compartments of the body. The mammalian cell membrane consists of a lipid layer sandwiched between two protein layers, with a combined thickness of about 100 Å. Large protein molecules, freely mobile in the plane of the membrane, can penetrate one or both faces, and small pores 2 to 4 Å in diameter traverse the membrane. There are thus three mechanisms by which a chemical can cross a membrane: simple diffusion of lipid-soluble substances through the membrane; filtration through the pores by small molecules that accompany the bulk flow of water; and binding by specialized carrier molecules, which transport polar molecules actively or passively through the lipid layer.

In a steady-state situation, the solute concentrations on the two sides of a membrane reach an equilibrium. This equilibrium is described by Fick's first law of diffusion, which states that the amount of solute (ds) that diffuses across an area (A) in time (t) is proportional to the local concentration gradient (dc/dx):

$$\frac{ds}{dt} = -DA \frac{dc}{dx}$$

The proportionality constant (D) is the diffusion coefficient. This constant is inversely proportional to the cube root of the molecular weight for a spherical molecule. Accordingly, many small molecules that ordinarily cross membranes without difficulty are unable to cross the same membranes once bound to large serum molecules. The diffusion coefficient also reflects the lipid/water partition coefficient. The result is an important generalization: molecules that are fat-soluble cross membranes far more readily and far more rapidly than compounds that are water-soluble.

This generalization not only describes the distribution of toxins in the body; it has clinical applications as well. Manipulating the pH on one side of a membrane can alter the extent of ionization of a solute, which, in turn, modifies its membrane solubility. This practice can be used to "trap" solute in a desired body compartment—in effect changing the flux by changing the diffusion coefficient. For example, patients who ingest large amounts of salicylates are treated with bicarbonate, in part because the resulting alkaline urine ionizes the filtered salicylate and prevents reabsorption by renal tubular cells.

Movement from one body compartment to another may not entail traversing membrane bilayers. Each of three morphologic forms of capillaries—continuous, fenestrated, and discontinuous—provides an alternative way for solutes to leave the bloodstream. Thus, various mechanisms exist by which membrane-insoluble substances and fluids can cross capillary walls, leave the vascular compartment, and reach target cells. The importance of these mechanisms is unclear, as most chemicals are thought to pass directly through capillary cells. However, in the face of local conditions such as acidosis, or in organs like the liver with discontinuous capillaries, these mechanisms may contribute significantly to the extravasation of toxins.

Two barriers to distribution deserve special attention. First, the *blood-brain barrier* hinders the passage of many toxins from central nervous system (CNS) capillaries into the brain. Its anatomic identity is not precisely known, but it probably involves the glial connective tissue cells (astrocytes), very tight junctions between endothelial cells, or an unusually low capacity for pinocytosis by endothelial cells. The blood-brain barrier is not uniform throughout the brain; for example, the cortex, lateral hypothalamic nuclei, area postrema, pineal body, and neurohypophysis are relatively less protected, perhaps due to a richer blood supply, a more permeable barrier, or both. Radiation, inorganic and alkyl mercury, and several other toxins and diseases can damage the blood-brain barrier and impair its performance.

Chemical passage across the blood-brain barrier is governed by the same rules that describe membrane crossing elsewhere in the body. Only molecules that are not bound to plasma proteins can cross into the brain. Greater fat solubility helps a molecule permeate the barrier; thus, nonionized molecules enter the brain at a rate proportional to their lipid/water partition coefficient, while ion-

ized molecules are essentially unable to leave the CNS capillaries. The blood-brain barrier, then, is distinctive mainly in its quantitatively greater protective effect compared to the body's other capillary beds.

The second barrier of particular interest is the *placenta*. In the placentas of humans and other primates, three layers of fetal tissue (trophoblast, connective tissue, and endothelium) separate the fetal and maternal blood. Some species such as the pig have six cell layers in the placental barrier, while others—the rat, rabbit, and guinea pig—have only one. These structural differences may correspond to differences in permeability, so animal data on transplacental transport must be interpreted with caution.

The placenta has active transport systems for vital materials like vitamins, amino acids, and sugars. However, most toxins appear to cross the placenta by simple diffusion. In addition, a variety of nonchemical agents can cross the placenta, including viruses (such as rubella), cellular pathogens (such as the syphilis spirochete), antibody globulins (IgG, but not IgM), fibers (including asbestos!), and even erythrocytes. There is evidence suggesting that the placenta actively blocks transport of some substances into the fetus, perhaps through chemical biotransformation mechanisms. Substances that do diffuse into the fetal circulation observe the laws discussed above, and in a steady state their maternal and fetal plasma concentrations are equal. Of course, since maternal and fetal tissues may have different affinities for some substances, the concentrations in specific kinds of tissues may differ. For example, the fetal blood-brain barrier is incompletely formed, and lead can accumulate in the fetal CNS far faster than in the maternal CNS; workplace exposure to lead thus poses a special problem for pregnant women.

STORAGE

Most foreign substances that reach the plasma water are excreted fairly promptly, either intact or following chemical modifications. However, some

BIRTH DEFECTS IN CHILDREN OF MOTHERS EXPOSED TO CHEMICALS AT WORK

Case A: A 19-year-old woman, who worked in the reinforced plastics industry and whose husband was a 26-year-old carpenter in the same factory, gave birth to her first child, a 3900-gm, 54-cm boy, 18 days before her predicted delivery date. The child was found to have congenital hydrocephalus, anomaly of the right ear, and bilateral malformations of the thoracic vertebral column and ribs. Antibody tests for rubella, toxoplasma, and listeria in mother and child, and mumps and *Herpes simplex* in the mother, were negative.

In the third month of pregnancy the mother had had bronchitis, and she was given 3 days sick leave and treated with penicillin. Otherwise her pregnancy was normal, and she had taken no drugs except for iron and vitamin preparations. The mother worked regularly during pregnancy; she ground, polished, and mended reinforced plastic products and was exposed to styrene, polyester resin, organic peroxides, acetone, and polishes. In her second trimester she was heavily exposed to styrene for about 3 days when she cleaned a mold without a face mask.

Case B: A 24-year-old woman, who worked in the reinforced plastics industry and whose husband was a 22-year-old welder-plater in the metal industry, gave birth to her first child, a 2200-gm, 47-cm girl, 6 weeks before her predicted delivery date. The baby died during delivery; anencephaly was diagnosed. Serological tests of the mother for toxoplasma and listeria, and placental culture for listeria, were all negative.

The pregnancy had been normal except for contractions during the second month. At that time 10 mg of isoxsuprine was prescribed three times a day for 7 days. Slight edema occurred in the seventh month of pregnancy, and 500 mg of chlorthiazide a day was prescribed for 7 days. The mother worked during most of her pregnancy. In the third month of pregnancy she did manual laminating for about 3 weeks with no face mask and was then exposed to styrene, polyester resin, organic peroxides, and acetone. After this period she did needlework in the same workshop for about 1 month and then laminated again at varying intervals [2].

These cases were identified during an investigation of congenital malformations in Finland. They were reported when the investigators found an overrepresentation of workers in the reinforced plastics industry among the parents of affected infants.

Teratogenesis due to industrial chemicals may well have occurred in these cases. Styrene (vinyl benzene) is metabolized to styrene oxide, a known bacterial mutagen. Styrene is also a structural analogue of vinyl chloride, which is associated with lymphocyte chromosomal aberrations and hepatic angiosarcomas among exposed workers (see Chap. 15). These molecules are sufficiently fat-soluble to cross membranes and could have passed from the maternal to the fetal circulation. Of course, the women had multiple chemical exposures, and the possibility of combined effects cannot be excluded.

However, as is typical when a chemical exposure is clinically associated with teratogenic or carcinogenic effects, no causal relation can be proven in these cases. In fact, for any particular substance it may be impossible ever to assemble a large enough group of exposed subjects to conduct an epidemiologic study that would yield statistically significant results (see Chap. 5). Health professionals must therefore use available toxicologic knowledge to evaluate case reports such as this one, identify potential hazards, and advise their patients on appropriate precautionary measures.

substances, while being distributed as described above, reach sites for which they have a high affinity, where they accumulate and persist. The result is storage depots.

These depots may occur at the sites of toxic action. For example, carbon monoxide has a very high affinity for its target molecule, hemoglobin, and the herbicide paraquat, which causes pulmonary fibrosis, accumulates in the lungs. But more commonly, the storage depot is different from the site of toxic action. For example, lead is stored in bone but exerts its toxic effects on various soft tissues. There is an equilibrium between plasma and depot concentrations of any stored substance, so a depot can slowly release its content into the bloodstream long after exposure has ended.

One important storage depot is adipose tissue. Most chlorinated solvents like carbon tetrachloride and chlorinated pesticides like DDT and dieldrin migrate from the blood to the fat due to their high lipid solubility. Storage of such substances appears to involve simple physical dissolution in neutral fats, which constitute about 20 percent of a lean individual's weight and up to 50 percent of an obese individual's weight. The fat reservoir can therefore protect an obese person by sequestering a toxin from circulation; conversely, a rapid loss of weight through illness or dieting might release toxic amounts of a stored substance back into the bloodstream.

A variety of proteins can bind exogenous molecules and thereby function as a storage depot. Probably the best known example is serum albumin, which binds and transports many pharmacologic agents. Recent evidence suggests that environmental agents such as DDE (the principal metabolite of DDT) and some dyes may compete for the albumin-binding sites. Molecules that are bound to albumin or to other plasma proteins like ceruloplasmin and transferrin are unavailable for toxic action elsewhere as long as they remain bound. A more deleterious form of protein binding occurs with mercury and cadmium: Both metals complex with renal tubular proteins, and mercury complexes with CNS proteins as well, causing dysfunction at these sites. Finally, carcinogenic hydrocarbons appear to complex with proteins on contact with the skin and lung wall, and they initiate transformation by their continued presence (see Chap. 15).

Several important toxins are stored as insoluble salts. Lead, strontium, and radium form phosphates, which are deposited in bone. Lead has a toxic effect on marrow (see Chap. 28), and it can be mobilized during acidosis to cause acute lead poisoning. Strontium, if deposited as a radioactive isotope (especially strontium 90), releases ionizing radiation, and radium is an alpha-emitter; both are associated with osteosarcomas and hematologic neoplasms (see Chap. 16). Finally, fluoride is stored in the bones and teeth as an insoluble calcium salt; high levels can lead to bone and joint distortion, joint dysfunction, and mottling of dental enamel in children.

An unusual example of storage is the lymphatic accumulation of crystalline silica in the lung. Macrophages that engulf the silica migrate to lymph nodes where they are destroyed. Continued irritation by the silica then induces inflammation and fibrosis (see Chap. 21).

PRINCIPLES OF BIOLOGIC EFFECTS

The aspect of toxic substances of greatest medical concern is their biologic effects. Several concepts have been developed to help classify and account for these effects.

Exposure to a toxic agent, and likewise the biologic response, may be *acute* or *chronic*. An acute exposure often evokes an acute response, and a chronic exposure a chronic response, but neither sequence is invariable. For example, a short-term exposure to asbestos may cause mesothelioma, a fatal neoplasm, to develop many years later.

A biologic effect may be *reversible* or *irreversible*, independent of its time course. Chronic lead poisoning can cause hematologic, renal, neurologic, gastrointestinal, and reproductive effects, and all but the late renal (and possibly some neurologic) effects are reversible. On the other hand, acute mercury poisoning can produce irritability, tremors, delirium, or outright psychosis, which may all be irreversible. Reversibility is a function of the nature of the damage done and the regenerative capacity of the damaged tissue.

Generally, higher levels of toxic exposure will lead to greater responses. They may occur within an individual—as when higher concentrations of inhaled carbon monoxide lead to higher concentrations of carboxyhemoglobin—or within a pop-

A CAR PAINTER EXPOSED TO ORGANIC SOLVENTS

During a routine medical examination a 24-year-old man reported problems with concentration: He frequently lost his train of thought, forgot what he was saying in mid-sentence, and had been told by friends that he seemed forgetful. He also felt excessively tired after waking in the morning and at the end of his workday. He had occasional listlessness and frequent headaches. At work he often felt drunk or dizzy, and several times he misunderstood simple instructions from his supervisor. These problems had all developed insidiously during the previous 2 years. The patient thought that other employees in his area of the plant had complained of similar symptoms. He had noted some relief during a recent week-long fishing vacation. He denied appetite or bowel changes, sweating, weight loss, fever, chills, palpitations, syncope, seizures, trembling hands, peripheral tingling, and changes in strength or sensation. He was a social drinker and denied drug use and cigarette smoking.

The patient had worked for 3½ years as a car painter in a railroad car repair garage. He had compiled a list of substances to which he had been exposed:

PAINT SOLVENTS	PAINT BINDERS	OTHER SUBSTANCES
Toluene	Acrylic resin	Organic dyes
Xylene	Urethane resin	Inorganic dyes
Ethanol	Bindex 284	Zinc
Isopropanol	Solution Z-92	Chromates
Butanol		Titanium
Ethyl acetate		dioxide
Ethyl glycol		Catalysts
Acetone		
Methyl ethyl ketone		

His plant had been inspected by OSHA one year previously, and the only citations issued were for minor safety violations.

Physical examination, including a careful neurologic examination, was completely normal. The erythrocyte sedimentation rate was 3 mm per hour. Routine hematologic and biochemical tests, thyroid function studies, and heterophile antibody assay were all negative, except for slight elevations of serum gamma glutamyl transpeptidase (SGGT) and alkaline phosphatase [3].

This case illustrates some of the many problems that confront a health professional in applying occupational toxicology. The patient reported vague, non-specific symptoms, which a busy clinician might easily dismiss. Unfortunately, many toxins have just such generalized effects. Furthermore, the patient had multiple chemical exposures, and no one toxin could be readily identified. This patient was unusual in that he was able to provide a list of his exposures, but even this list had its limitations. Note the presence of two (fictional) trade names on the list; their identities are unknown and may be off limits even to an inquiring physician (see the appendix to Chap. 3). The absence of OSHA citations a year earlier may mean that all exposures were currently at permissible levels, but one cannot be certain of this finding. The inspection might have been directed only at safety hazards; the plant may have been temporarily cleaned up for the inspectors' benefit; conditions could have deteriorated in the subsequent year; and new production processes could have been initiated. In any event, all the symptoms reported by this patient have been associated with "safe" levels of solvent exposure, so even a well-maintained plant might offer cause for concern.

The toxicology of organic solvents is complex and varied. Many solvents have their initial manifestations in the nervous system, in both acute and chronic poisoning. These can range from the generalized CNS symptoms described here to remarkably selective peripheral nerve involvements (see Chap. 25). Liver function is often affected, on either an acute or a chronic basis (see Chap. 29). Many organic solvents are efficient delipidizing agents, which can cause dermatitis physically and/or immunologically (see Chap. 23). Acute intoxications can lead to death from renal failure (see Chap.

30). Finally, an increasing number of solvents are being suggested as possible human carcinogens by animal and in vitro tests (see Chap. 15).

When a specific toxin has been identified, health professionals can sometimes utilize toxicology in their treatment plans. For example, ethylene glycol poisoning has been successfully treated with ethanol infusion, based on the knowledge that this substance is a substrate for the enzyme alcohol dehydrogenase. Often, however, assiduous inquiry fails to identify a specific toxin, and a physician's appropriate response must rely on common sense and general industrial hygiene improvements.

ulation—as when higher levels of benzidine dye exposure cause an elevation in the incidence of bladder cancer. Either relationship may be depicted with the familiar *dose-response curve* (Fig. 14-2).

The dose-response curve quantifies the dependence of biologic effects on dose levels. Note that the curve in Figure 14-2 has a sigmoidal shape. This shape is common. At the lower end the beginning of a linear increase reflects the existence of a *threshold dose* below which variations in exposure presumably have no effect. At the upper end the flattening of the curve reflects a *ceiling* level of maximal response that cannot be increased by greater doses. This level might correspond to death in an individual or to 100 percent incidence of disease in a population.

Several additional toxicologic concepts emerge from the dose-response curve. The LD_{50} is the dose that is lethal to 50 percent of a population; it is a measure of the *potency* of a compound, or the dose required to produce a certain effect. Potency should be distinguished from another pharmacologic measure, *efficacy,* which reflects the maximal effect a drug can produce (the ceiling on a dose-response curve). There are other standards that might be used. For example, cell killing by radiation is sometimes quantified by the "D_o" which corresponds to an LD_{63} on the exponential cell-kill curve.

Individual departures from the expected dose-response pattern can take several forms. *Hyper-susceptibility* indicates an unusually high response to some dose of a substance. This term requires very careful interpretation, however, since it is used in several different ways. It may refer to a genetic predisposition to a toxic effect; it may indicate a statistically defined deviation from the mean; it may reflect an observer's subjective impression; or it may be used, incorrectly, as a synonym for hypersensitivity. *Hypersensitivity* is one form of hypersusceptibility, characterized by an acquired, immunologically mediated sensitization to a substance. In workplace settings this sensitization is most commonly manifested in pulmonary or dermatologic responses with features of all four Gell and Coombs immunologic reaction types [6, 7]. For example, toluene diisocyanate (TDI), a major ingredient in polyurethane manufacture, will evoke asthmatic reactions in a small percentage of exposed workers even at permissible exposure levels (see Chap. 21), and workers exposed to nickel can develop a skin reaction that resembles chronic eczema (see Chap. 23). It is important to remember that such so-called hypersensitivities need not be aberrant or even unusual. Among epoxy workers, for instance, the incidence of skin sensitization to resins is approximately 50 percent, and at least 75 percent of long-term employees relate a history of dermatitis.

Hyposusceptibility, conversely, indicates an unusually low response to some dose of a substance, and it also is defined in a variety of ways. One form of hyposusceptibility is *tolerance,* a dimin-

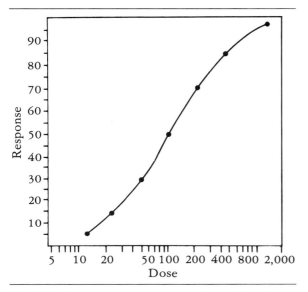

Fig. 14-2. The dose-response curve. (From J Doull, C Klaassen, M Amdur, eds. Casarett and Doull's Toxicology. 2nd ed. New York: Macmillan, 1980.)

sponsiveness that differs significantly from the mean of the larger population.

Many factors, some already mentioned, determine the *localization of effect* of a chemical exposure. These include translocation barriers such as membranes, which limit migration of the chemical; chemical affinities that concentrate the chemical on certain molecules; and regional differences in metabolic activity, in susceptibility to a given toxic effect, or in capacity for repair.

A useful classification of chemical-induced toxic effects, based in part on the work of Loomis [8], is as follows:

Normal (or expected) effects, depending on:
    Physical actions
    Nonspecific caustic or corrosive actions
    Specific toxicologic actions
    Production of pathologic sequellae
Abnormal (or unexpected) effects:
    Immune mechanisms
    Genetic susceptibility

ished response to a given dose of a chemical following repeated exposures. Tolerance classically involves an attenuation of the immune response to a specific antigen and appears graphically as a shift to the right of the dose-response curve. In experimental animals tolerance can be induced by administering antigen in certain forms or doses, and this process may well occur in workplace settings following chronic low-dose exposures. However, several equally conceivable events could yield an empirically similar result; these include the impairment of absorption, the induction of metabolizing enzymes, and the enhancement of excretion. Typically, such acquired resistance to a chemically induced response can be overcome with sufficiently large doses. *Tachyphylaxis,* in contrast, is a rapidly acquired resistance that persists even with a large subsequent dose. In view of the variety of mechanisms of hyper- and hyposusceptibility, an individual worker may readily show a dose-re-

Normal effects can be repeatedly induced, do not require preconditioning, and occur with an incidence that is primarily dose-dependent. These range from simple physical phenomena, such as the displacement of oxygen by asphyxiants, to more elaborate pathophysiological events. Immune mechanisms, in contrast, require preconditioning (sensitization) and may not be inducible in the majority of members of a population simply by increasing the exposure. Finally, genetic susceptibility is in most cases not based on sensitization and may be nothing more than a quantitatively greater propensity for developing some "normal" response. An example is the elevated risk of hemolysis among people with glucose-6-phosphate dehydrogenase (G6PD) deficiency following exposure to oxidants like naphthalene. Immune and genetic effects may coincide as inheritable immunodeficiency diseases. Further examples of each of these toxic effects appear in Appendix A at the back of this book.

NON-SPECIFIC SYMPTOMS IN AN AUTO ASSEMBLY WORKER

A 25-year-old man reported to his physician a one-month history of severe frontal headaches. They occurred daily, beginning in the early morning and lasting throughout the day. He said he felt nervous and had had a short temper for the past month. He had been sleeping normally, retiring at about 1:30 A.M. and not waking until about 7:00 A.M.

He had been seen for his headaches 3 weeks previously at an emergency room. At that time he was examined, had skull x-rays taken, and was treated with Fiorinal (a muscle relaxant containing butalbital, aspirin, phenacetin, and caffeine). Over the past month he had noted early satiety and constipation (a bowel movement every other day, whereas previously he had had a bowel movement daily), and he had noticed some weakness in his left hand.

He had never been hospitalized, had had no operations, injuries, or allergies, and was taking no medications. He had smoked a half pack of cigarettes daily for 6 years; he drank two six-packs of beer per week and one cup of coffee daily. He lived in a house in a large city, had made no repairs on it, and had not removed any of its paint; prior to that he lived with his parents in the same city. He had not traveled abroad.

Occupational History

The patient began working part-time at age 16, helping prepare new cars for a dealer. At age 21 he began full-time work in the parts department of another car dealership and remained at that job for 3 years.

Eight months previously he had begun work at an auto-body assembly plant. He worked at several jobs until his regular assignment, four months before, to the solder-grinding booth where he smoothed the solder joints between pieces of the auto bodies with a wire wheel. The job was performed by several workers within an enclosed part of the assembly line, which held four autos at a time. The solder consisted of lead and tin.

While working in this area, he used a helmet with a hood that draped down to his waist and included an air-supplied respirator. In order to communicate with him, a coworker would tap a flap on the front of the hood. At break time he removed the hood and blew the dust off his coveralls with an air hose. At the end of each day he washed up but did not shower and removed his coveralls, shoes, and socks.

He reported that the company had been testing his blood for lead at about 3-month intervals. His blood had been tested when he was hired and on two occasions since then.

The patient's wife reported that he had undergone a complete change of personality in the past several weeks and that he had not had a bowel movement for over a week. She insisted, "Something has to be done about these problems!"

Physical examination was completely normal. Blood lead was elevated at 87 µg per deciliter, and free erythrocyte protoporphyrin (FEP) was 770 µg per deciliter of packed red cells (normal 16–36) [4].

Lead is a malleable, corrosion-resistant metal with a tremendous variety of applications. Workers at risk of exposure include plumbers, solderers, and foundry workers, and those in battery, automobile, glass, ceramics, and paint manufacturing. In addition, children who eat flaking paint on walls and woodwork and consumers of "moonshine" whiskey, are at risk of lead poisoning. The addition of tetraethyl lead to gasoline increased ambient lead concentrations in the air of most cities. The toxicology of no other metal has been as thoroughly investigated.

Lead shares several characteristics with other metals. It exists in both organic and inorganic forms, and the two have markedly different effects. (The exposure in this case, like most industrial exposures, was to inorganic lead.) Most metals, including lead, exert their biologic effects through enzyme ligand binding, and for many metals excretion can be hastened by chelation therapy with agents such as dimercaprol (British antilewisite, or BAL) and ethylenediaminetetraacetic acid (EDTA). But beyond these generalizations metal toxicology is as varied as the metals themselves.

The major routes of lead absorption are the GI and respiratory tracts. The bones act as a virtually unlimited depot for lead, while soft tissue levels seem to reach a plateau. Equilibration with lead in the blood is quite rapid.

Lead was recognized as an occupational hazard as early as the first century A.D. Its early effects are non-specific: fatigue, malaise, sleep disturbance, headache, muscle and bone pain, constipation, abdominal pain, and decreased appetite. Later symptoms can be understood in terms of the five body systems principally affected: hematologic, neurologic, renal, GI, and reproductive. Lead inhibits the conversion of protoporphyrin IX to heme and increases red blood cell fragility, causing a sideroblastic anemia; erythrocytes show basophilic stippling (see Chap. 28). Lead encephalopathy causes severe CNS symptoms, which are often irreversible and sometimes fatal (see Chap. 25). Peripheral neuropathy affects motor more than sensory function; a characteristic "wrist drop" often reflects radial nerve involvement. Lead nephropathy may occur, with irreversible loss of renal function and progressive azotemia (see Chap. 30). Gastrointestinal effects include "lead colic," nausea, and constipation (or, occasionally, diarrhea). Lead toxicity has an adverse effect on pregnancy, manifested by increased stillbirths and miscarriages, and may affect male fertility (see Chap. 26). Finally, recent results suggest that lead may be a carcinogen.

Blood lead assays have traditionally been used to quantify body burden, but this parameter is less reliable than associated enzyme changes. Measurements now used in addition to blood lead include deltaaminolevulinic acid in blood and urine, erythrocyte protoporphyrin, and urinary coproporphyrin. As of 1982 OSHA required that lead-exposed workers be monitored with periodic blood tests.

Workers found to have in excess of 50 µg lead per deciliter of whole blood must be removed from exposure, at full pay, until their levels fall to below 40 µg per deciliter. (These cutoffs are accompanied by a limit on lead levels in workplace air.) Research with lead-exposed neonates and children has demonstrated neuropsychological impairment at levels below 25 µg per deciliter [5].

The patient in this case was admitted to the hospital and underwent chelation therapy with EDTA. He was discharged one week later with marked improvement in his symptoms. During the year following treatment his blood lead level gradually fell to normal. (At the time of admission the blood lead levels of the patient's wife and two children were checked; all were normal.)

This case was reported to the state health department and the state occupational health unit. An investigation of the patient's records showed that his blood lead level was 25 µg per deciliter 6 months prior to admission, 68 µg per deciliter 2 months prior to admission, and 74 µg per deciliter 1 month prior to admission. The patient had never been informed that his blood lead was elevated, and he had been permitted to remain at his job. Further investigation revealed that most of the workers in the lead solder booth had elevated blood lead levels. Subsequently, three other workers were hospitalized and treated for symptomatic lead poisoning.

METABOLIC TRANSFORMATIONS

Between initial absorption and final excretion many substances are chemically converted by the body. Although many different metabolic conversions have been described, they can be characterized by a few simple generalizations and divided into a small number of categories. Metabolic transformations are mediated by enzymes. The liver is rich in metabolic enzymes, and most biotransformation occurs there. All cells in the body, however, have some capacity for metabolizing xenobiotics (chemicals foreign to the body).

Any enzyme system has a finite capacity. When a preferred pathway is saturated, the remaining substrate may be handled by alternative pathways. (Most substrates can be metabolized by more than one enzyme system.) However, in some instances when a preferred metabolic pathway is saturated, the substrate may persist in the body and exert toxic effects. An example is dioxane metabolism. Dioxane (cyclic-$OCH_2CH_2OCH_2CH_2$) is a solvent with a variety of industrial applications, including painting, printing, and textile manufacturing. High-dose exposure in rats causes hepatocellular and renal tubular cell damage as well as hepatic and nasal carcinoma. Based on rat studies, the principal human metabolite of dioxane has been identified as β-hydroxyethoxyacetic acid (HEAA). HEAA is found in the urine of exposed workers at over 100 times the concentration of dioxane, suggesting that at low exposures the dioxane is rapidly converted to HEAA. However, the metabolic pathway from dioxane to HEAA can be saturated by high-dose exposure, and in rats this event has been correlated with toxicity. Thus, the effects of dioxane appear to be most pronounced when the ordinary metabolic pathway is saturated, allowing high levels of the solvent to accumulate. (All of this, however, does not prove that low-dose workplace exposure to dioxane is harmless, since dioxane is a carcinogen for which no safe threshold can be demonstrated.)

A particular form of enzyme saturation is *competitive inhibition,* which may be a mechanism of toxicity, as when organophosphate pesticides compete with acetylcholine for the binding sites on cholinesterase molecules, or when metals such as beryllium compete with magnesium and manganese for enzyme ligand binding. However, competitive inhibition is important as well in the metabolic processing of toxins. For example, methyl alcohol is oxidized by the enzyme alcohol dehydrogenase to the optic nerve toxin formaldehyde. This process can be blocked by large doses of ethanol, which competes for the binding sites of the enzyme and slows the formation of the toxic metabolite.

A less salutary example of competitive inhibition is the synergy demonstrated by two organophosphate pesticides, malathion and EPN (ethyl *p*-nitrophenyl phenylphosphonothionate). Although they are structurally similar, EPN is far more toxic than malathion. When the two pesticides are present together, the EPN competes for the enzyme that would ordinarily hydrolyze and thus detoxify the malathion. As a result malathion persists at unusually high concentrations, and the combined toxicity is far greater than would be expected. Other pairs of organophosphates that interact similarly are malathion and trichlorfon (Dipterex), and azinphos-methyl (Gusathion) and trichlorfon. Since most workplace exposures involve multiple substances, such synergistic effects are common but probably go unrecognized most of the time. This synergism is important to remember when evaluating reports on the toxicity of individual substances.

The enzyme systems that metabolize xenobiotics are not static. When the demand is high, their synthesis can be enhanced in a process called *enzyme induction.* The resulting increase in enzyme activity helps the organism respond to subsequent exposures not only to the original xenobiotic but to similar substances as well. DDT and methyl cholanthrene are examples of substances known to induce metabolic enzymes.

In general, metabolic transformations lead to products that are more polar and less fat soluble, consistent with the eventual goal of excretion. This process usually entails a change from more toxic to less toxic forms: For example, benzene is oxidized to phenol, and glutathione combines with halogenated aromatics to form nontoxic mercapturic acid metabolites.

However, metabolic transformations sometimes yield increasingly toxic products. One example, the oxidation of methanol to formaldehyde, has already been mentioned. Another example is the solvent methyl *n*-butyl ketone (MBK), which produces peripheral neuropathy ("cabinet finisher's neuropathy") in exposed workers (see Chap. 25). Animal toxicology studies have revealed that a γ-diketone metabolite of MBK, 2,5-hexanedione, is probably the actual neurotoxin. *N*-hexane is also oxidized to 2,5-hexanedione, which probably accounts for the neurotoxicity of that solvent (see

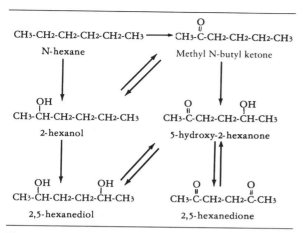

Fig. 14-3. The metabolic transformation of *n*-hexane. (From PS Spencer, et al. On the specific molecular configuration of neurotoxic aliphatic hexacarbon compounds causing central-peripheral distal axonopathy. Toxicol Appl Pharmacol 1978; 44:17. Modified from GD Divincenzo, et al. Characterization of the metabolites of methyl-*n*-butyl ketone, methyl isobutyl ketone, and methyl ethyl ketone in guinea pig serum and their clearance. Toxicol Appl Pharmacol 1976; 36:511.)

Fig. 14-3). In contrast, other hexacarbons such as methyl isobutyl ketone (MIBK) and methyl ethyl ketone (MEK) cannot give rise to 2,5-hexanedione and would thus be preferable to MBK as solvents.

The concept of toxic metabolites is especially salient with regard to carcinogens (see Chap. 15). Vinyl chloride, a causative agent of liver, lung, lymphatic, and central nervous system tumors, is oxidized to a reactive epoxide intermediate, which is actually the proximate carcinogen. The same is probably true for trichloroethylene, vinylidene chloride, vinyl benzene, and chlorobutadiene. In fact, a major mechanism of carcinogenicity of aromatic compounds is conversion to reactive epoxides, which in turn combine with cellular nucleophiles like DNA and RNA.

Classically, metabolic transformations are divided into four categories: oxidation, reduction, hydrolysis, and conjugation. The first three reaction types, which are known as phase I reactions, increase the polarity of substrates and can either increase or decrease toxicity. In conjugation, the only phase II reaction, polar groups are added to the products of phase I reactions. Most chemicals are handled sequentially by the two phases, although some are directly conjugated. The spectrum of reactions of each type can be found in any toxicology text, and only a few examples of occupational health interest will be presented here.

Oxidation is the most common biotransformation reaction. There are two general kinds of oxidation reactions: direct addition of oxygen to the carbon, nitrogen, sulfur, or other bond; and dehydrogenation. Most of these reactions are mediated by microsomal enzymes, although there are mitochondrial and cytoplasmic oxidases as well. Examples of oxidation include:

Hydroxylation:

Benzene   to   Phenol

N-Hydroxylation:

Aniline   to   Phenylhydroxylamine

Desulfuration:

Parathion   to   Paraoxon

The thiophosphate insecticides, such as parathion, are relatively nontoxic until the S is replaced by O through this reaction.

Deamination:

N-Butylamine   to   Butaldehyde and Ammonia

Reduction is a much less common biotransformation than oxidation, but it does occur with substances whose redox potentials exceed that of the body. Examples include:

Azo reduction:

O-aminoazotoluene   to   Aniline derivatives

The azo dyes have been known since the 1930s to include many mutagens and carcinogens. Reduction of the azo bond yields aromatic amines, such as aniline and benzidine, which are probably the active carcinogens. In mammalian test species, the principal target sites are the bladder and liver. Not all azo dyes are carcinogenic; extensive investigation of these compounds has yielded a rich body of information about structure-activity relationships.

Aromatic nitro reduction:

Nitrobenzene   to   Aniline

Conjugation involves combining a toxin with a normal body constituent. The result is generally a less toxic and more polar molecule, which can be more readily excreted. However, conjugation can be harmful if it occurs in excess and depletes the body of an essential constituent. Examples of conjugation reactions include:

Sulfation:

Phenol   to   Its sulfate conjugate

Sulfation is the major means of preparing phenol for excretion. It is also used for alcohols, amines, and other groups.

Acetylation:

Aniline   to   Its acetyl conjugate

The above two reactions exemplify the sequential processing of substances by phase I and phase II reactions. Phenol and aniline can themselves be metabolites of other toxins, as previously illustrated; they are then conjugated and excreted.

Mercapturic acid addition:

Naphthalene   to   Its mercapturic acid conjugate

The addition of mercapturic acid (*N*-acetylcysteine) is a multi-step process, which proceeds through the addition of glutathione and subsequent cleavage to cysteine derivatives. This reaction is extremely important in handling reactive electrophilic compounds, the products of exogenous exposure or of endogenous metabolic processes. Polyaromatic hydrocarbons (PAHs) and polyhalogenated hydrocarbons are predominantly excreted in this way.

Hydrolysis is a common reaction in a variety of biochemical pathways. Esters are hydrolyzed to acids and alcohols, and amides are hydrolyzed to acids and amines.

As mentioned above, various combinations of these reactions may be assembled in response to the same toxin. Metabolic strategies for a particular toxin may vary widely among species, so an animal study, to be applicable to humans, must use a species with pathways similar to those of humans. To a lesser extent there is also variation among people, based on general health, age, nutrition, sex, genetic, and other factors.

EXCRETION

Since biotransformation tends to make compounds more polar and less fat soluble, the happy outcome of this process is that toxins can be more readily excreted from the body. The major route

A FARMWORKER WITH PESTICIDE POISONING

A 34-year-old migrant farmworker was brought to a hospital emergency department by his friends. All spoke only Spanish, and no interpreter was available. However, the friends indicated that the patient had suffered from nausea, vomiting, diarrhea, weakness, and increased salivation for several hours.

The patient was a well-developed, well-nourished Hispanic man who seemed restless and anxious. His speech was slurred, and despite profuse sweating he appeared somewhat dehydrated. Blood pressure was 160/100, pulse 90, and respirations 24 and labored. Physical findings included bilateral pinpoint pupils, a watery nasal discharge, profuse salivation, and marked expiratory wheezing. Occasional, diffusely distributed muscular fasciculations were noted. The patient was oriented to place and day, but mental status could not be evaluated further due to the language barrier. He had moderate proximal and distal muscle weakness, and his deep tendon reflexes were delayed.

Serum electrolytes were normal, glucose was 190 mg per deciliter, and arterial blood gases showed mild respiratory acidosis. Naloxone was administered twice without improvement.

During the hour following his arrival the patient became progressively dyspneic and finally required intubation. When an interpreter arrived, she learned from the patient's friends that the patient had been accidentally sprayed by a pesticide applicator several hours earlier at the orchard where they all worked. He had sustained a concentrated exposure, both respiratory and percutaneous, to the pesticide. His friends were unable to identify the pesticide.

Within a half hour of the exposure the patient had begun to complain of chest tightness, nausea, and dysphagia. He vomited several times, passed three loose stools, and developed generalized muscular weakness over several hours. It was then that he had been brought to the emergency department.

A wide variety of pesticides is used in the United States and abroad. The most ubiquitous are insecticides, including:

Organophosphates: malathion, parathion, mevinphos
Carbamates: aldicarb (Temik), zectran, carbaryl
Organohalides: DDT, aldrin, dieldrin, lindane, methoxychlor, chlordecone (Kepone), methyl bromide
Botanicals: pyrethrum
Miscellaneous others: arsenicals, phenolic compounds

There are other forms of pesticides as well, including herbicides (such as dinitrophenols and bipyridyls), fungicides, and rodenticides. According to statistical accounts compiled by the California Department of Public Health, organophosphates are the most frequent cause of occupational pesticide poisonings. Specifically, parathion is the major cause of both occupational poisoning and pesticide-related deaths. Those at risk of occupational poisoning include production and application workers and field hands. Furthermore, the increasing home use of pesticides has been associated with an increasing number of childhood poisonings, and pesticides are frequently implicated in suicidal ingestions.

The worker in this case was acutely exposed to parathion. Like other organophosphates, parathion can be absorbed by respiratory, percutaneous, and gastrointestinal routes, the first two of which occurred here. It is then metabolized by hepatic microsomal enzymes. The first major conversion it undergoes is replacement of its sulfur by oxygen to form paraoxon, the actual anticholinesterase. Subsequent oxidation and hydrolysis result in detoxification.

Paraoxon binds with acetylcholinesterase molecules at cholinergic nerve endings, both centrally and peripherally. The organophosphates and the carbamates both act through this mechanism; a major difference is that the carbamate complexes dissociate spontaneously, while the organophosphate complex formation is virtually irreversible. Thus, organophosphate poisoning causes a predictable constellation of muscarinic, nicotinic, and central nervous system symptoms such as those described above. Severe cases can progress to coma and death.

Proper treatment entails thorough washing of an exposed patient, including eye cleaning and gastric lavage if appropriate, and provision of ventilatory assistance when necessary. Atropine blocks the excessive cholinergic stimulation, and pralidoxime (2-PAM) uncouples the cholinesterase-organophosphate complexes; the two seem to act synergistically. Most patients recover completely, although some may suffer residual motor neurotoxicity.

The patient described in this case went on to complete recovery. His poisoning was reported to the department of public health as required by law. A follow-up study of the farm workers at that orchard revealed that most had a moderate to marked inhibition of cholinesterase function as measured by erythrocyte cholinesterase levels. Many reported nausea, vomiting, diarrhea, and increased secretions during work. Under legal pressure, the grower soon introduced a series of procedural safeguards for pesticide application (see Chap. 33).

of excretion of toxins and their metabolites is through the kidneys (see Chap. 30). The kidneys handle toxins in the same way that they handle any serum solutes: passive glomerular filtration, passive tubular diffusion, and active tubular secretion. The daily volume of filtrate produced is about 200 liters—five times the total body water—in a remarkably efficient and thorough filtration process.

Smaller molecules can reach the tubules through passive glomerular filtration, since the glomerular capillary pores are large enough (40 Å) to admit molecules of up to about 70,000 daltons. However, this excludes substances bound to large serum proteins; these substances must undergo active tubular secretion to be excreted. The tubular secretory apparatus apparently has separate processes for organic anions and organic cations, and, like any active transport system, these can be saturated and competitively blocked. Finally, passive tubular diffusion out of the serum probably occurs to some extent, especially for certain organic bases.

Passive diffusion also occurs in the opposite direction, from the tubules to the serum. Like any of the membrane crossings discussed previously, lipid-soluble molecules are reabsorbed from the tubular lumen much more readily than polar molecules and ions, which explains the practice, already mentioned, of alkalinizing the urine to hasten the excretion of acids.

A second major organ of excretion is the liver (see Chap. 29). The liver occupies a strategic position, since the portal circulation promptly delivers compounds to it following gastrointestinal absorption. Furthermore, the generous perfusion of the liver and the discontinuous capillary structure within it facilitate its filtration of the blood. Thus, excretion into the bile is potentially a rapid and efficient process.

Biliary excretion is somewhat analogous to renal tubular secretion. These are specific transport systems for organic acids, organic bases, neutral compounds, and possibly metals. These are active transport systems with the ability to handle protein-bound molecules. Finally, reuptake of lipid-soluble substances can occur after secretion, in this case through the intestinal walls.

Marked variation in biliary secretion can exist. Liver disease can compromise the process, while some chemicals such as phenobarbital and some steroids, in addition to inducing hepatic metabolic enzymes, can actually increase bile flow and hence biliary excretion. The effects of different chemicals may have practical applications; certain steroids have been demonstrated to decrease mercury toxicity in animals, which is attributed, at least in part, to their effect on biliary excretion.

Toxins that are secreted with the bile enter the gastrointestinal tract and, unless reabsorbed, are secreted with the feces. Materials ingested orally and not absorbed and materials carried up the respiratory tree and swallowed are also passed with the feces. All of this process may be supplemented by some passive diffusion through the walls of the gastrointestinal tract, although it is not a major mechanism of excretion.

Volatile gases and vapors are excreted primarily by the lungs. The process is one of passive diffusion, governed by the difference between plasma and alveolar vapor pressure. Volatiles that are highly fat-soluble tend to persist in body reservoirs and take some time to migrate from adipose tissue to plasma to alveolar air. Less fat-soluble volatiles, on the other hand, are exhaled fairly promptly, until the plasma level has decreased to that of ambient air. Interestingly, the lungs can sustain alveolar and bronchial irritation when a vapor such as gasoline is exhaled, even if the initial exposure occurred percutaneously or through ingestion.

Other routes of excretion, although of minor significance quantitatively, are important for a variety of reasons. Excretion into mother's milk obviously introduces a risk to the infant, and since milk is more acidic (pH of 6.5) than serum, basic compounds are concentrated in milk. Moreover, owing to the high fat content of breast milk (3–5%), fat-soluble substances such as DDT can also be passed to the infant (see Chap. 31). Some toxins, especially metals, are excreted in sweat or laid down in growing hair, and these may be of use in diagnosis. Finally, some materials are secreted in the saliva and may then pose a subsequent gastrointestinal exposure hazard.

This chapter has presented basic principles of toxicology that are fundamental to the understanding of the effects of toxic substances and the treatment and prevention of these effects. In the chapters that follow (particularly Chapters 15, and 21 through 30), there will be detailed exploration of the types of biologic effects caused by

workplace toxins. Readers interested in particular toxins should refer to the appendix to Chapter 3 ("How to Research the Toxic Effects of Chemical Substances"), Appendix A at the back of the book (a detailed listing of many toxic substances), and the index at the back of the book.

REFERENCES

1. Centers for Disease Control. Morbidity and Mortality Weekly Report. June 8, 1979; 28:254.
2. Holmberg PC. Central nervous defects in two children of mothers exposed to chemicals in the reinforced plastics industry. Scand J Work Environ Health 1977; 3:212.
3. Husman K. Symptoms of car-painters with long-term exposure to a mixture of organic solvents. Scand J Work Environ Health 1980; 6:19.
4. Keogh J. University of Maryland Hospital, Baltimore, Md.
5. Bellinger D, Leviton A, Waternaux C, et al. Longitudinal analyses of prenatal and postnatal lead exposure and early cognitive development. N Engl J Med 1987; 316:1037.
6. Newman L, Storey E, Kreiss K. Immunologic evaluation of occupational lung disease. Occup Med: State of the Art Rev 1987; 2:345.
7. Coombs RAA, Gell PGH. Classification of allergic reactions responsible for clinical hypersensitivity and disease. In: Gell PGH, Coombs RAA, Lachmann PJ, eds. Clinical aspects in immunology. Oxford: Blackwell, 1963, p. 363.
8. Loomis T. Essentials of toxicology. Philadelphia: Lea & Febiger, 1974.

BIBLIOGRAPHY

Brain JD, Beck BD, Warren AJ, et al. Variations in susceptibility to inhaled pollutants: Identification, mechanisms, and policy implications. Baltimore: Johns Hopkins University Press, 1988.
Sophisticated discussion of biological variability in toxic responses, including statistical, biological, and policy considerations.
Brain JD, Valberg PA. Aerosol deposition in the respiratory tract. Am Rev Resp Dis 1979; 120:1325–73
The "classic" review article on airways deposit with a discussion of major classes of inhaled part and their effects on health.

Clayton GD, Clayton FE. Patty's industrial hygiene and toxicology. (4 vols, 3rd ed.). New York: Wiley, 1981.
An encyclopedic reference text of toxicology.
Klaassen CD, Amdur MO, Doull J eds. Casarett and Doull's toxicology: the basic science of poisons. 3rd ed. New York: MacMillan, 1986.
The standard toxicology text with chapters on general principles, individual body systems, and specific families of toxins.
Lauwerys RR. Industrial chemical exposure: guidelines for biological monitoring. Davis, CA: Biomedical Publications, 1983.
A review of the metabolism and excretion of various substances geared toward rational use of biologic monitoring tests.
Loomis T. Essentials of toxicology. Philadelphia: Lea & Febiger, 1974.
Slightly dated, but still the best short introductory toxicology text. Clear writing and lucid organization of basic principles.

15
Carcinogens

Howard Frumkin and Barry S. Levy

In early 1972, a 43-year-old patient with newly diagnosed lung cancer was referred to a young pulmonary physician in Philadelphia, Dr. William Figueroa. The patient had worked at a Philadelphia chemical company, and according to the referring physician, some of his coworkers had succumbed to lung cancer. Figueroa later described his first encounter with the patient: "He came in, told me that he believed he had lung cancer, the same thing that had killed 13 other men he'd worked with. What excited me was that he had oat cell carcinoma, which is very rare among nonsmokers, and he'd never smoked. Oat cell is the wild, undifferentiated kind. It spreads fast. It's usually found among smokers. But [the patient] swore he'd never smoked and neither had three of the other men who'd died. Most of the others were very light smokers, he said. They were young. Cancer is an old man's disease, usually among men in their fifties and sixties who've smoked at least a pack a day for 20 to 30 years" [1].

Figueroa recognized that an occupational carcinogen might be involved, and he decided to investigate further. Many of the workers, it turned out, were exposed to chloromethyl methyl ether (CMME), an intermediate in the manufacture of ion-exchange resins. CMME is invariably contaminated with bis(chloromethyl) ether (BCME); animal data suggesting that BCME was a carcinogen had appeared in 1967, and well-designed experiments verified this by 1971. Figueroa appealed to company management for the exposure records of a cohort of workers in order to determine if BCME was associated with human lung cancer. Unfortunately, the records were not made available to him.

Faced with a similar situation several years earlier, another Philadelphia physician had not pursued the matter. "I had a feeling that four cases in 125 was excessive . . ." he explained. "I didn't go any further because I didn't know if it was significant. [The company] said there was no exposure data and I didn't know what to do" [1]. Figueroa, however, turned to another source of data—his patient.

"I decided to trust the memory of this guy, of one honest American worker," recalled Figueroa. "We stood next to [his] bed as he lay there, dying of cancer, in an oxygen mask. I read him all the names and he told me which had been exposed and who had died." Through this investigation Figueroa was able to suggest that BCME exposure was associated with a marked elevation in lung cancer mortality. His results were soon published [2], and together with subsequent corroborating data, produced both local and national effects. In 1974, the widows of BCME victims were informed that they could file for workers' compensation benefits based on the work-relatedness of their husbands' deaths. That same year, the Occupational Safety and Health Administration (OSHA) promulgated a series of regulations designed to control exposure to 14 carcinogens, one of which was BCME [1].

The BCME story illustrates six important principles:

1. Alert clinicians have a valuable role to play in occupational health through both clinical observation and appropriate follow-up.
2. Accurate information about occupational etiologies can benefit not only populations affected by preventive measures but also individual patients and their families.
3. Accurate exposure histories are often difficult to obtain, especially in cancer cases—when exposure predates disease by many years—and in situations involving proprietary interests.
4. One of the best sources of information on occupational hazards is one of the most frequently overlooked—exposed workers.
5. Animal data on carcinogenicity correlate well with the human experience and are usually available before epidemiologic data can be developed.
6. Confounding variables, such as smoking, can obscure carcinogenic associations. If all of the BCME victims had been smokers, their oat cell carcinomas might have been attributed to smoking, and the carcinogenicity of BCME could have remained unnoticed.

In terms of morbidity and mortality, work-related malignancies are an important category of occupational disease. We probably underestimate the quantitative importance of occupational cancer since the occupational etiology of many cancers goes unrecognized. Certainly, few diseases have raised as much public concern as cancer. With few exceptions, progress in treating cancer has been disappointing, so public health interventions such as prevention and education are critical.

Health care providers confront occupational cancer in many ways. They have a vital role in recognition, as the BCME example illustrates. Similarly, they can educate and advise their patients on avoiding exposure to proven or suspected occupational carcinogens. Patients may ask their providers to evaluate whether their cancers resulted from workplace exposures. When an occupational cancer is discovered, the clinician can be a valuable source of information, not only to the patient seeking compensation but also to coworkers, managers and representatives of government agencies. Health professionals can actively contribute to efforts to prevent further exposure to carcinogens. Finally, the study and understanding of occupational carcinogens have important implications for the control of similar (although lower-dose) exposures in the general environment and consumer products.

THE PROCESS OF CARCINOGENESIS

A *carcinogen* is a substance that causes cancer. Carcinogens may be chemicals, physical agents such as ionizing radiation, or biologic agents such as viruses or aflatoxin. In some cases, such as in parts of the rubber industry, elevated rates of cancer have been detected, but a specific carcinogen has not been identified.

Current knowledge of the mechanisms of carcinogenesis remains incomplete. Based on experimental work with mouse skin in the 1940s, two stages in carcinogenesis were identified: *initiation* and *promotion*. More recently, this scheme has been expanded to a multistep sequence, beginning with initiation, proceeding to promotion, and culminating in one or more *progression* steps [3]. The multistage models accord with experimental observations of carcinogenesis, and mathematical models that incorporate sequential steps have been relatively successful in accounting for observed dose-response relationships.

During initiation, irreversible DNA damage, or *mutation,* occurs. Many initiators are metabolized to active forms, usually electrophiles, which then bind covalently with DNA. The resulting *DNA adducts* may be long-lived or short-lived and may vary greatly in form. The significance of the various kinds of adducts, of associated conformational changes in DNA, and of even grosser chromosomal alterations such as frame shifts and deletions, is not well understood. In addition, there is some evidence that covalent binding to DNA is not always necessary for initiation. It is likely, for example, that some carcinogens such as ionizing radiation act through a "hit-and-run" effect on DNA, without adduct formation. These points are important in considering screening programs for carcinogen-exposed populations.

Most cells are believed to have some capacity for repair. When an initiator alters DNA in some way, repair processes may supravene to correct the alteration. However, if cell replication occurs before repair is complete, the DNA damage may be permanently "fixed," setting the stage for propagation of the damage through future cell generations. For this reason cell replication is considered an essential part of initiation.

Promotion is the process by which initiated cells develop into focal proliferations such as nodules or papillomas. Current evidence suggests that promoters are not mutagens (substances that cause mutations). Instead, they seem to act through "epigenetic" mechanisms such as increases in macromolecule synthesis, through disrupting the normal control of cell proliferation and differentiation, or even through whole organ effects that somehow facilitate tumor development. The hallmark of promotion is the acquisition by the cell of some *autonomy,* so that continued evolution is independent of further environmental stimulus. During *progression,* the focal proliferation evolves into a more malignant cancer. The determinants and components of progression are among the least understood aspects of carcinogenesis [3].

Initiation and promotion differ in several ways. Initiators are mutagens whereas promoters are mitogens (inducers of cell division). Initiation is irreversible; promotion may be reversible early on, becoming irreversible only later. Initiation occurs a considerable time before the appearance of a tumor whereas promotion may occur relatively late. Based on these considerations, the concept of a *practical promoter* has been advanced [4]. Features of practical promoters include evidence of interaction with other risk factors, evidence that exposure acts relatively late, and evidence that removal from exposure decreases risk. These concepts have obvious practical application.

An important issue in carcinogenesis is *latency.* Latency refers to the period of time between the onset of exposure to a carcinogen and the clinical detection of resulting cancers. The latency period for hematologic malignancies is in the range of 4 or 5 years, whereas the latency period for solid tumors is at least 10 to 20 years, and possibly as long as 50 years. This period presumably corresponds to the stages of initiation, promotion, and progression between the first DNA mutation and the ultimate appearance of a malignant tumor. Because of latency considerations, screening of workers at risk of cancer should focus on the time *after* initiation and before clinical presentation (see Chap. 4). If surveillance is conducted too soon after the onset of exposure, no increase in risk would be expected. The yield of screening at this stage is low, the expense is avoidable, and there is a danger that negative results will be falsely reassuring.

The existence of *threshold* levels of exposure to carcinogens has been a controversial topic [5]. A threshold is suggested to be a "safe" level of exposure below which carcinogenesis does not occur. Since a single mutation in a single cell can theoretically give rise to a malignancy, it has been argued that there is no safe level of exposure. Moreover, both epidemiologic and animal studies are insensitive to effects at extremely low doses, so the presence of thresholds may be impossible to confirm. However, several arguments in favor of thresholds have been advanced. First, there are known repair mechanisms that correct DNA damage, at least at low levels of exposure. Second, certain carcinogens, such as trace elements and hormones, are ubiquitous and at low doses even essential to life; it is argued that these substances are carcinogenic only at higher doses. Third, if a substance is a promoter rather than an initiator, its effects may be reversible, at least at low doses, implying a threshold. Finally, certain empirical results have been interpreted as illustrating the existence of thresholds. The issue remains unsettled, and preventive strategies have generally taken a conservative approach, setting zero exposure to carcinogens as a goal. This approach has engendered considerable controversy.

Interaction is another important concept in occupational carcinogenesis. This phenomenon occurs when the joint effect of two or more carcinogens is different from what would have been predicted based on the individual effects [6]. *Synergy,* in which joint effects exceed the combined individual effects, and *antagonism,* in which joint effects are less than combined individual effects, are two examples of interaction. In some cases, interaction may be nothing more than the combined effects of an initiator and a promoter. Individually, these substances may be predicted to have a certain magnitude of effect, but following sequential exposure, a much more potent carcinogenic effect may result.

CLINICAL AND EPIDEMIOLOGIC EVIDENCE

The understanding of how environmental agents cause cancer developed through clinical and epidemiologic observation. The first modern report of environmental carcinogenesis was probably that of a London physician, Dr. John Hill, who in 1761 described the elevated prevalence of cancer of the nasal passages among tobacco snuff abusers. In 1775, a perceptive surgeon of the same city, Dr. Percival Pott, reported the first occupational cancer—an increased prevalence of scrotal skin cancer among chimney sweeps, who were heavily exposed to soot in their work. In the 1800s, skin cancer was linked with occupational exposure to inorganic arsenic, to tar, and to parrafin oils (now known to contain polycyclic aromatic hydrocarbons [PAHs]), and bladder cancer was linked with occupational exposure to certain dyes. In 1935, the first case report of bronchogenic carcinoma in a patient with asbestosis was published.

Clinical reports and numerous epidemiologic studies have provided further insight into how environmental agents cause cancer. Overall, these data have strongly supported the concept of environmental carcinogenesis. Several types of data are particularly suggestive.

Temporal trends are one example. The lung cancer mortality rate among U.S. males has increased tenfold during the past 50 years, a trend that can only be explained by a change in environmental factors, especially smoking.

Geographic comparisons reveal vast differences in cancer mortality among nations. For example, age-adjusted stomach cancer mortality rates in 1980 to 1981 were 63.1 per 100,000 in Japan, 40.2 in Poland, 23.6 in the Netherlands, 8.2 in the United States, and 2.2 in Thailand. This variability likely reflects differences among populations in exposure to environmental factors (including diet), although differences in genetic susceptibility, diagnosis, treatment, and reporting also play a role. Cancer mortality rates are found to vary markedly among regions of the United States (Fig. 15-1).

Gender comparisons may reveal quite disparate cancer rates between men and women in the same region. These differences may relate, in part, to different environmental exposures of men and women, including occupational exposures.

Migration studies have strongly implicated environmental factors, including diet, in cancer incidence. For example, native Japanese who migrate to the United States (Issei) experience a threefold increase in intestinal cancer mortality and a 36 percent decrease in gastric cancer mortality, compared to those Japanese who remain in Japan. The U.S.-born children of Japanese immigrants (Nissei) have rates that approximate U.S. rates even more closely.

Observations such as these have confirmed the role of environmental carcinogens. What about occupational carcinogens? Some of the highest environmental exposures occur in workplaces, and clinical and epidemiologic data have helped identify a number of occupational carcinogens causing a variety of tumors (Table 15-1). Examples include vinyl chloride (which caused a cluster of hepatic hemangiosarcomas in a chemical plant), benzene (which was linked with high leukemia rates in the Turkish shoe industry), and coke oven emissions (which were found to cause lung cancer elevations

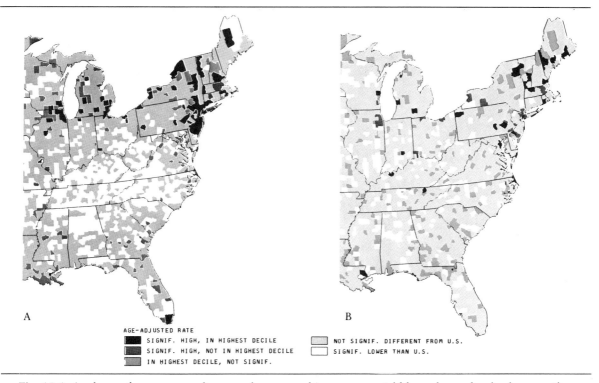

AGE-ADJUSTED RATE

■ SIGNIF. HIGH, IN HIGHEST DECILE	▨ NOT SIGNIF. DIFFERENT FROM U.S.
▨ SIGNIF. HIGH, NOT IN HIGHEST DECILE	☐ SIGNIF. LOWER THAN U.S.
▨ IN HIGHEST DECILE, NOT SIGNIF.	

Fig. 15-1. Analyses of cancer mortality rates by geographic area may yield hypotheses that lead to specific research studies on cancers of occupational and/or environmental origin. These maps show U.S. bladder cancer mortality by county from 1950–1969. There is a concentration in petrochemical industry centers for males (A) but not for females (B), consistent with an occupational etiology. (Abridged from TJ Mason et al. Atlas for cancer mortality for U.S. counties, 1950–69. Bethesda, MD: National Cancer Institute, 1975.)

among coke oven workers). Epidemiologic studies have also identified industries where cancer risks are present but no specific carcinogen has yet been identified (Table 15-2). A variety of epidemiologic methods has been applied to occupational cancer (see Chap. 5).

Occupational cancer epidemiology remains a challenging undertaking because of several unique limitations. One pertains to cohort definition and followup; these may be difficult when exposed groups underwent exposure years before the time of a study. Another set of limitations pertains to

exposure information; job designations and even direct measurements may not accurately reflect worker exposures. Still another set of limitations pertains to outcome information. Death certificates, the major source of diagnostic information in occupational cancer epidemiology, are notoriously inaccurate. A final problem is confounding. For many cancers of interest, both occupational and nonoccupational exposures may be causal, but information on the relevant nonoccupational exposures is often unavailable for study cohorts.

Table 15-1. Some occupational carcinogens

Carcinogen	Human cancer site	Industry setting
Acrylonitrile	?Lung, ?colon, ?brain, ?stomach, ?prostate	Acrylic fiber, chemical, and pesticide production
4-aminobiphenyl	Bladder	Formerly used as rubber antioxidant and dye intermediate
Arsenic and arsenic compounds	Lung	Smelting, metallurgy, pigment and glass production, and pesticide
Asbestos	Lung, pleura, peritoneum, larynx, gastrointestinal tract	Insulation; e.g., ships, buildings, pipes, brake shoes
Benzene	Leukemia	Multiple uses in chemical products: e.g., adhesives, rubber, petrochemicals
Benzidine and salts	Bladder	Plastic, rubber, dye, chemical industries
Beryllium and certain beryllium compounds	?Lung	Mining, electronics, chemical, electric, ceramics industries
Bis (chloromethyl) ether (BCME)	Lung	Contaminant of CMME
Chloromethyl methyl ether (CMME)	Lung	Ion exchange resin, organic chemical manufacturing
Chromium	Lung	Welding, etching, plating; steel and metal industries
Coal tars and coal tar pitches; soot	Lung, skin, ?kidney, ?prostate	Petrochemical and steel industries; fossil fuel combustion byproduct
Coke oven emissions	Lung, bladder, skin	Steel industry
1,2-dibromo-3-chloropropane (DBCP)	A	Former nematocide
1,2-dibromoethane, ethylene dibromide (EDB)	A	Gasoline additive, solvent, pesticide
3,3'-dichlorobenzidine and salts	A	Polyurethane and pigment workers
1,4-dioxane	A	Solvent, degreaser
Epichlorohydrin	A	Chemical production
Ethyleneimine	A	Paper, chemical, and organic chemicals
Ethylene oxide	A	Sterilizing agent
Formaldehyde	A	Manufacture of woods, resins, leather, rubber, metals
4,4'-methylene-bis-2-chloroaniline (MBOCA)	A	Polyurethane, epoxy resin, elastomer manufacturing
Mineral oils (certain ones)	Skin, scrotum	Lubricant in metal-working; solvents in printing
Alpha-naphthylamine	Bladder	Chemical, textile, dye, rubber industries
Beta-naphthylamine	Bladder	No longer in commercial use
Polychlorinated and polybrominated biphenyls (PCBs and PBBs)	A	Flame retardants (PBBs), transformer and capacitor fluids, solvents (PCBs)
Beta-propiolactone	A	Production and use of plastics, resins, and viricides
Vinyl chloride	Liver	Polyvinyl plastic production

Key: A = only animal evidence of carcinogenicity is currently satisfactory.

Table 15-2. Industries with cancer risk*

Auramine manufacture
Boot and shoe manufacture and repair (certain
 exposures)
Coal gasification (older processes)
Coke production (certain exposures)
Furniture manufacture (wood dusts)
Isopropyl alcohol manufacture (strong acid processes)
Nickel refining
Rubber industry
Underground hematite mining (with radon exposure)

*According to the International Agency for Research on
Cancer.

TESTING AND EVALUATION
OF CARCINOGENS

Several methods have emerged by which carcinogens are identified (Table 15-3). These methods include epidemiologic studies, animal studies, in vitro test systems, and analysis of structure-activity relationships.

Epidemiologic studies are potentially the most definitive source of information on human carcinogenicity since they are based on human exposures in "real-life" situations. However, limitations of epidemiologic studies sometimes make interpretation difficult (see Chap. 5). Most of these limitations bias results toward the null hypothesis, or a finding of no effect. For this reason, great caution is necessary in drawing conclusions [7].

Moreover, epidemiologic studies are expensive and time-consuming, and they demonstrate carcinogenicity only *after* humans have been affected. In addition, given the long latency period of most cancers, by the time the epidemiologic studies have "conclusively" identified a carcinogen, many thousands of workers may have been exposed. For these reasons, animal and in vitro studies have gained wide importance.

Animal studies for carcinogenicity use species that range from *Drosophila* to higher mammals. In accordance with National Cancer Institute guidelines, a substance is usually tested at two doses in both sexes of two strains of rodents, with at least 50 animals in each test group (2 doses × 2 sexes × 2 strains = 8 test groups). Therefore, at least 400 animals are usually studied, in addition to the 100 or more control animals that receive a placebo. The testing usually takes about 2 years, but 4 years can elapse from the initial planning of such a study until the final report has been completed, at a cost of several hundred thousand dollars.

Table 15-3. Relative advantages of the major methods of carcinogenicity testing[a]

Advantage	In vitro bioassay	Animal bioassay	Epidemiologic study
Low cost	+ + +	+ +	+
Rapidity	+ + +	+ +	+
Ease of performance	+ + +	+ +	+
Ability to control for multiple chemical exposures	+ + +	+ + +	+
Ability to demonstrate threshold level of carcinogen exposure	0	0	0
Validity of results as predictor of human carcinogenesis	+	+ +	+ + +
Validity of results in identifying locus of human carcinogenesis (i.e., organ specificity)	N.A.	+	+ + +
Provides absolute proof of human carcinogenicity	0	0	0[b]

[a]The grading scale used in this table is qualitative only. Specific methodologic features and appropriate applications of each method are discussed in the text.
[b]Although by formal standards there may be no "absolute proof" of carcinogenicity, evidence from multiple well-designed epidemiologic studies is generally accepted to be a functional equivalent of proof.

With test groups limited by cost to usually 50 animals each, small elevations in cancer incidence tend to be statistically insignificant. However, even a small elevation in incidence rate, when multiplied by a large exposed human population, could imply a substantial number of preventable cancers. Consequently, to ensure that positive results will not escape notice, every effort is made to detect the carcinogenic effect of a test substance. One way this is done is by using as one of the test doses the "maximum tolerated dose" (MTD), the highest dose that will not produce mortality or nonmalignant toxicity. (Often the other test dose is one-fourth of the MTD.) Critics have noted that the MTD introduces an element of unreality to bioassays: Such a large dose far exceeds human exposure levels, may create an unrepresentative biochemical milieu in test animals, and may overwhelm natural protective mechanisms such as detoxification and repair systems. However, even with the use of MTDs, most chemicals tested show no carcinogenic activity. This finding suggests that the use of high doses is reasonable and refutes the belief that "everything causes cancer."

Another controversial issue raised by animal testing is the existence of threshold levels of exposure. Since animal tests necessarily use high-dose exposures, our conclusions about the effects of low-dose exposures must come from downward extrapolation of observed dose-response patterns. Our uncertainty about the mechanisms of carcinogenesis make this extrapolation speculative (Fig. 15-2). It is largely for this reason and for analogous considerations in epidemiology that no safe threshold for carcinogen exposure can be established with certainty.

A related issue concerns the *potency* of a carcinogen. In animal testing, different chemicals vary quantitatively in their ability to induce tumors [8]. Such results can help identify the most worrisome human exposures, but they cannot quantitatively predict human cancer incidence following exposure.

The major questions about animal bioassays, of course, concern their accuracy at predicting

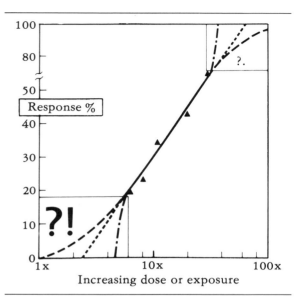

Fig. 15-2. Hypothetical dose-response curve for animal carcinogenicity study. These results are usually obtained at relatively high levels of exposure, as indicated by the triangles. The problem in estimating human risks is trying to determine what happens at lower exposures. As indicated on the diagram, there are several possible ways to extrapolate. In most cases, extrapolation of the observed results with a straight line will yield a result suggesting no response at low doses—that is, a threshold. Most scientists, however, now think that the actual response is indicated by the smooth curve passing through zero dose and zero response. (From PJ Gehring, Dow Chemical Co. Published in TS Maugh II. Chemical carcinogens: how dangerous are low doses? Science 1978; 202:37.)

human carcinogenesis. Some argue that animal studies are of limited value because animals and humans often have different sensitivities to carcinogens, and because the ability to activate and detoxify carcinogens may vary markedly among species. Of the several hundred chemicals that have been formally bioassayed, about half have given positive results [9]. Not all of these animal carcinogens have been shown to cause cancer in humans, but most have not been studied epidemiologically.

On the other hand, every human carcinogen, with the possible exception of benzene, is an animal carcinogen. In general, therefore, properly conducted and replicated animal bioassays are very good predictors of human cancer risk.

A final caveat concerns human organotropic effects seen in animal carcinogens. Although every animal carcinogen must be regarded as a potential human carcinogen, the target organ in a test species may differ from that in humans. Benzidine, for example, causes bladder cancer in humans, hepatomas in mice, and intestinal tumors in rats. A test species target organ, and probably its sensitivity as well, will vary with its metabolic pathways and concentrating mechanisms.

In vitro testing involves the use of bacterial or human tissue cultures. Suspected carcinogens are added to these systems, and endpoints that reflect DNA damage, such as DNA alteration, increased repair, or altered gene expression, are monitored. The prototype in vitro assay is the Ames test, first described in 1966 [10]. This test uses special strains of *Salmonella typhimurium* that cannot synthesize the amino acid tryptophan. Mutant strains synthesize tryptophan and show growth on a tryptophan-free medium, an endpoint easily detectable by examining the medium for bacterial growth.

In vitro assays, such as the Ames test, determine mutagenicity, not carcinogenicity. However, there is both theoretical and empirical basis for the concept that mutagenicity and carcinogenicity are closely linked processes. The theoretical link lies in the molecular event that is common to both: alteration of DNA. Empirically, the Ames test is over 90 percent sensitive in detecting carcinogens; false negatives include asbestos, some chlorinated hydrocarbons, hormones, and a few others [11]. It is slightly less specific. Sensitivity and specificity can be improved when the Ames test is used as part of a battery of in vitro assays, in which the strengths of various tests are combined.

Numerous modifications of the Ames test have been made, including the addition of liver microsomes to test systems in order to metabolize sub-

stances that may not be mutagenic in their original form. Other short-term in vitro assays include such tests as malignant transformation of cultured cells that produce tumors when inoculated into an appropriate host. Short-term assays, in addition to suggesting potential human carcinogenicity and helping set priorities for carcinogenicity tests in animals, are also used to help identify both mutagens in complex mixtures and active metabolites of mutagens in human body fluids, and to study mechanisms of chemical carcinogenesis.

Finally, *analysis of structure-activity relationships* is a review of the configuration of chemicals for their similarity to known carcinogens. Such analysis can direct suspicion to chemicals that may have carcinogenic potential; further testing will generally be necessary.

Based on these four methods of identifying carcinogens, regulatory and research agencies have developed standardized ways to classify chemical carcinogenicity. For example, the International Agency for Research on Cancer (IARC), a branch of the World Health Organization, designates three categories [12]. Group 1 includes chemicals established as human carcinogens, based on epidemiologic evidence. Group 2 includes chemicals that are "probably carcinogenic to humans." Since the evidence ranges from "limited" to "inadequate," two subgroups exist; group 2A reflects a higher level of certainty than group 2B. Group 3 includes chemicals that cannot be classified as to carcinogenicity. Using this classification, the IARC has evaluated over 700 chemicals, industrial processes, and personal habits. About 40 of these have been placed in Group 1, and about 70 have been placed in Group 2 [13]. The IARC policy has been to recommend treating these chemicals as if they presented a carcinogenic risk to humans. Over 200 chemicals, including most of the Group 1 and Group 2 entries, have been found to have "sufficient evidence of animal carcinogenicity." The American Conference of Governmental Industrial Hygienists (ACGIH), the National Toxicology Program (NTP), and the National Institute for Occupational Safety and Health (NIOSH) have all adopted analagous schemes. In addition, the generic carcinogen policy adopted in 1980 by OSHA is based on a similar scheme.

REGULATION OF CARCINOGENS IN THE WORKPLACE

OSHA's approach to carcinogen regulation was set forth in its generic carcinogen standard, "Identification, Classification, and Regulation of Potential Occupational Carcinogens" [14]. This document prescribes a standardized way of interpreting test data on carcinogenicity and classifying chemicals accordingly. It then provides a framework for the regulation of chemicals found to be carcinogens. In theory, any chemical with sufficient evidence of carcinogenicity is automatically regulated as a carcinogen. However, since its promulgation the standard has not been utilized by OSHA. Consequently, most known carcinogens that are regulated by OSHA are regulated through earlier consensus standards and not in accordance with the generic carcinogen standard (see Chap. 10).

A major concern in carcinogen regulation is the issue of *potency*. If two substances are both carcinogens, with one much more potent than the other, then some would argue that the two substances should be regulated differently, with more stringent restrictions applied to the more potent carcinogen. The same argument may be advanced when a greater population is exposed to one carcinogen than to another, when one carcinogen is felt to be more essential or irreplaceable than another, or even when control measures for two substances differ in cost. These considerations give rise to cost-benefit analysis in carcinogen regulation, a controversial but increasingly common practice.

CLINICAL ENCOUNTERS WITH CARCINOGENS

A clinician may confront carcinogenic exposures in several ways. The remainder of this chapter poses clinical situations and discusses responses to them.

"Is this chemical carcinogenic?" This question is best answered according to defined criteria, such as those discussed above. The primary animal and epidemiologic data on a chemical may be accessed through standard reference sources (see Appendix to Chap. 3). Formal evaluations of carcinogenicity may be found in the IARC monographs on the Evaluation of the Carcinogenic Risk of Chemicals to Humans, in annual reports of the NTP, and in NIOSH publications.

"I am exposed to a carcinogen. What should I do?" This query has two components: One pertains to the carcinogenic exposure and one to the patient.

Ideally, no worker should be exposed to a carcinogen. As previously discussed, safe "threshold" exposure levels cannot currently be demonstrated. A physician who becomes aware of an ongoing carcinogenic workplace exposure should take appropriate steps to end that exposure, which will often involve contacting responsible individuals at the workplace and government agencies. As discussed in Chapters 4 and 7, exposure may be ended through substitutions of the carcinogen, enclosure of the process or other engineering techniques, or, when necessary, personal protective equipment.

The worker who reports being exposed to a carcinogen should be advised to terminate the exposure, to avoid concomitant carcinogenic exposures such as smoking, and to seek appropriate medical follow-up as discussed later in the section on medical monitoring.

"Did my exposure cause my cancer?" Patients with cancer who have been exposed to carcinogens often inquire about the possibility that the exposures were causal. The question sometimes arises in the context of litigation or may simply reflect a patient's psychologic need to explain a catastrophic life event. The issue of cancer causation in an individual patient is difficult to address because it entails the application of epidemiologic and statistical data (which derive from groups) to individuals. The answers are not available from science alone [15].

Certain requirements must be met before it may be said that an exposure has "causally contributed" to a cancer. There must be evidence that the exposure has indeed occurred. The tumor type in question must be associated with the exposure, based on prior studies. Finally, the appropriate temporal relationship must hold; in particular, a sufficiently long latency period must have elapsed between the onset of exposure and the diagnosis of cancer. (Note that if a carcinogen acts as a promoter, late exposures may contribute to tumor development [4].) These requirements are necessary, but not sufficient, in the minds of most clinicians.

When these requirements have been met, further interpretation begins. Suppose that the baseline incidence of lung cancer in unexposed adult men is 80 cases per 100,000 per year. Suppose further that a particular occupational exposure has been associated with a relative risk of lung cancer of 1.8. Therefore, the incidence among exposed men would be 144 cases per 100,000 per year. If an exposed man develops lung cancer and wonders whether his exposure caused his cancer, what should he be told?

The simplest analysis is *qualitative*. Any exposure that markedly increases risk may be considered to contribute to the development of cancer in an exposed individual. A "marked" increase has no firm definition; relative risks as low as 1.3 have been considered in this category. By this analysis, the patient could be told that his exposure contributed to his cancer.

A second qualitative approach is to ask whether the patient's cancer would have occurred "but for" the exposure. In the above example, over half the cases of lung cancer in the exposed population would occur even without the exposure. It might then be concluded that any individual case is "more likely than not" to have occurred irrespective of exposure. Similarly, a relative risk of 2.2 would lead to the conclusion in any individual case that cancer would not have occurred "but for" exposure.

This approach is obviously unsatisfactory. It accounts for *no* cancer causation in individual cases when the relative risk is below 2.0, and it accounts for *all* cancer causation in individual cases when the relative risk exceeds 2.0. This violates common-sense notions of causation, and it places far too much weight on the precision of the relative risk estimate.

Finally, in the *quantitative* approach, causation is allocated to various causes, including occupational exposures. In the above example, the patient might be told that the occupational exposure was "responsible" for 44 percent (0.8/1.8) of his lung cancer. On the other hand, if he were a smoker, with a consequent tenfold increase in lung cancer risk, he might be told that smoking accounted for 83% (9/10.8) of his cancer and that the job exposure accounted for 7% (0.8/10.8).

This approach has intuitive appeal, since it confronts the multiplicity of exposures and attempts to quantify the relative importance of each. However, the data needed to employ this approach correctly are rarely available. Interaction of multiple exposures, such as synergy, often occurs but is rarely quantitated. Consequently, even if a population relative risk can be estimated for an occupational exposure, the relative causal contribution of several factors in an individual is usually impossible to quantitate.

The latter two approaches outlined above are often demanded in legal settings, but as noted, they generally have inadequate scientific basis. Until further data or analytical methods are available, the first approach is recommended. It accords with common sense, stays within the confines of available data, and is understandable to patients and their families.

"How should a medical monitoring program for cancer be designed?" The theory and practice of screening have advanced in recent years (see Chap. 6). With regard to cancer, three goals are sought by screening programs: (1) identifying susceptible individuals, presumably before exposure; (2) identifying markers of exposure (biologic monitoring); and (3) identifying early signs of disease (medical surveillance). Some screening tests fall between the second and third category, since they identify phys-

iologic changes related to exposure but of uncertain pathologic significance.

Efforts to identify susceptible individuals include both genetic and nongenetic tests. *Genetic* factors that may predispose to cancer include elevated aryl hydrocarbon hydroxylase, diseases such as xeroderma pigmentosum and familial polyposis, and a family history of certain cancers. For each of these factors, screening for susceptibles would either have low sensitivity, low specificity, or, given the low prevalence of these factors in the population, low predictive value (positive). *Nongenetic* factors that increase cancer susceptibility include behavioral patterns such as smoking, previous exposures to carcinogens, and others. There may be medical justification for preventing affected individuals from sustaining carcinogenic exposures, but if such a policy leads to job discrimination, significant ethical and legal problems arise. Moreover, screening for susceptibility to cancer implies that subsequent exposure to carcinogens will occur. Preventing such exposure is far more appropriate than selecting the most resilient workers.

Biological monitoring includes the measurement of carcinogens or their metabolites in body fluids or tissues. Such monitoring is available for several carcinogens [16]. For example, benzene exposure may be monitored through expired air, blood benzene levels, and urinary phenol levels. Exposure to the aromatic amine 4,4'-methylene-bis(2-chloroaniline) (MBOCA) may be monitored through urinary MBOCA levels. Biological monitoring, however, should never replace environmental monitoring. Rather, it should be used as a supplement. Most of these tests have important technical limitations and should be very carefully studied prior to use.

Monitoring of effects on genetic material combines elements of biologic monitoring with elements of conventional medical surveillance [17]. Examples include the measurement of carcinogen-DNA or carcinogen-protein adducts, the measurement of mutagenicity in body fluids of exposed workers, and the measurement of chromosomal alterations such as sister chromatid exchanges. A detailed review of these techniques is beyond the scope of this chapter. However, as of early 1988, each of them is in developmental stages, remains unstandardized, and is not yet suitable for routine use.

Cancer screening in occupational settings has been best explored with regard to bladder cancer and lung cancer. Among workers with a history of beta-naphthylamine and/or benzidine exposure, screening for bladder cancer using cystoscopy and/or urine cytology has had both low sensitivity and low specificity [18]. However, further study may reveal such screening to be beneficial. Lung cancer screening consists of sputum cytology tests and/or interval chest radiography. Extensive population-based studies of these tests in New York, Maryland, and Minnesota have demonstrated that screening yields earlier detection of lung cancer but no survival advantage, except possibly for squamous cell carcinoma [19–21]. However, one trial that focused on a high-risk population appeared to demonstrate improved survival through screening [22], and further research is clearly necessary.

"We have a cluster of cancer in our plant. How should we respond?" Suspected excesses of cancer, clustered in time or space, may be noted by workers or by the workplace medical department. These situations arouse a great deal of concern, and it is essential that they be handled openly, methodically, and expeditiously [23]. A multidisciplinary approach is necessary, drawing on the experience and knowledge of workers, physicians, epidemiologists, industrial hygienists, and managers. The following sequence is suggested:

First, the presence of a cluster should be confirmed or refuted. Each case of cancer should be confirmed, and tissue type, date of diagnosis, demographic data, and exposure data should be obtained. The worker population should be enumerated and subdivided into age, sex, and other pertinent categories. (If information on retirees is available, it should be included.) Age- and sex-specific cancer incidence rates for the state should be obtained from the state cancer registry, if one exists. With this information, an age-standardized cancer rate can be computed for the workplace and compared with the expected rate, based on state data. Confidence intervals can be calculated for the workplace cancer rate; these will usually be broad because of small numbers. However, even a statistically insignificant elevation in the cancer rate in the workplace should prompt further evaluation.

Next, the tissue types of the cancer cases should be reviewed. An excess of unusual tumors, or tumors known to be environmentally induced, should prompt further concern [24].

Then the latency periods of each cancer case should be reviewed. If many of the workers began their plant employment only shortly before diagnosis, an exposure-related cluster is less plausible.

Next, confounders should be reviewed. Other factors that may contribute to an elevation of cancer should be noted. However, care should be taken not to let the presence of confounders obscure one's view of an occupational carcinogen.

Next, the occupational histories of the cases should be reviewed. Detailed personnel histories of each affected worker may reveal that a particular job title is associated with cancer. It is important that jobs in the distant past, not just recent ones, be examined.

An industrial hygiene review should be made to determine whether any particular exposures are common among the affected workers. A variety of job titles may share a common chemical contact, which may help explain the cluster. Early exposures may need to be reconstructed, which may involve interviewing older workers or reviewing production records.

Next, the same analysis should be made with regard to worksites. If many of the cases arise from a single building or location, an environmental cause is suggested. Any worksites in question should be subjected to a thorough industrial hygiene evaluation, which should include both the production process and "incidental" exposures such as the heating, ventilation, and air-conditioning system (HVAC) and the drinking water.

Based on the above analysis, an initially suspected cancer cluster may be found to be (1) not actually present, (2) present but not consistent with occupational causation, (3) possibly related to occupational exposures, or (4) definitely related to occupational exposures. The results should be carefully and thoroughly communicated to all those concerned. If an occupational cause is implicated, aggressive corrective action is in order (see Chaps. 4 and 7). Whatever the conclusion, careful ongoing surveillance of both the workplace and the workforce should continue.

A physician who analyzes an apparent cancer cluster may require further assistance. The most appropriate sources are NIOSH or a qualified consultant group, such as a university-based occupational health program.

REFERENCES

1. Randall WJ, Solomon S. Building six: the tragedy at Bridesburg. Boston: Little, Brown, 1976.
2. Figueroa WG, Raszkowski R, Weiss W. Lung cancer in chloromethyl methyl ether workers. N Eng J Med 1973; 288:1096–7.
3. Farber E. The multistep nature of cancer development. Cancer Res 1984; 44:4217–23.
4. Hoover RN. Epidemiologic evidence of tumor promotion. Unpublished manuscript, available from Environmental Epidemiology Branch, National Cancer Institute, Room 3CO7 Landow Building, Bethesda, Md. 20205.
5. Van Duuren BL, Banerjee S. Thresholds in chemical carcinogenesis. J Am Coll Toxicol 1984; 2:85–100.
6. Rothman KJ. Interactions between causes. In: Rothman KJ, ed. Modern epidemiology. Boston: Little Brown, 1986. Chap. 15.
7. Wald NJ, Doll R. Interpretation of negative epidemiological evidence for carcinogenicity. Lyon, France: IARC, 1985. (IARC scientific publication no. 65). See especially Day NE, Statistical considerations, pp. 13–27.
8. Gold LS, de Veciana M, Backman GM, et al. Chronological supplement to the carcinogenic potency database: standardized results of animal bioassays published through December 1982. Environ Health Persp 1986; 67:161–200.

9. Huff JE, McConnell EE, Haseman JK. On the proportion of positive results in carcinogenicity studies in animals. Environ Mutagen 1985; 7:427–8.

10. Ames BN, McCann J, Yamasaki E. Methods for detecting carcinogens and mutagens with the Salmonella/mammalian-microsome mutagenicity test. Mutat Res 1975; 31:347–63.

11. Bartsch H, Malaveille C, Camus AM, et al. Bacterial and mammalian mutagenicity tests: validation and comparative studies on 180 chemicals. In: Molecular and cellular aspects of carcinogen screening tests. Lyon, France: IARC, 1980. (IARC scientific publication no. 27). pp. 179–241.

12. International Agency for Research on Cancer. IARC monographs on the evaluation of the carcinogenic risk of chemicals to humans, suppl. 4. Chemicals, industrial processes and industries associated with cancer in humans. Lyon, France: IARC, 1982.

13. Vainio H, Hemminki K, Wilbourn J. Data on the carcinogenicity of chemicals in the IARC monographs programme. Carcinogenesis 1985; 6:1653–65.

14. Occupational Safety and Health Administration. Identification, classification and regulation of potential occupational carcinogens. Federal Register 1980; Jan 22:45:5015.

15. Brennan T. Untangling causation issues in law and medicine: hazardous substance litigation. Ann Int Med 1987; 107:741–747.

16. Vainio H. Current trends in the biological monitoring of exposure to carcinogens. Scand J Work Env Health 1985; 11:1–6.

17. Bernard A, Lauwerys R. Present status and trends in biological monitoring of exposure to industrial chemicals. J Occup Med 1986; 28:558–62.

18. Cartwright RA. Screening workers exposed to suspect bladder carcinogens. J Occup Med 1986; 28:1017–19.

19. Martini N. Results of the Memorial Sloan-Kettering Lung Project. Recent Results Cancer Res 1982; 82:174–8.

20. Frost JK, Ball WC, Levin ML. Sputum cytopathology: use and potential in monitoring the workplace environment by screening for biological effects of exposure. J Occup Med 1986; 28:692–703.

21. Fontana RS, Sanderson DR, Woolner LB, et al. Lung cancer screening: the Mayo program. J Occup Med 1986; 28:746–50.

22. Kubik A, Polak J. Lung cancer detection: results of a randomized prospective study in Czechoslovakia. Cancer 1986; 57:2427–37.

23. Schulte PA, Ehrenberg RL, Singal M. Investigation of occupational cancer clusters: theory and practice. Am J Pub Health 1987; 77:52–6.

24. Rutstein DD, Mullan RJ, Frazier TM, et al. Sentinel health events (occupational): a basis for physician recognition and public health surveillance. Am J Pub Health 1983; 73:1054–62.

BIBLIOGRAPHY

Alderson M. Occupational Cancer. London: Butterworths, 1986.
A good general introduction.

Bailar JS, Smith EM. Progress against cancer? N Eng J Med 1986; 314:1226–32.
Argues that treatment results have been generally disappointing and calls for more emphasis on prevention.

Berlin A, Draper M, Hemminki K, Vainio H. Monitoring human exposure to carcinogenic and mutagenic agents. Lyon, France: IARC, 1984. (IARC scientific publication no. 59).
Especially informative with regard to biological monitoring.

Brandt-Rauf PW, ed. Occupational cancer and carcinogenesis. In: Occupational medicine: state of the art reviews. 1987. Vol. 2, no. 1.
Contains review articles on carcinogenic mechanisms, test methods, and specific tumor sites.

International Agency for Research on Cancer. Long-term and short-term screening assays for carcinogens: a critical appraisal. IARC monographs on the evaluation of the carcinogenic risk of chemicals to humans. Lyon, France: IARC, 1980.
A slightly dated but thorough and balanced review of test methods.

International Agency for Research on Cancer. Monographs on the evaluation of carcinogenic risks of chemicals to man.
The more than 30 volumes in this series include monographs on over 400 exposures with authoritative evaluations of the evidence for carcinogenicity.

J Occup Med 1986; 28:543–788, 901–1126.
These two issues of J Occup Med form the proceedings of a conference on medical screening and biologic monitoring for the effects of exposure in the workplace held in 1984. Papers were presented on cancer screening for specific tumors and on biologic monitoring including monitoring for genetic effects.

Maugh TH. Chemical carcinogens: the scientific basis for regulation. Science 1978; 201:1200–05. Chemical carcinogens: how dangerous are low doses? Science 1978; 202:37–41.

A useful pair of articles that clearly describes some of the controversy in carcinogen regulation.

National Toxicology Program. Fourth annual report on carcinogens. Washington, DC: U.S.D.H.H.S., P.H.S. (NTP 85-002).

This well-written and edited volume contains summaries of the evidence on a variety of carcinogens with the NTP assessment of the evidence for both human and animal carcinogenicity. Also contains a useful index of synonyms and trade names.

Nicholson WJ, ed. Management of assessed risk for carcinogens. Ann NY Acad Sci 1981. Vol. 363.

Papers presented at a 1981 conference on risk assessment, including many that are skeptical about this technique.

Pickle LW, Mason TJ, Howard N, et al. Atlas of U.S. cancer mortality among whites: 1950–1980. DHHS publication no. (NIH) 87-2900. Washington, DC: U.S. Government Printing Office, 1987.

This volume presents static maps of state economic area mortality rates for each of the three decades covered among whites: 1950–1980 for white males and females for 33 cancer sites, along with dynamic maps illustrating the trends in these cases over time. Other cancer mortality analyses are also included. A very useful volume indicating the value of monitoring mortality statistics on a small-area scale as a strategy for generating etiologic clues and targeting epidemiologic research.

Office of Science and Technology Policy. Chemical carcinogens: a review of the science and its associated principles. Federal Register 1985; 50:10372–442. Reprinted in Environ Health Perspect 1986; 67:201–82.

An excellent discussion of the relationship of carcinogen testing and identification to regulation.

Schottenfeld D, Fraumeni JF. Cancer epidemiology and prevention. Philadelphia: Saunders, 1982.

The standard text on this subject, covering basic concepts, descriptive epidemiology, specific causes (including occupation), and specific cancer sites.

Singer B, Grunberger D. Molecular biology of mutagens and carcinogens. New York: Plenum, 1985.

A detailed text.

Weinstein IB. Current concepts and controversies in chemical carcinogenesis. J Supramolec Struct Cell Biol 1981; 17:99–120.

With the Farber article cited in reference 3, a good review of mechanisms of carcinogenesis.

Williams GM. Batteries of short-term tests for carcinogen screening. In: Williams GM, Kroes R, Waaijers HW, van de Poll KW, eds. The predictive value of short-term screening tests in carcinogenicity evaluation. New York: Elsevier, 1980, pp. 327–46.

Explains the value of combining various short-term assays to improve their predictive power.

16
Ionizing Radiation

Arthur C. Upton

Chernobyl, USSR, April 27, 1986. An explosion and fire occurred in a large, uranium-fueled graphite power reactor during a test in which the emergency cooling, regulating, and shutdown systems had been deliberately turned off. The resulting damage to the reactor caused the release of large quantities of radioactive fuel and fission products, which contaminated the plant site and areas downwind from it for hundreds of miles. Two plant workers died immediately after the accident from burns and traumatic injuries, and hundreds were hospitalized later for radiation sickness, 29 of whom died within subsequent weeks.

Although no other radiation accident has been as serious as the one at Chernobyl, scores of other accidents have occurred, some of which have also caused fatalities [1]. Even in the absence of accidents, moreover, mortality from cancer and other diseases has been increased in radiation workers in the past. Today, even the smallest doses of radiation are considered to pose some risk of injury. Therefore, in view of the large number of workers at risk (Tables 16-1 and 16-2), the recognition, treatment, and prevention of radiation injury command an important place in occupational health.

NATURE AND MEASUREMENT OF IONIZING RADIATION

Ionizing radiations are of two main types: electromagnetic and particulate. The former include x-rays and gamma rays; the latter include electrons, protons, neutrons, alpha particles, and other corpuscular radiations of varying mass and charge (Table 16-3). Ionizing radiations are produced in the release of energy that occurs when atoms disintegrate. This process takes place in the disintegration of naturally unstable elements—such as uranium, thorium, and radium—and in the disintegration of elements that are disrupted by bombardment in an "atom smasher," atomic reactor, or other such device. After their release, x-rays and gamma rays travel with the speed of light, whereas particulate radiations vary in initial velocity, depending on their energy and mass.

As ionizing radiation penetrates matter, it collides with atoms and molecules in its path, disrupting them in the process, thereby giving rise to ions and free radicals, hence its designation *ionizing* radiation. The collisions tend to be clustered densely along the track of an alpha particle, causing the radiation to give up all of its energy in traversing only a few cells. With an x-ray, on the other hand, the collisions tend to be distributed so sparsely along its track that the radiation may traverse the entire body. The average amount of energy deposited per unit length of track (expressed in KeV/μ) is called the linear energy transfer (LET) of the radiation.

Radiations of high LET, such as alpha particles, tend to cause greater injury for a given total amount of energy deposited in a cell than do radiations of low LET, such as x-rays [2]. The high relative biologic effectiveness (RBE) of high-LET radiation results from the capacity of each densely ionizing particle to deposit enough energy in a critical site within the cell (for example, a DNA molecule or a chromosome) to cause biologically significant molecular damage. Hence, although alpha

231

Table 16-1. Estimated numbers of workers in the United States occupationally exposed to ionizing radiation

Types of work	Number of workers exposed annually	Average dose/year (mSv)
Nuclear energy (fuel cycle)	62,000	8.4
Naval reactor	36,000	2.2
Healing arts	500,000	1.2
Research	100,000	1.2
Manufacturing and industrial	7,000,000	0.07

Source: Department of Health, Education, and Welfare. Interagency task force on the health effects of ionizing radiation. Report of the work group on science. Washington, D.C.: Department of Health, Education, and Welfare, 1979.

Table 16-2. Types of workers who may be occupationally exposed to ionizing radiation

Atomic energy plant workers	Luminous dial painters
Cathode-ray-tube makers	Nuclear submarine workers
Dental assistants	Oil well loggers
Dentists	Ore assayers
Electron microscope makers	Petroleum refinery workers
Electron microscopists	Physicians
Electrostatic eliminator operators	Pipeline oil flow testers
Fire alarm makers	Pipeline weld radiographers
Gas mantle makers	Plasma torch operator
High-voltage television repairmen	Radar tube makers
High-voltage vacuum tube makers	Radiologists
High-voltage vacuum tube users	Radium laboratory workers
Industrial fluoroscope operators	Television tube makers
Industrial radiographers	Thickness gage operators
Inspectors using, and workers located near, sealed gamma ray sources (cesium-137, cobalt-60, and iridium-192)	Thorium-aluminum alloy workers
	Thorium-magnesium alloy workers
	Thorium ore producers
	Uranium mill workers
	Uranium miners
Klystron tube operators	X-ray aides
Liquid level gage operators	X-ray diffraction apparatus operators
	X-ray technicians
	X-ray tube makers

Source: MM Key, et al, eds. Occupational diseases: a guide to their recognition. Washington, D.C.: NIOSH, 1977: 471–472.

particles generally travel only a short distance (Table 16-3) and thus pose little risk if emitted outside the body, they are highly injurious to those cells that they penetrate.

When a radionuclide is taken into the body, its tissue distribution and retention depend on its physical and chemical properties. Radioactive iodine, for example, is normally concentrated in the thyroid gland, whereas strontium-90 is deposited primarily in bone. After deposition of a given amount of radioactivity, the quantity remaining in situ decreases with time through both physical decay and biologic removal. The time taken for a radionuclide to lose one-half of its radioactivity by physical decay varies from a fraction of a second in the case of some radionuclides to millions of years in the case of others. With iodine-131, for example, the physical half-life is seven days, whereas with plutonium-239 it is over 24,000 years. Biologic half-lives also vary, tending to be longer for bone-seeking radionuclides (for example, radium, strontium, and plutonium) than for radionuclides that are deposited predominantly in soft tissue (for example, iodine, cesium, and tritium).

SOURCES AND LEVELS OF RADIATION IN THE ENVIRONMENT

All living organisms have evolved in the presence of natural background radiation. This radiation consists of: (1) cosmic rays, which come from outer space; (2) terrestrial radiation, which emanates from the radium, thorium, uranium, and other radioactive elements in the earth's crust; and (3) internal radiations, which are emitted by the potassium-40, carbon-14, and other radionuclides

Table 16-3. Principal types and properties of ionizing radiation

Type of radiation	Relative mass	Charge	Range in soft tissue*
Gamma ray	0	0	Centimeters
X-ray	0	0	Centimeters
Beta particle (electron)	1/1840	−1	Millimeters
Neutron	1	0	Centimeters
Proton	1	+1	Microns
Alpha particle	4	+2	Microns

*Range depends on the energy of the radiation; values shown are typical for radiations commonly encountered in the workplace.

contained within living cells (Table 16-4). The average total dose received annually from all three sources by a person residing at sea level in the United States is about 0.80 mSv (80 mrem); however, a dose twice this size may be received by a person residing at a higher elevation, where cosmic rays are more intense, or by a person residing in an area where the radium content of the soil is comparatively high (Table 16-4). Also substantially higher is the average dose to the bronchial epithelium from inhaled radon and its daughters.

A nuclear power plant worker who measured his radioactivity immediately on entering the plant found it to be unexpectedly high. On investigation, the source of his radioactivity was found to be the radon in his home, which was present at concentrations thousands of times higher than average. The discovery that his house contained such high levels of radon prompted the worker to take steps to reduce the levels by improving the ventilation of the house and by blocking the entry of radon from the underlying soil. His discovery also prompted a survey of radon levels in other houses throughout the United States, preliminary results of which indicate radon levels to be well in excess of the recommended limits (4–8 pCi/liter) in a substantial percentage of houses.

People are exposed to radiation from artificial and natural sources. The major source of exposure to human-made radiation is the use of x-rays in medical diagnosis (Table 16-4). The average personal dose of radiation from medical and dental examinations in developed countries now exceeds that from natural background irradiation (Table 16-4). Smaller doses of human-made radiation are received from radioactive minerals in building materials, phosphate fertilizers, and crushed rock; radiation-emitting components of television sets, smoke detectors, and other consumer products; radioactive fallout from atomic weapons; and nuclear power.

To protect radiation workers against excessive occupational irradiation, their working conditions are generally designed to minimize exposure; nevertheless, the dose they receive occupationally varies, depending on their particular work assignment and operating conditions (see Table 16-1). The average dose of whole-body radiation received occupationally by workers in the United States is less than 5 mSv (0.5 rem) per year, and fewer than 1 percent of workers exposed to ionizing radiation approach or exceed the maximum permissible limit (50 mSv) in any given year [2, 3].

TYPES OF RADIATION INJURY

Irradiation can cause many types of effects on the human body, depending on the dose and the conditions of exposure. For purposes of radiologic protection, two types of radiation effects are distinguished: (1) *stochastic* effects—effects that vary in frequency but not severity with dose; and (2) *nonstochastic* effects—effects that vary both in frequency and severity with dose [4]. Since the production of nonstochastic effects requires doses large enough to kill many cells, there are thresholds for such effects. The production of stochastic effects, on the other hand, can conceivably result from random injury to a single cell, with the result that no threshold for such effects is presumed to exist [4].

Stochastic effects include mutagenic, carcinogenic, and teratogenic effects. Nonstochastic effects include erythema of the skin, cataract for-

QUANTITIES AND UNITS

The *amount of radioactivity* that is present at any one time in a given sample of matter is expressed in *becquerels;* one becquerel (Bq) corresponds to that quantity of radioactivity in which there is one atomic disintegration per second. Another unit that has been used for the same purpose is the *curie* (Ci). One Ci represents that quantity of radioactivity in which there are 3.7×10^{10} atomic disintegrations per second (1 Bq = 2.7×10^{-11} Ci).

The unit that is generally used for expressing the *dose of radiation* that is absorbed in tissue is the *gray* (Gy). Another unit used for the same purpose is the *rad* (1 Gy = 1 joule per kg of tissue = 100 rad).

The *sievert* (Sv) is the unit that expresses the so-called *dose equivalent*. This unit is used in radiologic protection to enable doses of different types of radiation to be normalized in terms of biologic effectiveness, since particulate radiations generally cause greater injury than x-rays or gamma rays for a given dose in Gy. Another unit that has been used for the same purpose is the *rem* (1 Sv = 100 rem). The dose equivalent of any radiation in sieverts is the dose in Gy multiplied by an appropriate RBE-dependent quality factor Q. In principle, therefore, one sievert of any radiation represents that dose which is equivalent in biologic effectiveness to one gray of gamma rays.

For expressing the *collective dose* to a population, the *person-Sv* (or *person-rem*) is used. This unit represents the product of the average dose per person times the number of people exposed. For example, 1 sievert to each of 100 people equals 100 person-sievert (= 10,000 person-rem).

For measuring *exposure* to x-rays, the classic unit is the *roentgen*. One roentgen (R), defined loosely, is the amount of x-radiation that produces one electrostatic unit of charge in one cubic centimeter of air under standard conditions of temperature and pressure. Exposure of the surface of the skin to 1 R of x-rays deposits a dose of slightly less than 10 mGy (1 rad) in the underlying epidermis.

mation, impairment of fertility, depression of hemopoiesis, and various other types of radiation-induced tissue injury. Both types of effects are end-results of radiation-induced changes at the cellular level, which are discussed briefly next.

EFFECTS OF RADIATION ON CELLS

At the cellular level, radiation injury may include inhibition of cell division, damage to chromosomes, damage to genes (mutations), neoplastic transformation, and various other changes, all of which result from macromolecular lesions initiated by radiation-induced ions and free radicals. Any molecule in the cell can be altered by irradiation, but DNA is the most critical target since damage to a single gene can profoundly alter or kill the cell.

A dose of x-radiation that is sufficient to kill the average dividing cell (for example, 1–2 Sv) produces dozens of strand breaks and other changes in the cell's DNA molecules. Most of the changes in DNA are reparable, but those that are caused by high-LET radiation are likely to be less reparable than those caused by low-LET radiation. The ultimate fate of the DNA, in any case, is likely to depend on the effectiveness of the cell's repair processes as well as on the nature of the initial lesions.

The susceptibility of cells to radiation-induced killing increases with their rate of proliferation. Dividing cells are thus radiosensitive as a class. The percentage of cells surviving, as measured by their ability to proliferate, tends to decrease exponentially with increasing dose. A rapidly delivered dose of 1 to 2 Sv generally reduces the surviv-

Table 16-4. Estimated average soft-tissue dose of whole-body radiation received annually by members of the U.S. population

Source of radiation	Dose/year (mSv)
Natural	
Environmental	
Cosmic radiation	0.28 (0.28–1.30)[a]
Terrestrial radiation	0.26 (0.30–1.15)[b]
Internal radioactive isotopes	0.26
Subtotal	0.80
Human-made	
Environmental	
Technologically enhanced	0.04
Global fallout	0.04
Nuclear power	0.02
Medical	
Diagnostic	0.78
Radiopharmaceuticals	0.14
Occupational	0.01
Miscellaneous	0.05
Subtotal	1.08
TOTAL	1.88

[a]Values in parenthesis indicate range over which average levels for different states in the United States vary with elevation.
[b]Values in parenthesis indicate range of variation attributable largely to geographic differences in the content of radium, thorium, uranium, and potassium-40 in the earth's crust. These values do not represent the dose to the bronchial epithelium from inhalation of radon and its daughters, which averages 20–30 mSv per year in the general population.
Source: National Academy of Sciences Advisory Committee on the Biological Effects of Ionizing Radiation (BEIR). *The Effects on Populations of Exposure to Low Levels of Ionizing Radiation.* Washington, D.C.: National Academy of Sciences, National Research Council, 1972, 1980.

ing fraction to 1/e, or 37 percent; however, if the same dose of low-LET radiation is divided into two or more exposures separated by several hours, fewer cells are killed because some of the sublethal damage is repaired between exposures [2].

DAMAGE TO CHROMOSOMES
Radiation-induced changes in chromosome number and structure are among the most thoroughly studied effects of radiation. These changes result from the breakage and rearrangement of chromosomes, as well as from interference with the normal segregation of chromosomes to daughter cells at the time of cell division. The majority of such aberrations interfere with mitosis, causing the affected cell to die when it attempts to divide.

The frequency of chromosomal aberrations increases in proportion to the radiation dose in the low-to-intermediate dose range, the increase being steeper with high-LET radiation than with low-LET radiation. Also increased in frequency by irradiation are sister chromatid exchanges. In human blood lymphocytes irradiated in culture, the frequency of chromosomal aberrations approximates 0.1 per cell per Sv. The frequency of acentric and dicentric aberrations in such cells is also increased in radiation workers and other irradiated populations, in whom it can serve as a crude biologic dosimeter [2]. Only a small percentage of all chromosome aberrations in members of the general population is attributable to natural background radiation; the majority result from other causes, including certain viruses, chemicals, and drugs.

DAMAGE TO GENES
Mutagenic effects of radiation have been investigated extensively in many types of cells, including human somatic cells, but heritable effects of radiation are yet to be documented in human germ cells. The increased frequency of mutations per locus amounts to about 10^{-6} per Sv in human lymphocytes and by about 10^{-5} Sv in mouse spermatogonia and oocytes, depending on the conditions of irradiation [5]. In view of the small magnitude of the increase per unit dose, it is not astonishing that no heritable abnormalities have been detectable in the children of atomic bomb survivors, given the limited number of such children (78,000) who have been available for examination and the relatively small average gonadal dose (0.5 Sv) that was received by their parents [5].

On the basis of the available data, the dose required to double the frequency of mutations in humans has been estimated to lie between 0.2 and 2.5 Sv. Hence, it is inferred that only a small percentage (0.1–2.0 percent) of all genetically related diseases in the human population is attributable to natural background irradiation [3, 5].

EFFECTS ON TISSUES

Effects of radiation on tissues include a wide variety of reactions, some that are delayed. Mitotic inhibition and cytologic abnormalities, for example, may be detectable immediately in irradiated tissues, whereas fibrosis and other degenerative changes may not appear until months or years after exposure. Tissues in which cells proliferate rapidly are generally the first to exhibit injury [2].

In tissues capable of rapid cell turnover, the killing of dividing cells by irradiation tends to elicit the compensatory proliferation of surviving cells. As a result, a given dose causes less depletion of cells when spread out in time than when received in a single brief exposure. By the same token, the effects of a given dose are generally less severe if only a fraction of the cells in the tissue are irradiated than if the entire tissue is exposed [6].

Depending on the specific tissue or organ irradiated and the conditions of exposure, the effects of irradiation may vary greatly. Since it is beyond the scope of this chapter to review such effects comprehensively, only those reactions that are particularly relevant to occupational irradiation are discussed briefly in the following section.

Skin

Because of its superficial location, the skin's response to radiation has been investigated more thoroughly than that of any other organ. Erythema is the earliest outward reaction of the skin, and it may occur within minutes or hours after exposure, depending on the dose. After rapid exposure to a dose of 6 Sv or more, the reaction typically lasts only a few hours, to be followed 2 to 4 weeks later by one or more waves of deeper and more prolonged erythema. After a dose of 10 Sv

or more, dry desquamation, moist desquamation, necrosis of the skin, and epilation may ensue, followed eventually by pigmentation. Sequelae, which may develop months or years later, include atrophy of the epidermis and its adnexae, telangiectasia, and dermal fibrosis [6].

Bone Marrow and Lymphoid Tissue

Hemopoietic cells are highly radiosensitive and show degenerative changes within minutes after a dose in excess of 1 Sv. If a dose as high as 2 to 3 Sv is received rapidly by the whole body, a sufficient percentage of such cells is killed so that the normal replacement of aging leukocytes, platelets, and erythrocytes is impaired. As a result, the blood count declines gradually, leading to maximal depression of the leukocyte and platelet counts in 3 to 5 weeks (Fig. 16-1). After rapid exposure to a dose above 5 Sv, leukopenia and thrombocytopenia are likely to be severe enough to cause fatal infection, hemorrhage, or both. Doses larger than 5 Sv can be tolerated only if they are accumulated gradually over a period of months, or delivered to only a small portion of the total marrow.

Lymphocytes are also highly radiosensitive, degenerating rapidly after intensive irradiation. A dose of whole-body irradiation in excess of 2 to 3 Sv thus causes severe aplasia of lymphoid tissues, with profound depression of the immune response.

Gastrointestinal Tract

In many respects, the reaction of the gastrointestinal tract to irradiation resembles that of the skin. Dividing cells in the mucosal epithelium of the small intestine are highly radiosensitive and are killed in sufficient numbers by a dose of 10 Sv to interfere with normal renewal of the epithelium. The resulting depletion of epithelial cells, if sufficiently severe, may lead within a few days to ulceration and, ultimately, denudation of the mucosa. Hence rapid delivery of a dose in excess of 10 Sv to a large part of the small intestine, as may happen in the event of a radiation accident, can cause a fatal dysentery-like syndrome.

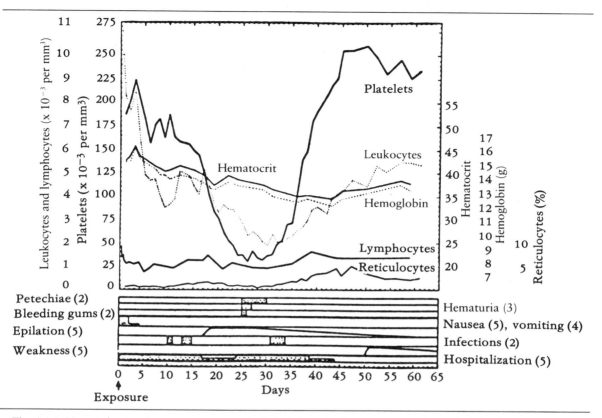

Fig. 16-1. Hematologic values, symptoms, and clinical signs in five men exposed to whole-body irradiation in a criticality accident. The blood counts are average values for the five men; the figures in parentheses denote the number showing the symptoms and signs indicated. (From GA Andrews, BW Sitterson, AL Kretchmar, et al. Criticality accidents at the Y-12 plant. In: Diagnosis and treatment of acute radiation injury. Geneva: World Health Organization, 1961:27–48.)

Gonads

Because of the high radiosensitivity of spermatogonia, the seminiferous tubules are among the most radiosensitive organs of the body. Acute exposure of the testes to a dose as low as 0.15 Sv suffices to depress the sperm count for months, and a dose of more than 2 Sv may cause permanent sterility [6].

Oocytes also are highly radiosensitive. Acute exposure of both ovaries to a dose of 1.5 to 2.0 Sv can cause temporary sterility, and to a dose of 2.0

to 3.0 Sv can cause permanent sterility, depending on the age of the woman at the time of exposure.

Lens of the Eye

Irradiation of the lens can cause the formation of lens opacities, or cataracts, which may not become evident until months or years later. The frequency, severity, and timing of the opacities depend on the dose and its distribution in time and space. The threshold for a vision-impairing opacity is estimated to vary from 2 to 3 Sv received in a single brief exposure, to 5.5 to 14.0 Sv received in repeated exposures over a period of months [6].

In the 1940s, a number of pioneer cyclotron physicists developed radiation cataracts as a result of their occupational exposure to neutrons. The occurrence of cataracts in these workers provided the first indication of the high relative biologic effectiveness of neutrons for injury to the lens [6].

RADIATION SICKNESS

Intensive irradiation of a major part of the hemopoietic system or the gastrointestinal tract can kill sufficient numbers of cells in these tissues to cause radiation sickness (acute radiation syndrome), as mentioned above. The associated prodromal symptoms characteristically include anorexia, nausea, and vomiting during the first few hours after irradiation, followed by a symptom-free interval until the main phase of the illness (Table 16-5) [6].

In the intestinal form of the syndrome, the main phase of the illness typically begins 2 to 3 days after irradiation, with abdominal pain, fever, and increasingly severe diarrhea, dehydration, disturbance of salt and fluid balance, prostration, toxemia, and shock, leading to death within 7 to 14 days [6].

In the hemopoietic form of the syndrome, the main phase typically begins in the second or third week after irradiation, with granulocytopenia, thrombocytopenia, and other complications of radiation-induced aplasia of the bone marrow. If damage to the marrow is sufficiently severe, death may ensue between the fourth and the sixth week after irradiation from septicemia, exsanguination, or other complications [6]. At mid-lethal dose levels, the probability of survival varies among indi-

Table 16-5. Symptoms of acute radiation sickness

Time after exposure	Lethal dose (6–10 Gy)	Median lethal dose (3–5 Gy)	Moderate dose (1–2 Gy)
First hours	Nausea and vomiting within several hours		
First week	Diarrhea, vomiting, inflammation of throat	No definite symptoms	
Second week	Fever, rapid emaciation, leading to death in all exposed		
Third to fourth weeks	Death	Loss of hair begins, loss of appetite, general malaise, fever, hemorrhages, pallor	
Fourth week		Leading to rapid emaciation and death for 50% of the exposed population	Loss of appetite, sore throat, pallor and diarrhea. Recovery begins (no deaths in absence of complications)

viduals, depending on differences in hemopoietic reserve, resistance to infection, and other variables.

Within hours after performing maintenance work in a large industrial radiography facility, which was subsequently found to have a defective safety interlock system, a pipefitter experienced transitory nausea and vomiting. One to two weeks later, he developed generalized erythema, followed within several days by loss of hair, sore throat, bleeding from the gums, diarrhea, and weakness. On examination, 3 weeks after his initial onset of symptoms, his lymphocyte count was 1,100 per mm³, leukocyte count 2,200 per mm³, platelet count 27,000 per mm³, hematocrit 40 percent, and reticulocyte count 1 percent. On cytogenetic analysis, his blood lymphocytes revealed an increased frequency of chromosomal aberrations, consistent with whole-body ionizing irradiation. Following treatment with platelet transfusions and antibiotics, his symptoms subsided in 2 to 3 weeks.

A third form of the acute radiation syndrome, the cerebral form, can result from acute exposure of the brain to a dose in excess of 50 Sv. In this syndrome, the same prodromal symptoms—anorexia, nausea, and vomiting—occur almost immediately after irradiation but are followed within minutes or hours by increasing drowsiness, ataxia, confusion, convulsions, loss of consciousness, and death [6].

EFFECTS ON GROWTH AND DEVELOPMENT OF THE EMBRYO

Embryonal and fetal tissues are extremely radiosensitive, in keeping with their highly proliferative character. Rapid exposure to 0.25 Sv during a critical stage in organogenesis has been observed to cause malformations of many types in experimental animals [7]. Comparable effects have been observed after larger doses in prenatally irradiated children. Mental retardation, for example, was greatly increased in frequency in children who were exposed to atomic bomb radiation at Hiro-

shima and Nagasaki between the eighth and fifteenth weeks of prenatal development [5].

EFFECTS ON CANCER INCIDENCE

Observations on atomic-bomb survivors, patients exposed to radiation for medical purposes, and early radiation workers (such as radiologists, radium dial painters, and pitchblende miners) indicate that many types of cancer can be increased in frequency by irradiation, depending on the conditions of exposure [2, 3, 7]. The cancers resulting from irradiation, however, do not appear until years or decades later and have no distinguishing features by which they can be recognized as radiation-induced. Hence, the occurrence of a given cancer in an irradiated individual cannot be attributed with certainty to previous irradiation.

The epidemiologic data come predominantly from observations at relatively high doses (0.5–2.0 Sv) and do not define the shape of the dose-incidence curve in the low-dose domain. Thus, the carcinogenic risks of low-level irradiation can be estimated only by interpolation or extrapolation, based on assumptions about the relationship between incidence and dose.

The most extensive dose-incidence data pertain to leukemia and cancer of the female breast. For leukemias other than the chronic lymphocytic type, the overall incidence increases with dose during the first 5 to 25 years after irradiation, by approximately 1 to 3 cases per year per 10,000 persons at risk per Sv to the bone marrow [8]. The relationship between the total cumulative incidence and the dose can be represented by various mathematical functions, including a linear-nonthreshold function, but interpretation of the dose-incidence data is complicated by unexplained variations among different types of leukemia in the magnitude of the increase for a given dose, age at irradiation, and time after exposure (Fig. 16-2). It is noteworthy that the incidence of chronic lymphocytic leukemia is apparently unaffected by irradiation [8].

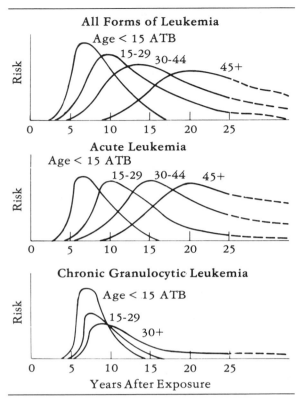

Fig. 16-2. Schematic representation of the tissue-distribution of the increase in absolute risk of leukemia in atomic bomb survivors in relation to age at time of irradiation. (ATB = at time of bomb.) (From M Ichimaru, T Ishimaru. A review of thirty years' study of Hiroshima and Nagasaki atomic bomb survivors. II. Biological effects. D. Leukemia and related disorders. J Radiat Res 1975; 16(Suppl):89–96.)

For cancer of the female breast, the incidence appears to increase in proportion to the dose (Fig. 16-3), and the magnitude of the increase for a given dose appears to be essentially the same whether the radiation is received instantaneously (as in the atomic bomb survivors), over 1 to 4 days (as in women treated with x-rays for acute postpartum mastitis), or over many months (as in luminous dial painters or women who received multiple fluoroscopic examinations of the chest in the treatment of pulmonary tuberculosis). The consistency of the dose-incidence relationship (Fig. 16-3) suggests that successive, small, widely-spaced exposures are fully additive in their cumulative carcinogenic effects on the breast and that the incidence thus increases as a linear, nonthreshold function of the cumulative dose [3, 8].

Two additional lines of evidence for carcinogenic effects at low doses are: (1) an increased incidence of thyroid cancer after 0.06 to 0.20 Gy of x-irradiation to the thyroid gland in childhood; and (2) an association between juvenile cancer and prenatal diagnostic x-irradiation [2, 3]. The latter has been interpreted to imply that exposure in utero to as little as 10 to 50 mGy may increase a child's risk of cancer by 40 to 50 percent [2, 3].

Other types of cancer also are increased in prevalence in irradiated populations (Table 16-6). The excess is generally dose-dependent, larger with high-LET radiation than with low-LET radiation, and of varying magnitude for a given dose, depending on the organ irradiated and the age at exposure (Table 16-6).

The total excess of all cancers combined approximates 0.6 to 1.8 cases per thousand persons per Sv per year, beginning 5 to 10 years after whole-body irradiation and continuing thereafter for the duration of life. The cumulative lifetime excess is thus estimated to approximate 20 to 100 additional cancers per 1,000 persons at risk per Sv, which corresponds to an increase of 10 to 60 percent per Sv in the average lifetime risk of cancer [2, 3, 8].

COMPARATIVE MAGNITUDE OF RADIATION RISKS

From the above risk estimates, the number of cancers attributable to occupational irradiation in radiation workers can be calculated to constitute less than 10 percent of the number expected to occur naturally in this population. Also, the average loss of life expectancy from all causes in radiation

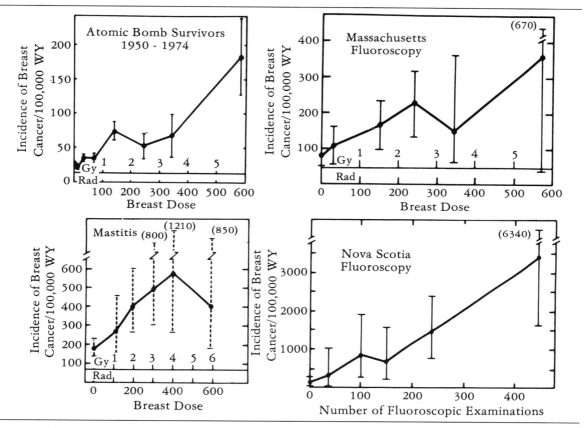

Fig. 16-3. Incidence of breast cancer in relation to dose in women exposed to atomic bomb radiation, women subjected to multiple fluoroscopic examinations of the chest in the treatment of pulmonary tuberculosis, and women given x-ray therapy to the breast for acute postpartum mastitis. (From JD Boice Jr, CE Land, RE Shore, et al. Risk of breast cancer following low-dose exposure. Radiology 1979; 131:589–597.)

workers is estimated to be no greater than that in occupations (such as construction and transportation work) that are generally considered to be relatively safe [9].

Nevertheless, since no amount of radiation is assumed to be entirely without risk, no dose in principle can be considered acceptable if it is readily avoidable. For this reason, the guiding rule in radiologic protection is the ALARA principle: The dose should be kept *as low as reasonably achievable.*

RADIATION PROTECTION

From the beginning of this century, increasing efforts have been made to prevent injury in radiation workers by limiting their occupational exposure. Initially, acute injuries were the main source of concern, and attempts were made to set "tolerance" doses, or threshold limit values (TLVs), to prevent such injuries. Gradually, however, it came to be suspected that genetic, carcinogenic, and teratogenic effects (stochastic effects) might have no threshold. Hence the concept of a "tolerance" dose

Table 16-6. Estimated annual excess radiation-induced cancers (per million per mSv[a]), by type of malignancy and age at exposure

Type of malignancy	Age at exposure (years)		
	20–34	35–49	50 +
Leukemia[b]			
Males	0.09	0.11	0.16
Females	0.05	0.07	0.10
Esophagus			
Both sexes	0.01	0.01	0.02
Stomach			
Both sexes	0.03	0.05	0.13
Colon			
Both sexes	0.02	0.03	0.09
Liver			
Both sexes	0.03	0.03	0.03
Pancreas			
Both sexes	0.02	0.03	0.08
Lung			
Both sexes	0.06	0.09	0.12
Breast			
Female	0.49	0.31[c]	0.08
Urinary tract			
Both sexes	0.02	0.04	0.07
Thyroid[d]			
Males	0.05	0.05	0.05
Females	0.15	0.15	0.15

[a]Risk expressed from tenth to thirtieth year after exposure unless otherwise specified.
[b]Risk expressed from fifth to twenty-sixth year after exposure.
[c]Value interpolated from figures in original report.
[d]Risk expressed from tenth to thirty-fourth year after exposure.
Source: J. E. Rall, G. W. Beebe, D. G. Hoel, et al. *Report of the National Institutes of Health Working Group to Develop Radioepidemiological Tables*. Washington, D.C.: U.S. Government Printing Office, 1985. (NIH publication no. 85-2748).

for the latter types of effects was eventually replaced by the concept of a "maximum permissible" dose—that is, a dose that was not intended to prevent stochastic effects altogether (since this would presumably be impossible without reducing the dose to zero) but that was intended to limit the frequency of such effects to levels that were ac-

ceptably low. At present, therefore, the system of protection for radiation workers involves two sets of dose limits; one of them is intended to prevent nonstochastic effects altogether, and the other is intended to limit the risks of stochastic effects to levels that are acceptably low [4].

To prevent the occurrence of nonstochastic effects, the recommended annual dose equivalent limit has been set at 0.5 Sv (50 rem) for all organs other than the lens of the eye; for the lens of the eye, the recommended annual dose equivalent limit has been set at 0.15 Sv (15 rem) [4, 6]. To limit the risks of stochastic effects to acceptable levels, the recommended annual dose equivalent limit for the whole body has been set at 50 mSv (5 rem); the annual dose equivalent limits for individual organs have been weighted in such a way that the combined risks of stochastic effects resulting from irradiation of any combination of organs separately do not exceed the overall risk of stochastic effects resulting from 50 mSv irradiation of the body as a whole [4]. This system of dose limitation is intended to protect radiation workers completely against radiation-induced cataracts, impairment of fertility, depression of hemopoiesis, and other nonstochastic effects, and to keep their combined risks of radiation-induced cancers, serious genetic diseases, and teratogenic effects from exceeding 1 per 10,000 per year, a rate of fatal work-related injuries encountered in many industries that are generally regarded as acceptably safe [4].

To minimize the radiation exposure of workers without unduly sacrificing their efficiency requires careful design of the workplace and work procedures, thorough training and supervision of workers, implementation of a well-conceived radiation protection program, and systematic health physics oversight and monitoring (Fig. 16-4).

Also needed are careful provisions for dealing with radiation accidents, emergencies, and other contingencies, systematic recording and updating of each worker's exposures, thorough labeling of all radiation sources and exposure fields, appropriate interlocks to guard against inadvertent ir-

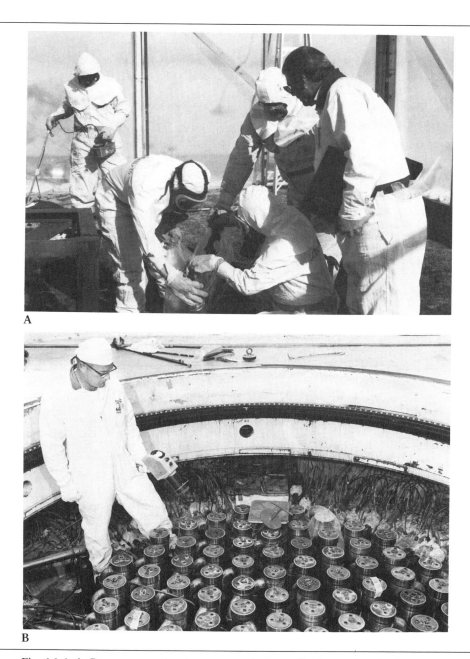

Fig. 16-4. A. Proper protection is necessary during collecting and packaging samples in the field with low-level radioactive contamination. B. Monitoring radiation levels atop a nuclear reactor. (Photographs courtesy of R. L. Kathren, Battelle Pacific Northwest Laboratory.)

radiation, and various other precautionary measures [1, 10, 11, 12].

General principles to be observed in every radiation protection program include the following [10]:

1. A well-developed, well-rehearsed, and updated emergency preparedness plan to enable prompt and effective response in the event of a malfunction, spill, or other radiation accident.
2. Appropriate use of shielding in facilities, equipment, and work clothing (such as aprons and gloves).
3. Appropriate selection, installation, maintenance, and operation of all equipment.
4. Minimization of exposure time.
5. Maximization of distance between personnel and sources of radiation (the intensity of exposure decreases inversely with the square of the distance from the source).
6. Appropriate training and supervision of workers to accomplish routine tasks with minimal exposure and to cope safely with irregularities.

MANAGEMENT OF THE IRRADIATED WORKER

In any workplace where employees may be exposed accidentally to radiation or radioactive material, plans for coping with such emergencies must be made in advance. These require delineation of lines of authority for managing accidents, knowledge in the workplace of the local health care facilities capable of evaluating and treating radiation accident victims, plans for transporting radioactive victims, and an understanding by the workers of the hazards of radiation.

In managing a radiation accident victim, good medical judgment and first aid should come first. Hence, even if the victim has been heavily irradiated or contaminated, he or she must also be evaluated for other forms of injury, such as mechanical trauma, burns, and smoke inhalation. To guard against self-contamination, those handling or examining the victim should wear gloves, masks, and other protective clothing.

The following general principles should also be observed [1, 10, 11, 12]:

General Emergency Medical Procedures
1. Apply emergency diagnostic and therapeutic maneuvers to assure stability of airway, respiration, and circulation as necessary.
2. Summon appropriate transport of the victim and inform attendants that the patient has been irradiated or contaminated.
3. Notify the appropriate medical facility personnel to expect the victim and inform them of the irradiation or contamination.
4. Keep detailed records concerning all examinations, measurements, findings, procedures, personnel, and times involved.

Procedures for Radioactive Contamination
1. Clothing should be removed promptly if contaminated, isolated in a plastic bag, and labeled to denote radioactivity.
2. Any contaminated parts of the body should be isolated with plastic or paper from the rest of the body and other surroundings and monitored for radioactivity.
3. Contaminated parts of the body should be thoroughly rinsed, contaminated rinse water isolated as "radioactive waste," and the part monitored again.
4. Care should be taken to avoid abrasion of contaminated skin during rinsing in order to minimize hyperemia and further absorption of radioactivity.
5. To expedite elimination of any inhaled radioactivity, the victim should rinse the oral and nasal cavities by gargling and snorting water.
6. Secretions should be collected in plastic bags, labeled, and isolated for future examination.
7. The victim should be isolated from others who are not essential for emergency care.
8. Precautions should be taken to avoid contamination of other people, objects, and areas. For

this purpose, the contaminated area should be sealed off as soon as possible.

REFERENCES

1. Huber CF, Fry S. The medical basis for radiation accident preparedness. New York: Elsevier, 1980.
2. United Nations Scientific Committee on the Effects of Atomic Radiation (UNSCEAR). Ionizing radiation: sources and biological effects. Report to the General Assembly, with annexes. New York: United Nations, 1982.
3. National Academy of Sciences Advisory Committee on the Biological Effects of Ionizing Radiation (BEIR). The effects on populations of exposure to low levels of ionizing radiation. Washington, DC: National Academy of Sciences, National Research Council, 1972, 1980.
4. International Commission on Radiological Protection (ICRP). Recommendations of the international commission on radiological protection. Oxford: Pergamon, 1977. (ICRP publication 26, Annals of the ICRP,vol. 1, no. 3).
5. United Nations Scientific Committee on the Effects of Atomic Radiation (UNSCEAR). Genetic and somatic effects of ionizing radiation. Report of the General Assembly, with annexes. New York: United Nations, 1986.
6. International Commission on Radiological Protection (ICRP). Nonstochastic effects of ionizing radiation. Oxford: Pergamon, 1984. (ICRP publication 41, Annals of the ICRP, vol. 14, no. 3).
7. United Nations Scientific Committee on the Effects of Atomic Radiation (UNSCEAR). Sources and effects of ionizing radiation. Report to the General Assembly, with annexes. New York: United Nations, 1977.
8. Rall JE, Beebe GW, Hoel DG, et al. Report of the National Institutes of Health Working Group to Develop Radioepidemiological Tables. Washington, DC: U.S. Government Printing Office, 1985. (NIH publication no. 85-2748).
9. Sinclair WK. Effects of low-level radiation and comparative risk. Radiology 1981; 138:1–9.
10. Kahn K, Ryan K, Sabo A, Boyce P. Ionizing radiation. In: Levy BS, Wegman, DH, eds. Occupational health. Boston: Little, Brown, 1983, pp. 189–206.
11. National Council on Radiation Protection and Measurements (NCRP). Management of persons accidentally contaminated with radionuclides. Washington, DC: National Council on Radiation Protection and Measurements, 1980. (NCRP report no. 65).
12. International Atomic Energy Agency. What the general practitioner (MD) should know about medical handling of overexposed individuals. Vienna, Austria: International Atomic Energy Agency, 1986. (IAEA-TECDOC-366).

BIBLIOGRAPHY

Huber CF, Fry S. The medical basis for radiation accident preparedness. New York: Elsevier, 1980.
A compendium of reports by recognized authorities on the causes, nature, consequences, and management of radiation accidents occurring in various countries prior to 1980.

International Commission on Radiological Protection (ICRP). Recommendations of the International Commission on Radiological Protection. Oxford: Pergamon, 1977. (ICRP publication 26, Annals of the ICRP, vol. 1, no. 3).
A detailed summary of the Commission's recommendations for limiting the exposure of workers and the public to ionizing radiation.

National Academy of Sciences Advisory Committee on the Biological Effects of Ionizing Radiation (BEIR). The effects on populations of exposure to low levels of ionizing radiation. Washington, DC: National Academy of Sciences, National Research Council, 1972, 1980.
A comprehensive review of the extent to which the U.S. population is exposed to ionizing radiation from various sources and of the resulting risks of carcinogenic and inherited effects of such irradiation.

Rall JE, Beebe, GW, Hoel DG, et al. Report of the National Institutes of Health Working Group to Develop Radioepidemiological Tables. Washington, DC: U.S. Government Printing Office, 1985. (NIH publication no. 85-2748.)
Report of a methodology for estimating the extent to which a developing cancer is likely to have been caused by previous radiation exposure.

United Nations Scientific Committee on the Effects of Atomic Radiation (UNSCEAR). Genetic and somatic effects of ionizing radiation. Report to the General Assembly, with annexes. New York: United Nations, 1986.
An updated version of parts of the report cited above including a review of the teratogenic effects of ionizing radiation.

United Nations Scientific Committee on the Effects of
Atomic Radiation (UNSCEAR). Ionizing radiation:
sources and biological effects. Report to the General
Assembly, with annexes. New York: United Nations,
1982.

*A comprehensive review of the sources, exposure lev-
els, and biomedical effects of ionizing radiation compiled by an international team of experts. Health effects surveyed include carcinogenic, inherited, and
nonstochastic effects.*

17
Noise and Hearing Impairment

Roger P. Hamernik and Robert I. Davis

Since the Industrial Revolution, the noise levels in our society have increased continually to such an extent that exposure to excessively loud sound now constitutes a serious hazard to hearing with profound impacts on the quality of life for the affected individual. Sound is ubiquitous. Excessive levels of noise are present in industrial and military work environments and permeate our social environments. The scope of the problem is large, with estimates of close to eight million civilian workers in the United States exposed to potentially damaging levels of noise, and many more exposed to such levels in the military and outside of work. Thus, an understanding of the mechanisms of noise-induced hearing loss (NIHL) and the strategies for combating the hazards of exposure are essential to public health and occupational health professionals.

To protect hearing from excessive noise exposure, we are required to answer what appears to be a fundamentally simple question: "How much noise is too much?" However, the answer to this question has eluded researchers. The answer is problematic, because it transcends scientific methodology and requires that important political and economic decisions be made. In this chapter, we are concerned primarily with the consequences of excessive noise exposure on our ability to hear.

The ear at the periphery is composed of three major components—the external ear, the middle ear, and the cochlea—and centrally, the ascending and descending auditory pathways of the central nervous system. To understand how noise affects hearing, some knowledge of the function of these structures is necessary. Also, some familiarity with the science of acoustics is needed before a meaningful examination of the various approaches to developing noise exposure standards is possible.

SOUND AS THE PHYSICAL STIMULUS—SOME DEFINITIONS

There are two broad classes of noise: continuous and impulsive. A noise is continuous if, once initiated, it continues for a prolonged period of time. Since, in some respects, our scaling of time is relative to the event being studied, this definition is not very precise, but for an industrial exposure situation we might consider an eight-hour period as representing a continuous exposure. However, the typical workday exposure is invariably broken up by rest periods and lunch. Thus, in reality, the exposure is interrupted. Experimental data on the effects of interruption are, in general, lacking. Impulsive noise is generally considered to be a "relatively" short (in duration), often intense presentation, which can occur at regular intervals throughout a workday or only sporadically.

Various intermediate types of noise and various combinations of different types can be defined. In many industrial situations, impulsive noise components are superimposed on a background continuous noise. Current measurement practice is not designed to accurately assess such combination exposures and will usually underestimate considerably the hazard potential of impulse-continuous noise combinations. In practice, some standards for continuous noise currently exist, but standards for impulsive noise exposures are still evolving, and little consideration is given to the interaction between different classes of noise or other causes of trauma to the ear, such as vibration, drugs, or disease processes.

Standards for exposure to noise, as well as hearing conservation manuals, use a variety of specialized terms from the science of acoustics that are not generally familiar. Therefore, understanding of commonly used terms is necessary before one can interpret information or instructions associated with hearing conservation measures with confidence (see box).

Complex industrial noise is often characterized by the Fourier spectrum computed or measured in terms of octave bands: that is, we can measure the sound pressure level (SPL) of consecutive octave frequency bands to determine how the SPL is distributed across the range of frequencies of interest. Figure 17-1 illustrates two typical frequency spectrums for a metal stamping mill. The spectra are somewhat typical of industrial noises with energy maxima in the 200 to 500 Hz region. Since the ear is differentially sensitive to sounds of different frequencies, such an analysis is an important step in the evaluation of the potential hazards of a noise environment. If the spectrum analysis shows that the energy of the noise in question is relatively uniformly distributed over a wide range of frequencies, the noise is called a broad band of noise. Prominent energy peaks in the spectrum in very narrow bands of frequencies may indicate the presence of pure tones or unusual concentrations of acoustic energy. In general, the more concentrated the acoustic energy is in the spectral domain, the greater the potential noise hazard is to the auditory system.

In addition to the variety of continuous noises, there is a large class of transient noises referred to as impulsive. Typically, these have high intensities and short durations (< 1 second). Both explosive discharges, such as gunfire, and industrial impacts produced by intermittent metal-to-metal contact fall in this category. Such noises are common in industrial and military environments. Im-

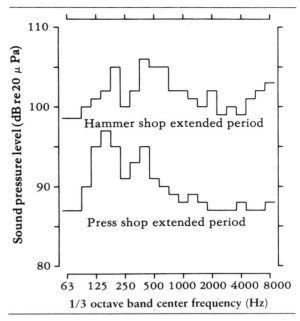

Fig. 17-1. An example of a ⅓ octave band spectrum of the noise in a forging industry. (From W Taylor, et al. J Acoust Soc Am 1984; 76(3):808.)

pulse noise exposures can, in general, be more hazardous than continuous noise exposures. Part of the reason for this is that, subjectively, we tend to underestimate the potential of an impulse for causing trauma because its transient nature makes it seem quieter than it truly is. Between the extremes presented above fall a myriad of intermediate types of noise.

When sound impinges on a surface, such as the walls of a room or the tympanic membrane, a part is reflected, a part is transmitted, and a part is absorbed by the surface. These properties of sound theoretically allow the engineer to control the sound environment: Suitable design of walls can contain the sound; suitable materials in the vicinity of the sound source can absorb the sound energy and convert it into harmless heat energy; suitable design of machinery can reduce or eliminate the source of the noise. Although engineering so-

SOUND DEFINITIONS

Sound, or *noise,* is a fluctuation of the ambient pressure that propagates in the elastic media, air. This longitudinally propagating disturbance, or wave, is capable of exerting a fluctuating force (pressure × area) on any surface on which it impinges. Thus, the magnitude of the pressure change above and below atmospheric pressure can be used as a measure of the strength of the sound wave and is given in units of Newtons per square meter (N/m^2), called *Pascals* (Pa). Because the ear is responsive to sound waves whose strength can cover a dynamic range on the order of more than 10^6, it is advantageous to use a logarithmic scale to measure the strength of a sound wave. A range of 10^6 on a linear scale converted into a logarithmic scale (Bel scale) is compressed into a range of 6 Bel units or a range of 60 units on a *decibel* (dB) scale. The dB scale is used in acoustical measurements where the strength of a sound wave can be defined in terms of a dB level. The *sound pressure level* (SPL) represents a ratio measure of the strength of the sound being measured relative to the reference pressure fluctuation. A sound wave that is twice as strong as the reference value produces a 6 dB increase in SPL over the reference value, which is still a very weak disturbance. The reference pressure is approximately equal to the smallest disturbance that the normal ear can just detect at its most sensitive frequency. If over time and space the disturbance of pressure follows a regular sine wave pattern, the sound is a *pure tone.* The rate at which the pressure fluctuations repeat in a sinusoidal fashion is called the *frequency* and is given in units of cycles per second, termed *Hertz* (Hz). Thus, a pure tone consists of a single frequency (f). The usual range of frequencies of interest in hearing science lies roughly between 20 and 20,000 Hz. The range of human conversation is from about 300 to 3,000 Hz. The speed at which the wave propagates through the environment is called the *speed of sound,* c meters per second (m/s), and is uniquely determined by the thermodynamic properties of the media in which the wave is traveling. In air, at standard conditions, c = 343 m/s. Therefore, the spacial extent of the disturbance created by a pure tone f, called the *wave length* (λ), is given by $\lambda = c/f$ (meters); the duration of the disturbance in time, the period T, is given as $T = 1/f$ (sec). (This formula is nothing more complex than velocity × time = distance.) In most industrial situations, pure tones are uncommon and the noise usually consists of a relatively complex temporal pattern of pressure fluctuations. *Fourier analysis,* which can be applied to most noises likely to be encountered in practice, is a mathematical means of decomposing a complex wave form into a series of pure tones having specific amplitudes, frequencies, and temporal relations to each other (phase). Thus, the temporal pattern of sound (amplitude versus time), which we intuitively feel that we are sensing with our ears, can be transformed uniquely into the frequency and phase domain to obtain a different, but equivalent, physical description of the sound. Fourier analysis has a wide application in noise research. Different types of sound can be more precisely classified in the frequency domain: For example, an octave band of noise contains all frequencies lying between upper and lower frequency limits such that the upper frequency is equal to two times the lower frequency. An octave band is usually defined by its center frequency—that is, the geometric mean of the upper and lower frequencies. Thus, an octave band of noise with a center frequency of 1,000 Hz would have 710 and 1,400 Hz as the approximate lower and upper frequency limits.

lutions can be difficult and expensive to implement, they still need to be considered in many situations.

Under field conditions, sounds are usually measured with a portable sound level meter, which is capable of converting the forces generated by the pressure fluctuations acting on a sensitive microphone element into an electrical signal. The electronics of the meter process this signal to produce a single number representing a mean SPL in dB or dB(A), the weighted scale, which will be discussed later. These meters can also be equipped with octave or $\frac{1}{3}$-octave band analyzers to obtain the SPL in consecutive bands of frequencies.

THE HEARING MECHANISM

Scientifically, much has been learned about the fundamental processes of hearing and how noise affects psychoacoustic performance, the basic physiology of the cochlea, and the morphology of the sensory elements of the cochlea [1, 2]. The need for the survival of the evolving species required that the sound-sensing organ be able to detect extremely low level stimuli in the presence of various masking noises, such as the approach of a predator masked by the rustle of leaves. Under such pressures, the ear has evolved into an exquisitely sensitive mechanoelectric transducer, which converts airborne sound energy impinging on the external ear into a micromechanical wave motion in the cochlea and, in turn, into a series of ordered electrical discharges (action potentials) that are transmitted via the eighth cranial nerve into the brainstem for subsequent information-processing in higher cortical centers. The ear was not designed for the types of contemporary noise environments to which it is being exposed.

The external ear and canal terminating at the tympanic membrane is the initial conducting pathway for sound entering the ear (Fig. 17-2A). Often modeled as a tube closed at one end, the external canal has resonance properties such that it can amplify certain regions of the environmental noise spectrum by more than 10 dB in the frequency range approximately 2,000 to 4,000 Hz, thus increasing the potential of that noise for producing hearing loss [3].

The middle ear, as a sound transmission line, is bound laterally by the tympanic membrane and medially by the oval window. Between these two membranes are fastened the three smallest bones of the body, the ossicles: the malleus, the incus, and the stapes. These bones are suspended by several ligaments and are under limited muscular control. The two smallest muscles of the body, the tensor tympani and the stapedius, attach to the malleus and stapes, respectively. These muscles are under voluntary control in some individuals, but normally, contractions of these muscles are initiated by excessively loud sounds (the acoustic reflex). For sound to reach the fluid-filled cochlea, it must first be conducted through the middle ear—that is, from the air environment of the external canal into the liquid environment of the cochlea. Because of the different physical properties of air and water, the ability of airborne sound to penetrate into a fluid environment is severely limited and some form of mechanical advantage (amplification) is necessary. Without amplification, more than 99 percent of the acoustic energy incident on a water surface is reflected. The middle ear performs this amplification in a frequency-selective manner, being most efficient in the 500 to 5,000 Hz region of the sound spectrum and least efficient at the extremely low or high frequencies.

The contraction of the muscles of the middle ear stiffens the tympanic membrane and ossicular chain and thereby reduces the transmission of sound energy to the cochlea. This reduction in transmission is achieved by an increase in the input impedance to the cochlea and is itself a frequency-dependent phenomena. Since the effects of stiffness on the impedance are inversely related to frequency, the acoustic reflex affects middle-ear transmission most strongly at low frequencies. Contraction in response to loud sounds is initiated at sound pressure levels in the range of 70 to 100 dB above the hearing threshold.

A number of theories have been proposed con-

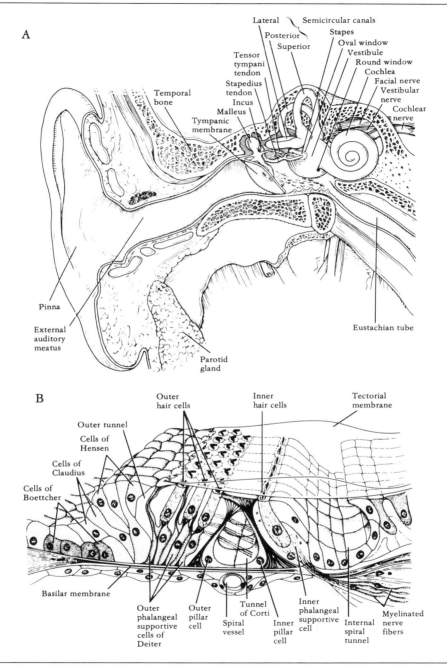

Fig. 17-2. A. Schematic representation of the relationships among the major anatomic components of the ear. (From LC Junqueira et al. Basic histology. San Mateo, CA: Lange, 1977.) B. A schematic of the organ of Corti illustrating the relation between sensory and supporting epithelia and the basilar membrane. (From WB Bloom and DW Fawcett. A textbook of histology. 10th ed. Philadelphia: Saunders, 1975.)

cerning the functional role of the acoustic reflex. One popular theory contends that since the reflex is elicited by sound levels that are potentially damaging to the auditory system, the primary purpose of the reflex is the protection of the cochlea. However, this "protection theory" is weakened by the fact that the latency and the rapid adaptation of the reflex cause it to respond too slowly to sudden sounds, such as impact noises, and make it ineffective against steady, continuous noises. Although the greatest reduction in sound transmission (20–30 dB) occurs for low frequencies, the protection offered by the reflex appears to be a beneficial side effect of a more functional purpose. Since the reflex mainly attenuates low frequencies, and since most of an individual's physiologic noises as well as environmental noises are of a low-frequency nature, the reflex response, when activated, should reduce both internal and external noise environments, resulting in an improved signal-to-noise ratio and subsequent improvement of speech intelligibility in high noise level environments.

The transmission characteristics of the external ear and middle ear therefore alter the spectrum of sound that is ultimately received by the cochlea. Hence, a knowledge of the free-field spectrum (assigned to the source alone) is important as a first estimate of its potential for causing hearing damage. For example, the relative lack of sensitivity of the cochlea to low-frequency sounds has led to the development of the dB(A) scale of sound pressure measurement. This A scale, in essence, biases the measurement of the sound against the low-frequency end of the spectrum. In this sense, it is a scale that mirrors the ear's sensitivity and thus is frequently used for measurements of noise environments where the hazard to hearing is to be evaluated.

The final peripheral receptor of the sound stimulus is the organ of Corti, which lies within the cochlea (Fig. 17-2B). Recently described as the most complex of mechanical systems, it has about 10^6 moving parts [4]. Packed into an organ the size of a housefly is a mechanical analysis system consisting of approximately 17,000 sensory cells or-

derly displayed on a membrane that possesses a mechanical frequency selectivity over a range of 20,000 Hz. The system at threshold is capable of detecting subangstrom level mechanical displacements with astonishing precision. Even more surprising, the cochlea performs this analysis over roughly a 10^6 dynamic range.

The primary mechanical sensing elements of the cochlea are the sensory hair cells, grouped into inner and outer hair cells. The pattern of innervation to these two classes of sensory cells is quite different; the inner hair cells are primarily responsible for the afferent flow of information, whereas the outer hair cells possess predominantly efferent synapses. The sensory cells are arranged within a supporting matrix of epithelial cells that rest on the mechanically active basilar membrane. The entire complex is referred to as the organ of Corti. The cilia of the sensory cells are capped by an acellular membrane, the tectorial membrane, which has its own mechanical properties [5]. The arrangement of the sensory cells on the basilar membrane is tonotopic: the lowest portions of the membrane are most sensitive to high-frequency disturbances, whereas the uppermost portions are most sensitive to low frequencies. The tonotopic organization is maintained throughout the ascending auditory pathways. This organization of cells on the basilar membrane allows for the correlation between stimulus, or noise frequency, and the location of sensory cell lesions.

The cochlea is of particular concern because once damaged, its normal functioning cannot be completely regained. In a sense, the cochlea has two Achilles' heels: structural fragility and metabolic frailty. Excessive disturbances on the basilar membrane, caused by noise, can directly damage the cilia on the sensory cells and can alter the integrity of the tight cell junctions of the epithelial linings. The epithelial tight cell junctions within the cochlea confine and maintain unique fluid environments necessary for proper sensory cell function. Any change in these tight cell junctions can result in a change in the microhomeostasis of the organ of Corti. Such changes can lead to the ulti-

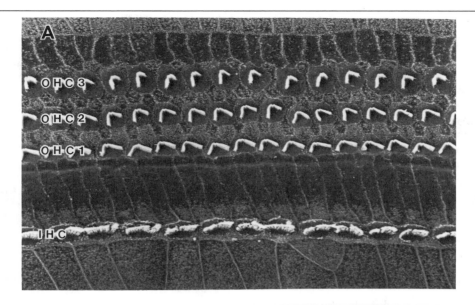

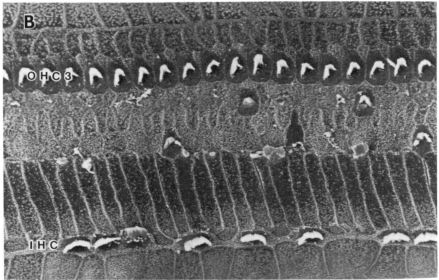

Fig. 17-3. A. A scanning electron micrograph of the surface of the organ of Corti. The W-shaped arrangement of the cilia on the outer hair cells (OHC) and the linear arrangement of the cilia on the inner hair cells (IHC) is easily distinguished. Noise-induced mechanical damage to these delicate cilia will result in abnormal function of this transducing sensory element. B. Scanning electron microscopic view of the surface of the organ of Corti, which has lost most of the first and second rows of OHCs and has scattered losses of inner hair cells. Compare this sparse population of sensory cells with the population in the normal appearing organ of Corti in (A).

mate loss of sensory cells. Also any changes that alter vascular physiology can lead to changes in the capillary beds of the cochlea (stria vascularis), which drive the metabolism of the cochlea. If these vessels are compromised, the normal functioning of the sensory cells can be altered or the cells permanently damaged. Typically, noise-induced lesions of the cochlea result in an irreplaceable loss of sensory cells (Fig. 17-3), changes in the capillary network, and a loss of first-order neurons of the spiral ganglion associated with the hair cells.

The auditory component of the eighth cranial nerve, which links the cochlea to the brainstem, consists of a bundle of approximately 30,000 myelinated afferent nerve fibers. Ninety-five percent of the afferent fibers innervate the inner hair cells, while a much smaller number of afferent fibers (about 5 percent) innervate the outer hair cells, which outnumber the inner hair cells by approximately 3 : 1. A smaller group of efferent fibers also enters the cochlea, terminating mostly on the outer hair cells. A series of nuclei beginning with the cochlear nucleus convey the coded cochlear signals through several brainstem nuclei eventually to the temporal lobe of the cortex. Lesions of the sensory cells in the cochlea can result in changes in the ascending auditory pathways. Such central changes can have additional implications for what we hear or for the efficacy of prosthetic devices used to help correct hearing deficits.

BEHAVIORAL AND AUDIOLOGIC MANIFESTATIONS OF NOISE-INDUCED HEARING LOSS

Sufficiently intense sounds have the potential of disrupting all parts of the peripheral and central auditory system. Noise can have direct mechanical effects on the middle ear, such as ossicular discontinuity, tympanic membrane perforation, or fistula of the oval window (Fig. 17-4) and on cochlear structures [1]. The outer hair cells are particularly vulnerable to the effects of excessive noise exposure, followed in vulnerability by the inner hair cells. The cochlea, once damaged, cannot be re-

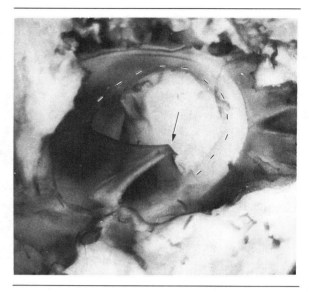

Fig. 17-4. An example of a pig middle ear damaged by high levels of impulse noise. The tip of the manubrium of the malleus is broken (arrow), and there is a very large tear (dashed line) in the tympanic membrane.

paired; the subsequent loss of sensory cells and neural changes produces an auditory pathology that represents the morphologic substrate for the loss of hearing threshold, referred to as a noise-induced sensorineural hearing loss, or simply a noise-induced hearing loss (NIHL). A similar set of cochlear changes can be induced by lower levels of noise that continuously stress the metabolic processes of the cochlea. While these changes may initially produce a temporary loss of threshold, with repeated exposures they may lead to permanent changes [2].

Hearing loss resulting from noise exposure can be separated into three distinct categories: acoustic trauma, temporary threshold shift (TTS), and permanent threshold shift (PTS). A single, relatively intense noise exposure is referred to as an acoustic trauma and is usually followed by tinnitus and a change in hearing threshold. While hearing may improve slightly over time, if the exposure is sufficiently intense a PTS will result. One or both ears may be involved. Those who experience an acoustic trauma may also suffer from tympanic membrane perforation(s) and disarticulated or fractured ossicles. Such middle-ear disorders are more likely to appear, if at all, once the peak noise exposure level exceeds approximately 160 dB SPL. In general, however, any acute sound exposure that causes any of the following symptoms represents a hazard to the auditory system and could result in an acute acoustic trauma: immediate pain, a tickling sensation in the ears often occurring if the SPL exceeds approximately 120 dB, vertigo, tinnitus, hearing loss, or reduced communication skills.

Lower levels of noise (< 85 dB[A]) are potentially hazardous and may result in a NIHL if, following exposure, there is a transient shift in the threshold of hearing that recovers gradually (a TTS). While the onset of hearing loss in acute acoustic trauma is instantaneous, the onset and progression of NIHL is far more insidious since it accumulates, usually unnoticed, over a period of many years of exposure to noise on a daily basis. During the initial stages of NIHL, the temporary hearing loss recovers within a few hours or days following removal from the noise. However, if the exposure to this noise is repeated often enough, the hearing loss may not recover completely (that is, permanent sensorineural hearing impairment will begin).

The following is a typical case history of an individual with permanent NIHL:

A 48-year-old man had chief complaints of constant, high-pitched tinnitus and progressive hearing loss in both ears over the previous 2 years. He reported some difficulty hearing in quiet surroundings but noticed marked difficulty understanding speech in noisy environments. He did not report any previous serious illnesses, accidents, atypical drug use, or problems with his ears. For the past 8 years, he had worked in a noisy textile mill, where he said that he "occasionally" wore hearing protective devices. The patient had not been exposed to other hazardous noises off the job, such as gunfire or motorbikes.

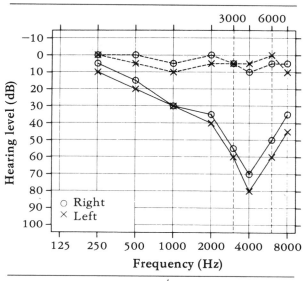

Fig. 17-5. An example of a typical audiogram from a normal individual (dashed lines) and an individual with a bilateral sensorineural hearing loss resulting from excessive noise exposure. Note the maximum loss at 4000 Hz and the spread of loss to the lower frequencies.

The diagnosis of a NIHL comes under the domain of the audiologist, whose primary responsibility is the identification and measurement of hearing loss and the rehabilitation of those with hearing impairment. By measuring auditory thresholds in decibels (relative to a normal hearing level or 0 dB HL) for pure tones as a function of frequency, an audiogram (a frequency-intensity graph) is generated. Hearing level (HL) is a term used to designate an individual's hearing threshold at a given test frequency, referenced to an audiometric zero level. The audiogram will help answer the following questions: (1) Is there evidence of a hearing loss? (2) If so, what is the severity of the loss? (3) What is the nature of the loss (conductive, sensorineural, or mixed)? and (4) Can the use of a hearing aid(s) benefit the hearing-impaired individual? A typical normal audiogram and an audiogram from an individual with a NIHL are shown in Figure 17-5.

Hearing loss induced by most industrial noise characteristically produces a bilateral symmetrical loss that is progressive in nature so long as the individual is continuously exposed to hazardous noise levels (Fig. 17-5). In the initial stages of development, the loss usually occurs at frequencies lying between 3,000 and 6,000 Hz [6]. The maximum loss is usually centered at 4,000 Hz. The audiometric configuration, therefore, is characterized by a downward slope with greater loss in the high-frequency region (3,000–6,000 Hz) than in the low- and mid-frequency regions (250–2,000 Hz). As the NIHL accumulates following further exposure, the 4,000 Hz loss increases in magnitude and the adjacent (higher and lower) frequencies also become increasingly affected. The progressive nature of NIHL may eventually result in a moderate to severe impairment across most of the usable hearing frequency range (250–8,000 Hz) unless preventive measures are taken to reduce the degree of hazard imposed by the noise.

Although the diagnosis of a permanent NIHL may be indicated by the audiometric configuration of the hearing loss (the 4,000 Hz notch), it would be premature to make a definitive diagnosis unless additional factors are considered, such as: (1) What is the duration, type, and time-weighted average of the individual's noise exposure? (2) What is the individual's hearing both before and after exposure? (3) What is the age and general health of the individual? (4) Are there any other disorders that may result in hearing impairment (such as middle-ear disorders, congenital factors, Ménière's disease, an eighth cranial nerve lesion, ototoxicity, and presbycusis)? Consideration of these questions provides important information as to whether the cause and degree of impairment can be solely attributable to noise exposure. Two major diagnostic problems are distinguishing NIHL from hearing loss associated with presbycusis or ototoxic agents and determining the degree of impairment attributed to the aging process. A reported history of tinnitus or "muffled" hearing occurring immediately after any noise exposure or after leaving the work environment and a characteristic 4,000 Hz notch on the audiogram strongly suggest an occupational NIHL hearing loss. Complaints of vertigo are also common.

People usually do not report any difficulty in hearing until a hearing loss of more than 25 dB HL occurs at a frequency at or below 4,000 Hz. Difficulty in hearing the high-frequency sounds of speech (such as s, f, k, t, and sh) may provide the only clue to the individual of a NIHL. Performance on speech intelligibility tasks varies considerably depending on the magnitude of the loss and the affected frequencies [6]. If the hearing loss is confined to frequencies above 3,000 Hz, speech intelligibility measured in quiet surroundings is usually within normal limits. As the frequencies below 3,000 Hz become involved, intelligibility decreases in relation to the degree of impairment. Given that approximately 95 percent of the frequency components in speech lie between 300 and 3,000 Hz, it should not be surprising to find a deterioration in speech intelligibility performance once the NIHL extends into this range of frequencies. Also, individuals with sensorineural hearing loss, due either to noise exposure or other factors, usually have greater difficulty understanding speech against a competing background noise environment than in a quiet environment. This common complaint may be minor if the hearing loss is restricted to frequencies at or above 3,000 Hz but may present marked difficulty for those with losses below 3,000 Hz. Since the usual pattern of progressive NIHL is one in which the speech frequencies are affected last, it is important to identify NIHL during its initial stages to help prevent future deterioration of hearing sensitivity and speech discrimination abilities.

Occupational health nurses and physicians involved in assessing and monitoring hearing status in hearing conservation programs should refer the worker to an audiologist if a significant change in hearing level ($\geq$ 10 dB at any frequency in either ear) is observed after the worker has had a minimum of 48 hours to recover from environmental noise exposure. Audiologic management of the individual with NIHL may include the use of hearing aids, aural rehabilitation, and assistive listening devices to help improve some of the communication dysfunction experienced in certain listening situations. What, if any, strategies are implemented depends largely on the severity of the communication handicap produced by the noise exposure and the listening needs of the individual.

The nature of hearing impairment is determined by conventional audiometric techniques (air-conduction [AC] and bone-conduction [BC] thresholds, impedance audiometry, speech discrimination, and site-of-lesion test procedures) [6]. Bone conduction audiometry is used in conjunction with air conduction audiometry to determine the nature of hearing impairment. In the former procedure, the stimulus is conducted directly to the cochlea by a source of vibration attached to the mastoid process of the temporal bone, thus bypassing the conventional route through the middle ear. "Normal" hearing is evident by an air-bone gap (the difference in dB between AC and BC thresholds of the same frequency) of 10 dB or less and a BC threshold less than 15 dB. If, for example, an air-bone gap of more than 10 dB is observed with normal BC threshold values, the loss is considered conductive (due to a defect of the sound-conducting mechanism: external auditory canal or middle ear). A sensorineural loss (a defect in the inner ear or auditory nerve) is characterized by similar, but elevated ($\geq$ 15 dB) AC and BC thresholds. If, on the other hand, there is an air-bone gap of 11 dB or more and BC thresholds are poorer than normal ($>$ 15 dB), the nature of the loss is considered mixed (conductive and sensorineural). Consider the following examples:

SUBJECT	AC THRESHOLD (dB)	BC THRESHOLD (dB)	AIR-BONE GAP (dB)	NATURE
1	40	10	30	Conductive
2	40	35	5	Sensorineural
3	40	25	15	Mixed

Each individual's AC threshold is the same, but their BC thresholds are different. Subject 1, for ex-

ample, has a pure conductive hearing impairment since an air-bone gap ($>$ 10 dB) is present with a normal BC threshold ($<$ 15 dB). Subject 2 has a pure sensorineural impairment since there is no significant air-bone gap ($<$ 10 dB), which rules out the presence of a conductive component, but an elevated BC threshold (35 dB HL). Subject 3 has a mixed impairment, given the presence of both an air-bone gap ($>$ 10 dB) and an elevated BC threshold ($\geq$ 15). Although the use of threshold criteria is a valuable aid in determining the degree and nature of the loss, the audiologist will often use additional diagnostic test procedures to more accurately define the location of pathology within the auditory system. A normal audiometric pattern, however, does not necessarily indicate an absence of pathology to the auditory system (either peripherally or centrally in the nervous system).

HEARING CONSERVATION

Prevention of NIHL is the concern of workers and managers. In both industrial and nonindustrial noise environments, the control of NIHL is primarily through prevention, stressing a decrease in existing noise, a decrease in exposure noise levels, or both. No present medical therapy can restore the permanent changes in the inner ear (sensorineural hearing impairment) that have resulted from excessive noise exposure.

OSHA regulations limit the occupational noise exposure according to duration of exposure and intensity of sound. A daily average exposure of 90 dBA over 8 hours is the current limit; however, the regulations also permit sounds of greater intensity for shorter periods. Workplaces in many industries sometimes exceed the 90 dBA OSHA limit: noises associated with grinding, drilling, or stamping of metal to manufacture metal products and machinery (Fig. 17-6), sawing of wood in lumber mills, printing machines in publishing and newspaper companies, air hoses in many industries, and looms in textile mills frequently approach or exceed the 90 dBA level. (See Chap. 7 for a discussion of noise control principles and measures.)

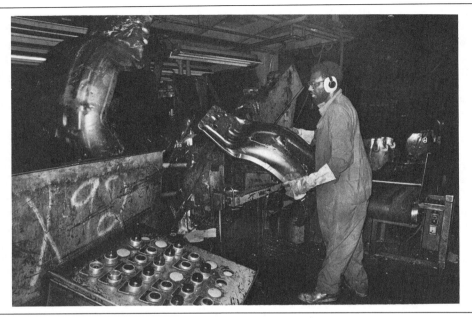

Fig. 17-6. Noise production in a stamping operation may be difficult to control at the source.
(Photograph by Earl Dotter.)

Federal law also mandates the institution of a hearing conservation program (HCP) if a noise exposure equals or exceeds a time-weighted average (TWA) of 85 dB(A) over an 8-hour period. Industries should, however, consider such programs if employees complain of either communication difficulty while working in the noise environment, tinnitus, or temporary hearing loss after leaving the working environment, even if the measured noise exposure is below a TWA of 85 dB(A). For purposes of protecting the rights of the employer and the rights and hearing health of the employee, OSHA requires employers to obtain a baseline measurement of hearing (reference audiogram) within 6 months of an employee's first exposure to noise levels of at least 85 dB(A) for 8 hours a day [7]. A HCP should, therefore, include a pre-placement hearing test and periodic repeat tests (air conduction thresholds at 500, 1,000, 2,000,

3,000, 4,000, and 6,000 Hz in each ear via binaural earphones). Periodic monitoring of hearing levels should also be carried out, preferably on Monday mornings or whenever the employee has had approximately 48 hours of limited noise exposure in order to recover.

The reference audiogram (1) detects the presence of existing hearing loss; (2) determines if cochlear injury due to noise exposure has occurred, by comparison to future tests; and (3) documents properly any claims that noise exposure was the main cause of an individual's hearing loss. If a significant change in hearing level is observed ($\geq$ 10 dB) at any frequency in either ear, workplace managers, in order to prevent further hearing loss, should consider: (1) providing and encouraging the use of ear protection devices; (2) reducing the noise level at the source(s); and (3) limiting the employee's exposure time or re-

Time of test		Date	Time and date of last exposure	Type of noise
Hour of day	Day of week			
9:00	Monday	4/27/1987	5:00—4/24/1987	Continuous TWA of 95 dB

Audiometer	Calibration	Date last calibrated		
MAICO MA-12	ANSI—1969	1/20/1987		

HEARING THRESHOLD LEVEL

Right ear						Left ear					
500	1,000	2,000	3,000	4,000	6,000	500	1,000	2,000	3,000	4,000	6,000
15	20	30	45	55	40	10	25	35	50	65	45

EAR PROTECTION

Type plugs	Type muffs	Protection	
Neoprene inserts	None	3	1. Satisfactory 2. Unsatisfactory 3. Questionable

COMMENTS: Hearing levels have become progressively poorer from 500 to 4,000 Hz with some recovery at 6,000 Hz in each ear. These levels are approximately 10 dB poorer than those obtained one year ago at frequencies of 3,000 to 6,000 Hz in each ear. Recommend complete audiologic evaluation to determine nature of hearing loss and a reappraisal of adequacy of hearing protection currently used.

Fig. 17-7. Typical audiometric sheet used in hearing conservation programs.

moving the employee from the noise environment. A complete audiologic and otologic evaluation should also be made to specify the nature of the hearing loss and the primary cause of its progression. Managers should be responsible for monitoring hearing levels by providing a retest 3 months after the reference audiogram or earlier if the employee reports a change in hearing or tinnitus. If no significant change is seen at this later time, then periodic retests may be performed on an annual basis, or sooner if these symptoms occur.

Hearing tests conducted for industrial workers are usually performed by an audiologist, nurse, or audiometric technician using a calibrated pure-tone audiometer. The test environment and audiometer must meet the criteria proposed by the American National Standards Institute [8]. Also, OSHA regulations specify that "audiometric tests shall be performed by a licensed or certified audiologist, otolaryngologist, or other physician, or

by a technician who is certified by the Council of Accreditation in Occupational Hearing Conservation or by other technicians" [7]. Audiometric technicians are trained to perform only air-conduction pure-tone tests. An example of the kind of information that might be required on an individual is shown in Figure 17-7.

Medical management of a HCP is also highly desirable since diagnosis, prevention, and treatment of hearing loss are medical responsibilities. A physician, occupational health nurse, or audiologist should be responsible for (1) organizing and administering the hearing test program, (2) evaluating and validating hearing test records for compensation claims, (3) reporting inadequacies of noise control methods, and (4) providing ear protectors to employees and promoting attitudes that will benefit the program.

The success of a HCP depends on the cooperation of managers, workers, and others concerned with the health and safety of workers.

NOISE STANDARDS

Much noise research has as its final objective the creation of a damage risk criterion (DRC) for human exposure to noise. As in all public health criteria, there are not only scientific questions that must be answered, but numerous social, economic, and legal considerations. In the scientific realm, we must first answer the question, "What do we want to protect?" Hearing is a multi-dimensional ability. "Do we protect hearing thresholds? Discrimination ability? The ability to understand speech? In quiet? In noise? Do we protect all aspects or only some? Which aspects and how much?" There is, as yet, no uniform agreement on such issues. Even the issue of how a hearing handicap is to be defined is unresolved. The most common, although debatable, approach is to protect against permanent threshold shifts and to accept some hearing loss as an inevitable compromise if that hearing loss is less than that considered to represent the beginning of a hearing handicap.

Currently, an average hearing level of 26 dB at 500, 1,000, and 2,000 Hz is taken as the onset of handicap, although this approach is not uniformly agreed on. At this point, social and legal issues begin to arise. A shift in the 26 dB fence upward represents a tremendous economic advantage to institutions that must compensate for handicap, but it may also represent a significant decrease in the quality of life for affected individuals. If the 26 dB fence is lowered 5 dB or if other frequencies are taken into consideration, the advantage goes to the affected individuals. Note that the higher frequencies are omitted from the above definition of handicap. Frequencies such as 4,000 Hz are usually the first and most affected frequencies in the audiogram of an individual exposed to noise (the classic 4,000 Hz dip or notch) and thus incorporating 4,000 Hz into the handicap definition would make it not only a more sensitive index (or liberal definition) but also a more expensive one for employers. The most common rationale for incorporating only 500, 1,000, and 2,000 Hz in the definition is that these frequencies contribute most toward understanding speech (in the quiet). Since

handicap is equated with losses in ability to communicate, this group of frequencies has gained acceptance, although agreement is not unanimous.

Over the past 30 years, considerable efforts have been made by a number of government regulatory agencies to establish the permissible levels of noise that an individual may be exposed to during a working lifetime without developing NIHL. For a long time, the central argument focused around the efficacy of an 85 dB(A) versus a 90 dB(A) upper limit criterion for an 8-hour workday. OSHA, for example, proposed keeping the allowable level of 90 dB(A), as recommended in the Walsh-Healey amendments, while the Environmental Protection Agency (EPA) suggested a reduction to 85 dB(A). The EPA criterion was established with the health and welfare effects of noise on humans in mind, with relatively less concern for the economic concerns of industry. OSHA, reluctant to comply with the EPA criterion, argued that only two percent of the population is at risk for NIHL under a 90 dB(A) standard, citing the American Academy of Ophthalmology and Otolaryngology-American Medical Association (AAOO-AMA) [9] low fence of a 26 dB average for frequencies 500, 1,000, and 2,000 Hz as the beginning of impairment. At present, the final OSHA rule, which became effective in 1983, maintains that a hearing conservation program must be introduced if a noise exposure equals or exceeds a time-weighted average (TWA) of 85 dB(A) over an 8-hour period. In addition, employers must provide hearing protection devices to (1) workers exposed to an 8-hour TWA of 90 dB(A), and (2) those who have experienced a threshold shift of 10 dB or more from a baseline audiogram at the frequencies 2,000, 3,000, and 4,000 Hz—if exposed to an 8-hour TWA of 85 dB(A).

The determination of the acceptable noise exposure limits for less than an 8-hour exposure was also adapted from the Walsh-Healey Act. The "5 dB rule" was accepted; that is, 90 dB(A) of continuous noise exposure is equivalent to 4 hours of 95 dB(A) or 2 hours of 100 dB(A) exposure in an 8-hour day, with a maximum upper limit of 115 dB(A) for one-fourth of an hour or less. If the daily exposure is a mixture of different intensities, then a fractional method is specified for determining if the exposure exceeds the allowable limit. Impact noises are not to exceed 140 dB peak SPL, with no further specification of the parameters of the exposure, such as number of impulses or presentation rate.

REFERENCES

1. Hamernik RP, Henderson D, Salvi R, eds. New perspectives on noise-induced hearing loss. New York: Raven, 1982.
2. Lipscomb DM, ed. Noise and audiology. Baltimore: University Park, 1978.
3. Pickles JO. An introduction to the physiology of hearing. New York: Academic, 1982.
4. Hudspeth AJ. The cellular basis of hearing: the biophysics of hair cells. Science 1985; 230:745–52.
5. Zwislocki JJ. Sound analysis in the ear: a history of discoveries. Am Scientist 1981; 69:184–92.
6. Katz J. Handbook of clinical audiology. Baltimore: Williams and Wilkins, 1985.
7. Federal Register 48, March 8, 1983. (no. 46: 9738–85).
8. American National Standards Institute. American National Standards Institute criteria for permissible ambient noise during audiometric testing. New York: Acoustical Society of America, 1977. (ANSI 53.1).
9. AAOO guide for the evaluation of hearing impairment. Trans Am Acad Opth and Otol 1959; 235–8. Recommended, but not generally accepted alternative: Guide for the evaluation of hearing handicap. American Council of Otolaryngology. JAMA 1979; 241:2055–9.

BIBLIOGRAPHY
Davis H, Silverman SR, eds. Hearing and deafness. New York: Holt, Rhinehart and Winston, 1970.
An extensive review of hearing and hearing conservation, auditory disorders, diagnosis, and rehabilitation.
Kryter KD. The effects of noise on man. New York: Academic, 1970.
A comprehensive reference volume on virtually all aspects of the human psychophysical response to noise.
Martin FN, ed. Medical audiology. New Jersey: Prentice Hall, 1981.
Presents state-of-the-art information on the basic elements requisite to understanding medical conditions of the ear.
Newby HA, Popelka GR. Audiology. New Jersey: Prentice Hall, 1985.
Current treatment of basic and advanced hearing test procedures and hearing conservation.
Northern JL, ed. Hearing disorders. Boston: Little, Brown, 1984.
An orientation to the evaluation, manifestations, diagnosis, treatment, and management of hearing disorders.
Salvi RJ, Henderson D, Hamernik RP, Colletti V, eds. Basic and applied aspects of noise-induced hearing loss. New York: Plenum, 1986.
An up-to-date reference manual that emphasizes the physiologic and anatomic aspects of noise-induced hearing loss.

18
Other Physical Hazards and Their Effects

Howard Hu

In this chapter, several types of physical exposures and environments are discussed that may be hazardous to workers. These include *nonionizing radiation* (ultraviolet, visible light, infrared, microwave/radiofrequency, and laser radiation); *vibration; atmospheric variations* (hot and cold environments and hyperbaric [compression/undersea] and hypobaric [high altitude] environments); *electric and magnetic fields;* and *ultrasound.* Some of these have well-recognized health effects, but others are controversial and are still being studied.

NONIONIZING RADIATION

Nonionizing radiation (see Chap. 16 on ionizing radiation) refers to emissions from those parts of the electromagnetic spectrum where emitted photons generally have insufficient energy to produce ionization of atoms. These forms of radiation include microwaves, television and radio waves, visible light, and infrared and ultraviolet (UV) radiation, among others (Fig. 18-1). Laser radiation is an amplified form of nonionizing radiation.

All types of nonionizing radiation obey certain general laws of electromagnetic radiation. The equation that fundamentally characterizes electromagnetic radiation is

$$\lambda = c/f$$

where λ = wavelength in meters, c = velocity (usually the velocity of light, 3×10^8 meters per second), and f = frequency in cycles per second.

Nonionizing radiation has other important characteristics shared by all forms of electromagnetic radiation: (1) it travels in straight lines and can be bent or focused: (2) the energy delivered is directly proportional to the frequency (and therefore inversely proportional to the wavelength); and (3) this energy occurs in small units, or quanta, that can be measured in electron volts.

When nonionizing radiation strikes matter, energy is absorbed. Nonionizing radiation is of lower frequency than ionizing radiation and therefore contains less energy. Instead of causing ionizations, this energy is usually transformed into heat, which accounts for many of its important physiologic effects. Absorption in the UV and visible portions of the spectrum can also produce photochemical reactions or fluorescence; this occurrence depends on the absorption spectrum of the molecule that has been struck and the efficiency of the specific radiation wavelength in producing this effect.

Ultraviolet Radiation

Ultraviolet radiation (UVR) is an invisible form of radiant energy produced naturally by the sun in a *low-intensity* form and artificially by incandescent, fluorescent, and discharge types of light sources.* In industrial work settings, *high-intensity* UVR exposure occurs primarily from expo-

---

*The UV radiation spectrum can be further subdivided, based on wavelength, into UV-A ($4.0–3.2 \times 10^{-7}$m, black light) and UV-B ($3.2–2.8 \times 10^{-7}$m) radiation, which are the two principal radiations of sunlight; and UV-C ($2.8–2.0 \times 10^{-7}$m) radiation, which is germicidal.

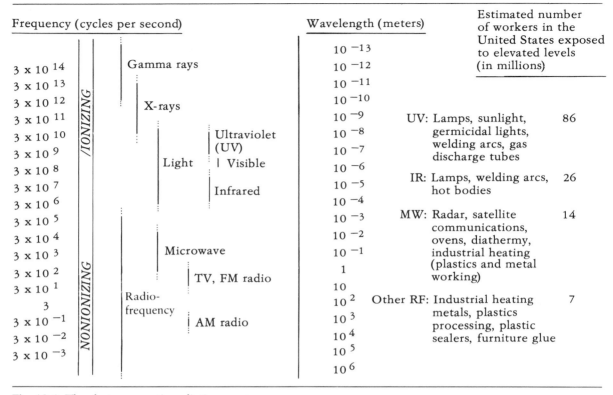

Fig. 18-1. The electromagnetic radiation spectrum.
(From M. M. Key, et al. *Occupational Diseases—A Guide to Their Recognition.* Cincinnati: NIOSH, 1977.)

sure to arc welding* (see Fig. 24-6). Other industrial sources include plasma torches, which are used in heavy industrial cutting processes, electric arc furnances, germicidal and black-light lamps, and certain types of lasers. UV light is also being used by some coal processing and refining companies to detect coal tar residues on the skin of workers and equipment (due to coal tar's fluorescence under UV).

The skin and the eyes absorb UVR and are particularly vulnerable to injury (primarily due to UV-B radiation). The common sunburn is a well-known result of acute over exposure to solar UVR. Long-term, low-intensity UVR exposure from the sun is also responsible for a number of other skin conditions, including solar elastosis, solar keratosis, and skin cancer (see Chap. 23). These effects are intensified in areas with greater solar UV exposure (few clouds, equatorial location, or high altitude).

Recent epidemiology studies have also called into question whether long-term exposure to nonsolar UVR in the form of fluorescent lighting can pose a slightly elevated risk for the development of melanoma [1]. The data are equivocal, and additional investigation is needed [2].

UVR health effects can be potentiated by several *photosensitizing agents.* When ingested, certain

*Arcs are high-temperature sources generated between electrodes; during the welding process, they appear as blinding flashes of light and emit UV radiation.

drugs (such as chlorpromazaine, tolbutamide, and chlorpropamide) as well as many plants containing furocoumarins and psoralens (such as figs, lemon and lime rinds, celery, and parsnips) can increase susceptibility to UVR [3]. Locally applied coal tar is also a photosensitizer. Photosensitization can lead to an immediate sunburn-type effect on exposure to a small dose of radiant energy. Individuals vary in their susceptibility to this reaction, depending on their tendency to concentrate sufficient quantities of the photosensitizing agent in the skin.

Protection from the effects of low-intensity UV radiation simply entails covering the skin and avoiding prolonged exposures. Benzophenone and anthranilate sunscreens absorb UVR and offer some protection to bare skin. Opaque sunscreens, such as titanium dioxide, offer the best protection and may be essential if there is photosensitization.

Ultraviolet radiation from arc-welding operations has not been associated with skin cancer, probably because these high-intensity exposures are of an acute, short-term nature, and operators usually wear protective clothing. High-intensity acute exposures, however, can result in eye damage. Eye damage most commonly occurs with exposure to arc-welding, but it can also occur through exposure to direct or reflected radiation from UV lamps, such as those used in laboratories as bacteriocidal agents. The end result is conjunctivitis or keratitis (inflammation of the cornea), a work-related condition commonly referred to as "ground-glass eyeball," "welder's flash," or "flashburn" (see Chap. 24). The welder or bystanders can be affected by just a brief moment of exposure to unprotected or underprotected eyes. Prevention requires the isolation of high-intensity UV sources and the use of goggles and other shields with proper filters.

Ultraviolet radiation also has an indirect impact on health through its ability to cause photochemical reactions. UVR, as encountered in welding operations, converts small amounts of oxygen and nitrogen into ozone and nitrogen oxides, which are respiratory irritants. At certain wavelengths, UVR can also decompose solvent vapors into toxic gases (for example, perchloroethylene and trichloroethylene into hydrogen chloride and phosgene, respectively). Control of these hazards requires proper local exhaust ventilation and isolation of high-intensity UV sources from solvent processes.

Visible Radiation

Visible light plays an important role in determining working conditions. A considerable amount of literature in the field of ergonomics deals with the proper use of different lighting systems for different tasks. Types of illumination may also play a role in ocular health (see Chap. 24).

Infrared Radiation

An epidemiologic investigation on the prevalence of cataracts in glass workers was performed. The study included 209 workers over 50 years of age exposed to infrared radiation (IR) in the Swedish manual glass industry for 20 years or more and 298 non-IR-exposed controls. . . . In the same age group the risk for an IR-exposed worker to have his vision reduced by cataracts to 0.7 or less was 2.5 times as high as for nonexposed controls (95% confidence interval 1.4–4.4). The risk that he would have to be operated for cataracts was 12 times as high (95% confidence interval 2.6–53) [4].

In industry, significant levels of IR are produced directly by lamp sources and indirectly by sources of heat. The primary effect of IR on biologic tissue is thermal; it can cause skin burns, although one is generally warned of IR exposure by the sensation of heat before skin burns can occur. The lens of the eye, however, is particularly vulnerable to damage because the lens has no heat sensors and a poor heat-dissipating mechanism. Cataracts may be produced by chronic IR exposure at levels far below those that cause skin burns (see Chap. 24). Glass blowers as well as furnace workers have an increased incidence of all types of cataracts (particularly posterior cataracts) after chronic IR exposure for over 10 years. Other workers potentially at risk of harmful IR exposure include those involved in handling molten metal (such as foundry workers, blacksmiths, and solderers), oven operators, workers in the vicinity of baking and drying heat lamps, and movie projectionists. Control of IR hazards requires the use of shielding of the IR source, eye protection with IR filters, and reliance on distance to reduce the intensity of the IR source.

Microwave/Radiofrequency Radiation

Microwave/radiofrequency radiation (MW/RFR) encompasses a wide range of wavelengths used in radar, television, radio, and other telecommunications systems (see Fig. 18-1). It is also used in a variety of industrial operations including the heating, welding, and melting of metals, the processing of wood and plastic (radiofrequency sealers), and the creation of high-temperature plasma. There may be as many as 21 million workers in the United States exposed to MW/RFR, and the commercial use of MW/RFR is expected to increase; thus, any health effect could have a very significant public health impact.

The heating effect of MW/RFR depends on the amount of energy absorbed from MW/RFR, which, in turn, depends on the frequency of the radiation and the position, shape, and other properties of the exposed object. In general, detectable tissue heating requires relatively high power MW/RFR at power densities above 100 watts per square meter. This mechanism is responsible for some of the better-known adverse health effects of MW/RFR, some of which have been reported in humans, such as cataract formation, testicular degeneration, and at extremely high intensities, death from hyperthermia [5, 6, 7].

Recognition of this phenomenon prompted the institution of federal exposure guidelines, which currently limit MW/RFR power to 100 watts per square meter ($10 \, \text{mW/cm}^2$), as averaged over any 6-minute period.

However, controversy exists as to whether adverse health effects can be caused by chronic exposure to MW/RFR at power densities *below* this standard. Laboratory studies of animals have demonstrated that MW/RFR, at intensities that are too low to cause thermal effects, can result in other significant biologic effects that are primarily of a neurologic and immunologic nature, such as alterations in electroencephalograms (EEGs) and behavior, and impairment of immune cell function [8]. Some published reports suggest a link between low-level MW/RFR and neurobehavioral effects in humans, such as headaches, depression, cataracts [9], and cancer [10]. Establishing the validity of these associations currently awaits well-designed epidemiologic and experimental studies.

Importantly, many workers may be exposed to MW/RFR at levels above the federal standard [11, 12]. Thus, a high priority must be given to establishing work guidelines, especially shielding and engineering controls, which will bring compliance to the existing standard, in addition to doing research on low levels of exposure.

Finally, microwaves and high-power radio waves can interfere with medical electronic devices, especially cardiac pacemakers of the ventricular-synchronous type. Implanted pacemaker dysfunction has been observed near electrocautery and diathermy machines, radar and communications systems, electric shavers, spark coils, gasoline ignition systems, and microwave ovens. These devices can generally be protected from microwave interference by thorough shielding of the microwave source. Such precautions must be taken wherever workers are exposed to microwaves.

Laser Radiation

Laser is an acronym for Light Amplification by the Stimulated Emission of Radiation, a special category of manufactured nonionizing radiation. Laser radiation is produced by forcing atoms of a particular gas media to emit a stream of photons that are monochromatic and in phase with each other. These photons are emitted at specific wavelengths that depend on the source medium. The many and increasing applications of laser radiation derive from its ability to concentrate a large amount of energy in a small cross-sectional area in a highly coherent and minimally divergent manner. Lasers of various types are widely used as reference lines in surveying, instrumentation, and alignments; as a heating agent in welding; as a cutting instrument in microelectronics and microsurgery; and for a variety of functions in communications; and in the military, where their application is expected to increase dramatically.

The eye, including the retina, lens, iris, and cornea, is extremely vulnerable to injury from laser radation in the near-UV, near-infrared, infrared, and visible frequency ranges (see Chap. 24). Ocular damage can occur not only directly from intrabeam viewing, but also indirectly by exposure to diffuse reflections from a high-power laser. Lasers of wavelengths that fall outside the visible portion of the electromagnetic spectrum can be particularly hazardous, since exposure to the beam may not be readily apparent. Skin burns are caused by direct exposure to high-energy lasers.

Laser installations should be isolated wherever possible, and the laser beam should be terminated by a material that is nonreflective and fireproof. Special goggles can be helpful but must afford specific protection to the wavelength of laser being used. Care must be paid to minimizing diffuse reflected radiation that may not be visually detectable. Finally, proper worker education and a baseline eye exam must be included in the preventive program.

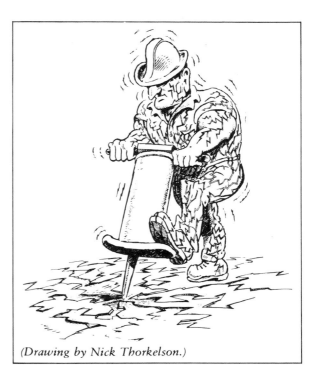

(Drawing by Nick Thorkelson.)

VIBRATION

A 40-year-old man, 12 years before examination, started work as a copper stayer using a hammer weighing 12 lb with a frequency of 2,300 vibrations a minute (38 Hz*). He also wore a glove on the left hand. After he had been working for 2 years he noticed his finger would go white; the first one involved was the index finger on the left hand. The whiteness was associated with paresthesias. Gradually the right hand became involved and soon all the fingers on both hands would go white. He found the hands very awkward to use and had difficulty with buttons. It often took 2 hours for the sensation to return. At the start the syndrome occurred only in winter, but after 4 years it occurred in summer as well. After 6 years' work with the hammer he had to

*1 Hz = 1 hertz = 1 cycle per second; 1 KHz = 1,000 Hz

change jobs because of the symptoms and is now working as a laborer in the boiler shop [13].

Vibration refers to the mechanical oscillation of a surface around its reference point. Health hazards of interest generally stem from vibration at frequencies of 2 to 1,000 Hz. Occupational health effects of vibration stem from prolonged periods of contact between a worker and the vibrating surface. It has been estimated that 8 million workers in the United States are exposed to occupational vibration—either whole-body vibration or segmental vibration to a specific body part. Truck, tractor, bus, and other vehicle drivers and certain heavy-equipment operators are subject to chronic whole body vibration transmitted through the seat or floor of their workposts that is generally of lower frequency (2–100 Hz). Chain-saw, chipping hammer and other pneumatic-tool operators, and grinders are exposed to segmental vibration, usually through the hands, that is of higher frequency (20–1,000 Hz).

Whole-Body Vibration

Little is known about the chronic effects of low-frequency whole-body vibration. Several epidemiologic studies, including ones conducted by NIOSH, have suggested an association with changes in bone structure, gastrointestinal disturbances involving secretion and motility, prostatitis, and changes in nerve conduction velocity [14]. Vibration at the resonating frequency of the eyeballs (60–90 Hz) has been associated with disorders of vision.

Although adequate proof of causality in the form of epidemiologic and experimental evidence has been lacking, it would seem wise to limit exposure to whole-body vibration as much as possible.

Segmental Vibration

Chronic exposure to segmental vibration at low frequencies of 20 to 40 Hz, such as encountered with the operation of heavy pneumatic drills, has been associated with degenerative osteoarticular lesions in the elbows and shoulders. These lesions are thought to represent a "wear and tear" process from repetitive impulse loading; however, epidemiologic proof of causality has so far been lacking.

At frequencies between 40 and 300 Hz, the use of vibratory hand tools (such as chain saws, grinders, and pneumatic hammers and drills) has been well known to elicit Raynaud's phenomenon, also known as "vibration syndrome," "dead hand," "vibration white fingers" (VWF), or "traumatic vasospastic disease." Raynaud's phenomenon* consists of blanching and numbness of the fingers and is often accompanied by loss of muscular control, reduction of sensitivity to temperature and pain, and in severe cases, ulcerations of the finger-

*Raynaud's phenomenon, also known as Raynaud's syndrome, can also occur with other diseases or conditions. When it occurs for unknown reasons, it is called Raynaud's disease.

tips. Work under cold conditions, as commonly experienced by loggers working with chain saws, can increase the predisposition to this condition. A serious case of Raynaud's phenomenon with frequent episodes can greatly interfere with a worker's performance and other activities. Moreover, many cases can progress to a chronic condition, with permanent disability. Other possible effects of vibration in this range include a long-term diminution in grip strength, tenosynovitis (such as carpal tunnel syndrome), Dupuytren's contractures (flexion contractures of the fingers), bone cysts, and hearing loss [15].

Little is known about the physiologic basis for Raynaud's phenomenon. While it is commonly agreed that arterial vasospasm is the cause of blanching, the mechanism relating the roles of the neurologic, vascular, and vasomotor systems is unclear. Early diagnosis must rely on a history of typical symptoms, such as numbness or tingling of the fingers, which is precipitated by exposure to vibration and persists for progressively longer periods of time. Finger blanching is often the next symptom to occur with continued chronic exposure.

It is difficult to confirm a diagnosis objectively unless an attack is occurring. Physiologic tests, such as ice water provocation, plethysmography (a measurement of circulation as reflected by changes in volume), and others are still being investigated but appear to have limited sensitivity and specificity. Clinicians may follow a set of criteria recently developed to grade the progressive stages of vibration syndrome [16].

Preventing these health effects requires minimizing exposure to segmental vibration and surveillance for early health effects. NIOSH has published a set of recommendations that include engineering controls, medical surveillance and worker education, work practices, and personal protective equipment [17]. Among these are recommendations to (1) alter production methods to minimize the need for vibratory hand tools; (2) redesign tools to reduce hand-arm vibration; (3) give adequate maintenance to vibratory hand tools, since those that do not receive it show higher vibration levels; (4) provide preplacement medical exams and physician evaluations if workers experience tingling, numbness, or blanching; and (5) keep hands warm with gloves (claims concerning the anti-vibration properties of some gloves are unproven).

Once vibration-associated health problems begin to arise, exposure must be terminated. Most associated symptoms disappear with early removal from exposure.

No federal standard currently exists that limits exposure to vibration or the use of vibrating tools. Thus, workers, managers, and clinicians have crucial roles in the early recognition of segmental vibration-induced problems and the prevention of their progression.

ATMOSPHERIC VARIATIONS

Heat

A 24-year-old laborer was brought to the emergency room after collapsing during work. Several hours before, he became extremely irritable and, for no apparent reason, provoked arguments with several of his coworkers. He had been working on an incentive basis next to a blast furnace in a metals factory on a day when the temperature had not been more than 90°F, but the humidity exceeded 60 percent. Physical examination showed a stocky man who was totally unresponsive with hot, flushed, moist skin. He had dilated, equally sized pupils that were unresponsive to light. Fundi were normal. Rectal temperature was greater than 41°C (105.8°F), pulse rate was 160, blood pressure was 80/0 mm Hg, and respirations were deep at a rate of 30 per minute. Despite rapid cooling in an ice bath with decrease in core temperature and aggressive care in the intensive care unit, the patient suffered a series of grand mal seizures followed by marked metabolic acidosis, rhabdomyolysis, acute respiratory distress syndrome, and acute renal failure. Following emergency hemodialysis, the patient had another grand mal seizure followed by cardiac arrest that was refractory to all therapy.

Heat is a potential physical hazard that can exist in almost any workplace, especially during summer. Hot industrial jobs requiring heavy work afford the greatest potential for problems because they add to the worker's heat load by generating more metabolic heat (Fig. 18-2). When a worker's physiologic capacity to compensate for thermal stress is exceeded, heat can lead to impaired performance, an increased risk of accidents, and clinical signs of heat illness.

Internal temperature is regulated within narrow limits, predominantly by sweat production and evaporation. To a lesser extent, temperature regulation is accomplished by (1) physiologic control of blood flow from muscles and other deep sites of heat production to the cooler surfaces of the body where heat is dissipated by convective exchange with air; and (2) evaporative cooling from the lungs.

The relationship between heat loss/gain variables and internal heat production is described by a simple heat balance equation:

$$S = (M - W) \pm C \pm R - E$$

in which S = net amount of heat gained or lost by the body; M = heat produced by metabolism; W = external work performed; C = heat transfer by convection; R = heat transfer by radiation; and E = body heat loss by evaporation (in kcal/hour). Should S be greater than zero, heat imbalance occurs, leading to manifestations of heat stress. Convection refers to heat transfer between skin and the immediately surrounding air, assuming that air is being circulated. Its value is a function of the difference in temperature between skin and air and the rate of air movement over the skin. Radiation in this context refers to the direct transfer of heat between surfaces of differing temperature—that is, the skin surface and immediate solid surroundings, such as an oven furnace or a cold floor.

The quantity (M − W) describes the total amount of body heat produced. The C and R variables can be positive or negative because convection and radiation may work in both directions. Ordinarily, with ambient temperature lower than surface body temperature (< 95°F, 35°C), convec-

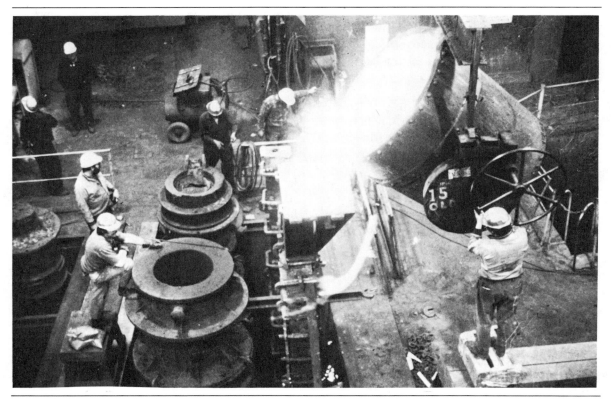

Fig. 18-2. Foundry workers with exposure to excessive heat at work.
(Photograph by Earl Dotter.)

tion and radiation promote transfer of body heat to the environment; however, if the environment is hotter than surface body temperature, radiation and convection can increase the body's heat load.

The heat loss/gain variables (C, R, and E) are influenced by environmental factors encountered in the workplace. In general, industrial heat exposures may be classified as either hot-dry or warm-moist. Hot-dry situations may prevail in a hot desert climate or near any furnace operation (for example, in metallurgical, glass, or ceramic industries) radiating high levels of heat. Heat absorption in these circumstances may overwhelm the cooling effect of sweat evaporation, leading to heat imbalance.

The most troublesome situation usually arises in warm-moist environments, as found in tropical climates, and in such industries as canning, textiles, laundering, and deep metal mining. High humidity and still air impede evaporative and convective cooling. Heat imbalance may occur despite an only moderate increase in ambient temperature; when this happens, thermal stress begins and can result in a variety of illnesses.

The mildest form of heat stress is discomfort. Prolonged exposure to a moderately hot climate may also cause irritability, lassitude, decrease in morale, increased anxiety, and inability to concentrate.

Heat rash (prickly heat) is common in warm-moist conditions due to inflammation in sweat glands plugged by skin swelling. Affected skin bears tiny red vesicles and, if sensitive, can actually impair sweating and greatly diminish the worker's ability to tolerate heat.

Prolonged exposure to heat may result in *heat cramps,* especially when there is profuse sweating and inadequate replacement of fluids and electrolytes. As net-retained body heat increases, *heat exhaustion* may occur, evidenced by pallor, lassitude, dizziness, syncope, profuse sweating, and clammy, moist skin. An oral temperature reading may or may not reveal mild hyperthermia, whereas a rectal temperature is usually elevated (37.5–38.5°C, 99.5–101.3°F). Heat exhaustion usually occurs in the setting of sustained exertion in hot conditions with dehydration from deficient water intake.

Finally, there is *heat stroke,* a medical emergency that often occurs in a setting of excessive physical exertion. The underlying physiologic disturbance is failure of the central nervous system sweat control, thus leading to loss of evaporative cooling. The uncontrolled accelerating rise in core temperature that follows is manifested by signs and symptoms including dizziness, nausea, irritability, severe headache, hot, dry skin, and a rectal temperature of 40.5°C (104.9°F) or higher. This process quickly leads to confusion, collapse, delirium, and coma. Cooling of the body must be started immediately if vital organ damage and death are to be averted. Workers who are not acclimatized (see below) are especially prone to heat stroke; other predisposing factors include obesity, recent alcohol intake, and chronic cardiovascular disease.

Heat rash can be treated with mild drying lotions, but it generally can be prevented by allowing the skin to dry in a cooler environment between heat exposures. Heat cramps are alleviated by drinking electrolyte-containing liquids (such as juices) or intravenous fluid administration of such liquids, if necessary. Workers with heat exhaustion or heat stroke must be removed to a cooler environment immediately. Heat exhaustion can be treated with rapidly administered saline fluids and

observation, whereas heat stroke must be treated with immediate supercooling by immersion in ice water with massage, or, if ice water is not readily available, by wrapping the person in a wet sheet with vigorous fanning with cool, dry air. Meanwhile, the victim of heat stroke must be closely monitored for signs of shock or overcooling.

Monitoring a workplace environment for heat exposure is a task that involves measuring heat-modifying factors and assessing work loads. Industrial hygienists commonly employ a measurement called the Wet Bulb Globe Temperature (WBGT) index, which takes into account convective and radiant heat transfer, humidity, and wind velocity. It is calculated by integrating the readings of three separate instruments that indicate the "dry" bulb temperature, the natural "wet" bulb temperature (which takes into account convective and evaporative cooling), and the "globe" temperature (which, through the use of a black copper sphere, registers heat transfer by radiation). The WBGT index has been used by NIOSH and the American Conference of Governmental Industrial Hygienists as an indicator of heat stress in a recommended set of guidelines that suggest maximum permissible standards of heat exposure, depending on the level of work performed in the hot environment [18, 19] (Table 18-1).

Ideally, prevention of heat stress should be accomplished by isolating workers from hot environments through engineering design. However, as this is often not possible, heat stress is usually averted by a combination of engineering controls, work practice changes, personal protective clothing, and the education of those who work under conditions of excessive heat.

In addition to guidelines regarding heat exposure, NIOSH has made other recommendations regarding heat exposure, including: (1) *medical surveillance* supervised by a physician and paid by the employer for all workers if exposed to heat stress above the "action" level, to include comprehensive history-taking, physical exams, and overall assessment of a worker's ability to tolerate heat; (2) *posting of warning signs in hazardous areas;* (3)

Table 18-1. Permissible heat exposure threshold limit values (values are given in °C wet bulb globe temperature)

Work-rest regimen	Work load		
	Light	Moderate	Heavy
Continuous work	30.0	26.7	25.0
75% Work			
25% Rest, each hour	30.6	28.0	25.9
50% Work			
50% Rest, each hour	31.4	29.4	27.9
25% Work			
75% Rest, each hour	32.2	31.1	30.0

Source: American Conference of Governmental Industrial Hygienists. Threshold limit values and biological exposure indices for 1985–86. Cincinnati: ACGIH, 1985: 69.

protective clothing and equipment; (4) *worker information and training;* (5) *control of heat stress* with engineering controls, work and hygienic practices that specify time limits for working in hot environments, the use of a buddy system, and provision of water; and (5) *recordkeeping* of environmental and medical surveillance data [18].

One of the recommended work practices is an acclimatization program for new workers and for workers who have been absent from the job for longer than 9 days. *Acclimatization* is a process of adaptation that involves a step-wise adjustment to heat; it usually requires 1 week or more of progressively longer periods of exposure to the hot environment while working. Some workers may fail to acclimatize and consequently cannot work in such environments. Unfortunately, the heat-intolerant worker cannot be easily distinguished from the heat-tolerant worker, except by a trial of exposure to high-heat load. A baseline VO_2-max less than 2.5 liters/minute provides suggestive evidence for heat-intolerance. Finding a short and easily administered screening test that can reliably predict heat intolerance has been listed as an important research need [18].

NIOSH also recommends (1) the reduction of peaks of physiologic strain during work; (2) the establishment of frequent, regular, short breaks for replacing water and electrolyte losses; and (3) preplacement and periodic medical examinations.

Workers must be trained to replace fluid losses systematically. During the course of a day's work in a hot environment, a worker may lose up to 1 liter per hour of fluid and electrolytes in sweat. This loss should be replaced by drinking fluids every 15 to 20 minutes in greater amounts than are necessary to satisfy thirst. (Thirst is an inadequate stimulus for fluid replacement in stressful heat conditions.)

The recent findings that heat-acclimatized workers lose less salt in sweat than previously thought, together with recognition of the high salt content in the average American diet and concern over exacerbating hypertension, has led experts to discourage the routine use of salt tablets to replace electrolyte losses [20]. If salt replacement is required in a nonemergent setting (such as strenuous work on a hot, dry day), adding extra salt to food is recommended. Workers on a low-sodium diet for cardiovascular or other reasons require close medical supervision if working in a hot environment.

Decreasing heat stress can involve engineering measures, such as devising heat shielding or insulating and ventilating with cool, dehumidified air. Workers should be provided with a cooled rest area close to the work station. Although clothing impedes the evaporation of sweat, it can reduce heat exposure in situations where the ambient air temperature is higher than the skin temperature and the air is relatively dry, or when a worker is near a strong heat-radiating source. Some types of industrial heat exposure require special protective equipment, such as gloves, aluminized reflective clothing, insulated and cooling jackets, and even self-contained air-conditioned suits.

Cold

Cold stress is an environmental hazard that confronts cold-room workers, dry-ice workers, liquefied-gas workers, divers, and outdoor workers during cold weather. The body maintains thermal homeostasis in a cold environment by decreasing skin heat loss through peripheral vasoconstriction and increasing metabolic heat production through shivering. Harmful effects of cold include frostbite, trench foot, and general hypothermia.

Frostbite is actual freezing of tissue due to exposure to extreme cold or contact with extremely cold objects. It ranges from erythema and slight pain to painless blistering, deep-seated ischemia, thrombosis, cyanosis, and gangrene. Windchill (loss of heat from exposure to wind) can play an important role in accelerating frostbite.

Trench foot (immersion foot) is a condition resulting from long, continuous exposure to damp and cold while remaining relatively immobile. It may involve not only the feet but the tip of the nose and ears as well; it typically occurs in a worker who has just experienced prolonged immersion in cold water or exposure to cold air. The clinical changes in affected tissue can progress from (1) an initial vasospastic, ischemic, hyperesthetic (oversensitive), pale phase to (2) a later stage equivalent to a burn with hyperemia, vasomotor paralysis, vesiculation, and edema; and finally to (3) gangrenous stage.

General hypothermia usually occurs in an individual subjected to prolonged cold exposure and physical exertion. When a person becomes wet, either from exposure or sweating, body heat is lost even faster. Most cases occur in air temperatures between minus 1°C (30°F) and plus 10°C (50°F); however, it can also occur in air temperatures as high as 18°C (65°F) or in water at 22°C (72°F), especially in the setting of fatigue. As exhaustion sets in, the vasoconstrictive protective mechanism becomes overwhelmed, resulting in sudden vasodilation and acute heat loss. Coma and death can ensue rapidly. The danger of hypothermia is increased by the consumption of sedatives and alcohol.

Finally, many workers handle cold metal objects that can cause local freezing and metal to skin adhesions. The use of silk gloves makes it possible both to handle cold metals (up to minus 40°C, which happens also to be minus 40°F) without freezing to them and to retain good manual dexterity.

In general, cold hazards are well recognized and preventable by the use of insulated clothing and protective barriers. However, one should note that at temperatures below 15°C (59°F), the hands and fingers become insensitive long before these described cold injuries take place, thereby decreasing manual dexterity and increasing the risk of accidents.

Hyperbaric Environments

In a handful of occupational environments, the ambient air pressure exceeds one atmosphere absolute (ATA), the atmospheric pressure found at sea level; these include certain caisson* operations, underwater tunneling†, and diving. Pressures encountered generally range from 2 to 5 ATA, although commercial divers often dive to depths greater than 100 meters at 11 ATA pressure (a 10-meter increase in depth below seawater adds 1 ATA pressure).

The most common health problems stemming from work in a hyperbaric environment are caused by unequal distribution of pressure in tissue air spaces, which are incurred during compression (descent) or decompression (ascent). For example, when the eustachian tube becomes blocked as a result of inflammation or failure of a diver to clear the ears, descent compression causes negative middle-ear pressure with inward deformation of the tympanic membrane and possible rupture. Sinus

---

*Caissons, tubular steel structures submerged in a river or sea bed or water-bearing ground, are used for construction or repair of bridges and piers and in excavation work. The pneumatic type of caisson has a closed top and is entered through an airlock; the bottom is open, allowing workers to excavate the ground, and water is excluded by the maintenance of a pressurized (hyperbaric) environment.

†In tunneling operations, compressed air is used to keep out water and to aid in supporting the structure.

cavities also experience pressure build-up. The lungs can become compressed in a breath-holding dive; conversely, if a diver with compressed air holds in breath during an ascent or during decompression in a chamber, the lungs can expand beyond their capacity, leading to rupture and pneumothorax, mediastinal emphysema, or even air embolism.

In addition to these mechanical hazards, workers in these environments encounter problems due to toxicity of the gas components of air at elevated partial pressures. At 4 ATA or greater, gaseous nitrogen induces a narcosis ("diver's high" or "rapture of the deep") marked by mood changes and euphoria. Oxygen inhalation at a high partial pressure can cause a toxic reaction with tingling, hallucination, confusion, nausea, vertigo, and sometimes seizures. These reactions can be avoided by limiting the depth of descent as well as the proportion of oxygen in a compressed air mixture.

Another common problem arises when ascending too rapidly from a medium depth. As nitrogen becomes less soluble, bubbles are formed in blood and other tissue that impair circulation and lead to a variety of effects commonly known as "the bends" or "decompression sickness." Symptoms include dull, throbbing joint pain and deep muscle or bone pain, usually occurring within 4 to 6 hours. Occasionally, bubbles forming in the spinal cord can lead to paralysis. Treatment of decompression illness requires immediate recompression followed by prolonged decompression, which is also the method of preventing the syndrome. A decompression rate of at least 20 minutes for each atmosphere (ATA) is recommended.

Most of these problems have been prevented through the use of decompression work practices. Well-standardized procedures for medical surveillance and emergencies involving divers and other workers in hyperbaric environments are available in the literature.

Probably the major hazard associated with compressed-air work that is still not completely addressed involves chronic exposure to hyperbaric environments with repeated decompression:

Workers so exposed have been found to have aseptic bone necrosis, mostly of the articular heads of long bones. The pathophysiology is believed to involve the occlusion of small arteries by nitrogen bubbles with platelet aggregation acting as microemboli during decompression. It is still uncertain whether this disease can be prevented by firm adherence to recommended decompression schedules. Meanwhile, compressed-air workers should undergo routine exams to try to identify early aseptic bone necrosis and to prevent its potentially crippling sequelae. Several experts recommend bone radiography, at a frequency of every 2 or 3 years, for workers performing normal diving or compressed-air work and annually for workers regularly exposed to conditions that may potentially provoke decompression sickness. Bone-scanning, though useful as a confirmatory diagnostic test, is not more sensitive as a screening tool than bone radiography.

Finally, it is important to recognize an indirect hazard associated with hyperbaric environments: the potential contamination of compressed-air sources. Carbon monoxide is probably the most common contaminant of compressed air, particularly if a compressor is powered by a gasoline engine; other potential contaminants include carbon dioxide, oil vapor, and particulates.

Hypobaric and Hypoxic (High Altitude) Environments

A 41-year-old man was dead on arrival at a hospital. He had flown from 1,500 to 2,750 meters, and during the next few days had climbed to 4,270 meters where he rapidly lost consciousness, dying 5 days after leaving 1,500 meters. Autopsy about 5 hours after death revealed severe cerebral edema, multiple petechial hemorrhages throughout the brain, bilateral pulmonary edema, bilateral bronchial pneumonia, dilatation and hypertrophy of the heart, and moderate arteriosclerosis of coronary arteries [21].

Workers in high altitude, mountainous regions and pilots in unpressurized cabins experience occupational exposure to hypobaric (low-pressure) and hypoxic environments. At high altitudes, decreased pressure reduces the gradient for oxygen absorption, leading to a fall in arterial pO_2, although the percentage of oxygen remains at 21 percent. At 5,500 meters (18,000 ft) the partial pressure of oxygen is half that at sea level. Illness associated with high altitude is rarely experienced below 2,000 meters; it becomes common, however, above 3,000 meters, especially in persons who venture to this altitude without taking time for acclimatization.

The most common health problem at high altitudes is *acute mountain sickness* (AMS), an illness characterized by headache, nausea, vomiting, depression, and loss of appetite. Almost all people undergoing an abrupt altitude changes by venturing into the mountains experience one of these symptoms to a degree within 24 hours; however, acclimatization usually occurs in a few days and symptoms disappear over 4 to 6 days of exposure. The pathophysiology has been suggested to involve the imbalance occurring between the cerebral vasodilatation from hypoxia and the cerebral vasoconstriction from hypocarbia. Acclimatization with few symptoms is best achieved by slow ascent (350 m or 1,000 ft/day) and gradually progressive activity for several days. Some climbers who are required to reduce acclimatization time have lessened AMS symptoms by using acetazolamide (Diamox), which results in a metabolic stimulus to increase the rate and depth of breathing.

More serious is *high-altitude pulmonary edema* (HAPE), which also strikes unacclimatized people, usually within 24 to 60 hours, especially if they engage in vigorous activity soon after arrival at high altitude. Onset is usually insidious. Symptoms include shortness of breath, cough, weakness, tachycardia, and headache. This condition characteristically progresses to cough productive of bloody sputum, low-grade fever, and evidence of increasing pulmonary congestion, with rales and cyanosis. If untreated, coma may ensue from hypoxia or cerebral edema (see below). The pathophysiology is unclear; clinical studies seem to suggest a process involving hypoxic vasoconstriction and pulmonary capillary leakage. It is treated ideally with descent to a lower altitude, rest, and administration of oxygen. Sometimes diuretics, positive pressure breathing, and aggressive pulmonary intervention are necessary. Lack of recognition of this syndrome is probably most responsible for serious morbidity and mortality.

Cerebral edema is a rare but often fatal consequence of high altitude. The presence of neurologic signs and symptoms of headache, confusion, ataxia, and hallucination in a person who has had an altitude change should make one consider this diagnosis. Treatment, as in HAPE, centers on rapid descent and oxygen administration. Scattered case reports have suggested a beneficial effect using dexamethasone in the same manner as for other forms of cerebral edema [22].

Most cases of altitude-related illnesses can be prevented by slow acclimatization. The physiologic mechanism of acclimatization involves an increase in red blood cell production and hematocrit, increases in intraerythrocytic 2,3-diphosphoglycerate (2,3-DPG, leading to a favorable shift in the oxyhemoglobin dissociation curve), and mild hyperventilation [23]. Exercise can be a part of this program, especially if heavy physical work is expected. The lack of a previous history of altitude-related illness while at high altitudes does not preclude the possibility of its occurrence.

Electric and Magnetic Fields

The ubiquitous use of electricity for a multitude of purposes has led to exposure of the general population and occupational groups to high-voltage electricity. While the hazards of electrocution and burns due to direct electrical exposure are well known, long-term effects, if any, due to exposure to electric and magnetic fields associated with the use and transmission of electricity have not been determined.

An *electric field* exists around an electric particle. If an electric particle moves, as in an electric current, these lines of electric force set up a *magnetic field,* whose lines of force are perpendicular

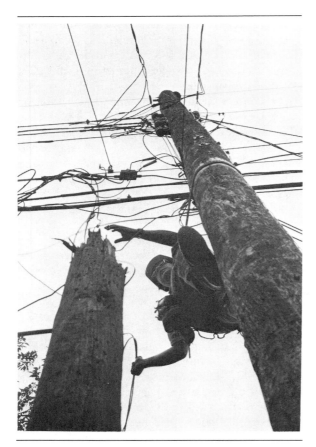

Fig. 18-3. Linemen working on high-voltage electric lines are being studied for disease potentially induced by electromagnetic fields.
(Photograph by Earl Dotter.)

to the particle's direction of movement. A variable electric field is always accompanied by a magnetic field; this interplay is often referred to as an *electromagnetic field* (E/MF).

In general, workers who potentially sustain exposure to high-intensity E/MFs include those working in proximity to high-voltage electrical lines (Fig. 18-3), such as streetcar and subway drivers, power station operators, power and telephone line workers, and electricians, movie projec-

tionists, welders, and other groups of technicians and electrical workers.

Concern has been raised by several recent epidemiology studies that have suggested a small increase in leukemia risk among occupational and residential groups exposed to high-intensity E/MFs [24, 25]. Criticism of the methodologies and interpretation of these studies has been intense. However, there is reason to believe that E/MFs may have an impact on health because within all organisms there exist endogenous electric currents that play crucial roles in physiologic processes, such as neural activity, tissue growth and repair, glandular secretion, and cell membrane function. Indeed, some basic biologic effects due to E/MF exposure have been observed, such as altered cellular metabolism and growth rate [26]. Experiments on the chronic health effects of E/MFs on animals have been fewer and more difficult to interpret [27].

More basic scientific and epidemiologic research is required to determine whether E/MFs encountered in industry and the home pose a serious health risk. Such an effort is currently being undertaken by several governmental and private investigators. In the meantime, it would seem prudent to minimize high-intensity E/MF exposure of workers and residents through work-scheduling as well as workplace and residential engineering.

Ultrasound

The term *ultrasound* is used to describe mechanical vibrations at frequencies above the limit of human audibility (approximately 16 KHz*). These vibrations, like sound, are pressure waves and unrelated to electromagnetic radiation. Ultrasound has many industrial and other uses, depending on the frequency of its generation. (With increasing frequency, ultrasound has a tendency to be absorbed by the transmitting medium and consequently has less penetrating ability.) Low-frequency (18–30 KHz), high-power ultrasound is

---

*1 KHz = 1 Kilohertz = 10^3 cycles per second.

used in industry for its penetrating and disruptive abilities to facilitate drilling, welding, and cleaning operations, and to help emulsify liquids. It is also a component of noise generated by a variety of high-power engines. High-frequency (100–10,000 KHz) ultrasound has many analytical and medical uses, and diagnostic ultrasound is widely used in obstetrics.

Low-frequency ultrasound can cause a variety of health problems, either by its transmission through air or by bodily contact with the ultrasound generator or target, as the immersion of hands in an ultrasound cleaning bath. A worker with such exposure may complain of headache, earache, vertigo, general discomfort, and possible irritability, hypersensitivity to light, and hyperacusia (sensitivity to sound). Exposure through bodily contact may eventually cause peripheral nervous system lesions, leading to autonomic polyneuritis or partial paralysis of the fingers or hands (see previous *Vibration* section).

High-frequency ultrasound may result in the same spectrum of problems; however, since high-frequency ultrasound is absorbed by air and poorly penetrating, excessive exposure is only obtained in cases of direct contact between the ultrasound generator and a part of the worker's body. Under these circumstances, the mechanism of harmful effects is similar to that of segmental vibration. Recent evidence has suggested a reduction of vibration perception in the fingers of ultrasonic therapists [28].

Protection from the harmful effects of ultrasound is primarily an engineering problem requiring insulation and isolation of the ultrasound process. Ear protective devices are also helpful. Workers with ultrasound exposure should undergo yearly audiometric and neurologic examinations.

REFERENCES

1. Maxwell KJ, Elwood JM. Could melanoma be caused by fluorescent light? A review of relevant physics. In RP Gallagher, ed. Recent results in cancer research: epidemiology and malignant melanoma. 1986; 102:137.
2. Elwood JM. Could melanoma be caused by fluorescent light? A review of relevant epidemiology. In RP Gallagher, ed. Recent results in cancer research: epidemiology and malignant melanoma. 1986; 102:127.
3. The Medical Letter. Drugs that cause sensitivity. Med Let 1986; 28:51.
4. Lydahl E, Philipson B. Infrared radiation and cataract. II. Epidemiologic investigation of glass workers. Acta Ophthalmologica 1984; 62:976.
5. Cleary SF. Microwave cataractogenesis. Proc. I.E.E.E. 1980; 68(1):49.
6. Lancranjan I, Maicanescu M, Rafaila E, et al. Gonadic function in workmen with longterm exposure to microwaves. Health Phys. 1975; 29:381.
7. McLaughlin JT. Tissue destruction and death from microwave radiation (radar). Calif. Med. 1957; 86:336.
8. Izmerov NF. Current problems of nonionizing radiation. Scand J Work Environ Health 1985; 11:223.
9. Zaret MM, Kaplan IT, Kay AM. Clinical microwave cataracts. In: Cleary SF ed. Biological effects and health implications of microwave radiation, symposium proceedings, Richmond, Va.: BRH/OBE, 1970. (BRH/OBE report no. 70-2). p. 84.
10. Cunningham DS, Kleinstein BH. Carcinogenic properties of ionizing and nonionizing radiation. Cincinnati: NIOSH, 1977. Vols. 1 and 2.
11. Moss E, Conover D, Murray W, et al. Estimated number of U.S. workers potentially exposed to electromagnetic radiation. Reprinted in Radiation health and safety; hearing before the Senate Committee on Commerce, Science and Transportation, 95th Congress, 1st session, 1977. p. 633–7.
12. Curtis RA. Occupational exposures to radiofrequency radiation from FM radio and TV antennas. In: Proceedings of an ACGIH topical symposium. Cincinnati: Nov. 26–28, 1979. p. 211–22.
13. Hunter D, McLaughlin AIG, Perry KM. Clinical effects of the use of pneumatic tools. Br J Ind Med 1945; 2:10.
14. Helmkamp JC, Talbott EO, Marsh GM. Whole body vibration—a critical review. Am Ind Hyg Assoc J 1984; 45(3):162.
15. Pyykkö I, Starck J, et al. Hand-arm vibration in the aetiology of hearing loss in lumber jacks. Br J Ind Med 1981; 38:281.
16. NIOSH. Vibration syndrome in chipping and grinding workers. J Occup Med 1984; 26(10):765.
17. NIOSH. Current intelligence bulletin 38: vibration

syndrome. Washington, DC:NIOSH/DHHS, March 29, 1983. (pub. no. 83–110).

18. NIOSH. Criteria for a recommended standard . . . occupational exposure to hot environments. (Revised Criteria) Washington, DC: NIOSH, 1986. (NIOSH, DHHS publication no. 86–113).

19. ACGIH. Threshold limit values and biological exposure indices for 1986–1987. American Conference of Governmental Industrial Hygienists. Cincinnati: ACGIH, 1986, 1987. (ISBN:0-936712-69-4).

20. Greenleaf JE, Harrison MH. Water and electrolytes. In: Layman DK, ed. Exercise, nutrition and health. American Chemical Society, 1985.

21. Houston CS, Dickinson J. Cerebral form of high-altitude illness. Lancet 1975; 2:758.

22. Johnson TS, Rock PB, Fulco CS, et al. Prevention of acute mountain sickness by dexamethasone. N Engl J Med 1984; 310: 683.

23. Frisancho AR. Functional adaptation to high altitude hypoxia. Science 1975; 187:313.

24. Savitz DA, Calle EE. Leukemia and occupational exposure to electromagnetic fields: review of epidemiologic surveys. J Occup Med 1987; 29:47.

25. Wertheimer N, Leeper E. Adult cancer related to electrical wires near the home. Int J Epi 1982; 11:345.

26. National Academy of Sciences. Biological effects of electric and magnetic fields associated with proposed Project Searfarer. Report of the committee on biosphere effects of extremely-low frequency radiation. Washington, DC: National Research Council, 1977.

27. Delgado JMR, Leal J, et al. Embryological changes induced by weak extremely low frequency electromagnetic fields. J Anat 1982; 134:533.

28. Lundstrom R. Effects of local vibration transmitted from ultrasonic devices on vibrotactile perception in the hands of therapists. Ergonomics 1985; 28(5):793.

BIBLIOGRAPHY
Nonionizing Radiation

ULTRAVIOLET

NIOSH. Criteria for a recommended standard: occupational exposure to ultraviolet radiation. Washington, DC: U.S. Government Printing Office, 1972. (DHEW publication no. (NIOSH) HSM 73-11009).
A good in-depth review.

VISIBLE LIGHT

Cogan DG. Lighting and health hazards. In: the occupational safety and health effects associated with reduced levels of illumination. Proceedings of a Symposium. Cincinnati, OH: (HEW [NIOSH] publication no. 75-142). 1974, p. 28.
A good review of ergonomic considerations and other potential hazards.

INFRARED

Lydahl E, Philipson B. Infrared radiation and cataract. I. Epidemiologic investigation of iron and steel workers. II. Epidemiologic investigation of glass workers. Acta Ophthalmoligca 1984; 62:961.
A recent epidemiological review.

MICROWAVE/RADIOFREQUENCY

Foster KR, Guy AW. The microwave problem. Scientific Am 1986; 225(3):32.
A history of recent controversy and less technical review of science.

NIOSH/OSHA. Current intelligence bulletin 33—radiofrequency (RF) sealers and heaters: potential health hazards and their prevention. Washington, DC: NIOSH and OSHA, 1980.
A discussion specific to the workplace.

Roberts NJ Jr, Michaelson SM. Epidemiological studies of human exposures to radiofrequency radiation. A critical review. Int Arch Occup Environ Health 1985; 56:169.
A review of epidemiology of low-level MW/RFR effects.

LASER

Sliney DH. Safety with lasers and other optical sources. New York: Plenum, 1980.
Preventive measures.

Wolfe JA. Laser retinal injury. Military Med 1985; 150:177.
A review of pathology.

Vibration

WHOLE-BODY

Helmkamp JC, Talbott EO, Marsh GM. Whole body vibration—a critical review. Am Ind Hyg Assoc J 1984; 45(3):162.
As stated in title, a somewhat skeptical discussion.

SEGMENTAL

NIOSH. Vibration syndrome in chipping and grinding workers. J Occup Med 1984; 26(10):765.
A good review with 66 references.

NIOSH. Current intelligence bulletin 38. vibration syndrome. Cincinnati, OH: NIOSH, 1983. (DHHS (NIOSH) publication no. 83–110).
A discussion of effects and appropriate work practices.

Starck J, Pyykkö I, eds. Fourth international symposium on hand-arm vibration. Scand J Work Env Health vol. 12, 1986.
An entire volume devoted to clinical and research aspects of this problem.

Atmospheric Variations

HEAT

NIOSH. Criteria for a recommended standard . . . occupational exposure to hot environments revised criteria. 1986. Cincinnati, OH: NIOSH, 1986. (DHHS/CDC/NIOSH publication no. 86–113).
A good review of known effects.

NIOSH. Working in hot environments. Washington, DC: NIOSH, revised 1986. (DHHS/NIOSH publication no. 86–112).
An overview of hazards and recommendations in plain language.

COLD

Ramstead KD, Hughes RG, Webb AT. Recent cases of trench foot. Postgrad Med J 1980; 56:879.
A good review of this less-well known entity.

HYPERBARIC

Hills BA. Decompression sickness. New York: Wiley, 1977. Vols. 1 and 2.
Includes detailed discussion of aseptic bone necrosis.

Strauss RH. Diving medicine. New York: Grune & Stratton, 1976.
A review of treatment and safety procedures.

HYPOBARIC

Foulks GE. Altitude-related illness. Am. J. Emerg. Med. 1985; 3(3):217.
A review of clinical syndromes, treatment, and prevention.

Special Topics

VDTS (see also Chap. 31)

Marriott IA, Stuchly MA. Health aspects of work with visual display terminals. J Occup Med 1986; 28(9):833.
A comprehensive review with 62 references, stemming from 1985 World Health Organization conference.

FLUORESCENT LIGHTS AND MELANOMA

Gallagher RP. ed. Epidemiology of malignant melanoma. Recent results in cancer research. Vol. 102, 1986.
A comprehensive review of melanoma epidemiology with several chapters focusing on fluorescent lights.

ELECTRIC AND MAGNETIC FIELDS

Florida Electric and Magnetic Fields Science Advisory Commission. Biological effects of 60 Hz power transmission lines. Report to the Florida State Dept. of Environmental Resources, Tallahassee, FL.: March 1985.
A comprehensive review, except a somewhat limited discussion of epidemiology.

Savitz DA, Calle EE. Leukemia and occupational exposure to electromagnetic fields: review of epidemiologic surveys. J Occup Med 1987; 29:47.
A review of proportionate morbidity/mortality studies.

19
Infectious Agents

Nelson M. Gantz

Work-related infectious diseases are caused by all categories of infectious agents. As with other types of disorders, the occupational history often provides the key clue to identifying the cause of a puzzling infectious disease.

Occupations associated with a risk of an infectious disease (Table 19-1) are divided into two categories: health care occupations, either with direct patient contact or laboratory exposure to infective material; and non-health-care occupations, primarily those involving contact with animals or animal products, ground breaking or earth moving, or travel into endemic areas. Table 19-2 presents the number of potentially work-related cases of selected infectious diseases reported to the Centers for Disease Control in 1985; it is not known how complete these data are or what percentage of these cases is actually work-related.

INFECTIOUS DISEASES IN HEALTH CARE WORKERS

The hazards of hospital-acquired (nosocomial) infectious diseases have been well recognized since the mid-nineteenth century, when Semmelweiss discovered the cause of puerperal fever. The risk of nosocomial infection exists both for hospitalized patients and for workers involved in their care. (Table 19-3 lists some infectious agents that have been transmitted from patients to health care workers.) Such problems exist not only for hospital workers but also for those in out-patient settings such as dentists' offices. The risk of infection is also present for personnel working in out-pa-

tient renal dialysis centers, laboratories where there is contact with blood, nursing homes, institutions for the retarded, and prisons.

Hepatitis B

A 25-year-old intensive-care-unit nurse reported to the employee health service at her hospital. She complained of nausea, weakness, malaise, loss of appetite, dark urine, and jaundice of about 1 week's duration. She had not eaten any raw shellfish, never had a blood transfusion, did not know of any friends with hepatitis, and denied use of drugs. She recalled having been stuck with a needle 8 weeks before while caring for a patient having a cardiac arrest, but she took no precautionary measures. Abnormal liver function tests and a positive blood test for hepatitis B surface antigen (HB$_s$Ag) confirmed the diagnosis of hepatitis B. Because of persistent vomiting and markedly abnormal liver function tests, she was hospitalized for 2 weeks. After this, she convalesced at home for 2 more weeks. She then thought she was ready to return to work. The cost of her illness, including hospital charges and lost wages, was approximately $8,000.

Viral hepatitis, type B (hepatitis B), is probably the most frequent work-related infectious disease in the United States. It continues to be a major problem for physicians, nurses, dentists (especially oral surgeons), and laboratory workers (especially those having direct contact with blood). Evidence of past hepatitis B virus (HBV) infection, based on the presence of antibody to HB$_s$Ag (anti-HB$_s$), is present in about 18 percent of physicians, over four times that reported for volunteer blood do-

Table 19-1. Selected work-related infectious diseases by occupation

Occupation	Selected work-related infectious diseases
Bulldozer operator	Coccidioidomycosis, histoplasmosis
Butcher	Anthrax, erysipeloid, tularemia
Cat and dog handler	Cat-scratch disease, *Pasteurella multocida* cellulitis, rabies
Cave explorer	Rabies, histoplasmosis
Construction worker	Rocky Mountain spotted fever, coccidioidomycosis, histoplasmosis
Cook	Tularemia, salmonellosis, trichinosis
Cotton mill worker	Coccidioidomycosis
Dairy farmer	Milkers' nodules, Q fever, brucellosis
Delivery personnel	Rabies
Dentist	Hepatitis B
Ditch digger	Creeping eruption (cutaneous larva migrans), hookworm disease, ascariasis
Diver	*Mycobacterium marinum* (swimming pool granuloma)
Dock worker	Leptospirosis, swimmers' itch (Schistosoma species)
Farmer	Rabies, anthrax, brucellosis, Rocky Mountain spotted fever, tetanus, leptospirosis, plague, tularemia, coccidioidomycosis, histoplasmosis, sporotrichosis, hookworm disease, ascariasis
Fisherman, fish handler	Erysipeloid, swimming pool granuloma
Florist	Sporotrichosis
Food-processing worker	Salmonellosis
Forestry worker	California encephalitis, Lyme disease, Rocky Mountain spotted fever, tularemia
Fur handler	Tularemia
Gardener	Sporotrichosis, creeping eruption (cutaneous larva migrans)
Geologist	Plague, California encephalitis
Granary and warehouse worker	Murine typhus (endemic)
Hide, goat hair, and wool handler	Q Fever, anthrax, dermatophytoses
Hunter	Lyme disease, Rocky Mountain spotted fever, plague, tularemia, trichinosis
Laboratory worker	Hepatitis B
Livestock worker	Brucellosis, leptospirosis
Meat packer and slaughterhouse (abattoir) worker	Brucellosis, leptospirosis, Q fever, salmonellosis
Nurse	Hepatitis B, rubella, tuberculosis
Pet shop worker	*Pasteurella multocida* cellulitis, psittacosis, dermatophytoses
Physician	Hepatitis B, rubella, tuberculosis
Pigeon breeder	Psittacosis
Poultry handler	Newcastle disease, erysipeloid, psittacosis
Rancher	Lyme disease, rabies, Rocky Mountain spotted fever, Q fever, tetanus, plague, tularemia, trichinosis
Rendering plant worker	Brucellosis, Q fever
Sewer worker	Leptospirosis, hookworm disease, ascariasis
Shearer	Orf, tularemia
Shepherd	Orf, plague
Trapper	Leptospirosis, Lyme disease, tularemia, rabies, Rocky Mountain spotted fever
Veterinarian	Anthrax, brucellosis, erysipeloid, rabies, leptospirosis, *Pasteurella multocida* cellulitis, salmonellosis, cat-scratch disease, orf, tularemia, psittacosis
Wild animal handler	Rabies
Zoo worker	Psittacosis, tuberculosis

Table 19-2. Annual U.S. incidence (1985) of
infectious diseases that are sometimes work-related*

Diseases	Number of reported cases
Anthrax	0
Brucellosis	133
Hepatitis, viral, type B	25,808
Leptospirosis	34
Plague	16
Psittacosis	106
Rabies	1
Tetanus	70
Tuberculosis	21,106
Tularemia	163
Typhus fever, murine	25

*Actual number of cases that are work-related is unknown;
data include both work- and non-work-related cases.
Source: Centers for Disease Control. *Morbidity and Mortality Weekly Report* 34:774, 1986.

nors; rates are highest for pathologists and surgeons.

Blood is the major source of infective virus. Only minute amounts are required: One milliliter of blood from a chronic carrier diluted to 10^{-8} still retains infectivity. HB_sAg is present not only in blood and blood products but also in saliva, semen, and feces; however, non-blood sources of infection are probably rare. The presence of HB_sAg in serum correlates well—but not perfectly—with infectivity. All patients who are HB_sAg-positive, however, should be considered as potentially infectious.

Transmission of HBV may occur from an accidental percutaneous stick from a contaminated needle or other instrument. Infection may also develop after contaminated blood enters a break in the skin, splatters onto a mucous membrane, or is ingested, such as in a pipetting accident. Airborne transmission has not been reported.

Health care workers who are positive for HB_sAg or anti-HBs usually have had substantial contact with blood or blood products. Patient contact seems to be less important than direct contact with patients' blood. The incidence of hepatitis B infec-

tion for health care workers is increased in certain work areas, including hemodialysis units, hematology and oncology wards, blood banks and clinical laboratories (especially where personnel have contact with blood), operating rooms, dental offices and oral surgery suites, and wash areas for glassware and other equipment.

In the hospital the major sources of HBV are patients with acute hepatitis B infection, patients with chronic liver disease, patients on chronic hemodialysis, immunosuppressed patients, parenteral drug abusers, and multiple blood transfusion recipients. In many hospitals the chronic hemodialysis unit is the highest risk area. Patients on chronic hemodialysis who become HB_sAg-positive have up to a 60 percent chance of becoming chronic carriers. Other individuals at high risk of becoming chronic carriers are male homosexuals and residents of institutions for the retarded. Parenteral drug abusers have a HB_sAg carrier rate of 1 to 5 percent, compared with a rate of 0.1 percent for volunteer blood donors.

Although certain features help distinguish hepatitis B from other forms of acute viral or toxic hepatitis, often they are not distinguishable clinically, and serologic studies are required for a specific diagnosis. Some patients are asymptomatic; others have malaise, fatigue, anorexia, nausea, vomiting, distaste for cigarettes, fever, abdominal pain, dark urine, light-colored stools, and other symptoms. Laboratory studies show abnormally high serum aminotransferases (such as serum glutamic-oxaloacetic transaminase [SGOT] and serum glutamic-pyruvic transaminase [SGPT]), often an increased serum bilirubin, and, in severe cases, a prolonged prothrombin time.

HB_sAg can be detected in the blood of a hepatitis B patient usually 6 to 12 weeks after exposure and for about 1 to 6 weeks after onset of clinical illness. Five to 10 percent of hepatitis B patients will become chronic carriers of HBV and serve as potential sources of infection for personnel. If a patient remains HB_sAg-positive for 5 months, the probability of becoming a chronic carrier increases to 88 percent. Most chronic HB_sAg carriers are

Table 19-3. Some infectious agents that are occupational risks for health care workers

Viruses	Bacteria	Others
Creutzfeldt-Jakob agent	*Bordetella* species	*Chlamydia psittaci*
Cytomegalovirus	*Campylobacter* species	*Coxiella burnetti*
Hepatitis B	*Corynebacterium diphtheriae*	*Cryptosporidium* species
Non-A, non-B hepatitis	*Mycobacterium tuberculosis*	*Mycoplasma pneumoniae*
Herpes simplex	*Neisseria meningitidis*	*Sarcoptes scabiei*
Human immunodeficiency virus (HIV)	*Salmonella* species	
Influenza	*Shigella* species	
Lassa fever	*Yersinia pestis*	
Measles		
Mumps		
Parainfluenza		
Poliovirus		
Respiratory syncytial virus		
Rotavirus		
Rubella		
Rubeola		
Varicella-zoster		

asymptomatic; a subgroup of these carriers will have mild to moderate elevations in their liver function tests. Chronic active hepatitis will occur in 30 percent of chronic carriers and may result in cirrhosis.

Recommendations for preventing hepatitis B in health care workers include surveillance of staff in high-risk areas, employee education, appropriate sterilization and disinfection procedures, designation of a specific person responsible for safety, use of protective clothing and gloves, and avoidance of eating or smoking in laboratory work areas. (For an update on hepatitis B prevention, see *Morbidity and Mortality Weekly Report,* June 19, 1987.) Health care personnel should minimize their contact with potentially infectious patient secretions. Patients and staff in high-risk areas like hemodialysis units can be screened for HB_sAg and anti-HB_s. HB_sAg-positive patients can be separated from HB_sAg-negative patients and dialyzed by staff who have anti-HB_s (or who are HB_sAg-positive). Personnel must carefully avoid needle sticks and contact of mucous membranes and skin

with potentially contaminated blood or other secretions; wearing gloves is one means of achieving this. All blood specimens should be handled as if potentially infectious. HBV-contaminated reusable equipment should be autoclaved before reuse, and HBV-contaminated disposable material should be disposed of in closed systems (Fig. 19-1). Hepatitis B immune globulin (HBIG) is recommended for prophylaxis within 1 week following either parenteral or mucosal contact with HB_sAg-positive blood. Clinical hepatitis developed in 2 percent of HBIG recipients following a needle-stick exposure to HB_sAg-positive blood compared with a rate of 8 percent in immune serum globulin recipients. The HB_sAg and anti-HB_s status of the exposed health care worker should be determined. If either test is positive, HBIG has no value and should not be given. If both tests are negative, HBIG should be given in two doses spaced 25 to 30 days apart.

Hepatitis B vaccine is a killed virus vaccine consisting of the virus surface antigen (HB_sAg) particles. The vaccine was approved by the Food and Drug Administration in 1981. The vaccine induces

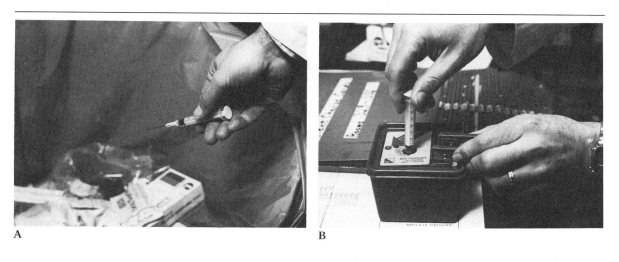

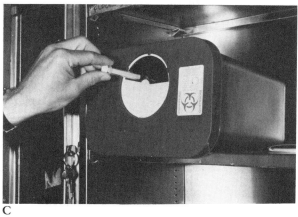

Fig. 19-1. Incorrect disposal of a blood-contaminated needle in (A) a trash barrel and (B) cutting device. C. Correct method of disposal. Proper disposal of needles is an important means of reducing the risk for hospital and other health care workers of hepatitis B and non-A, non-B hepatitis.
(Photographs by Marilee Caliendo.)

a protective antibody (anti-HB$_s$). Three doses at 0, 1, and 6 months with hepatitis B vaccine are recommended. The vaccine has been studied in high-risk pre-exposure situations among male homosexuals and dialysis staff. The results of the vaccine trials have been impressive with efficacy rates from 71 to 92 percent. The vaccine has also been given in post-exposure situations to sexual partners or spouses of those with hepatitis B and following needlestick exposures. In the United States the two major target populations for the vaccine are individuals with occupational exposures, such as surgeons, and those with sexual exposures.

Despite the proven safety of the hepatitis B vaccine, about one-third of surgeons, almost two-thirds of family practitioners and internists, and over three-quarters of pediatricians have not yet been immunized with the vaccine. In July 1986, a new hepatitis B vaccine manufactured by recombinant DNA techniques, called Recombivax HB, was licensed. It is hoped that the availability of this new vaccine will increase the frequency of immunization of health care workers, although it is no more effective or safe than the previously developed hepatitis B vaccine. For recommendations on vaccine use, see *Morbidity and Mortality Weekly Report,* June 7, 1985.

The case of hepatitis B at the start of this section raises several questions concerning prevention of this disease: How should a needle stick be managed? When should HBIG be given? When (and should) this nurse return to work? If the needle has been in contact with a known individual ("donor"), then the HB$_s$Ag status of that person can be determined. If the donor is HB$_s$Ag-positive or has a history of multiple blood transfusions and the worker is susceptible to hepatitis B (negative HB$_s$Ag and negative anti-HB$_s$), then the worker stuck by the needle is at risk of developing hepatitis B and should be given HBIG. If the status of the "donor" is unknown and the worker is susceptible, then either HBIG or regular gamma globulin (immune serum globulin) can be given. The nurse should be able to return to work when she is clinically well, but if she remains HB$_s$Ag-positive she should not draw blood from patients (or donate blood). Had this nurse reported her needle stick to the employee health service, the "donor" been found to be HB$_s$Ag-positive, and the nurse given HBIG, her clinical manifestations of hepatitis B might have been prevented. In this context it is disappointing that most health care workers do not take such preventive measures after sticking themselves with needles possibly contaminated with HBV.

Hepatitis A

Infection with hepatitis A virus is a risk for health care workers in institutions for the retarded where personal hygiene is poor and for certain animal caretakers, especially those with close exposure to chimpanzees. This virus is mainly transmitted by the fecal-oral route. Maximal viral shedding in the stool occurs during the 2-week period before onset of jaundice (and usually before diagnosis). Virus persists in the stool for about 7 to 15 days after the onset of jaundice. There is no chronic carrier state of hepatitis A virus in the stool or blood.

Careful hand washing by health care personnel is probably the most important measure for preventing in-hospital spread of hepatitis A virus. Immune serum globulin (ISG) may be indicated for selected personnel working in institutions for the retarded within 1 to 2 weeks of contact with residents with hepatitis A virus infection. Nonhuman primates, which may be a source of hepatitis A virus, should be quarantined for 2 months after importation.

Non-A, Non-B Hepatitis

About 90 percent of transfusion-induced hepatitis cases are designated as non-A, non-B. This entity, which conceivably might be caused by more than one virus, is diagnosed by excluding other causes of hepatitis. Its epidemiology resembles to some extent that of hepatitis B. Disease in health care personnel has occurred following a needle stick, but the extent of this infection as an occupational hazard is unknown. The clinical course of the disease resembles that of hepatitis B. About one-third of patients will become chronic carriers.

Delta Hepatitis

Delta hepatitis infection is caused by a unique RNA virus that requires HB$_s$Ag for its replication. Hepatitis caused by the delta agent occurs only in patients having a simultaneous hepatitis B infection or as a superinfection in a chronic HB$_s$Ag carrier. Diagnosis can be established by demonstrating the presence of either IgM or IgG delta antibody (anti-HD) or delta antigen in the serum. Delta infection occurs most often in intravenous drug addicts and patients with hemophilia. Nosocomial transmission of the delta agent among hemodialysis patients has been reported and the potential for acquisition of delta hepatitis by health care personnel exists. Clinically, delta agent can cause fulminant hepatitis and chronic carriage of delta agent may be found. Measures aimed at limiting the spread of hepatitis B will prevent the transmission of delta agent.

Tuberculosis

Transmission of tuberculosis (TB) from patients—often undiagnosed—to hospital workers and health care profession students remains a significant hazard. Unfortunately, as TB incidence declines, the clinical acumen of physicians to diagnose it diminishes. In one study TB was not initially suspected in one-half the patients admitted with pulmonary TB, and in nearly one-third the diagnosis was not established by the time of discharge. The diagnosis was often missed because of a declining incidence of TB in this country and a low index of suspicion of this diagnosis by today's physicians. The incidence of tuberculin skin test positivity in U.S. physicians is at least twice the expected rate; in one study personnel exposed to patients with unsuspected TB had a sixfold increase in the rate of positive tuberculin skin tests compared with a group of unexposed personnel. Employees in nursing homes, mental health hospitals, and prisons are also at an increased risk of developing TB.

Prevention of TB in hospital employees requires that physicians have a high index of suspicion and institute respiratory isolation precautions pending confirmation of the diagnosis. Employees with nonreactive tuberculin skin tests should be screened with a tuberculin test once a year; tuberculin skin testing of exposed personnel is also indicated. Indications for isoniazid (INH) prophylaxis include household contacts of patients with active TB, recent converters, tuberculin reactors with an abnormal chest x-ray, special clinical situations such as patients who are tuberculin reactors on high-dose corticosteroids, and tuberculin reactors under 35 years of age. Use of BCG (bacillus Calmette-Guérin) vaccination is not currently recommended for hospital personnel: the use of BCG vaccine would make skin testing less helpful in identifying tuberculin reactors. However, the vaccine is suggested for health care workers if the annual skin test conversion rate exceeds 1 percent.

Rubella and Cytomegalovirus

Rubella infection may be transmitted from hospital employees to patients and from patients to susceptible personnel. In one outbreak 47 cases of rubella occurred among hospital personnel (a dietary worker was the suspected index case); this outbreak resulted in one pregnancy being terminated and 475 workdays being lost. The major hazard of rubella is infection in pregnant women, with the possibility of congenital rubella syndrome resulting in the offspring. School teachers are also at an increased risk of acquiring rubella since they are likely to have contact with persons with the illness. About 15 percent of women in the childbearing age group are susceptible to rubella. Rubella vaccine is the most effective means of preventing disease, and susceptible personnel should be immunized. The vaccine is well tolerated and in the work setting results in minimal absenteeism. Pregnancy should be avoided for 3 months in vaccinated individuals.

Cytomegalovirus (CMV) is another potential threat for pregnant women, but nurses who practice good personal hygiene are at no greater risk of acquiring this infection than their peers in the community. Transmission of CMV appears to require prolonged intimate contact. The use of gloves when handling potentially contaminated wastes as well as handwashing after each patient contact are the appropriate infection control measures to prevent acquisition of CMV.

Acquired Immunodeficiency Syndrome

Transmission of the acquired immunodeficiency syndrome (AIDS) agent, the human immunodeficiency virus (HIV), occurs only by sexual contact, by blood or blood products, and perinatally from an infected mother. There is no evidence for transmission of this virus by casual contact, such as by hand shaking or face-to-face conversation. Although initial panic occurred among many health care workers assigned to care for patients with AIDS, these fears have proved excessive. There have been few cases of AIDS to date in health care workers. Also, seroconversion after a needle-stick injury has been documented. The risk of a seroconversion to the AIDS virus following a needle-stick injury is estimated to be less than 1 percent, which is much lower than the risk (6–30%) of acquiring hepatitis B after a needle-stick injury. Guidelines to prevent the transmission of AIDS to health care workers have been developed (see *Morbidity and Mortality Weekly Report,* August 21, 1987). Measures that will prevent transmission of hepatitis B should be effective for AIDS. Health care workers should take precautions to prevent needle-stick injuries and exercise care when handling blood, tissues, or mucosal surfaces of all patients.

Laboratory-Associated Infections

A 23-year-old hospital bacteriologist was admitted with a 1-week history of chills, fever, headache, and diarrhea. She had a pulse of 80 beats per minute, temperature of 105°F, and a few macular areas on her abdomen. After blood cultures were obtained, she was given ampicillin and became afebrile. The blood cultures were positive for *Salmonella typhi.* The patient was diagnosed as having laboratory-acquired typhoid fever when further history revealed that she had been working with this organism 3 weeks earlier as part of a state laboratory proficiency-testing program. She admitted to smoking in the laboratory and occasionally eating her lunch there. The risk of infection from this organism can be reduced by immunizing laboratory personnel with typhoid vaccine as well as by enforcing basic laboratory safety procedures.*

More than 6,000 cases of laboratory-associated infections and over 250 fatalities have been reported in the literature. The most frequently identified laboratory-associated infections are brucellosis, tuberculosis, tularemia, typhoid fever,

*Adapted from MB Holmes, et al. Acquisition of typhoid fever from proficiency-testing specimens. N Engl J Med 1980; 303:519.

hepatitis B, Venezuelan equine encephalitis, Q fever, coccidioidomycosis, dermatomycosis, and psittacosis. The Centers for Disease Control has classified infectious agents by risk hazard. Class 1 agents are the least hazardous; they include *Tinea capitis* (which causes ringworm of the scalp) and mumps virus. Class 4 agents pose the most risk and require the highest degree of containment; two examples are *Herpes simiae* B virus and Lassa fever virus. Smallpox, a major threat to health care workers in the past, is still a concern for the few laboratory workers who still work with the virus.

Laboratory-acquired infections usually result from accidents. Syringes and needles, either as a result of self-inoculation or causing a spray, have been involved in 25 percent of these infections; another 25 percent are related to spilling or spraying the infectious material. Other accidents result from injuries due to broken glass or other sharp objects, aspirating material by mouth pipetting, and animal bites and scratches. The source of many laboratory-associated infections is obscure, although many of these are probably transmitted by aerosols. Air sampling techniques have shown that many laboratory procedures release organisms into the air.

Several approaches are available to prevent infection in laboratory personnel. Since inhalation of an infectious aerosol is probably the major mode of transmission, the use of biological safety cabinets with filters and laminar air flow has been recommended to help protect against this hazard. Similarly, material being centrifuged should be put in tubes with sealable lids. Hand-pipetting devices should be used for pipetting infectious materials; mouth pipetting should always be avoided.

Extreme care is required in the use and disposal of needles and syringes to decrease this frequent source of accidental infection. Experimentally infected animals are another important source of infection, and attention should be given to the animal quarters to minimize airborne spread of infection (see following section). In addition, measures must be employed to prevent animal biting and scratching accidents; vaccination to prevent rabies, tetanus, or plague may be indicated for persons at risk. Sera should be collected from employees and stored to be used diagnostically as acute phase sera if an illness develops. Other measures to decrease the risk of infection include use of biohazard signs; limited access to laboratories; restrictions for pregnant employees working with cytomegalovirus, herpes virus, and rubella virus; and educational programs for personnel regarding possible hazards and preventive measures. Laboratory safety must receive each employee's highest priority at all times.

Recently, considerable interest has developed in the use of monoclonal antibodies for diagnosis as well as therapy. Rat immunocytomas have been used in this work and the cell lines may be infected with various viruses. In one report, laboratory workers developed hemorrhagic fever from contact with rat cell lines infected with hantavirus. Prevention of these infections requires screening of the rats prior to their use.

INFECTIOUS DISEASES
IN NON-HEALTH-CARE WORKERS

Most work-related infectious diseases among non-health-care workers are zoonoses, diseases primarily of animals that are transmitted to man. Although these diseases occur infrequently, they are occupational hazards for workers who have contact with animals, such as farmers, veterinarians, butchers, and slaughterhouse workers. Some zoonoses also can result from recreational exposures. Examples of these diseases are listed in Table 19-4.

Bacteria

A sheep shearer became ill with fever and a headache. On examination he was found to have a 2-cm ulcerative skin lesion on his right hand and enlarged right epitrochlear and axillary lymph nodes. A gram's stain of the skin ulcer drainage showed polymorphonuclear leukocytes but no organisms. Because of his occupation and the clinical presentation, tularemia was suspected. Isolation of the organism was not attempted because of

the risk of creating an infectious aerosol in the bacteriology laboratory. The patient responded to oral tetracycline therapy and recovered in 10 days. The diagnosis of tularemia was later confirmed serilogically by a fourfold rise in antibodies to tularemia agglutinins between the initial ("acute") and convalescent sera.

Tularemia, like most other work-related bacterial diseases in non-health-care workers, is an uncommon disease. However, the disease should be considered in the differential diagnosis of a patient with the appropriate work history who presents with a skin lesion and lymphadenopathy. Laboratory workers and others whose work requires repeated exposure to tularemia are candidates for tularemia vaccine.

Other work-related bacterial diseases affecting non-health-care workers include anthrax, brucellosis, erysipeloid, leptospirosis, Lyme disease, *Pasteurella multocida* cellulitis, plague, non-typhoid salmonellosis, and swimming pool granuloma. Prevention of bacterial zoonoses is summarized in Table 19-4 and includes vaccination when available and use of protective clothing.

Viruses

Viral infections acquired occupationally by non-health-care workers fall into two categories:

Arthropod-borne: Yellow fever; Colorado tick fever; and Venezuelan, California, St. Louis, and Western and Eastern equine encephalitis are in this group. A human vaccine is available only for yellow fever; other preventive measures involve use of protective clothing, insect repellents, and vector control programs.

Non-arthropod-borne: These diseases include orf, milkers' nodules, Newcastle disease, and, most important, rabies. Orf is a skin disease caused by a poxvirus of sheep. Reddish-blue papules develop at sites of contact within 6 days of exposure to infected sheep; spontaneous recovery occurs. Milkers' nodules is another viral skin disease transmitted to the hands of milkers from the udders of infected cows; the nodules resolve within 4 to 6 weeks. Newcastle disease virus,

Table 19-4. Examples of occupational zoonoses in the United States

Diseases	Clinical manifestations	Common animal sources	Mode of acquisition	Workers at risk	Prevention
BACTERIAL DISEASES					
Anthrax	Malignant pustule, regional lymph-adenopathy, or pneumonia	Cattle, sheep, horses, goats (usually in form of imported animal products)	Direct contact or inhalation of spores, scouring of hides	Farmers, butchers, veterinarians	Vaccination, identification of infected animals
Brucellosis	Fever, headache, profuse sweating, anorexia, arthralgias, fatigue	Cattle, pigs, goats, sheep, dogs	Direct contact, ingestion, or inhalation	Meat packers, livestock workers, rendering plant workers, veterinarians	Animal vaccines, protective clothing and glasses
Cat-scratch disease	Regional lymph-adenopathy, fever, primary skin papule	Cats, dogs	Direct contact	Veterinarians, cat and dog handlers	Avoidance of cat scratches
Erysipeloid (not to be confused with the acute cellulitis erysipelas)	Localized purplish-red skin lesions	Fish, other wild and domestic animals	Direct contact (often after skin abrasions)	Fishermen, butchers, fish handlers, poultry handlers, veterinarians, homemakers	Gloves, hand washing
Leptospirosis	Chills, fever, myalgias, headache, hepatitis, conjunctival suffusion, skin rash	Rodents, dogs, cats, cattle, pigs, wild animals	Contact with urine-contaminated soil or water or direct contact with infected animal	Veterinarians, trappers, farmers (of sugar and rice), slaughterhouse workers, sewer workers, dock workers	Animal vaccines, avoidance of contact with contaminated water, rat control
Pasteurella multocida cellulitis	Localized cellulitis (pain, swelling, and redness)	Cats and dogs (part of normal nasopharyngeal flora)	Animal bite	Veterinarians, pet shop workers	Prevention of animal bites

Disease	Symptoms	Reservoir/Source	Transmission	Occupations at Risk	Prevention
Plague	Chills, high fever, regional lymphadenopathy, septicemia, or pneumonia	Ground squirrels, rabbits, hares, prairie dogs, rats, mice, coyotes	Direct contact with infected animal, rat flea bite, or respiratory droplets of infected patients	Farmers, ranchers, hunters, geologists in Southwest and West	Rat and vector control, vaccination
Salmonellosis	Chills, fever, headache, diarrhea	Poultry, cows, horses, dogs, cats, turtles	Direct contact with infected animal or its feces, or ingestion of infected food	Veterinarians, cooks, food processing and abattoir workers	Vaccination for laboratory workers, improved food processing and preparation
Swimming pool granuloma	Skin ulceration	Fish (marine and freshwater)	Direct contact	Fishermen, tropical fish store workers, divers	Pool disinfection, gloves
Tularemia	Red skin, papule that becomes ulcer, regional lymphadenopathy, pneumonia, or conjunctivitis with chills and fever	Rabbits, hares, ticks	Direct contact with infected animal, ingestion, aerosolization, or tick bite	Trappers, fur handlers, ranchers, butchers, cooks	Vaccination, gloves, insect repellents
VIRAL DISEASES					
Encephalitis (for example, California encephalitis)	Lethargy, fever, headache, disorientation	Rodents, horses	Mosquito or tick bite	Agriculture and forestry workers, geologists, geographers, entomologists	Protective clothing, insect repellents
Rabies	Fever, headache, agitation, confusion, seizures, excessive salivation	Raccoons, dogs, cats, skunks, bats, foxes	Animal bite	Veterinarians, cave explorers, ranchers, trappers, farmers, wild animal handlers	Avoid animal bites, local wound care, pre- and post-exposure immunization

Table 19-4 (continued)

Diseases	Clinical manifestations	Common animal sources	Mode of acquisition	Workers at risk	Prevention
RICKETTSIAL DISEASE					
Murine typhus (endemic typhus)	Headache, fever, skin rash, myalgias	Rats	Direct contact	Granary and warehouse workers	Rodent and vector control
CHLAMYDIAL DISEASE					
Psittacosis	Fever, headache, pneumonia	Parakeets, parrots, pigeons, turkeys	Inhalation of organism	Pet shop workers, pigeon breeders, zoo workers, veterinarians, poultry handlers	Tetracycline, chemo-prophylaxis of fowl

which causes pneumoencephalitis in fowl, may produce a self-limited conjunctivitis in exposed workers.

Rabies is a good example of a possibly work-related viral disease for which prevention is available. High-risk groups include veterinarians, animal handlers, and laboratory personnel working with the virus. Of course, not all cases are work-related. Rabies prevention has been successful and has resulted in a decrease in the United States from an average of 22 cases per year in the period from 1946 to 1950 to only one to five cases per year presently. Prevention of rabies includes local wound care, avoiding of animal bites, and immunization with vaccines or immune globulins. Persons at high risk of rabies should be immunized before exposure with multiple doses of human diploid-cell rabies vaccine. Post-exposure prophylaxis with human rabies immune globulin (HRIG) and the human diploid rabies vaccine is also recommended.

Rickettsia

Rocky Mountain spotted fever (RMSF), Q fever, and murine typhus can be work-related. RMSF is a potential risk for workers exposed to ticks in endemic areas such as the South Atlantic states; disease may occur, for example, in foresters, hunters, and construction workers. Q fever occurs commonly in cattle, sheep, and goats; dairy farmers, ranchers, stockyard and slaughterhouse workers, and hide and wool handlers are at risk of inhaling the organism and acquiring pneumonia or hepatitis. Murine typhus occurs in persons working in rat-infested areas; granary and warehouse workers are at risk. (Most of the cases in the United States occur in Texas.)

Chlamydia

Psittacosis, which is caused by a strain of *Chlamydia psittaci* and usually takes the form of a pneumonia, is an occupational hazard for pet shop employees, pigeon breeders, zoo workers, and veterinarians. In addition, several outbreaks have been reported in turkey-processing plants.

FEVER AND "FLU" MAY NOT BE INFECTIOUS

Two work-related syndromes, metal fume fever and polymer fume fever, are characterized by fever and influenza-like symptoms but are noninfectious in origin.

Metal fume fever produces chills, increased sweating, nausea, weakness, headache, myalgias, and cough. It often begins with thirst and a metallic taste in the mouth. The white blood cell count is often elevated. Metal fume fever results from exposure to oxides of various metals, usually zinc, copper, or magnesium; aluminum, antimony, cadmium, copper, iron, manganese, nickel, selenium, silver, and tin have also been implicated. Welding, melting of copper and zinc in electric furnaces, and zinc smelting and galvanizing are work processes that have often been associated with this syndrome.

Polymer fume fever is characterized by dry cough, tightness in the chest, a choking sensation, and shaking chills. It is caused by exposure to unknown breakdown products of fluorocarbons, which are among the substances formed when polytetrafluoroethylene (PTFE, also known as Teflon or Fluon) is heated above 300°C. Since the first description of this syndrome in the 1950s, its control has been accomplished by preventing exposure to the heated fluorocarbon. In a workplace where there is PTFE exposure, however, cigarettes may become contaminated by PTFE on a worker's hands or in workplace air. Within the cigarette, PTFE is heated to temperatures high enough to convert it to substances that are strong respiratory irritants. Therefore, even when the fluorocarbon is not directly heated to sufficient temperature, if smoking is allowed at the workplace the classic syndrome may still occur.

Both syndromes often occur after a delay of several hours from initial exposure. Both syndromes resolve within 24 to 48 hours with as yet no known long-term sequelae.

Parasites

Some parasites are occupational hazards for non-health-care workers in the United States; many more, not listed here, are hazards for workers in other countries. Schistosome dermatitis or "swimmers' itch" is an infrequent hazard for water workers, such as skin divers, lifeguards, clam diggers, and rice field workers. Workers having direct contact with the soil, such as barefoot farmers, ditch diggers, sewer workers, and tea-plantation workers, may infrequently develop hookworm disease, ascariasis, cutaneous larva migrans (creeping eruption), and visceral larva migrans. Cooks are at risk of acquiring taeniasis, trichinosis, or toxoplasmosis if they taste uncooked meats. Mites, chiggers, and ticks that infest poultry and substances such as straw, dust, and grains may affect workers who handle them. Prevention of occupational parasitic diseases usually involves wearing protective clothing and shoes, health education, and measures to improve the standard of living.

Fungi

Workers involved in earth-moving jobs such as bulldozer operators are at risk of acquiring deep fungal infections. Infection usually results from inhalation of spore-containing dust in endemic areas. Occupational fungal infections include histoplasmosis, coccidioidomycosis, and sporotrichosis. Superficial fungal infections can also result from occupational exposures; for example, ringworm in dogs, cats, cattle, and other animals is common and therefore animal handlers are at increased risk. Superficial candidal infection may be a hazard for workers such as bakers whose hands are often wet.

Histoplasmosis is a well-recognized occupational pulmonary disease; the organism is found in certain soils, and its growth is stimulated by bat or bird guano. In the United States the peak incidence of disease is in the Ohio and Mississippi River Valleys. At great risk are cave explorers, bridge scrapers, excavators, bulldozer operators, and grave diggers. Earth-moving activities at sites of chicken coops or bird roosts in endemic areas such as Tennessee or Kentucky should be preceded by appropriate soil cultures for fungi. A 5 percent formalin solution sprayed on contaminated soil prior to earth-moving operations may be effective in preventing disease where a disease risk has been documented.

Coccidioidomycosis is caused by *Coccidioides immitis,* a fungus found in the soil in the Southwest. Infection is associated with earth-moving activities. Rarely, infection may be transmitted via inanimate objects (fomites) such as fruits, cotton, and vegetables that contain spores that can become airborne. Archeologists, geologists, bulldozer operators, and farm workers are at greatest risk. Prevention of naturally acquired disease is difficult at present, and workers involved in earth-moving activities should be aware of the risks. Before earth moving in an endemic area, one should consider obtaining soil cultures.

Sporotrichosis infection usually results from traumatic inoculation of the organism into the skin. Sphagnum moss is often implicated as the source of the organism although timber and other plant material are potentially a risk. Florists, nursery workers, farmers, berry pickers, and horticulturists are at greatest risk. Spraying sphagnum moss with a fungicidal solution may help prevent infection.

INFLUENZA CONTROL IN THE WORKPLACE

Influenza and other respiratory viruses are responsible for considerable morbidity and days lost from work for workers in both health care and non-health-care settings. Hospital personnel may transmit influenza to elderly patients, those with underlying heart, lung, or metabolic diseases, or immunosuppressed patients, resulting in morbidity and mortality. Control measures include use of antiviral compounds such as amantadine and influenza vaccines. Use of influenza vaccine in the work setting for health care personnel should be considered, depending on the recommendations of the Centers for Disease Control for that year.

There are relatively few industry-based influenza immunization programs.

BIBLIOGRAPHY

Balfour CL, Balfour HH Jr. Cytomegalovirus is not an occupational risk for nurses in renal transplant and neonatal units: results of a prospective surveillance study. JAMA 1986; 256:1909.
CMV was not an occupational risk for health care workers; hand washing should be emphasized.

Barrett-Connor E. The epidemiology of tuberculosis in physicians. JAMA 1979; 241:33.
A good review.

Berenson AS, ed. Control of communicable diseases in man. Washington, D.C.: American Public Health Association, 1985.
A very useful handbook on the prevention and control of communicable diseases.

Conte JE. Infection with human immunodeficiency virus in the hospital: epidemiology, infection control, and biosafety considerations. Ann Intern Med 1986; 105:730.
A review that should decrease the fears of health care workers.

Elliot DL, Tolle SW, Goldberg L, Miller JB. Pet-associated illness. N Engl J Med 1985; 313:985,
A review of illnesses acquired from dogs and cats.

Geiseler PJ, Nelson KE, Crispen RG, Moses VK. Tuberculosis in physicians: a continuing problem. Am Rev Respir Dis 1986; 133:773.
Risk still exists for medical students and physicians.

Hagen MD, Meyer KB, Pauker SG. Routine preoperative screening for HIV: does the risk to the surgeon outweigh the risk to the patient? JAMA 1988; 259:1357–1359.

Maynard JE. Viral hepatitis as an occupational hazard in the health care profession. In: Vyas GN, Cohen SM, Schmid R, eds. Viral hepatitis: a contemporary assessment of epidemiology, pathogenesis and prevention. Philadelphia: Franklin Institute, 1978: 321–331.
A very good review.

Patterson WB, Craven DE, Schwartz DA, Nardell EA, Kasmer J, Noble J. Occupational hazards to hospital personnel. Ann Intern Med 1985; 102:658.
A review that emphasizes measures to prevent these problems.

Schwartz J, Kauffman CA. Occupational hazards from deep mycoses. Arch Dermatol 1977; 113:1270.
An excellent review of occupational fungal diseases.

Steele JH. Occupational health in agriculture. Arch Environ Health, 1968; 17:267.
A comprehensive review of occupational zoonoses.

20
Occupational Stress

Dean B. Baker

A 54-year-old taxicab driver develops unstable angina after a 10-year history of hypertension and two episodes of bleeding duodenal ulcers. He does not drink alcohol or smoke cigarettes.

A 21-year-old video display terminal operator develops visual discomfort, headaches, backaches, irritability, and trouble sleeping.

A 46-year-old automobile assembly-line worker calls in sick on a Monday for the fourth time in the past 2 months.

A 39-year-old investment banker with an exceptional record of achievement no longer seems able to complete projects on time. He reports feeling fatigue to the point where he has given up his regular recreational activities.

Consideration of stress in the evaluation, prevention, and treatment of potential occupational diseases substantially expands the range and complexity of the medical practitioner's task. Despite much research, the stress phenomenon remains elusive. In fact, there is still no consensus about the definition of the term *stress*. Unlike other occupational hazards that tend to be specific for tasks, stress is ubiquitous and, to a varying extent, is associated with all work. Because stress is affected by the nature of the work process, yet modified by perceptions of the individual worker, it is inherently a psychosocial phenomenon with organizational and economic ramifications. These latter factors generally are outside of the medical practitioner's realm of expertise.

The exact magnitude of stress-related disorders is not known, although it is large. With regard to stress at work, the National Council of Compensation Insurance indicates compensation claims for stress-related disorders are growing while all other disabling work injuries are decreasing [1]. Stress may contribute to the development of heart and cerebrovascular disease, hypertension, peptic ulcer and inflammatory bowel diseases, and musculoskeletal problems [2, 3, 4]. Recent evidence suggests that stress alters immune function, possibly facilitating the development of cancer [4, 5]. Anxiety, depression, neuroses, and alcohol and drug problems clearly are associated with stress [6, 7]. These latter conditions contribute to the incidence of accidents, homicide, and suicide. Considered together, all these disorders that are affected by stress are responsible for the great majority of mortality, morbidity, disability, and medical care use in the United States.

The etiologic contribution of stress to chronic health disorders has not been determined since most are complexly multifactorial and no consensus has developed on the measurement of stress. Although assessment of stress remains problematic, awareness of the role of stress in these conditions has increased during the past two decades. It is now generally recognized that stress plays an important role in the etiology of work-related disorders. The medical practitioner should be able to recognize stressful working conditions, to evaluate stress-related disorders, and to manage stress in the individual.

DEFINITION OF TERMS

The term *stress* is used in a number of ways: as an environmental condition, as an appraisal of an environmental condition, as a response to an environmental condition, and as a form of relationship between environmental demands and a person's abilities to meet the demands [2].

The first two uses are found in the popular literature where one reads that an environment is "full of stress" or a person experiences stress at home or work. The influence of this literature is demonstrated by recent studies of public beliefs about causes of heart attacks. The most frequently cited causes, ahead of accepted biologic risk factors, were "stress, worry, nervous tension, pressure." Unfortunately, these popular uses of *stress* are not specific enough to assist the medical practitioner in identifying and managing stress-related disorders.

The third use of *stress* as a response to an environmental condition is found widely in primary care medical literature and in the stress management literature. This definition is based on Selye's original concept of stress as "the nonspecific response of the body to any demand made upon it" [8]. Selye first conceived of the notion of biologic stress over 50 years ago. Within this paradigm, stress is a nonspecific neuroendocrine response related to the process of homeostasis. Identification of stress is tautologic—that is, stress is present whenever a stress response is observed. Furthermore, stress can be either good (eustress) or bad (distress), depending on whether the adaptive response is overwhelmed and homeostasis is no longer achieved. The Selye definition of stress has much utility for the general management of stress, but it has not proven to be useful for the evaluation of occupational stress. In particular, the definition of stress as a nonspecific response has tended to obviate the need to identify environmental factors responsible for stress. Consequently, stress management programs have emphasized strategies to increase adaptive resources, rather than to decrease causes of stress.

Notwithstanding the general popularity of the Selye definition, the most common definition among stress researchers is the fourth definition, in which stress is seen as arising at the interface between the environment and the person. McGrath's definition of stress as "a (perceived) substantial imbalance between demand and response capability, under conditions where failure to meet demand has important (perceived) consequences" is the most widely cited [9]. This definition differs from that of Selye in that stress is (1) a function of both the environment and the person and must be evaluated in regard to both; (2) fundamentally a psychosocial as well as a biologic phenomenon linked to the perceptions of the individual; and (3) an undesirable phenomenon (what Selye would call "distress"). Constructive adaptation of workers to environmental challenges is not typically considered stress and is subsumed within the notion of "quality of working life."

Despite continuing ambiguity about the term *stress*, general agreement has been reached about related terms (see box). Thus, "stressors" interact

---

DEFINITIONS RELATED TO STRESS

Stress   A (perceived) substantial imbalance between demand and response capability under conditions where failure to meet demand has important (perceived) consequences [9]. Alternatively, many clinicians define *stress* more generally as a rubric encompassing the sequence from stressors to stress reactions and long-term consequences.

Stressor   Environmental event or condition that results in stress.

Stressful   Pertaining to an environment that has many stressors.

Strain (or stress reaction)   Short-term physiologic, psychologic, or behavioral manifestations of stress.

Modifier   Individual characteristic or environmental factor that may act on each stage of the stress response to produce individual variation.

with the individual to cause "strain" or short-term stress reactions. Unresolved stress reactions lead to stress-related disorders. "Modifiers" are factors that can act on each stage of the stress response to produce individual variation in the sequence from stressors to stress reactions to long-term consequences.

CONCEPTUALIZATION OF STRESS

The complexity of the stress phenomenon has defied attempts at concise conceptualization. The most common approach has been for investigators to provide an enumeration of environmental factors that are considered to be stressors. These factors include objective conditions, such as overtime, shift work, and unemployment, and subjective job attributes, such as overload, role conflict, and role ambiguity. Many of the subjective attributes were obtained through post hoc analysis of responses to questionnaires. Although initial questions may have been based on psychologic or sociologic precepts, the resultant constructs often have not reflected the theoretical precepts. In addition, labels for the constructs have tended to be used by different investigators in reference to different assessment instruments. Thus, for example, "role ambiguity" reported by one investigator may not be based on the same questions as "role ambiguity" reported by other investigators. This confusion over conceptual definition of stressors has contributed to the inconsistent results reported in the stress research literature. It also makes it difficult for the medical practitioner to place much reliance on any particular stress management instrument.

Some investigators have presented enumerations of stressors with conceptual groupings. For example, McGrath groups stressors into task, role, behavior setting, physical environment, social environment, and personal characteristics [9]. Shostak lists the major stressors among blue-collar workers to be anxieties over job loss, safety and health risk, and self-esteem erosion [10]. These groupings may be useful to the practitioner in pro-

viding a framework for evaluation of potential stressors. This approach is used below to review recognized stressors.

Other investigators have attempted to define the essential characteristics of stressful work. A notable example is the list provided by Kasl: (1) the stressful work condition tends to be chronic rather than intermittent or self-limiting; (2) there is external pacing of work demands, such as that created by machines, payment mechanisms, or competition; (3) habituation or adaptation to the chronic situation is difficult and, instead, some form of vigilance or arousal must be maintained; (4) failure to meet demands leads to drastic consequences (regarding equipment, lives, and money); and (5) there is a "spillover" effect of the work role to other areas of functioning (such as family and leisure) so that daily impact of the demanding job situation becomes cumulative and health threatening, rather than being defused or eased daily [4]. Kasl cites the jobs of air-traffic controllers, sea pilots, and train dispatchers as prototypes.

Two models have been developed that attempt to conceptualize the etiologic dynamics of stress: the Person-Environment (PE) fit model and the Job Demands-Control (JD-C) model. Both models are based on McGrath's concept of imbalance between the environment and the person. These models have the greatest influence on current occupational stress research.

Person-Environment Fit Model

The PE fit model posits that strain develops when there is a discrepancy (1) between the demands of the job and the abilities of the person to meet those demands (demand-ability dimension), or (2) between the motives of the person and the environmental supplies to satisfy the person's motives (motive-supply dimension) [6, 11]. Demands include workload and job complexity. Motives include income, participation, and skill-utilization. Supplies refer to whether the job, for example, provides sufficient income to satisfy the motives of the individual. The model distinguishes the *objec-*

tive environment and person from the *subjective* environment and person, where subjective refers to the perceptions of the individual. It assumes that strain arises due to poor fit between the sub-

jective person and subjective environment (Fig. 20-1).

According to the model, strain results from an excess in demands over abilities. An excess of abil-

Fig. 20-1. The Person-Environment fit model indicating that strain results from the fit between the subjective person and the subjective environment. (From R Van Harrison. Person-environment fit and job stress. In CL Cooper and R Payne eds. Stress at work. Chichester: Wiley, 1978. Reprinted with permission of John Wiley & Sons Inc.)

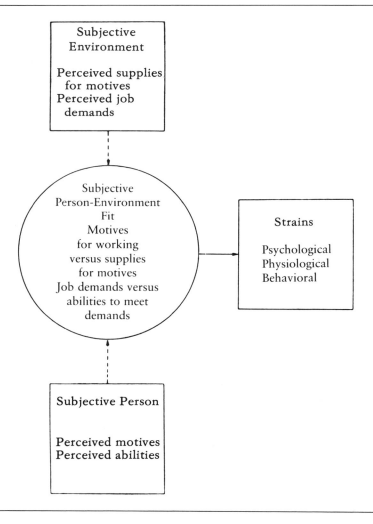

ities over demands may result in no change in the level of strain, decreased strain, or increased strain. On the motive-supply dimension, strain results from insufficient supplies for motives. Excess supplies for motives may result in no change in the level of strain, decreased strain, or increased strain. The unpredictability of strain outcomes when abilities exceed demands and when supplies exceed motives is that misfit on these dimensions may create misfit on other relevant dimensions. For example, an excess of ability may lead to important motives, such as the need for skill-utilization. When this need is not being met, strain may increase.

A difficulty with the PE fit model is its limited utility for predicting what objective work conditions are likely to result in stress [2, 12]. The model states that stress may result from a misfit between the person and the environment in either direction of two possible dimensions, but the relationship between the dimensions of the model has not been clarified. Also since interpretation of stressors is subjective, stress becomes a function primarily of individual perceptions. A strength of the model is its emphasis on the need for flexibility in job design and consideration of workers as individuals with varying abilities, motives, and perceptions.

A major test of the PE fit model was a cross-sectional evaluation of 2,010 workers in 23 occupations [6, 11]. PE fit was assessed by asking questions about environmental stressors and then questions about preferences on the stressors. Misfit was the amount of difference between the scaled responses to the paired questions. The investigators found clear differences in the degree of PE fit across occupations. Quantitative workload was highest for family physicians, administrative professors, and train dispatchers. Demand for concentration was high for air-traffic controllers, train dispatchers, and family physicians but low for machine-paced assembly-line workers. Several job stressors tended to have similar levels in any given job: low utilization of abilities, low participation, and low complexity. The occupations highest on

these stressors were assembly-line workers, forklift drivers, and machine tenders. The investigators concluded that "assemblers and relief workers on the machine-paced assembly lines have the highest stress and strain of any of the 23 occupations." While the model emphasizes subjective misfit between person and environment, the systematic differences in fit between occupations suggest that the work environment was a significant source of the perceived misfit.

Job Demands-Control Model

The JD-C model views strain as arising primarily due to the characteristics of work. It states that strain arises due to an imbalance between demands and decision latitude (control) in the workplace, where lack of control is seen as an environmental constraint on response capabilities [13, 14]. Job demands and decision latitude represent the instigators of action and the constraints on alternative resulting actions, respectively. If no or inadequate actions can be taken, the unreleased stress will result in strain (Fig. 20-2). This model is consistent with the McGrath definition of PE fit model, but the emphasis is on control since most

Fig. 20-2. The Job Demand-Control model indicating the combined effects of job demands and decision latitude on strain. (From DB Baker. The study of stress at work. Reproduced, with permission, from *Ann. Rev. Public Health* 6:367. © 1985 by Annual Reviews Inc.)

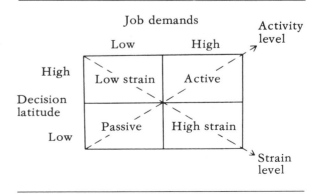

workers are physically and intellectually capable of responding to demands arising in the workplace. Thus, most imbalance between demands and response capabilities is due to environmental constraints on response capabilities.

The JD-C model characterizes jobs by their combination of demands and control. Jobs with high demands and low control, such as those of waiters, video display terminal operators, and machine-paced assemblers, will result in strain. These characteristics are found typically in occupations with a high division of labor and deskilling of tasks. Studies using the JD-C model have demonstrated significant associations between job demands, decision latitude, and strain [3, 14]. In general, investigators have concluded that decision latitude acts both as a modifier of demands and as an independent risk factor for strain. The amount of control over the job is now recognized as a decisive factor in the development of occupational stress.

The PE fit and JD-C models provide a conceptual framework for understanding the dynamics of the stress process. Research is underway to test and refine these models further. In the meantime, the medical practitioner is faced with the need to identify and manage stress-related disorders in individuals. Such practical matters necessitate that we return to a more pragmatic presentation of the stress process.

COMPONENTS OF THE STRESS PROCESS

Major components of the stress process include stressors, stress responses (strain) and long-term outcomes, and modifiers of the stress process (Table 20-1). The causal linkages between these components are dynamic and complex. Although epidemiologic studies of large populations have been able to demonstrate some specificity in associations between stressors and stress responses, it is not possible to determine specific etiologic relationships between stressors and health effects for

Table 20-1. Components of the stress process

Stressors
  Job structure—overtime, shiftwork, machine pacing, piecework
  Job content—quantitative overload, qualitative underload, lack of control
  Physical conditions—unpleasant, threat of physical or toxic hazard
  Organization—role ambiguity, role conflict, competition and rivalry
  Extra-organizational—job insecurity, career development, commuting
  Other sources—personal, family, community
Outcomes
  Physiologic:
    Short-term—catecholamines, cortisol, blood pressure increases
    Long-term—hypertension, heart disease, ulcers, asthma
  Psychologic (cognitive and affective):
    Short-term—anxiety, dissatisfaction, mass psychogenic illness
    Long-term—depression, burnout, mental disorders
  Behavioral:
    Short-term—job (absenteeism, reduced productivity and participation), community (decreased friendships and participation), personal (excessive use of alcohol and drugs, smoking)
    Long-term—"learned helplessness"
Modifiers
  Individual—behavioral style and personal resources
  Social support—emotional, value or self-esteem, and informational

one individual or in a small group of workers. One cannot analytically separate the effects of many coexisting stressors when examining one or a few individuals. Thus, from a practical clinical perspective, the relationship between stressors and health outcomes is nonspecific. The medical practitioner only can assess the presence of stressors and stress responses and make a judgment as to the likelihood that the former caused the latter.

Stressors

Stressors may be divided into those relating to the individual's job (structure, content, and physical conditions), to the organization (role, structure, and interpersonal relations), and to extra-organizational factors.

Job Structure. Job structure stressors include the amount and scheduling of work hours and the objective structure of the job. Several studies have reported associations between working excessive hours or holding down more than one full-time job and coronary heart disease morbidity and mortality [2, 15]. Lack of control over work hours exacerbates this stressor; required overtime has been associated with low job satisfaction and indices of poor mental health.

Substantial evidence indicates that the temporal scheduling of work can have a significant impact on physical, psychologic, behavioral, and social well-being. Shift work exists when a facility has working periods other than the normal day shift. Workers may stay on fixed shifts or rotate through shifts. Over one-fourth of workers in the United States work on shifts. Rotating shift and permanent night work, in particular, have been linked to a variety of disturbances [16]. Major complaints include sleep disturbances, nervous troubles, and disturbances of the alimentary tract. Shift workers also have disruptions in their family and social lives.

A primary structural factor is whether the work pace is controlled by the individual or is externally determined. Machine pacing is when the pace of the operation and the work output are controlled to some extent by a source other than the operator. There are numerous varieties of pacing systems that require different amounts of cognitive and motor activity from the workers. In general, this work presents a deleterious combination of short-interval demands with lack of control. It requires vigilance, yet it is monotonous and repetitive. Research has indicated that machine-paced assembly-line work is highly stressful [6, 13, 17] (Fig. 20-3).

Piecework is when the worker's remuneration is based on the quantity of products produced. This system has been shown to induce stress responses similar to those of machine pacing. Individuals on piecework may increase their work pace even to the point of discomfort. For example, one study found that when invoicing clerks were put on piecework, as opposed to their usual hourly rate, they doubled their work rate but also increased their urinary epinephrine and norepinephrine levels by about one-third.

Job Content. Job content has been a central focus of stress research. Gardell suggests three groupings of task characteristics: (1) quantitative overload (too much to do, time pressure or deadlines, repetitious fast-cycle work flow); (2) qualitative underload (too narrow job content, lack of stimulus variation, and no demands on creativity or problem solving); and (3) lack of control, especially in relation to pace and work methods [15]. Although these task characteristics are generally thought to relate only to industrial assembly lines, modern office environments share many of them (Fig. 20-4). Lack of control can lead to the paradoxical situation where a worker simultaneously experiences both quantitative overload and qualitative underload. Labels vary somewhat among investigators, but these characteristics consistently have been shown to be stressors.

Changes in job content also may be a source of stress. Transfers, demotions, and even promotions can be stressful. The potential for change to act as a stressor is affected by the predictability of the event and the control the individual or work group has over the transition process.

Physical Conditions. Unpleasant working conditions include improper lighting, excessive noise, inadequate work space, depressing surroundings, and unsanitary conditions. Investigators have found poor mental health to be associated with unpleasant working conditions [4]. Investigations of complaints among office workers have found

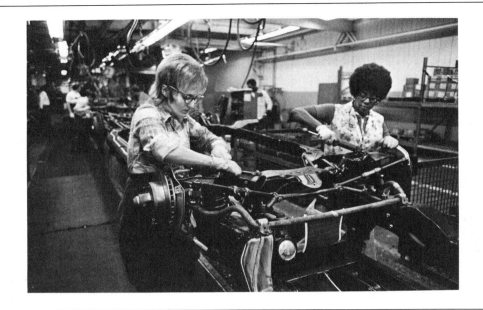

Fig. 20-3. Assembly line workers have machine-paced jobs in a fractionated and dehumanizing work environment.
(Photograph by Earl Dotter.)

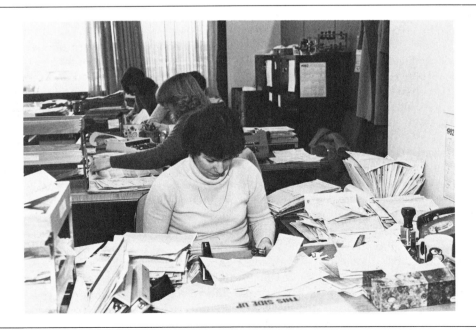

Fig. 20-4. Secretaries are among the most highly stressed workers.
(Photograph by Marilee Caliendo.)

that uncomfortable work stations, crowding, and inadequate ventilation and temperature control are associated with stress responses.

Noise causes physiologic stress reactions at levels below those that lead to hearing loss. It is difficult to study the effect of noise per se since one cannot separate noise from an individual's interpretation of the sound. Nevertheless, it is clear that control over the noise source can modify the stress response. A laboratory study showed that the perception of an ability to control noise eliminated the adverse effects of unpredictable high-intensity noise on task performance, even though none of the subjects ever actually exercised the option of turning off the noise [18].

The threat of physical or toxic hazard can act as a stressor. Certain workers have an increased risk of physical danger; these include police, mine workers, and fire fighters. Chronic stress reaction among workers in these types of occupations is well recognized. Other studies have revealed that among workers in the trade and service sectors the potential for abuse or violence from clients is a significant source of stress. However, stress induced by the uncertainty of physical danger is substantially relieved if the worker feels adequately trained and equipped to cope with emergency situations.

For each of these work-condition stressors, it appears that increased control over the condition ameliorates the stress response. Thus, the demand-control paradigm applies to physical conditions as well as to job content.

Organization. Work is a social process that occurs within an organization (see Chap. 2). Major organizational stressors include role in the organization, organizational structure, and interpersonal relationships. Role ambiguity results from lack of clarity concerning the requirements of the job; the worker does not know the objectives, scope, and responsibilities of the job. Studies have indicated that between 35 and 60 percent of workers are affected by role ambiguity [19]. This stressor may lead to job dissatisfaction, feelings of tension, and lowered self-confidence. Role conflict occurs when conflicting demands are made on the worker by different groups in the organization or when the worker is required to do work that he or she dislikes or believes to be outside of the requirements of the job. One survey indicated that 48 percent of workers in the United States are affected by role conflict [19].

Large organizations with a "flat" structure (relatively few job levels) are associated with greater job dissatisfaction, absenteeism, and accidents. Jobs at the boundaries of organizations have increased stress. For example, a supervisor who is at the interface between union and management, could be considered in a boundary job. Elevated rates of peptic ulcer disease and, in some industries, of heart disease have been demonstrated in supervisors.

Competition and rivalry are sources of stress for many workers. Poor work relationships are "those which include low trust, low supportiveness, and low interest in listening to and trying to deal with problems that confront the organizational member" [20]. Conflict tends to occur when inadequate information is provided to designate responsibilities, job roles, and the means of carrying them out. Poor interpersonal relationships can have a debilitating effect, not only on individuals, but also on the organization.

Extra-Organizational Stressors. Extra-organizational stressors are factors that are related to work but extend beyond the specific job or organization. These stressors include factors related to career and commuting.

Several conditions associated with career development or job future (lack of job security, under-promotion, overpromotion, and fear of job obsolescence) have been related to adverse behavioral problems, psychologic effects, and poor physical health. Lack of job security is a primary stressor for many workers. In the evaluation of career as a stressor, anticipated changes associated with the stage of the worker's career must be considered. Lack of change may be a stressor if it represents

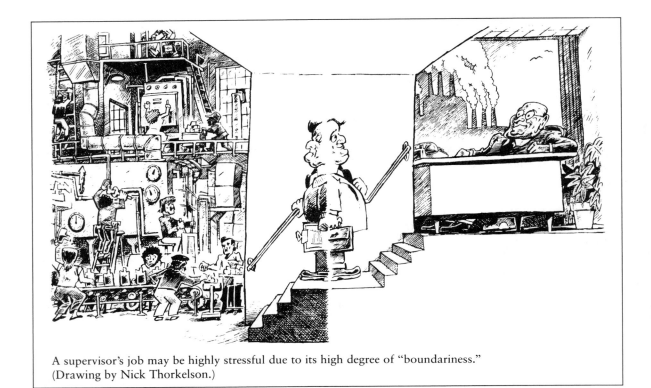

A supervisor's job may be highly stressful due to its high degree of "boundariness." (Drawing by Nick Thorkelson.)

thwarted ambition or "inadequate forward mechanisms" (that is, personal recognition, promotion, or financial return). Retirement can be a stressor. This anticipated change is modified to the extent that the individual requires work for self-image and has potential for constructive activity outside of work. Stress reactions may begin long before retirement.

An evaluation of work stress also must consider sources of stress related to preparing for and going to and from work. In many cities, commuting can be an arduous task taking as long as 3 hours daily. Among shift workers, public transportation may not be provided late in the evening or at night.

Sources Other Than Work. Finally, sources of stress other than work must be considered in an evaluation of the stress process. The boundary be-

tween work and non-work stressors is not distinct, and certainly they interact in causing stress responses. Personal, family, and community factors can be stressors. These potential sources of stress should be more familiar to the reader and are not reviewed in this chapter.

Outcomes
Stress responses can be divided into short-term reactions and long-term consequences. Long-term consequences develop following chronic, unresolved short-term reactions or "strain." Most investigators consider three major categories of stress responses: physiologic, psychologic, and behavioral. Effects on the organization should also be considered.

The multifactorial relationship between work stress and health outcomes has engendered some confusion among health professionals. Many practitioners confuse the concept of psychosocial factors as etiologic agents with the notion of work-related mental health. One should be clear that psychosocial *factors,* such as stress, may cause both psychological and physiological disorders. On the other hand, work-related psychological *disorders* may be caused by both psychosocial factors and toxic chemical exposures. Intoxication due to solvents and mood disturbances due to chronic mercury poisoning are examples of the latter.

Physiologic. Work-related stressors have been shown to induce a variety of short-term physiologic reactions. Much of this work derives from Selye's initial concept of stress as a neurendocrine response. A classic example is a study that demonstrated that serum cholesterol increases and blood coagulation accelerates among tax accountants as tax deadlines approach [21].

Substantial advances in understanding have occurred in recent years as telemetry and biochemical measurement techniques have evolved [3]. Bioelectric measures of stress reactions include the heart rate and rhythm, electromyogram, and galvanic skin response. Increases in galvanic skin response were found to be a sensitive index to behavioral changes related to boredom, fatigue, and monotony. Biochemical measures include catecholamines, corticosteroids (such as cortisol), cholesterol, uric acid, free fatty acids, glucose, thyroxin, and growth hormone. Measurement of metabolites of the catecholamines and corticosteroids in the blood and urine has received much attention in the past few years. It is now possible to demonstrate short-term physiologic responses to work stressors. The significance of these short-term responses for chronic health outcomes remains to be determined, although the relationship makes intuitive sense.

The chronic pathophysiologic effects of stress are generally considered within the rubric of psychosomatic disorders. Depending on one's perspective, this category may be as narrow as including only headache and gastritis or may encompass such diseases as hypertension, cardiovascular disease, ulcers, asthma, and musculoskeletal disorders. Unfortunately, the label *psychosomatic* has developed the deprecatory connotation of being unreal and probably should be avoided. Some researchers have suggested replacing the term *psychosomatic* with *psychophysiologic.* In any case, the association between work stress and this group of health outcomes is strongly suggestive but difficult to prove in cause-effect terms.

Much research has focused on the potential effect of stress on coronary heart disease [2, 3]. However, methodologic limitations have made it difficult to quantify the contribution of stress. Some experts have concluded that the ambiguity of earlier research may be traced to incomplete models of stress that did not evaluate the role of job control [13]. Recent studies based on the JD-C model have shown significant associations between high-strain (high-demand, low-control) occupations and subsequent development of angina pectoris and myocardial infarction after analytically controlling for other potential risk factors such as age, smoking, education, and obesity [14].

Psychological. A large body of research has demonstrated the association between job stress and adverse short-term psychological effects, including anxiety, situational depression, and job dissatisfaction [2]. Association with chronic mental illness is not as well documented.

Causes of depression and job dissatisfaction follow the predictions of the PE fit and JD-C models. Among blue-collar workers, major stressors tend to be lack of job complexity, role ambiguity, and job insecurity. Particularly among clerical and service workers, low self-esteem arises due to lack of respect from supervisors. For white-collar workers, major stressors are responsibility for people, high job complexity, and high and variable workload.

Behavioral. Short-term behavioral responses to stress include deleterious personal behaviors such as escapist alcohol drinking and increased tobacco and drug use. Quantitative workload has been directly associated with cigarette smoking and an inability to quit smoking. It also has been related to escapist drinking, absenteeism, low work motivation, lowered self-esteem, and lack of interest in contributing suggestions to management.

The work organization also is affected. Deleterious personal behaviors, such as absenteeism, alcoholism, and accidents, have a negative impact on the organization. Stress decreases productivity through reduced output, production delays, and poor work quality, which leads to lost time, equipment breakdown, and wasted material. Poor morale can lead to labor unrest, excessive number of grievances, sabotage, and increased turnover. Thus, both the individual and the organization suffer from the manifestations of job stress.

The long-term behavioral manifestations of job stress include what Seligman has referred to as "learned helplessness" [13, 15]. In essence, the individual gives up on the possibility of controlling one's own destiny. This attitude leads to escapism and passive behavior. Studies based on the JD-C model have shown that workers with little control at work eventually become passive at home and in their community, with decreased participation in union, recreation, social, and religious activities.

Specific Stress-Related Disorders. For the effects just described, job stress is one of multiple factors in the etiology of the conditions. For some disorders, stress is recognized as the primary etiologic agent; examples include burnout, post-traumatic stress disorder, and mass psychogenic illness.

Burnout is a phenomenon that has been recognized mostly in professional settings, although it can affect any worker [22]. It may occur after years of high-quality performance when the individual suddenly seems unable to perform work. Behavioral manifestations include decreases in efficiency and initiative, diminished interest in work, and an inability to maintain work performance. Symptoms characterizing the syndrome are fatigue, intestinal disturbances, sleeplessness, depression, and shortness of breath. Other symptoms include irritability, decrease in frustration tolerance, blunting of affect, suspiciousness, feelings of helplessness, and increased risk taking. There is a tendency to self-medicate with tranquilizers, narcotics, and alcohol, all of which may lead to addiction. When away from the job, the individual is unable to relax and often reports giving up recreation and social contacts.

Burnout does not emerge spontaneously; it progresses in stages beginning during the initial stages of employment. Because burnout-prone individuals often start out as enthusiastic overachievers, the organization tends to heap more and more responsibilities on them. Failure to recognize the connection between constant overachievement and burnout and to exercise proper preventive measures can lead to an exhausted workforce whose achievements, desires, and creative talents are defunct [22].

Post-traumatic stress disorder (PTSD) is a specific anxiety disorder that occurs following a stressful or traumatic event [23]. The disorder may occur among workers who have had occupational toxic exposure or injury. Any situation that evokes feelings of intense fear, helplessness, loss of control, or annihilation may precipitate the disorder. The trauma may be massive and discrete like an accident or may be comprised of episodes of exposure to a dangerous chemical or work process. The cardinal feature is repeated reexperiencing of the traumatic event. Typically, any stimulus that resembles the initial event will evoke the reexperience of the event. Patients may believe they are allergic to everything. Other symptoms include emotional blunting, detachment from others, sleep disturbances, and trouble concentrating. The recurrent symptoms and anxiety experienced by individuals with PTSD may be disabling. It is important to recognize the psychologic effect of the initial trauma to avoid costly, unnecessary, and sometimes reinforcing medical diagnostic evaluations.

Mass psychogenic illness is the label applied to

apparent group anxiety reactions in industrial establishments [24]. A number of workers simultaneously become ill at the worksite. As rumors of the illness spread through the plant, worker anxiety and general confusion may escalate to such an extent that it becomes necessary to close the facility. The outbreak usually is triggered by a physical stimulus, such as an odor, that the workers believe to be harmful. Specific symptoms may vary across incidents, but typically consist of somatic complaints, such as headache, nausea, and chills. Evaluation of these outbreaks is difficult because specific complaints often have resolved by the time an investigative team can reach the site. Studies have indicated that these outbreaks tend to occur among industrial workers who experience substantial underlying psychosocial stressors and physical strain. The triggering event is the last straw that exhausts the adaptive resources of the individuals and organization. Treatment involves demonstrating that the triggering event does not represent an ongoing risk and reducing the level of underlying stressors (see Chap. 25).

Modifiers

The association between stressors and stress responses is modified by characteristics of the individual and the environment. This notion is intrinsic to all models of psychosocial stress. Stressors, individual characteristics, and social environment are specific instances of the generally recognized medical triad: agent, host, and environment.

Individual. Individual characteristics that affect vulnerability to stressors include emotional stability, conformity (versus innerdirectedness), rigidity (versus flexibility), achievement orientation, and behavioral style. A behavioral style that has received much attention as a risk factor for coronary heart disease is the type A, coronary-prone behavior, characterized by a sense of competitiveness, time urgency, and overcommitment [25]. Despite substantial research since Friedman and Rosenman originated the concept two decades ago, no one has been able to identify and reliably measure the precise aspects of the type A behavior pattern that engender the heart disease risk.

An unfortunate side effect of the research on type A is that it has tended to focus attention on individual vulnerability rather than on environment stressors. In fact, occupational stress does not affect an identifiable subpopulation of vulnerable individuals (for example, as one might say for atopic individuals who are exposed to some workplace allergens). Thus, the primary prevention strategy should be the identification and reduction of environmental stressors and not the identification, treatment or removal of possibly vulnerable individuals.

Environment. Many investigators have concluded that the most important factor ameliorating the stress response is social support. Social support includes emotional, informational, and instrumental support. Emotional support and understanding lead workers to believe they are cared for and valued, and belong to a network of communication and mutual obligation. Informational support depends on the clarity and effectiveness of communication patterns in the organization. Instrumental support includes such factors as having adequate instructions and tools to complete the task. A large amount of research has demonstrated that social support can reduce the adverse health effects of stress [4, 26]. A prime strategy of stress management is to encourage and develop supportive networks on the job.

MANAGEMENT OF STRESS

The phrase *stress management* typically denotes worksite programs that address employee stress; however, management of work stress should occur in multiple settings, including the medical office or clinic. A comprehensive approach should encompass assessment, treatment, and prevention of stress in the individual worker, family, and organization. This effort requires the expertise of a multidisciplinary team of professionals working in a variety of settings. Stress management should be

Table 20-2. Approaches to the prevention and control of stress

Treat the individual:
  Medical treatment—hypertension, backache, depression
  Counseling services
  Employee assistance programs—alcohol, drugs
Reduce individual vulnerability:
  Counseling—individual, group programs
  Training programs—relaxation, meditation, biofeedback
  General support—exercise programs, recreational activities
Treat the organization:
  Diagnosis—attitude surveys, rap sessions
  Develop flexible and responsive management style
  Improve internal communications
Reduce organizational stress:
  Variable work schedules
  Job restructuring—enlargement, enrichment, increased control
  Supervisor training and management development

Source: Adapted from JJ Warshaw. Managing stress. In LW Krinsky, SN Kieffer, PA Carone, et al. eds. Stress and productivity. New York: Human Sciences, 1984:15–30.

considered in this broader sense. Table 20-2 provides an overview of stress management approaches.

Principles
While any effort to ameliorate stress will have some beneficial effect, certain strategies are more likely to lead to long-term success. Programs should view prevention and stress control as a shared responsibility between the health professional, worker, and organization. In the past, program approaches have covered the range from "stress is a personal problem" to superpaternalism [27]. Neither extreme has achieved lasting success. Rather, programs should develop a balance between requiring some responsibility for self-help, while providing a variety of support mechanisms. All parties should work together to identify and control stressors.

Effective control of stress requires an appreciation of the dynamic, multifactorial nature of stress. Programs should take an ecologic systems approach that recognizes the inherent interrelationship of physical, biologic, chemical, psychologic, and social factors in the determination of health status. In particular, it is inappropriate to dichotomize etiologic factors into "toxic" or "psychosocial" and relegate the latter to a secondary level of consideration. One must be aware that potential stressors range from the microenvironment of the individual work station to the broad socioeconomic context of the work organization. Assessment (as described below) requires parallel consideration of multiple stressors since it is unlikely that any one stressor would be a sufficient etiologic agent. Assessment of interaction among factors is even more critical than for other workplace exposures. Since stress is a dynamic process, stress management must be a continuous cycle of assessment, intervention (treatment and prevention), and evaluation of the intervention. Control of stress requires ongoing feedback from the individual and the organization.

Long-term prevention strategies should be based on an understanding of the etiology of stress. The PE fit model suggests that every job must be designed to supply rewards at the same time it presents demands. The balance between motives-supplies and demands-abilities may be particular for each worker. Thus job requirements and stress management efforts should be flexible and individualized. The JD-C model demonstrates that the fundamental source of imbalance between the person and the work environment is due to environmental constraints on the worker. Ultimately, primary prevention strategies must be directed toward modification of stressors in the environment, and in particular, increasing the control workers have over their work environment.

A statement of principles for control of stress based on these precepts is worth noting. The National Institute for Occupational Safety and Health (NIOSH) recently presented its proposed national strategy for the prevention of work-re-

Table 20-3. Recommendations for job design proposed by NIOSH

Work schedule— Work schedules should be designed to avoid conflicts with demands and responsibilities outside of the job. When rotating shift schedules are used, the rate of rotation should be stable and predictable.

Participation/control—Workers should be able to provide input to decisions or actions affecting their jobs and the performance of their tasks.

Workload—Demands should be commensurate with the capabilities and resources of individuals. Work should be designed to allow recovery from demanding physical or mental tasks.

Content—Work tasks should be designed to provide meaning, stimulation, a sense of completeness, and an opportunity for the use of skills.

Work roles—Roles and responsibilities at work should be well defined.

Social environment—Opportunities should be available for social interaction, including emotional support and actual help as needed in accomplishing tasks.

Job future—Ambiguity should be avoided in matters of job security and career development opportunities.

Source: National Institute for Occupational Safety and Health. A proposed national strategy for the prevention of work-related psychological disorders (draft). Cincinnati: NIOSH, October 1986.

lated psychologic disorders [7]. In the proposal, a committee of experts recommended that the Occupational Safety and Health Administration (OSHA) mandate guidelines for job design (Table 20-3). The report also recommended improved government and industry surveillance of work-related stressors and disorders; improved training of workers, managers, and health professionals; and enrichment of mental health components of industry health services. The report concluded, "In general, psychological health services need to evolve to a higher state of awareness and practice, exploiting methods offering a more holistic view of the workers, sorting out occupational as well as nonoccupational factors that are influential to health, and offering opportunities for individual-

ized interventions" [7]. This NIOSH statement of principles should guide the manager and health professional in developing a strategy for the control of work stress.

Assessment

The initial step in the prevention and control of stress is an assessment of potential stressors, stress reactions, and modifiers. For many factors, there are no indicators that can be measured by purely objective methods, and this is not even needed. Subjective indicators are indispensable for identifying components of the stress process. Both objective and subjective indicators should be collected simultaneously.

Measuring Stressors. Evaluation of physical and chemical agents should include environmental measurement and toxicologic assessment together with an assessment of psychosocial impact. Knowledge of workplace exposures is an important aid in the interpretation of psychosocial stressors. Questionnaires or interviews should be used to determine whether the workers perceive the existence of the hazards and to what extent they are concerned about their effects.

Analysis of the work environment should include monitoring of tasks and work organization. Sources of information other than the workers may be used after these indicators have been demonstrated to predict stressors reliably. Examples include objective descriptions of job structure (such as overtime, shift work, and machine pacing), task analysis, and organizational structure. Since perceptions of workers must be taken into account, the assessment should include a questionnaire or interview with them. Structured questionnaires are available to assess task and organizational characteristics. A Job Content Survey (JCS) based on the JD-C model has been developed and validated [28].

The JCS was designed to measure the "content" of a respondent's work task in a general manner that is applicable to all jobs and jobholders. Primary scales based on defined combinations of questions are used to measure the JD-C model of stress, but other aspects of work (such as physical workload, job insecurity, and social interaction on the job) and the individual can be assessed. The instrument comes in several-length formats, ranging upward from the minimum "core" of 27 questions and the recommended standard instrument of 50 questions. Approximately 60 percent of the questions were derived from the U.S. Department of Labor's Quality of Work Surveys of 1969, 1972, and 1977. Use of these questions has allowed the generation of nationally standardized scales for comparison with small study populations.

Measuring Stress Reactions and Health Outcomes. Practically, assessment of stress effects must be based on diagnostic skills already familiar to the health professional. Many of the more specific and reliable stress diagnostic instruments developed in recent years remain too expensive or time consuming to be of practical use outside of the research setting. Examples include measurement of urinary metabolites of catecholamines, galvanic skin response, or mental health status using extensive structured-interview instruments [3, 29]. The medical practitioner may have to make a diagnosis based on the results of several nonspecific but accessible indicators, rather than relying on the results of one definitive test.

A minimum assessment should include the following observations: (1) complaints of "distress"—symptoms and motivation related to work conditions; (2) emotional reactions—anxiety, depression, and other reactions; (3) cognitive function and work performance—psychometric testing and performance evaluations at work; (4) behavioral changes—such as sleep disturbances and drug and alcohol use; (5) physiologic function—such as heart rate, blood pressure and serum cholesterol; and (6) symptoms and diseases that may be due to stress. One also should consider behavioral characteristics that may affect suscepti-

bility or resistance and the worker's family, community, and cultural environment.

Diagnosis. The large number and complexity of factors involved in the stress process virtually preclude exhaustive documentation of each factor using definitive instruments. There is no simple yet comprehensive instrument for measuring stressors and stress reactions. Consequently, the medical practitioner must inventory the range of factors discussed above and ultimately make a judgment as to the likelihood that the identified stressors were responsible for the observed stress reactions. This judgment must take into consideration the following issues: (1) presence of potential workplace stressors; (2) presence of potential nonoccupational stressors; (3) physical, psychologic, and behavioral health status (consistency with known patterns of stress reactions); (4) presence of other accepted risk factors for observed health conditions; (5) individual characteristics and social factors that may affect vulnerability to stress; and (6) presence of similar health conditions among co-workers.

Stress Treatment and Prevention for the Individual

Control of stress involves treatment for individuals already suffering from stress, identification and secondary prevention for individuals who demonstrate early stress reactions, and prevention through reducing individual vulnerability and increasing social support. Treatment of clinically apparent stress effects follows the traditional medical model as in the treatment of, for example, hypertension, depression, or excessive use of alcohol. At the same time, it is necessary to reduce exposure to stressors and increase individual resistance in order to prevent future sequelae.

Efforts to reduce individual vulnerability can take place individually in the practitioner's office or through group counseling, courses, and workshops. The common denominators of successful programs include: (1) training in self-awareness and problem analysis so that the individual is better able to detect signs of increasing stress and to identify the stressors that may be producing it; (2) assertiveness to become more dynamic in controlling stressors; and (3) techniques that will reduce the stress to more tolerable levels [27]. Examples of the latter include meditation, relaxation programs, exercise programs, and biofeedback. The following components for teaching individual control of stress have been recommended (adapted from reference 22):

1. Increasing awareness of particular stressors that cause distress.
2. Teaching how to avoid unnecessary stressors.
3. Teaching how to react more positively to unavoidable stressors.
4. Demonstrating and providing practice in techniques to reduce the physical and psychologic effects of stress.
5. Pointing out how to minimize dysfunctional coping responses and maximize those that tend to help achieve personal equilibrium, such as dealing with the problem head-on but with a constructive attitude and rethinking the problem carefully to see new possible solutions.

These approaches have been implemented most widely for white-collar workers, although the basic principles apply to blue-collar workers as well. Teaching styles and materials may need to be adapted for the educational level and past experiences of the individuals. A key first step is to introduce the program in a way that gains acceptance and motivates individuals to participate.

Control of Stress in the Organization
A 1985 survey by the United States Public Health Service revealed that nearly two-thirds of private worksites with 50 or more employees were supporting at least one health-promotion activity. More than one-fourth had stress management programs. The number of these programs is increasing rapidly. Thus, it is likely that many medical prac-

titioners will be asked to assist employers or unions in the development and implementation of these programs.

A three-step process for implementing a stress management program has been suggested. First, use a stress diagnostic test, such as worker attitude surveys that can provide information on stress levels and sources. An attitude survey may be counterproductive if it offers no feedback on the results of that survey and, even more important, if it is not followed by demonstrable actions to address some of the problems that are uncovered [27]. Second, once stress diagnoses have defined problem areas, top management must become involved in the effort to relieve worker stress, instituting and supporting corrective and preventive programs. Interventions may include developing variable work schedules, job restructuring (enlargement, rotation, and enrichment), supervisor training, management development, changing management style, improving internal communications, and encouraging organizational development. Some stress managers state that the most important strategy is to increase social support through the organization of cohesive work groups, development of improved communication patterns, and provision of recreational facilities for employees. Third, there should be an evaluation of the effort. Follow-up surveys permit comparison with baseline conditions.

Finally, the health professional may be asked to make a recommendation on which program should be implemented. One expert states that it does not really matter because all of the approaches will work, at least to some extent, and for a time [27]. Virtually every kind of program will provide some benefit to at least some of the people exposed to it. However, the correct approach is more complicated. Each organization must be treated as if it were a living system that has its own personality and vulnerability; it operates in a context of the industry, community, and society of which it is a part. Long-term success requires a true commitment from the organization to do something about stress and allocation of re-sources. The desires and characteristics of the workers and the types and severity of stress-related problems influence the type of program. The intensity and timing of the program may vary depending on whether the organization is in a short-term crisis situation, whether there is a high level of stress on a continuing basis, or whether there is a low level of stress most of the time. As with individual stress management, the process of assessment, intervention, and evaluation must be ongoing.

REFERENCES

1. National Council of Compensation Insurance. Emotional stress in the workplace—new legal rights in the eighties. New York: NCCI, 1985.
2. Kasl SV. Epidemiological contributions to the study of work stress. In: Cooper CL, Payne R, eds. Stress at work. Chichester, England: Wiley, 1978.
3. Sharit J, Salvendy G. Occupational stress: review and reappraisal. Hum Factors 1982; 24:129–62.
4. Kasl SV. Stress and health. Annu Rev Public Health 1984: 5:319–41.
5. Fox BH. Psychosocial factors and the immune system in human cancer. In: Adler R, ed. Psychoneuroimmunology, New York: Academic, 1981: 103–57.
6. Caplan RD et al. Job demands and worker health. Washington, D.C.: NIOSH, 1977. (Publication no. 75-160).
7. NIOSH. A proposed national strategy for the prevention of work-related psychological disorders (draft). Cincinnati: NIOSH, October 1986.
8. Selye H. The stress concept: past, present and future. In: Cooper CL, ed. Stress research issues for the eighties. Chichester, England: Wiley 1983: 1–20.
9. McGrath JE. A conceptual formulation for research on stress. In: McGrath JE, ed. Social and psychological factors in stress. New York: Holt, Rinehart, Winston, 1970: 22–40.
10. Shostak AB. Blue-collar stress. Reading, MA: Addison-Wesley, 1980.
11. French JR Jr, Caplan RD, Van Harrison R. The mechanisms of job stress and strain. Chichester, England: Wiley, 1982.
12. Baker DB. The study of stress at work. Annu Rev Public Health 1985; 6:367–81.
13. Karasek RA. Socialization and job strain: the implications of two related psychosocial mechanisms for job design. In: Gardell B, Johansson G, eds. Working life. London: Wiley, 1981.
14. Karasek RA, Baker DB, Marxer F, Ahlbom A, Theorell T. Job decision latitude, job demands, and coronary heart disease: a prospective study of Swedish men. Am J Public Health 1981; 71:694–705.
15. Gardell B. Scandinavian research on stress in working life. Int J Health Serv 1982; 12:31–41.
16. Maurice M. Shift work. Geneva: International Labour Office, 1975.
17. Salvendy G, Smith AJ. Machine pacing and occupational stress. London: Taylor & Francis, 1981.
18. Kryter KD. Non-auditory effects of environmental noise. Am J Public Health 1972; 62:389–98.
19. LaDou J. Occupational stress. In: Zenz C, ed. Developments in occupational medicine. Chicago: Yearbook, 1980: 197–210.
20. French JR Jr, Caplan RD. Organizational stress and individual strain. In: Manow AJ, ed. The failure of success. New York: AMACOM, 1973.
21. Friedman MD, Rosenman RD, Carrol V. Changes in serum cholesterol and blood clotting time in men subjected to cyclic variation of occupational stress. Circulation 1958; 17:852–61.
22. Fielding JF. Corporate health management. Reading, MA: Addison-Wesley, 1984: 309–31.
23. Schottenfeld RS, Cullen MR. Occupation-induced postraumatic stress disorder. Am J Psychiatry 1985; 142:198–202.
24. Colligan MJ, Murphy LR. Mass psychogenic illness in organizations: an overview. Occup Psychol 1979; 52:77.
25. Rosenman RH, Brand RJ, Sholtz RI, Friedman M. Multivariate prediction of coronary heart disease during 8.5 year follow-up in the Western Collaborative Group Study. Am Cardiol 1976; 37:903–10.
26. LaRocco JM, House JS, French JR Jr. Social support, occupational stress, and health. Health Soc Behav 1980; 21:202–18.
27. Warshaw JJ. Managing stress. In: Krinsky LW, Keiffer SN, Carone PA, Yolles SF, eds. Stress and productivity. New York: Human Sciences, 1984: 15–30.
28. Karasek RA, Gordon G, Pietrokovsky C et al. Job content instrument: questionnaire and user's guide. Los Angeles: University of Southern California, Department of Industrial and Systems Engineering, 1985.

29. Kalimo R. Assessment of occupational stress. In: Kaovonen M, Mikheev MI, eds. Epidemiology of occupational health. Copenhagen: WHO Regional Publications. 1986: 231–50. (European series no. 20).

BIBLIOGRAPHY

Addison-Wesley Series on Occupational Stress

This series of monographs, each written by an expert in the field, is oriented toward a general audience. Each book stands on its own as a review of an aspect of the stress phenomenon. The following titles are recommended:

House JS. Work stress and social support. Reading, MA: Addison-Wesley, 1981.
  A clear presentation on the role and importance of social support.
Levi L. Preventing work stress. Reading, MA: Addison-Wesley, 1981.
  Principles to prevent work stress as seen from the perspective of a leading researcher in Sweden; it discusses the relationship between work stress and social policy.
McLean A. Work stress. Reading, MA: Addison-Wesley, 1979.
  A simplified overall introduction to the topic by the editor of the series. Newer developments in stress research (such as the Job Demand-Control model) are not covered in the 1979 publication.
Warshaw LJ. Managing stress. Reading, MA: Addison-Wesley, 1979.
  This monograph provides an introduction to the principles and practice of stress management by a recognized expert.

Wiley Series on Studies in Occupational Stress

This is another series of monographs on occupational stress. These monographs tend to be more technical than the Addison-Wesley series but still provide an excellent source of material. Selected titles include:

Cooper CL, Payne R, eds. Stress at work. Chichester, England: Wiley, 1978.
  A collection of chapters reviewing research on work stress and role of person, environment, and person-environment fit.
Cooper CL, Payne R, eds. Current concerns in occupational stress. Chichester, England: Wiley, 1980.
Beech HR, Burns LE, Sheffield BF. A behavioral approach to the management of stress. Chichester, England: Wiley, 1981.
Cooper CL. Stress research: issues for the eighties. Chichester, England: Wiley, 1983.
  A collection of chapters by leading researchers covering topics such as the relationship between cancer and stress, type A behavior, and the Person-Environment Fit model. A chapter by Selye reviews his initial conceptualization of the stress phenomenon.
Krinsky LW, Kieffer SN, Carone PA, Yolles SF, eds. Stress and productivity. New York: Human Sciences, 1984.
  A collection of chapters based on a national conference on stress. Authors represent varying views, which provides for a broad overview. One volume in a series: Kieffer SN, ed. Problems of industrial psychiatric medicine New York: Human Sciences, 1984
Murphy LR, Schoenborn IF. Stress management in work settings. NIOSH Publication No. 87-111. Washington, DC: US Government Printing Office, 1987.
  A multiauthor report that summarizes scientific evidence and reviews conceptual and practical issues relating to worksite stress management.

IV
Occupational Disorders by System

21
Respiratory Disorders

David H. Wegman and David C. Christiani

A 60-year-old male, a sandblaster for 23 years, was hospitalized for the third time in the past 4 months for shortness of breath (SOB). Three years ago he began having respiratory problems, first mild SOB and increased heart rate when walking in snow and climbing steps and with heavy exertion at work. These symptoms increased moderately over the next several months. He was seen by the company physician, who told him that he had "bad lungs" but gave him no treatment. Two years ago he sought therapy at a community hospital due to increasing SOB while walking at normal speed on level ground for one to two blocks. He was hospitalized. Resting room-air arterial blood gases were PaO_2 = 87 and $PaCO_2$ = 31. A chest x-ray showed multiple interstitial nodules without evidence of hilar disease. Pulmonary function tests revealed a reduced forced vital capacity (73% of predicted) with normal diffusing capacity. Tuberculosis culture and cytology of bronchial washings were negative. The patient was sent home without therapy. He was told not to return to work; he has not worked since.

Seven months ago, he developed a cough occasionally productive of clear-to-grayish, thin sputum. Three more hospital admissions for increasing SOB occurred with no new findings reported. Since the last hospitalization, 1 month ago, he has been on oxygen continuously and stays in bed most of the day. He has also had dysuria and some trouble initiating his urinary stream, which seems to make his SOB worse.

The patient had smoked one pack of cigarettes per day for 5 years, until he quit 20 years ago. He has no history of asthma, pneumonia, surgery, or allergies.

Occupational history revealed a 23-year period of operating a sand-blasting machine located in a basement room (20 × 40 ft). Dust escaped continuously through crevices of the sandblasting unit; every time the patient opened the door to remove and install a piece to be blasted, much fine dust escaped. The windows were closed; there was an exhaust fan in the wall that did not seem to help. A room fan, installed to circulate the air in the room, was often out of order. The patient wore a helmet with a cloth apron on the bottom, covering his shoulders, and, when the room was especially dusty, a compressed air supply.

Physical examination revealed a slim male in moderate respiratory distress, sitting hunched over, gasping for breath, with grunting expirations. The pulse was 110, respiratory rate 40, blood pressure 110/80, and temperature 98° F. Pulmonary and cardiac exams were normal, except for a systolic ejection murmur and an increased second heart sound over the pulmonic area.

His extremities revealed clubbed fingernails and cyanosis. The rest of the exam was normal. Resting arterial blood gases on room air revealed PaO_2 = 39 and $PaCO_2$ = 38. Chest x-ray showed diffuse interstitial small rounded densities throughout both lung fields with hilar fullness. These were judged to be "q"-sized with a 2/2 profusion in all lung fields, using the International Labor Organization (ILO) nomenclature for chest x-rays. The diagnosis of silicosis was made. He remained completely disabled and died 3 months later.*

This case is characteristic of severe occupational respiratory disease. Workplace exposure responsible for such chronic disabling lung disease occurs gradually over long periods of time; exposures do not result in any obvious acute symptoms, but once symptoms do appear, in many instances little can be done beyond making the worker comfort-

*Case courtesy of Stephen Hessl, Daniel Hryhorczuk, and Peter Orris, Section on Occupational Medicine, Cook County Hospital, Chicago.

able. Unless discovered very early in their course, most work-related respiratory diseases are not curable; it is for this reason that disease prevention is so important.

Occupational lung disease is recorded in accounts of ancient history. Case reports exist in the writings of Hippocrates, and evidence of silicosis is present in pictographs from Egypt. Yet today some of those chronic diseases are still an important problem for workers. Recently, attempts have been made to quantify the amount of occupational respiratory disease, but few data exist for estimates of its actual magnitude. Estimates suggest that less than 5 percent of chronic occupational respiratory disease is correctly identified as associated with work.

Pneumoconiosis and occupational asthma are two work-related respiratory diseases that are often not correctly diagnosed. For example, approximately 3 percent of Americans suffer from what physicians diagnose as asthma, but a much larger proportion of people report either having asthma or episodes of wheezing; physicians who see workers who report wheezing should determine if a work-related bronchoconstrictive response is occurring.

EVALUATION OF INDIVIDUALS
Evaluation of pulmonary response to toxic exposures is important because work-related respiratory disease is frequently a contributory cause— and commonly a primary cause—of pulmonary disability. Complete evaluations can generally be performed effectively in a physician's office.

The clinical evaluation of pulmonary disease includes a minimum of four elements: (1) a complete history including occupational and environmental exposures, a cigarette-smoking history, and a careful review of respiratory symptoms; (2) a physical examination with special attention to breath sounds; (3) a chest x-ray with appropriate attention to parenchymal opacities; and (4) pulmonary function tests.

History
Review of symptoms should include questions on chronic cough, chronic sputum production, degree of shortness of breath (dyspnea), wheezing unrelated to respiratory infections, chest tightness, chest pain, and reports of allergic or asthmatic responses to work or non-work environments. For example, one peculiar characteristic of several types of occupational asthma and of pulmonary edema is that the symptoms may peak in intensity approximately 16 hours after exposure has ended. The symptoms will often occur at night as shortness of breath or cough. In assessing acute airway disease, one should question the patient about the principal symptoms: chest tightness, wheezing, dyspnea, cough; a formal survey questionnaire for systematic respiratory effect studies is available [1] (see Chap. 3 for information on the occupational history).

Physical Examination
The physical examination is helpful when abnormal. The most remarkable finding in most patients with occupational lung diseases is the relative absence of physical signs; however, certain conditions are associated with physical signs and the presence or absence of such abnormalities should be noted.

Auscultation can reveal important diagnostic clues. Fine rales at the bases are more common in asbestosis than in other interstitial lung diseases. Wheezes and their relationship to exposure are helpful in evaluating a suspected case of work-related asthma. A pleural rub can occur with pleural reaction due to acute, chronic, or long-distant asbestos exposure.

Clubbing of the digits occurs in asbestosis and usually appears after other evidence of the disease has become apparent. It does not usually occur in other mineral pneumoconioses or in hypersensitivity pneumonitis. The most common nonoccupational causes of clubbing are bronchial carcinoma and idiopathic pulmonary fibrosis.

Examination of the heart is important since left

ventricular failure can present as dyspnea alone, and right ventricular failure may indicate severe lung disease.

Chest X-Ray

A chest x-ray should be taken and, in addition to a standard interpretation, it should, if possible, be interpreted according to the ILO classification for pneumoconiosis [2]. Although this classification is only now beginning to be used in radiology departments, it serves an important extra function in the general x-ray interpretation. The standard technique permits semiquantitative interpretation of x-rays to identify early evidence and progression of parenchymal and pleural disease; it focuses on size, shape, concentration, and distribution of small parenchymal opacities as well as distribution and extent of pleural thickening or calcification. For example, rounded opacities in the upper lung fields are associated with silicosis, whereas linear (irregular) opacities in the lower lung fields are associated with asbestosis (Figs. 21-1 and 21-2). The ILO system has the distinct advantage of a standardized set of comparison x-ray films, which can be used to classify x-rays at one point in time or to follow an individual or a population for change over time. Even though chest x-rays present evidence of abnormality, they do not provide information on disability or impairment and do not necessarily correlate well with pulmonary function test findings. An individual with severe obstructive disease may show little evidence of it on chest x-ray. In contrast, an individual exposed chronically to iron oxide or tin oxide may show a dramatically abnormal chest x-ray (Fig. 21-3); but iron or tin oxide in the lung causes little, if any, pulmonary reaction or lung function abnormality.

Pulmonary Function Tests

A critical element in determining respiratory status is an evaluation of pulmonary function. In a well-equipped pulmonary function laboratory, spirometry, lung volume determinations, gas exchange analyses, and exercise testing can be performed with relative ease. In a physician's office, only the spirometry is readily and inexpensively performed; it does, however, provide a surprising amount of information. Pulmonary function tests, required for medical surveillance by some Occupational Safety and Health Administration (OSHA) standards, are commonly used and are easy to perform, reliable, and reproducible. Most lung disease will yield abnormal results well before onset of clinical symptoms, especially if individuals are followed at regular 1- to 3-year intervals. The tests have the advantage of being polyvalent, each demonstrating several types of abnormalities; as a result, however, they are not highly discriminatory in determining etiology by themselves. The hospital-based tests (lung volume determinations, gas exchange analyses, exercise tests, and bronchial challenge tests) can contribute to a refined diagnostic evaluation once work-related disease is suspected.

The basic tests of ventilatory function can be obtained with a simple portable spirometer. Test results are derived from the forced expiratory curve (Fig. 21-4). Many types of equipment are currently being marketed to provide these tests, yet several have been inadequately standardized and are either insufficiently or overly sensitive. The National Institute for Occupational Safety and Health (NIOSH) has evaluated spirometers and can provide information on which ones are most reliable and accurate [3]. Although many measures are possible from the forced expiratory curve, the simplest and generally most useful ones for evaluating work-related respiratory disease are forced vital capacity (FVC), forced expiratory volume in the first second of a forced vital capacity maneuver (FEV_1), and the ratio of these two measurements (FEV_1/FVC). A simple model of the interpretation of these tests is shown in Table 21-1 and Figure 21-4. Results are compared to Knudson's expected values, derived from a normal population of nonsmoking adults [4], and are expressed as a percentage of the expected value.

No reliable race-specific expected values are

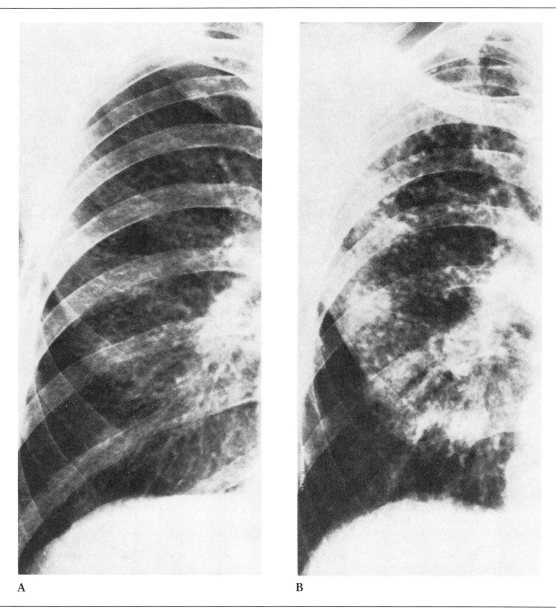

A   B

Fig. 21-1. Progression of discrete nodules of silicosis over 10 years in a slate quarry worker. (From WR Parkes. *Occupational Lung Disorders*. 2nd ed. London: Butterworth, 1982.)

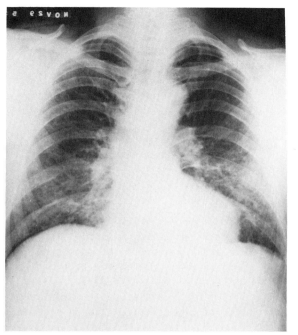

A

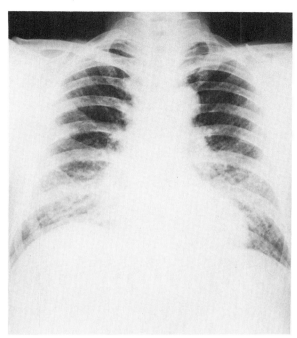

B

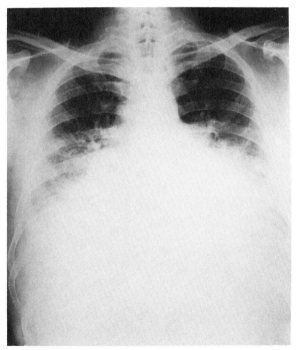

C

Fig. 21-2. Chest x-rays showing early (A), moderate (B), and advanced (C) fibrosis in asbestosis, especially in lower lung fields. (Courtesy of Benjamin G. Ferris, M.D.)

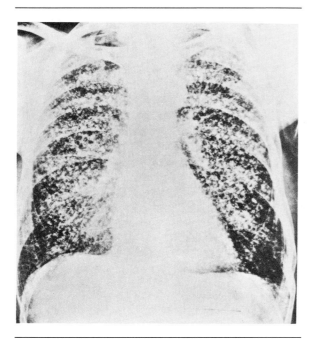

Fig. 21-3. Chest x-ray demonstrating stannosis, the benign pneumoconiosis due to the inhalation of tin oxide, in a man who worked as a furnace charger in a smelting works for 42 years. (From WR Parkes. *Occupational Lung Disorders*. 2nd ed. London: Butterworth, 1982.)

available; OSHA recommends multiplying Knudson's values by 0.85 for blacks. Criteria for the proper evaluation of spirometry are based on American Thoracic Society recommendations.

Pneumoconioses, including silicosis, asbestosis, and coal worker's pneumoconiosis, are considered restrictive diseases because there is reduction in lung volume. In the absence of significant airways disease, flow rates will be maintained and may be above normal due to decreased lung compliance with increased elastic recoil. Occupational asthma is considered an obstructive disease because there is obstruction of air flow without reduction in lung volume. Of course, with cigarette smoking and multiple environmental exposures, a mixed condition is frequently present, and precise discrimination is not possible. Nevertheless, the basic distribution of ventilatory function abnormalities (see Table 21-1) is useful in considering the general characteristics of work-related respiratory disease.

EVALUATION OF GROUPS

If the physician is able to examine several workers from the same work environment, careful attention should be directed toward evaluation of the grouped results in addition to those of each individual. For an individual, emphasis is on the work history and collection of information to explain specific symptoms and signs. It should be recognized, however, that absence of basilar rales does not exclude asbestosis, wheezes do not necessarily diagnose occupational asthma, opacities on chest x-ray do not specify their pathology, and pulmonary function tests may be falsely considered "normal" because of the wide variation of "normal" in standard populations. In fact, it may not be until a group of coworkers is evaluated that pulmonary disease can be recognized as associated with work. Group evaluations have the benefit that results can be subdivided according to duration of work or types of exposure. Chest x-ray findings, pulmonary function tests, and symptom histories can be examined by subgroups to evaluate previously unrecognized work effects (see examples in Chap. 5). Furthermore, the average value of a group of tests has less variability than an individual test result. For example, measurements of FEV_1 and FVC in individuals that vary between 80 and 120 percent of the population standards are still considered normal; a group of 10 or 20 individuals, however, should have a mean result much closer to the standard values (100%). If the difference is as little as 10 percent lower (that is, 90% of the predicted value), then an adverse health effect in that population should be seriously considered.

Comparisons to baselines should be performed whenever possible to permit evaluation of change

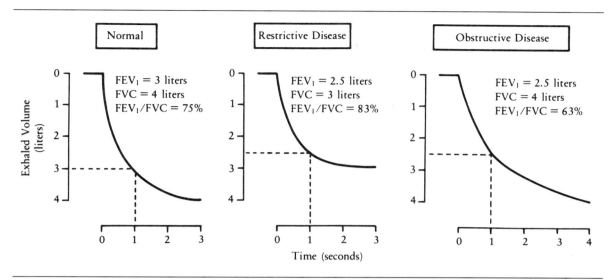

Fig. 21-4. Spirographic results in normal and disease states. (Adapted from JA Nadel. Pulmonary function testing. *Basics of RD* [American Thoracic Society] 1973; 1(4):2.)

Table 21-1. Spirometry interpretation

| Type of response | Percent predicted[a] | | $\dfrac{FEV_1}{FVC}\%$ | Response to inhaled bronchodilators |
	FEV$_1$	FVC		
Normal	≥ 80	≥ 80	≥ 75	−
Obstructive	< 80	≥ 80[b]	< 75	±
Restrictive	< 80	< 80	≥ 75	−
Mixed	< 80	< 80	< 75	±

[a]Predicted FEV$_1$ and FVC based on RJ Knudson et al. The maximum expiratory flow volume curve. Am. Rev. Respir. Dis. 1976; 113:581.
[b]Severe obstruction can result in reduction of FVC also.

over time in individuals or a group compared to a known—not a predicted—value. Accelerated decrements in lung function and accelerated development of abnormal chest x-rays or respiratory tract symptoms are far more significant when the comparison is based on earlier examinations rather than on expected population experience. These evaluations can be done effectively and completely in a physician's office. Any worker potentially ex-

posed to respiratory hazards at work should have a baseline ventilatory function test included in the medical record.

The major types of respiratory response to external agents discussed in this chapter are summarized in Table 21-2. Occupational lung cancer and work-related infectious diseases of the respiratory tract are discussed in Chapters 15 and 19, respectively.

Table 21-2. Major types of occupational pulmonary disease

Type	Occupational disease example	Clinical history	Physical exam	Chest x-ray	Pulmonary function tests	
Restrictive (fibrosis)	Silicosis	Dyspnea on exertion, shortness of breath	Clubbing, cyanosis	Nodules	↓ FEV ↓ FVC	→ FEV/FVC
	Asbestosis	Dyspnea on exertion, shortness of breath	Clubbing, cyanosis, rales	Linear densities, pleural calcifications	↓ FEV ↓ FVC	→ FEV/FVC ↓ Diffusion
Obstructive	Byssinosis, isocyanate asthma	Cough, chest tightness, shortness of breath, asthma attacks	Respiratory rate ↑, breath sounds ↑	Usually normal	→ FVC ↓ FEV	↓ FEV/FVC
Granulomata	Beryllium disease	Cough, weight loss, shortness of breath	Respiratory rate ↑	Interstitial fibrosis	↓ FVC ↓ FEV	↓ Diffusion
Pulmonary edema	Cadmium poisoning	Frothy, bloody sputum production	Coarse, bubbly rales	Hazy, diffuse infiltrate	↓ FEV ↓ FVC	↓ Diffusion

Key: ↑ = increase; ↓ = decrease; → = no change; FEV = FEV_1.

ACUTE IRRITANT RESPONSES

Irritation in the upper respiratory tract, in contrast to the mid- or lower tract, is frequently associated with work-related symptoms. Acute symptoms are often due to regional inflammation, which a patient perceives as irritation. With nasal and paranasal sinus irritation there is congestion that can result in violent frontal headache, nasal obstruction, runny nose, and occasionally nosebleed. Throat inflammation is commonly reported as a dry cough. Laryngeal inflammation can cause hoarseness and, if severe, may result in laryngeal spasms associated with glottal edema, presenting dramatic symptoms: shortness of breath, cyanosis, and anxiety.

In the mid-respiratory tract, the acute reaction is characteristically bronchospasm. The extreme case is asthma, which is histologically distin-guished by a thickened basement membrane, increased number of goblet cells with secretions, mucus plugging, and increased smooth muscle at preterminal bronchioles. Asthma associated with work is being recognized with increasing frequency; precipitating agents include isocyanates, detergent enzymes, and Western red cedar dust (Table 21-3). In addition to asthma caused by exposure to agents listed in this table, many irritant substances not usually associated with asthma can produce bronchial hyperreactivity when high levels of exposure have occurred. Single high-dose exposure and episodic low-dose exposure to irritants such as ammonia or chlorine can result in nonspecific bronchial reactivity, referred to by some authors [5] as reactive airways dysfunction syndrome (RADS), which may persist for undetermined lengths of time.

Table 21-3. Selected causes of occupational asthma*

Agents	Jobs
High molecular weight compounds	
Animal products: dander, excreta, serum, secretions	Animal handlers, laboratory workers, veterinarians
Plants: grain dust, flour, tobacco, tea, hops	Grain handlers, tea workers, bakers and workers in natural oil manufacturing and in tobacco and food processing
Enzymes: *B. subtilis,* pancreatic extracts, papain, trypsin, fungal amylase	Bakers and workers in the detergent, pharmaceutical, and plastic industries
Vegetable: gum acacia, gum tragacanth	Printers and gum-manufacturing workers
Other: crab, prawn	Crab and prawn processors
Low molecular weight compounds	
Diisocyanates: toluene diisocyanate (TDI), methylene-diphenyldiisocyanate (MDI)	Polyurethane industry workers, plastics workers, workers using varnish, and foundry workers
Anhydrides: phthallic and trimellitic anhydrides	Epoxy resin and plastics workers
Wood dust: oak, mahogany, California redwood, Western red cedar	Carpenters, sawmill workers, and furniture makers
Metals: platinum, nickel, chromium, cobalt, vanadium, tungsten carbide	Platinum and nickel-refining workers and hard-metal workers
Soldering fluxes	Solderers
Drugs: penicillin, methyldopa, tetracyclines, cephalosporins, psyllium	Pharmaceutical industry workers
Other organic chemicals: urea formaldehyde, dyes, formalin, azodicarbonamide, hexachlorophene, ethylene diamine, dimethyl ethanolamine, polyvinyl chloride pyrolysates	Workers in chemical, plastic, and rubber industries; hospitals; laboratories; foam insulation manufacture; food wrapping; and spray painting

*Mechanism believed allergic except for some low molecular weight compounds.
Source: Adapted from M Chan-Yeung, S Lam. Occupational asthma. Am Rev Respir Dis 1986; 133:686–703.

The conditions deriving from acute irritation of the deep respiratory tract are pulmonary edema and pneumonitis. With pulmonary edema there is extravasation of fluid and cells from the pulmonary capillary bed into the alveoli. Primary pulmonary edema is due to direct toxic action on the capillary walls. For example, exposure to ozone and oxides of nitrogen is common in industrial settings; both agents can cause pulmonary edema either when there are delayed effects of overexposure or when a trapped worker cannot escape exposure. Pneumonitis, on the other hand, is an inflammation of the lung parenchyma in which cellular infiltration rather than fluid extravasation predominates. Beryllium and cadmium can cause acute pneumonitis.

Factors Involved in Toxicity
The most widespread causes of acute responses are irritant gases. Water is a major constituent of the respiratory tract lining, and solubility of these gases in water is the most significant factor influencing their site of action. Gases with high solubility act on the upper respiratory tract within seconds. For example, fatal epiglottic edema has been associated with irritants of high solubility, such as ammonia, hydrogen chloride, and hydrogen fluoride. The moderately soluble gases act on both the

upper and lower respiratory tract within minutes. Chlorine gas, fluorine gas, and sulfur dioxide are irritants of this type, producing upper respiratory irritation as well as symptoms of bronchoconstriction. The low-solubility irritants are most insidious; they penetrate to the deep portions of the respiratory tract and act predominantly on the alveoli 6 to 24 hours after exposure. Because of the considerable delay in onset of symptoms, large doses can be delivered without any irritant symptoms to serve as warnings. Pulmonary edema is the major effect of overexposures to materials such as ozone, oxides of nitrogen, and phosgene.

Other factors influencing the site of action of an irritant gas are intensity and duration of exposure. The amount of exposure depends not only on air concentrations but also on work effort: A worker with a sedentary job exposed to a given concentration of a respiratory irritant will receive a much lower dose than one with an active job requiring rapid breathing and a high minute volume.

A final element that influences the site of action is interaction—both synergism and antagonism. Sulfur dioxide and particulates of water are synergistic; they combine to deliver a sulfuric acid-like vapor to the respiratory tract. Ammonia and sulfur dioxide, however, are antagonistic and together produce less response than either can individually. The presence of a carrier such as an aerosol may increase the effect of an irritant gas: Sulfur dioxide may cause a moderate effect and a sodium chloride aerosol no effect on the respiratory tract, whereas animal studies indicate that the two combined may result in a marked effect because the aerosol delivers the sulfur dioxide more deeply into the lung.

Highly Soluble Irritants
Primary examples of highly soluble irritants are: (1) ammonia, used as a soil fertilizer, in the manufacture of dyes, chemicals, plastics, and explosives, in tanning leather, and as a household cleaner; (2) hydrogen chloride, used in chemical manufacturing, electroplating, and metal pickling; and (3) hydrogen fluoride, used predominantly for etching and polishing of glass, as a chemical catalyst in the manufacture of plastics, as an insecticide, and for removal of sand from metal castings in foundry operations.

The primary physical effects of highly water-soluble irritants are first the odor and then eye and nose irritation; throat irritation is slightly less frequent. In high doses, the respiratory rate can increase and bronchospasm can occur. Lower respiratory tract effects, however, do not occur unless the individual is severely overexposed or trapped in the environment. The irritant effects are powerful and generally provide adequate warning to prevent overexposure of individuals free to escape from exposure. The history and physical exam are the most important parts of irritant exposure evaluation. Reflex bronchoconstriction may be evident on pulmonary function tests shortly after exposure. Chest x-rays are not helpful unless there is pulmonary edema.

Management of reactions to these irritants is immediate removal of the worker and, if breathing is labored, provision of oxygen. If severe exposure or unconsciousness occurs, observation in a hospital for development of pulmonary edema is advisable.

Prevention of exposures relies on proper industrial hygiene practices with local exhaust ventilation as an essential component. If respirators are required to prevent overexposure, then workers must be trained in their proper use and maintenance.

A 25-year-old man came to the emergency room with acid burns. Prior to taking a job as an electroplater 5 weeks before admission, he was in perfect health. On the first day at this job, he developed itching. Subsequently, he developed sores, which healed with scars, at sites of splashes of workplace chemicals. After 4 days on this job, he had a runny nose, throat irritation, and a productive cough. He also noted some shortness of breath at work.

His work involved dipping metal parts into tanks containing chrome solutions and acid. He wore a paper mask, rubber gloves, and an apron, but no eye protection. Although heavy fumes were present in the 60 × 20 × 14 ft. room, no respirator or ventilation was provided. Apparently none of the other eight workers in the room had similar medical problems.

Past history revealed three prior hospitalizations for pneumonia but not asthma or allergies. He smoked about four cigarettes per day.

From age 16 to 18, he worked as a sheet-metal punch-press operator for a tool and die company. From age 18, he worked as a drip-pan cleaner for a soup company. He was a student in an auto mechanics' school from age 19 to 21. From age 23 to 24, he occasionally worked as a gas station attendant.

Physical examination was normal, except for multiple areas of round, irregularly-shaped, depigmented 1-mm atrophic scars on both forearms and exposed areas of anterior thorax and face; a 4-mm, rounded, punched-out ulcer, with a thickened, indurated, undermined border and an erythematous base on his left cheek; an erythematous pharynx; and bilateral conjunctivitis. There was no perforation of the nasal septum. Patch tests with dichromate, nickel, and cobalt were all negative. A chest x-ray was normal.

The diagnoses were irritation of the upper respiratory tract and an irritant contact dermatitis, both due to chromic acid mist. His symptoms resolved with removal from exposure. Periodic medical surveillance was advised to provide early diagnosis of a possible malignancy of the nasal passages for which he may be at risk as a result of the chromium exposure.*

Many small electroplating firms have no local ventilation over open vats of chromic and other acids. Frequently a high level of chrome or other metals in the fumes is liberated as metal parts that are being plated are immersed. Chrome and chromic acid mist are local irritants and chromates (hexavalent forms especially) are considered to be carcinogens, although it is not known whether electroplaters have a special cancer risk.

Moderately Soluble Irritants

The moderately soluble irritants commonly encountered in industrial settings are chlorine, fluorine, and sulfur dioxide. Chlorine is widely used in the chemical industry to synthesize various chlorinated hydrocarbons, whereas outside the chemical industry its major use is in water purification and as a bleach in the paper industry. Fluorine is used in the conversion of uranium tetrafluoride to uranium hexafluorides, in the development of fluorocarbons, and as an oxidizing agent. Fluoride is used in the electrolytic manufacture of aluminum, as a flux in smelting operations, in coatings of welding rods, and as an additive to drinking water. Sulfur dioxide is commonly used as a disinfectant, a fumigant, and a bleach for wood pulp, and is formed as a byproduct of coal burning, smelter processes, and the paper industry.

These irritants, like the highly soluble ones, initially cause mucous membrane irritation often manifest by a persistent cough. Acute symptoms are usually of short duration. Low levels of continuous exposures, which are better tolerated than exposures to highly soluble irritants, may cause obstructive respiratory disease.

In addition to causing respiratory symptoms, these irritants lead to other health problems. Chlorine gas contributes to corrosion of the teeth, while fluorine is a significant cause of chemical skin burns. Chronic exposure to fluoride is associated with increased bone density, cartilage calcification, discoloration of teeth in the young, and possibly rheumatologic syndromes. Sulfur dioxide, in particular, is associated with bronchospasm, especially in asthmatics, with some epidemiologic studies suggesting a possible role in chronic obstructive pulmonary disease.

Again the history and physical exam are most important in evaluating an industrial case. Management and prevention are similar to those for highly soluble irritants. Pulmonary function tests, especially the FEV_1, are indicated in surveillance programs for workers with chronic exposure.

Irritants of Low Solubility

Usually the effects of irritants with low solubility are mild throat irritation and occasionally headache. Much more significant is pulmonary edema,

*Case courtesy of Stephen Hessl, Daniel Hryhorczuk, and Peter Orris, Section of Occupational Medicine, Cook County Hospital, Chicago.

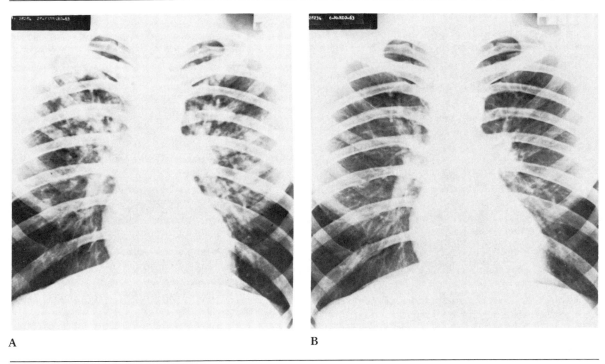

A   B

Fig. 21-5. Chest x-rays in a copper miner. A. Twenty-four hours after overexposure to oxides of nitrogen. Pulmonary edema is evident. B. One week after exposure, showing resolution of pulmonary edema. (Courtesy of Benjamin G. Ferris, M.D.)

which manifests itself 6 to 24 hours after exposure, preceded by symptoms of bronchospasm (chest tightness and wheezing) (Fig. 21-5). Ozone and oxides of nitrogen are the two low-soluble irritants most commonly encountered. Both occur in welding fumes and therefore are found in many work environments. Ozone is used as a disinfectant, as a bleach in the food, textile, and pulp and paper industries, and as an oxidizing agent; oxides of nitrogen are used in chemical and fertilizer manufacture and in metal processing and cleaning operations.

Chronic exposure to oxides of nitrogen may result in bronchiolitis obliterans. In addition to the history, physical exam, and the acute obstructive defect evident on pulmonary function tests, the chest x-ray can be examined for evidence of early pulmonary edema and the appearance of bronchiolitis obliterans. A specific syndrome associated with oxides of nitrogen is silo filler's disease, which results from exposures to this gas in the upper chambers of grain silos where it forms in the anaerobic fermentation of green silage. The brownish color of nitrogen dioxide is an important warning sign for farmers. Numerous instances of acute overexposures and death have resulted from inadequately ventilated silos.

Although management and prevention are similar to that for highly soluble irritants, overnight observation is frequently necessary when excess exposures have occurred due to the insidious onset of pulmonary edema.

OCCUPATIONAL ASTHMA

An 18-year-old woman arrived at an emergency room complaining of SOB. Eight weeks previously, she had consulted her physician about daytime wheezing and cough productive of white phlegm. She was treated with antibiotics and an expectorant and remained at home for 3 days with significant improvement. A week later, she again developed a cough and SOB. Again she was treated with antibiotics, an expectorant, and bed rest with significant improvement. She had an exacerbation of coughing, SOB, and cyanosis of her fingertips the day prior to her visit.

Her occupational history revealed that she had begun working at a tool supply and manufacturing company 9 weeks previously, a week before her symptoms began. Her usual job there was grinding carbide-steel drill bits. In her work she used one of four machines that sharpened drill bits. Her machine generated much metal dust, often covering the machines and her face, hands, and clothes. There was no exhaust system to draw dust away from her breathing zone, and no respiratory protection was provided.

After being treated the first time 8 weeks previously, she was temporarily assigned to cleaning drill bits in a solvent bath. On this job she felt lightheaded but had no difficulty breathing. After a long holiday weekend, she was again assigned to drill-bit grinding and after several hours developed a cough. The next day the cough increased and she developed SOB, prompting a second visit to her physician. When she improved from that episode, she returned to work again and experienced exacerbation of coughing and SOB. This prompted her emergency-room visit.

Past medical history revealed occasional seasonal rhinitis as a child but no asthma, eczema, or other allergies. There was no family history of allergies or asthma.

Physical examination was normal, except for a pulse rate of 128 and a respiratory rate of 40. She had cyanosis of lips and fingertips. Chest exam revealed diffuse bilateral wheezes and use of accessory muscles for breathing.

Arterial blood gases on room air at rest revealed a PaO_2 of 39. Spirometry showed normal forced vital capacity but markedly abnormal FEV_1 (53% of predicted). Chest x-ray was normal. White blood cell count was 11,200, with 10 percent eosinophils.

She was treated with oxygen, bronchodilators, and steroids. She improved clinically; by the second day, her FEV_1 improved to 82 percent of predicted.

A later call by her physician to the state occupational safety and health agency revealed that carbide-steel bit alloys contain nickel, cobalt, chromium, vanadium, molybdenum, and tungsten. Grinding such bits can produce cobalt and tungsten carbide dusts, which are recognized pulmonary sensitizers.*

The diagnosis in this case was occupational asthma. No specific agent was proved responsible, but the presence of tungsten carbide and cobalt dusts suggest possible agents. Since changing jobs, she has felt well and has not had further bronchospasm.

Many occupational asthma cases are not seen by physicians or other health care providers, probably because workers recognize the association between exposure and asthma and thus avoid further contact.

Individual responses may be so clear and occur so early in a new job that those workers who respond adversely may leave quite soon after being hired. Thus, in population surveys very few workers may be identified with immediate sensitivity because most of those who had experienced adverse effects had already left the job to avoid the asthma-producing exposure. A wide variety of materials and circumstances have been shown to cause occupational asthma (see Table 21-3).

Diagnosis of Occupational Asthma

Diagnosis of occupational asthma depends greatly on the occupational history. Major or minor constituents of substances as well as accidental by-products can incite attacks. Most individuals who suffer occupational asthma have a history of atopy, although those without such a history may become sensitized after prolonged exposure to specific environmental agents such as diisocyanates. Suspicion of this diagnosis should be aroused even

*Case courtesy of James Keogh, School of Medicine, University of Maryland, Baltimore (unpublished curriculum materials).

when a worker has had no previous history of asthma. Often the worker will report wheezing, chest tightness, or severe cough developing in the evening or at night with recovery overnight or over a weekend away from work. However, if exposure and its effects have been prolonged, the symptoms may persist at home or over the weekend. Specific questioning about nocturnal symptoms may elicit responses otherwise not volunteered. The physical exam of an acutely ill worker will reveal wheezing and rhonchi. While atopic individuals are more likely to develop occupational asthma, anyone can.

A particularly useful test for bronchoconstriction of occupational origin is the timed vital capacity (FEV_1) before and after a work shift. A drop of 300 ml or 10 percent or more of FEV_1 (measured as the mean of three values each time) between the beginning and end of the first shift of the work week suggests a work-related effect. (It should be noted that an acute drop in FEV_1 as large as 1.8 liters has been measured without the worker reporting symptoms.) Excessive eosinophils in the sputum or blood may distinguish asthma from bronchitis. Reliance should not be placed on skin tests for allergic reactions. Bronchoprovocation testing may be necessary to confirm reversible airways disease or identify the offending agent, although it should be noted that skin and bronchial responses do not always correlate well. Since virtually any chemical substance can precipitate an asthma attack, health professionals should rely heavily on the patient's medical and work histories even in the absence of a documented association between a given exposure and asthma.

Acute care of those with attacks of occupational asthma is the same as for any case of asthma. Long-term management, however, probably requires removal from exposure, since very small levels of exposure can trigger an asthmatic response. Close monitoring of symptoms and lung function should be maintained for an individual who must continue exposure to a suspected offending agent.

HYPERSENSITIVITY PNEUMONITIS

Hypersensitivity pneumonitis refers to reactions associated with the most picturesque of all occupational disease names (Table 21-4). This response results from organic materials, commonly fungi or thermophilic bacteria, that are present in a surprising variety of settings. In contrast to asthma, this response is more focused in the lung parenchyma (respiratory bronchioles and alveoli). Characteristics of this kind of reaction are antibodies (precipitins) present in serum and the collection of lymphocytes in pulmonary infiltrates. Activation of pulmonary macrophages with an increased number of T-lymphocytes and probably a change in their function appear to be the underlying cellular mechanisms. The end result can be fibrosis, yet the responses are much less dose-dependent than those for primary fibrosis due to inorganic dusts. Once hypersensitivity is established, small doses may trigger episodes of alveolitis. It should be emphasized that this disease is a complex inflammatory response often to bacterial or fungal material, not an infection, nor a true allergic response. Therefore, the commonly used clinical term *hypersensitivity pneumonitis* is actually inaccurate. A term proposed by some authors is *organic dust chronic toxic syndrome*, which is felt to be a more accurate description of the pulmonary cell reactions to organic dust constituents.

The worker suffering hypersensitivity pneumonitis will experience shortness of breath and nonproductive cough. In contrast to asthma, wheezing is not a large component. In acute episodes, the sudden onset of the respiratory symptoms along with fever and chills is dramatic. Physical exam may show rapid breathing and fine basilar rales. Pulmonary function tests can show marked reduction in lung volumes consistent with restrictive disease. The FEV_1 is reduced, but in proportion to the decreases in FVC and total lung capacity; generally, there is a normal or increased FEV_1/FVC ratio. Arterial blood-gas measurements show an increased alveolar-arterial oxygen difference [(A-a) DO_2] and a reduced diffusing capacity. Chest x-ray can be quite helpful in the acute episodes in re-

Table 21-4. Examples of hypersensitivity pneumonitis

Disease	Antigenic material	Antigen
Farmer's lung	Moldy hay or grain	Thermophilic actinomycetes
Bagassosis	Moldy sugar cane	
Mushroom worker's lung	Mushroom compost	
Humidifier fever	Dust from contaminated air conditioners or furnaces	
Maple bark disease	Moldy maple bark	*Cryptostroma* species
Sequoiosis	Redwood dust	*Graphium* species, Pallularia
Bird breeder's lung	Avian droppings or feathers	Avian proteins
Pituitary snuff user's lung	Pituitary powder	Bovine or porcine proteins
Suberosis	Moldy cork dust	*Penicillium* species
Paprika splitter's lung	Paprika dust	*Mucor stolonifer*
Malt worker's lung	Malt dust	*Aspergillus clavatus* or *A. fumigatus*
Fishmeal worker's lung	Fishmeal	Fishmeal dust
Miller's lung	Infested wheat flour	*Sitophilus granarius* (wheat weevil)
Furrier's lung	Animal pelts	Animal fur dust
Coffee worker's lung	Coffee beans	Coffee bean dust
—	Urethane foam and finish	Isocyanates (TDI, HDI)

vealing patchy infiltrates or a diffuse fine-micro-nodular shadowing.

If the individual is removed from exposure, symptoms and signs generally disappear in 1 to 2 weeks. If repeated exposures are experienced, especially at levels low enough to result in only mild symptoms, a more chronic disease may ensue. The worker may be unaware of the work association, as the low-level effects may appear symptomatically like a persistent respiratory "flu." Over a period of months, however, the gradual onset of dyspnea develops, which can be accompanied by weight loss and lethargy. The physical exam is similar to that in the acute episode, although the patient may appear less acutely ill and may demonstrate finger clubbing. Chest x-ray, however, is more suggestive of chronic interstitial fibrosis, and the pulmonary function tests show a restrictive defect. The disease may progress to severe dyspnea and the end result resembles, even histologically, chronic interstitial fibrosis of unknown etiology. Sometimes an asymptomatic patient without an episode of acute pneumonitis in the past will develop interstitial fibrosis.

Prevention rests on removal from exposure. This can be more readily accomplished than with asthma since environmental controls can focus on the elimination of conditions that foster bacterial or fungal growth. Process changes may also be necessary to prevent antigen production, and local exhaust ventilation rather than respiratory protective equipment should be relied on.

BYSSINOSIS AND OTHER DISEASES OF VEGETABLE DUSTS

Some types of airway constriction are believed not to be immunologic in origin but due to direct toxic effect on the airways. This has been referred to as pharmacologic bronchoconstriction, although for byssinosis, the pathogenesis is still poorly understood.

Byssinosis (meaning "white thread" in Greek) is associated with exposure to cotton, hemp, and flax processing. It has been popularly called "brown lung" (a misnomer since the lungs are not brown) to compare its severity to "black lung."

Byssinosis has been shown to develop in response to dust exposure in cotton processing. It is especially prevalent among cotton workers in the initial, very dusty operations where bales are broken open, blown (to separate lint from impurities), and carded (to arrange the fibers into parallel threads). A lower rate of disease occurs in workers in the spinning, winding, and twisting areas where dust levels are lower. The lowest prevalence rate of byssinosis has been found among weavers, who experience the lowest dust exposure. Byssinosis has also been described in other than textile sectors where cotton is processed, such as cottonseed oil mills, the cotton waste utilization industry, and the garnetting or bedding and batting industry. The same syndrome has been shown to occur in workers exposed in processing hemp, flax, and (probably) sisal.

Byssinosis is characterized by shortness of breath and chest tightness. These symptoms are most prominent on the first day of the work week or after being away from the factory over an extended period of time ("Monday morning tightness"). No previous exposure is necessary for symptoms to develop.

Symptoms are often associated with changes in pulmonary function. One characteristic of the acute pulmonary response to cotton dust exposure is a drop in the FEV_1 during the Monday work shift or the first day back at work after at least a 2-day layoff. Since workers do not normally lose lung function during a workday, an acute loss of 10 percent or 300 ml or more (whichever is greater) in an individual, or 3 percent or 75 ml (whichever is greater) in a group of 20 or greater, can be considered significant enough to require further investigation. Over time, cotton dust workers have an accelerated decrement in FEV_1 consistent with fixed air-flow obstruction and chronic obstructive lung disease. Diagnosis is based mainly on symptoms; no characteristic exam or chest x-ray findings are associated with

byssinosis. Therefore, the patient should be questioned systematically about symptoms.

It is assumed that progression of disease occurs if duration of exposure to dust levels is sufficiently high and prolonged. Mild byssinosis probably is reversible if exposure ceases, but severe disease is irreversible. Individuals with severe byssinosis are rarely seen in an industrial survey since they are too disabled to be working. Byssinosis seems more severe when it is associated with chronic bronchitis. The end stage of the disease is fixed airway obstruction with hyperinflation and air trapping. Cigarette smokers are at increased risk of irreversible byssinosis.

Much research has been done on possible etiologic mechanisms and effects. Extracts of cotton bract have been shown to release pharmacologic mediators, such as histamine, as well as prostaglandins. Cotton components also have a rather marked effect on the adrenergic nervous system with lowering of cAMP levels (or antagonizing intrinsic cAMP) and leading to bronchospasm or release of mediators. Finally, gram-negative bacterial endotoxin contaminates cotton fiber, and aqueous extracts of endotoxin have produced acute symptoms and lung function declines. Endotoxin is currently receiving much attention as a major cause of the byssinosis syndrome.

Two other respiratory conditions associated with work in the cotton industry are:

Mill fever: This self-limited condition usually happens on first exposure to a cotton gin environment. It lasts for 2 or 3 days and has no known sequelae. It is characterized by headache, malaise, and fever. A flu-like illness, it has symptoms similar to metal fume fever and polymer fume fever. Gin mill fever is probably related to gram-negative bacterial material in mill dust; it usually afflicts workers only once, except that after prolonged absence from a mill, reexposure may trigger another attack (see box in Chap. 19).

Weaver's cough: Weavers have suffered outbreaks of acute respiratory illness characterized by a dry cough, although their dust exposure is comparatively low. It may result from sizing material or from mildewed yarn that is sometimes found in high-humidity weaving rooms.

CHRONIC RESPIRATORY TRACT RESPONSES

Pneumoconiosis

Pulmonary fibrosis is the most readily recognized work-related chronic pulmonary reaction. This condition, which varies according to inciting agent, intensity, and duration of exposure, is generally referred to as a pneumoconiosis. It is usually due to an inorganic dust that must be of respirable size (< 5 microns) to reach terminal bronchioles and alveoli; dust of this size is not visible and so its presence may not be recognized by a worker. There are two basic types of fibrosis: localized and nodular, usually peribronchial fibrosis (such as silicosis); and diffuse interstitial fibrosis (such as asbestosis). The clinical features of all the pneumoconioses are similar: initial nonproductive cough, shortness of breath of increasing severity, and, in the later stages, productive cough, distant breath sounds, and signs of right heart failure.

Silica-Related Disease

Crystalline silica (SiO_2) is a major component of the earth's crust. Therefore, exposure occurs in a wide variety of settings: mining, quarrying, and stone cutting (see Fig. 7-4); foundry operations; ceramics and vitreous enameling; and in fillers for paints and rubber.

Estimates of the prevalence of silicosis in the United States vary, ranging from 30,000 to 100,000 current cases. No distinct clinical features can be cited beyond the ones listed above, but there is distinct pathology. Silicosis occurs more frequently in the upper rather than the lower lobes, with nodules 2 to 6 mm in diameter. In severe cases, nodules aggregate and become fibrotic masses several centimeters in diameter. Nodules are firm and intact with a whorled pattern and

rarely cavitate (Fig. 21-6). Microscopically, the nodules are hyalinized, with a well-organized circular pattern of fibers within a cellular capsule. The amount of fibrosis appears proportional to the free silica content and to the duration of exposure. One notable characteristic of this disease is that fibrosis progresses even after removal from exposure. Except in acute silicosis, symptoms generally do not occur until after 10 to 15 years of exposure. Evidence of pathologic response to silica exposure exists well before symptoms occur.

Evaluation of workers exposed to silica includes lung function tests (which may show reduced FVC or total lung capacity early), a chest x-ray (which may appear more abnormal than the lung function tests), and determination of (a reduced) hemoglobin oxygen saturation. As the disease progresses, there is decreased oxygen saturation and reduced total lung capacity. The x-ray shows rounded opacities, localized initially to the upper lung fields (see Fig. 21-1). The size and distribution of these opacities will increase over time, and "egg shell" calcification of hilar lymph nodes occurs in 20 percent of cases.

Chronic silicosis is classified either as simple or complicated, although there is a continuum between these two forms of the disease. The simple form is noted on the chest film by the presence of multiple small, round opacities, usually in the upper zones. The concentrations of these opacities are used in classifying simple silicosis (grades 1 to 3). Although simple silicosis alone is not a common cause of disability, it can contribute to disability as well as progress to complicated silicosis. In complicated silicosis, several of the simple nodules appear to aggregate and produce larger conglomerate lesions, which enlarge and encroach on the vascular bed and airways (ILO categories A, B, C). The extent of lung function impairment appears directly related to the radiographic size of the lesions and is most severe in categories B and C.

An important complication of silicosis is tuberculosis, which persists today as an added hazard peculiar to this pneumoconiosis. Treatment of

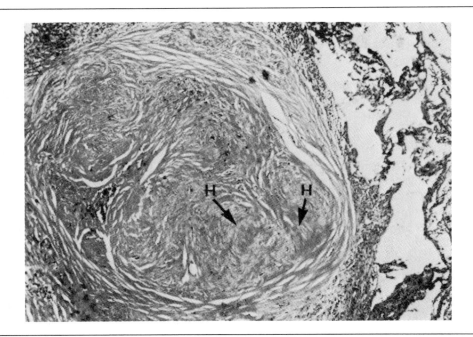

Fig. 21-6. Microscopic section of a typical silicotic nodule showing the concentric ("onion skin") arrangement of collagen fibers, some of which are hyalinized (H); lack of dust pigmentation; and the cellularity of the periphery. The lesion is clearly demarcated from adjacent lung tissue, which is substantially normal. (From WR Parkes. *Occupational Lung Disorders.* 2nd ed. London: Butterworth, 1982.)

such cases may require more vigorous drug treatment than tuberculosis without silicosis. More recently, atypical mycobacteria have supplanted *M. tuberculosis* as the important infectious complication of silicosis. To date, no interaction of silicosis has been shown with cigarette smoke effects.

Prevention of silicosis focuses on reduction of exposure through wet processes, isolation of dusty work, and local exhaust ventilation. Annual tuberculosis screening by PPD or, if the PPD is positive, chest x-ray is essential in silica-exposed workers.

Acute silicosis, a distinct entity, is a devastating disease. It is due to extraordinarily high exposures to small silica particles (1—2 μ). These exposures currently occur in abrasive sand blasting and in the production of silica flour. Symptoms include shortness of breath progressing rapidly over a few weeks, weight loss, productive cough, and sometimes pleuritic pain. Diminished resonance on percussion of the chest and also rales on auscultation can be found. Lung function tests will show a marked restrictive defect, with impressive decrement in total lung capacity. The x-ray has a diffuse ground-glass or miliary, TB-like appearance, rather than the classic nodular silicosis. The pathology in this disease shows a widespread fibrosis, with diffuse interstitial rather than nodular macroscopic appearance, and microscopic appearance resembling pulmonary alveolar proteinosis, but with doubly refractile particles of silica lying free within the alveolar exudate. Disease onset can occur 6 months to 2 years after initial exposure. Acute silicosis is often fatal, generally within 1 year.

Diatomaceous earth is an amorphous silica material mined predominantly in the western United States. It is used as a filler in paints and plastics, as a heat and sound insulator, as a filter for water and wine, and as an abrasive. In contrast to the various forms of crystalline silica, amorphous silica has relatively low pathogenicity. However, some processes using diatomaceous earth include heating (calcining) it to remove organic material. This heating process can produce up to 60 percent crystalline silica as cristobalite, which is highly fibrogenic. Exposure to this form of diatomaceous earth, therefore, must be treated the same as exposure to crystalline silica described above.

Silicate-Related Diseases, Including Asbestosis

Silica appears in a wide variety of minerals in different combined forms known as silicates. Many of these silicates (such as asbestos, kaolin, and talc) also cause pneumoconiosis, but the forms they produce have features distinct from those of silicosis. Asbestos is the most widespread and best known of the silicates and is responsible for asbestosis as well as several types of cancers (see Chap. 15).

Asbestos appears in nature in four major types (chrysotile, crocidolite, amosite, and anthophyllite) with relatively similar chronic respiratory reactions. All four types are characterized by their being fibrous and are indestructible at temperatures as high as 800°C. Use and production of these materials has greatly increased in the past century; more than 3,000,000 tons of asbestos are produced in the world annually. It is used in a variety of applications: asbestos cement products (tiles, roofing, and drain pipes), floor tile, insulation and fireproofing (in construction and ship building), textiles (for heat resistance), asbestos paper (in insulating and gaskets), and friction materials (brake linings and clutch pads). Probably

the most hazardous current exposures occur in repair and demolition of buildings and ships and in a variety of maintenance jobs where exposures may be unsuspected by the workers (Fig. 21-7). The construction industry is the major consumer of asbestos in the United States.

As with silicosis, the predominant symptoms of asbestosis are cough and SOB (the latter may be more severe than the appearance of the chest x-ray would indicate). Although not common, pleuritic pain or chest tightness may occur, and these are more frequent than in other pneumoconioses. In 20 percent of those affected, basilar rales are present, and pleural rubs and pleural effusions can occur. Pleural effusion in a person with a history of asbestos exposure even many years earlier should be considered evidence of mesothelioma until proven otherwise.

Pathologically, the macroscopic appearance of the lung is a small, pale, firm, and rubbery-like organ with a fibrotic adherent pleura. The cut surface shows patchy to widespread fibrosis and the lower lobes are more frequently affected than the upper. Microscopic appearance shows interstitial fibrosis. Chest x-ray shows widespread irregular (linear) opacities more common in the lower-lung fields (see Fig. 21-2) in contrast to the round opacities seen in silicosis, which occur first in the upper-lung fields.

A great deal of attention has focused on asbestos (or ferruginous) bodies in sputum and lung tissue. These are dumbbell-shaped bodies from 20 to 150 μ in length and 2 to 5 μ in width that appear to be fibers covered by a mucopolysaccharide layer. Iron pigment (from hemoglobin breakdown) gives them a golden-brown appearance. Although they are more frequent in individuals exposed to asbestos, they are present in most urban dwellers. They are not diagnostic of asbestos-related disease, but when present in large numbers in sputum or tissue sections, they indicate substantial exposure to airborne fibers. Asbestos bodies may also be found in other parts of the body besides the lungs, forming round fibers transported by lung lymphatics into the circulation.

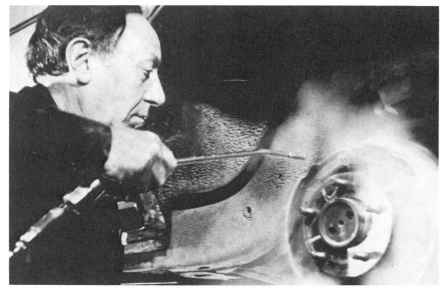

A

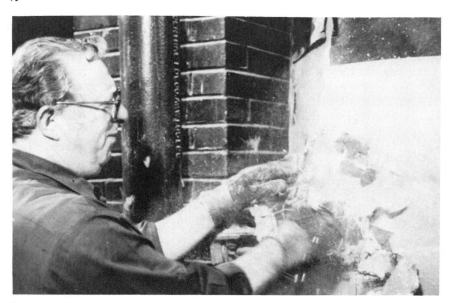

B

Fig. 21-7. Asbestos exposures. A. Brake mechanic exposed to asbestos fibers while using compressed air to clean brake drum. B. Boilermaker exposed to asbestos fibers while repairing insulation. Improper protection is illustrated. In both instances, local exhaust ventilation or personal protective equipment should be vigorously employed.
(Photographs by Nick Kaufman.)

A particular feature of asbestos exposure, unlike the other pneumoconioses, is the frequent presence of pleural plaques, which are sometimes the only evidence of exposure. These plaques, which can calcify, may be bilateral, and are located more commonly in the parietal pleura. In fact, the evidence for prior asbestos exposure or the explanation of abnormal pulmonary function tests may sometimes be found because of the calcified pleural plaques seen on chest x-ray (Fig. 21-8).

Pleural plaques are one manifestation of the rather marked pleural reaction to asbestos fibers. Other such evidence seen on the chest x-ray is a "shaggy"-appearing cardiac or diaphragmatic border. An early nonspecific sign is a blunted costophrenic angle. Diffuse pleural thickening also occurs probably less commonly than the more specific pleural plaques.

The evaluation of a worker suspected of having asbestosis includes determining if there has been a history of exposure; a physical exam to ascertain if rales are present; a chest x-ray, which may show irregular linear opacities and a variety of pleural reactions; and pulmonary function tests, which may show evidence of an interstitial type of abnormality—that is, restrictive disease and diminished diffusing capacity (DL_{CO}).

Asbestosis, like silicosis, may progress after removal from exposure. Asbestos exposure even without asbestosis carries with it the added risk of cancers of the lung, pleura and peritoneum (mesotheliomas), gastrointestinal tract, and other organs (see Chap. 15). Prevention focuses on substitution with materials such as fibrous glass, use of wet processes to reduce dust generation, and local exhaust ventilation to capture the dust that is generated. Exposed patients who smoke should be advised to stop smoking for the rest of their lives.

Talc is a hydrated magnesium silicate that occurs in a variety of forms in nature. The two major types are nonfibrous and fibrous. The nonfibrous forms, such as those found in Vermont, are free of both crystalline silica and fibrous asbestos tremolite; the fibrous forms, such as those found in New York State, can contain up to 70 percent fibrous material, including amphibole forms of asbestos. Talc exposures occur mainly during its use as an additive to paints and as a lubricant in the rubber industry, especially in inner tubes. Current evidence suggests that high doses of nonfibrous talc or moderate doses of fibrous talc accumulated over a long time will result in chronic respiratory disease known as talcosis, with the same symptoms as other pneumoconioses.

Pathologically, the macroscopic appearance of the lung is of poorly structured nodules, unlike the firm nodules of silicosis and the diffuse fibrosis of asbestosis. The microscopic appearance consists of ill-defined nodules with some diffuse interstitial fibrosis. Evaluation of persons exposed to talc includes pulmonary function tests and a chest x-ray. The chest x-ray could show both nodular and linear opacities and also pleural plaques. The possibility of a cancer risk associated with fibrous talc exposure has been addressed in several studies. Early reports found an increased risk of lung cancer in New York State talc miners, and follow-up of this group confirmed a fourfold increase in risk. However, it is now felt that the increased risk seen in that group was due to radon exposure, not asbestos-free talc. Animal studies with asbestos-free talc also have not revealed an increased cancer potential.

Kaolin (China clay) is a hydrated aluminum silicate found in the United States (in a band from Georgia to Missouri), India, and China. It is used in ceramics; as a filler in paper, rubber, paint, and plastic products; and as a mild soap abrasive. Kaolin is not particularly hazardous in the mining processes since it is generally a wet ore and mined by jet-water mining techniques.

The pneumoconiosis resulting from chronic exposures to kaolin dust produces no unique clinical features. Pathologically, the macroscopic appearance is of immature silicotic nodules, although conglomerate nodules may appear. Pleural involvement occurs only if the lung is massively involved. The microscopic appearance shows nodules with randomly distributed collagen.

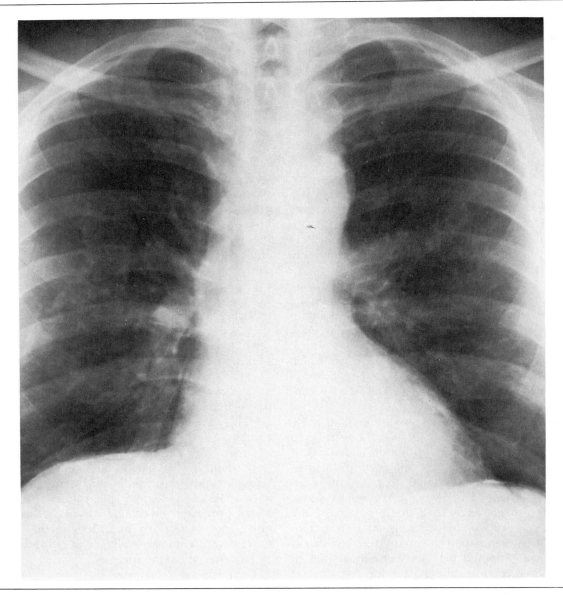

Fig. 21-8. Asbestos exposure is suggested by the presence of calcified pleural plaques seen in this AP chest x-ray, particularly on the right diaphragmatic border. (Courtesy of L. Christine Oliver, M.D.)

Coal Workers' Pneumoconiosis

In the United States until the 1960s, coal workers' respiratory disease was considered a variant of silicosis and was often known an anthracosilicosis. Now it is clear that coal workers' pneumoconiosis (CWP), popularly called "black lung," is an etiologically distinct entity, which both coal dust and pure carbon can induce. CWP exists both in simple and complicated forms; the latter, known as progressive massive fibrosis (PMF), is the most severe form of the disease. Although exposure to coal dust occurs most commonly in mines, there is some exposure in surface work. Significant exposure also occurs in the trimming or leveling of coal in ships when preparing material for transport.

Simple CWP, especially ILO profusion grade 3 (on a scale of 1 to 3), increases the likelihood for future development of the complicated form, which is generally agreed to be a disabling condition. Simple CWP is not clearly a disabling condition. The diagnosis of simple CWP has, to date, relied primarily on the chest x-ray, which shows nodular opacities of less than 1 cm (mostly < 3 mm) in diameter. PMF, in contrast, is seen on chest x-ray as the development of conglomerations of these small opacities to a size of greater than 1 cm in diameter.

In the early stages CWP is asymptomatic. The initial symptoms are breathlessness on exertion with progressive reduction in exercise tolerance. As nodular conglomeration begins and PMF is diagnosed, symptoms become more severe with marked exertional dyspnea, severe disability, or total incapacity. There is general agreement that PMF leads to premature disability and death. No such agreement, however, exists presently for the impact of simple CWP of grade 2 or less.

Coal dust also independently contributes to the disability observed in coal workers through the production of chronic bronchitis. The bronchitis is dose-related to coal dust in both smokers and nonsmokers.

Pathologically, simple CWP appears as soft, black indurated nodules. Microscopic observations show dust in and around macrophages near respiratory bronchioles. Nodules show random collagen distribution and the lung shows centrilobular emphysema. Chest x-ray shows widely distributed small, round opacities. In PMF, the large conglomerate masses have variable shape and do not respect the architecture of the lung. The surfaces are hard, rubbery, and black, and cavitation often occurs (Fig. 21-9). Copious, black sputum is often produced. Microscopically, the appearance is not distinct from the simple nodules. Chest x-ray shows large conglomerate opacities (Fig. 21-10). A separate condition called Caplan's syndrome, or rheumatoid CWP, is PMF accompanied by rheu-

Fig. 21-9. Gough section of lung of coal worker with 18 years of mining experience completed 20 years before death. It shows cavitation as well as centrilobular emphysema, which was present in both lungs. (Courtesy of J. C. Wagner, MRC Pneumoconiosis Unit, Llandough Hospital, Penarth, Wales.)

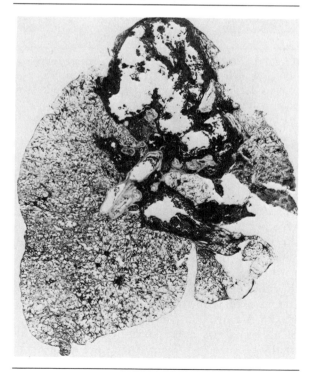

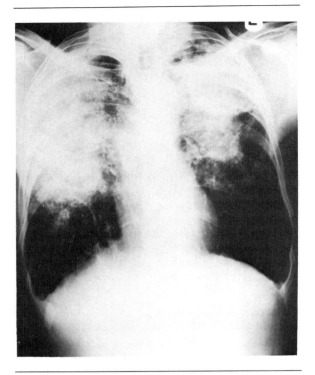

Fig. 21-10. Chest x-ray of coal worker whose lung section appears in Figure 21-9. It was taken 2 weeks before his death. The appearance is classic for progressive massive fibrosis (PMF) with larger conglomerate masses in both lung fields. (Courtesy of J. C. Wagner.)

matoid arthritis. There is a different pathologic appearance: alternate black and gray-white bands of material in the conglomerate masses. The conglomerate masses frequently cavitate or calcify. Whether there is a different clinical course for individuals with PMF accompanied by rheumatoid arthritis is not known.

Although evaluation for CWP is the same as for the other pneumoconioses, a particular feature affecting evaluation is the federal Mine Safety and Health Act of 1977, which prescribes what types of abnormalities make an individual eligible for disability benefits. Since these are subject to continuous revision, consultation with the Mine

Safety and Health Administration in the U.S. Department of Labor is advisable.

Miscellaneous Inorganic Dusts
Many questions have been raised about the potential pathogenicity of fibrous glass. At present, there is little evidence that long-term exposures to even small-particle fibrous glass produce significant nonmalignant pathologic response in the lung, although obviously marked upper respiratory tract irritation can occur. Animal experiments have shown some lung parenchymal reaction. Epidemiologic studies have suggested some chronic pulmonary effect, including lung cancer, associated with fibrous glass exposures, but a number of studies are still in progress and longer-term follow-up is necessary. Long-term studies of employment in industries using the respirable sizes of fibrous glass are now being performed.

Individual exposures to iron dusts, particularly those resulting from steel-grinding operations, welding, or foundry work, are common. The only clinical effect of pure iron oxide exposure is a reddish-brown coloring of the sputum. Lung function tests on individuals show no clinical abnormality, while the chest x-ray shows many small (0.5–2.0 mm) opacities without confluence (as with stannosis; see Fig. 21-3). Lung sections show macrophages laden with iron dust but without fibrosis or cellular reaction. With removal from further iron oxide dust exposure, the x-ray abnormalities slowly resolve. Similar results can be seen in exposures to tin, barium, and antimony.

Chronic Bronchitis
Probably the most common of the chronic responses of the respiratory tract is chronic bronchitis, which results from excessive mucus production in the bronchi. Diagnosis is made strictly on clinical grounds. *Chronic bronchitis* is a formally defined term, which must meet criteria of the American Thoracic Society: recurrent productive cough occurring 4 to 6 times a day at least 4 days out of the week, for at least 3 months during the year, for at least 2 years. The definition of simple bronchitis

("the production of phlegm on most days for as much as 3 months out of the year") can be used to distinguish those with probably important symptoms from those without. Chronic bronchitis is not a unique occupational pulmonary response; it is frequently superimposed on other respiratory diseases due to occupational toxins and most often cigarette smoke. Occupational toxins that can cause chronic bronchitis include mineral dusts and fumes (such as from coal, fibrous glass, asbestos, metals, and oils), organic dusts (such as from cotton, grains, and wood), gases (such as ozone and oxides of nitrogen), plastic compounds (such as phenolics and isocyanates), acids, and smoke (such as experienced in fire fighting).

Emphysema

Emphysema is a chronic response that depends more specifically on a pathologic description: It is the enlargement of air spaces distal to terminal (nonrespiratory) bronchioles, which includes destruction of the alveolar walls and results in air trapping. Occupational examples of this response are not well studied, but evidence suggests that fixed airway obstruction is the end stage of disease due to chronic coal dust or chronic cadmium exposure.

Granulomatous Disease

Another type of chronic response not commonly described as work-related is granuloma formation. In a granuloma many cells responding to an inciting agent become surrounded by bundles of collagen. The foreign-body granuloma in the skin is an analogous kind of tissue reaction. The best occupational example of pulmonary granulomas is chronic beryllium disease; workers who make metal alloys containing beryllium are exposed when dust control is poor. The disease appears as a restrictive pneumoconoisis although the pulmonary reaction is out of proportion to the amount of metal dust in the lungs. It is very similar to sarcoid and can be impossible to distinguish without measuring tissue levels (in lung and lymph nodes) of beryllium. Recently, a more specific test became

available: measurement of the lymphocyte blast transformation on peripheral or lavaged lymphocytes. It is difficult to perform, its sensitivity is unknown, and it is available at only a few academic medical centers.

REFERENCES

1. Ferris BG. Epidemiology standardization project. Am Rev Respir Dis 1978; 118:1–120 (part 2 of 2).
2. ILO. Guidelines for the use of the ILO international classification of pneumoconioses. Geneva: International Labor Office, 1980.
3. Gardner RM, Hankinson JL, West BJ. Evaluating commercially available spirometers. Am Rev Respir Dis 1980; 121:73.
4. Knudson RJ, et al. The maximum expiratory flow volume curve. Am Rev Respir Dis 1976; 113:587.
5. Brooks SM, Weiss MA, Bernstein IL. Reactive airways dysfunction syndrome (RADS). Persistent airways hyperreactivity after high level irritant exposure. Chest 1985; 88:376–84.

BIBLIOGRAPHY

American Lung Association. Lung disease—state of the art 1975–1976. New York: American Lung Association 1976.
   The first three articles are reviews of the epidemiology and implications for clinical practice for silicosis, respiratory disease in coal miners, and asbestos-related diseases of the lung and other organs. Although dated, these are still quite good references.
Anderson JM. Occupational lung disease. New York: American Lung Association, 1979.
   An 80-page primer in lay language that may be useful for educational programs for workers and management.
Chan-Yeung M, Lam S. Occupational asthma. Am Rev Resp Dis 1986; 133:686–703.
   A recent "state of the art" review of the subject.
Chatfield EJ, Elms PC, Muhle H, et al. Short and thin mineral fibers: identification, exposure and health effects. Solna, Sweden: National Board of Occupational Safety and Health, 1983.
   A recent summary of developing knowledge and research needs for the mineral fibers believed to be most biologically active.
Lewis BM. Pitfalls of spirometry. J Occup Med 1981; 23:35–9.
   A very functional summary of the actual procedures

for administering pulmonary function tests and some good guidelines for the interpretation of the results on individuals.

Merchant JA, Bodhlecke BA, Taylor GT. Occupational respiratory diseases. Washington, DC.: U.S. Government Printing Office, 1986. (DHHS [NIOSH] publication no. 86–102).

An inexpensive and well-written review of much of the major occupational respiratory conditions. Includes useful chapters on methods of study and evaluation of occupational respiratory disease, including environmental sampling, radiology, pulmonary function, and laboratory studies.

Morgan WKC, Seaton A. Occupational lung diseases. 2nd ed. Philadelphia: Saunders, 1984.

A readable review of occupational respiratory disease. Not as in-depth as the Parkes text, below, but somewhat better organized for reading rather than reference.

Parkes, WR. Occupational lung disorders. 2nd ed. London: Butterworths, 1982.

Excellent, detailed summary of occupational respiratory disease. Includes clinical and pathologic details. Some terminology is British but this does not cause a significant problem. Best used as a reference.

22
Musculoskeletal Disorders

Stover H. Snook, Lawrence J. Fine, and Barbara A. Silverstein

Work-related musculoskeletal disorders commonly involve the back, cervical spine, and upper extremities. Understanding of these problems has developed rapidly during the past decade. The two sections of this chapter provide an overview of these problems and a framework for recognition and prevention of them.

Low Back Pain

Stover H. Snook

A 30-year-old married auto mechanic had occasional bouts of low back pain without radiation since the age of 25. Early one morning at work, he bent forward and to the side to pick up a tire. He experienced sudden back discomfort. He continued to work, but, as the day went on, his back progressively stiffened. Toward the end of the day, he was unable to bend, was in much discomfort, and was sent home. He rested in bed and was unable to return to work the next day. After 3 days his pain subsided, and he returned to work, but he found that he had persistent discomfort and stiffness.

Two weeks later he bent over again and the back pain returned, with left thigh radiation. He was unable to finish the workday, went home again, and remained in bed. His family physician advised him to remain in bed for 2 weeks and to take aspirin and diazepam.

After 2 weeks at home the mechanic still had persistent pain. He was referred to an orthopedic surgeon, who found no evidence of neurologic impairment; there was tenderness over his lower lumbar spine and sacroiliac area, and his straight-leg raising was mildly limited. The orthopedist indicated that the mechanic had a low back sprain that might be related to a disc herniation, and he recommended continued bed rest and a structured exercise program.

A week passed. The pain subsided and the patient started exercises but could not tolerate them. He returned to the orthopedist, who took an x-ray and found no abnormalities; again, he was advised to have further bed rest. After another week had passed, he was able to walk about for short periods but had difficulty sitting, bending, and lifting and required much time lying in bed. Six weeks had now elapsed since the mechanic had stopped working; he returned to work, improved but not feeling back to normal.

The mechanic remained in relative comfort until 6 months later, when he again experienced the sudden onset of low back pain. Again he could not work, and again he sought the advice of the orthopedist and was put to bed for 2 weeks. A month later he could tolerate some activity during the day, but was unable to return to work. A second month passed; the mechanic then returned to work but could not work the entire day, and was unable to resume his former job.

He asked the orthopedist for a statement of disability and was given one, but he was informed by his supervisor that he could not keep even the available job if he did not work a normal day. He took a medical absence for another 3 weeks. His financial situation worsened. He was receiving disability pay, but many of the payments were overdue. He was very depressed. His wife was irritated with his grouchiness and his disinterest in sex.

The patient sought advice from his family physician, who said that he really did not know what he could do for him and referred him back to the orthopedist, who again found no neurologic abnormalities but thought that surgery might be indicated. But first, the orthopedist wanted the mechanic to see a psychiatrist.

This case is not unusual. Work-related back problems are common and often lead to persistent or recurrent pain with complex medical, psychologic, occupational, and legal implications. Treatment is uncertain.

Low back pain is one of the oldest occupational health problems in history. In 1700 Bernardino Ramazzini, the "founder" of occupational medicine, referred to "certain violent and irregular motions and unnatural postures of the body by which the internal structure" is impaired. Ramazzini examined the harmful effects of unusual physical activity, such as the sciatica caused by constantly turning the potter's wheel, lumbago from sitting, and hernias among porters and bearers of heavy loads. Before Ramazzini, physicians in ancient Egypt used leg-moving exercises to diagnose sciatica, recognized then as being connected with ver-

tebral problems. Authorities now believe that low pack pain existed before humans stood up on their hind legs—and that many four-legged animals suffer from this problem.

In addition to being one of the oldest occupational health problems, low back pain is one of the most common. Approximately 80 percent of the working population will experience low back pain sometime during their active working life. At any given moment, 14 percent of the adult U.S. population experiences low back pain [1]. Approximately 11 percent of Americans report low back impairment, or a reduced ability to function. Every year, about 2 percent of the employed population loses time from work because of low back pain, and approximately half of these people receive compensation for lost wages. Lost time from low back pain averages 4 hours per worker per year,

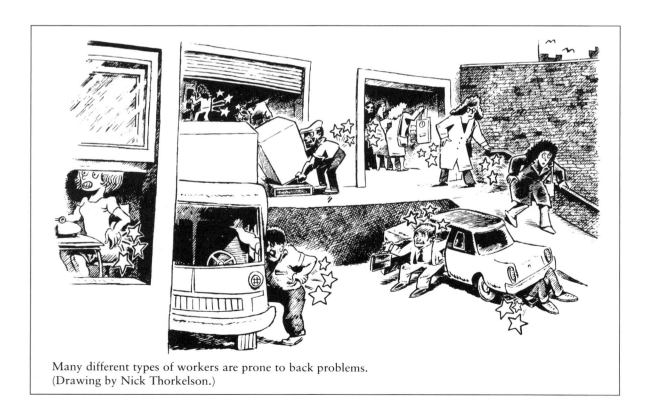

Many different types of workers are prone to back problems.
(Drawing by Nick Thorkelson.)

and among medical reasons for absence, it is second only to upper respiratory infections.

Low back pain is clearly the most costly occupational health problem. An estimated $16 billion is spent each year on the treatment and compensation of low back pain in the United States [1]. However, back pain expenses are not equally distributed; they are highly biased toward the more expensive cases. Twenty-five percent of the low back cases account for about 90 percent of the expenses. Most of the cases are relatively inexpensive. Psychologic impairments accompany many cases, either preceding or in response to the physical disability. Therefore, in cases of low back pain, one must attend to both the medical and the psychological aspects.

PATHOPHYSIOLOGY

Pain in the lumbosacral spine can result from inflammatory, degenerative, neoplastic, gynecologic, traumatic, metabolic, and other types of disorders. However, the great majority of low back pain is nonspecific and of indeterminate cause. Many theories regarding the origin of nonspecific low back pain have been proposed, but so far no one has been able to prove how and where the pain arises. There is no definite proof that nonspecific low back pain is associated with fasciitis, fibrositis, myositis, ruptured or degenerated ligaments, strain or sprain, degenerative joint disease, synovitis of the apophyseal joints, or hypertrophied ligamentum flavium. The intervertebral disc is the largest avascular structure in the body, devoid of directly penetrating vessels after 20 years of age (Fig. 22-1). Nutrition apparently is accomplished by diffusion of solutes through the endplates and the anulus fibrosus. Studies have shown that the boundary zone between the nucleus pulposus and anulus fibrosus is exposed to relative nutrient deficiency with respect to small solutes. This is the same location that biomechanical studies have indicated as an area of the highest tensile strain on the anular lamellae. No conclusive evidence confirms the role of abnormalities of the intervertebral disc, although the following indications suggest its involvement: [2, 3].

1. Herniation of the disc is often preceded by one or more attacks of nonspecific low back pain.
2. Disc degeneration, as seen on x-rays, is found significantly more often in people with low back pain.
3. Intradiscal injection of hypertonic saline or contrast medium often produces symptoms similar to those of nonspecific low back pain in both patients and controls.
4. Investigations have been performed in which thin nylon threads were surgically fastened to various structures in the lower back. Three to four weeks after surgery, these structures were irritated by pulling on the threads. Low back pain symptoms were produced only by irritating the anulus fibrosus and the nerve root.
5. Pathologic radial tears and ruptures are first seen in the outer anulus fibrosus at approximately age 25, the same age when low back symptoms become clinically important. When subjected to small amounts of pressure, these abnormal discs burst posteriorly or posterolaterally through the anulus fibrosus. Normal discs, on the other hand, burst inferiorly or superiorly through the vertebral endplates—and only under much higher pressures. Morphologic studies have found central posterior buttonhole protrusions of nuclear material, which have burst through the anulus fibrosus and that lie just beneath the posterior longitudinal ligament—a site where pain receptors have been found; this possible source of low back pain would be difficult to detect in the living patient.

Although the specific cause of low back pain is unknown, most authorities believe that low back pain is basically caused by changes in the spine, usually as one gets older. It is thought that these changes lower the resistance of the spine to heavy workloads; consequently, heavy workloads merely trigger the occurrence or onset of low back symp-

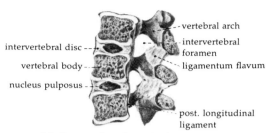

Median section through three successive vertebrae.

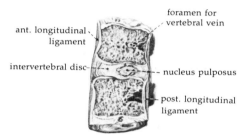

Median section through the intervertebral disc.

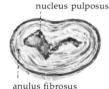

The intervertebral disc seen from above.

Fig. 22-1. The intervertebral disc. Movements in the vertebral column occur at the intervertebral joints, but the intervertebral discs also play an important role. These discs consist of an anulus fibrosus composed of fibrocartilage and a nucleus pulposus consisting of a gelantinous material that contains much water. The discs serve as shock absorbers and allow the vertebral bodies to move in relation to each other, as in flexion and extension of the spine.

The intervertebral discs are of great clinical importance. If the discs are exposed to sudden shocks or extreme compression, as in lifting heavy loads, the posterior part of the anulus fibrosus may be ruptured. This rupture occurs most frequently in the lumbar and cervical regions but rarely in the thoracic area. The nucleus pulposus is then forced through the ruptured area and protrudes (herniates) either into the vertebral canal or, more laterally, into the intervertebral foramen. Depending on the site of herniation, a spinal nerve or part of the spinal cord may be compressed. (From J Langman and MW Woerdeman. *Atlas of Medical Anatomy.* Philadelphia: Saunders, 1978.)

toms. The spinal changes related to injury include the following [4]:

1. The cartilaginous endplate undergoes fibrillation without evidence of repair; fissures form progressively with loss of integrity, subsequent thinning, calcium salt deposition, and ultimate necrosis that causes loss of the endplate.
2. The anulus fibrosus initially contains distinct fibers. During disc degeneration, it progressively becomes hyalinized and less cellular. It also becomes coarse with fissuring, shows signs of cell death and deposition of pigment, and, ultimately loses its lamellar distinction with shortened and thickened fibrils and hypocellularity.
3. The nucleus pulposus begins as a gelatinous, fairly acellular material at maturity, but with degeneration, it loses its mucoid appearance, and a fibrillar network appears. With time, the distinction between the nucleus and anulus becomes obscured, and fibrous change ensues, accompanied by pigment formation, desiccation, and cleft formation.
4. The intervertebral disc loses its blood supply by age 20. With increasing age, water content is decreased, collagen exhibits polymorphism, proteoglycan molecules decrease in size, and keratin sulfate increases.

With all these changes, the disc no longer behaves in a hydrostatic fashion, and the biomechanics of the entire motion segment are altered.

SIGNS AND SYMPTOMS
The most common types of low back pain have been classified as lumbar insufficiency, lumbago, and sciatica [5].

Lumbar insufficiency is defined as fatigue, stiffness, or pain in the lower back. These symptoms, frequently described as a "tight band across the small of the back," are often provoked by certain forms of exertion—particularly work in a bent-forward position. Symptoms are sometimes experienced when getting up in the morning or when sitting or standing for long periods. It is often difficult to straighten the back when standing up. The intensity of the symptoms can vary greatly; periods of pronounced discomfort usually alternate with periods of little or no discomfort. Lumbar insufficiency may or may not incapacitate the worker, depending on the nature of the job.

Lumbago (or nonspecific low back pain) is a more intense pain in the lower back that usually incapacitates the worker, especially the worker with an active or physically demanding job. The lumbago attack may begin in three different ways:

1. The worker experiences sudden, intense pain in the lower back and can barely move from the place where the attack occurs. Frequently there is pain fixation or locking of the back in an oblique or forward-flexed position. The attack almost always occurs in connection with a movement of the lumbar spine. The movement may be simply bending or stooping; it may be a sudden or unexpected twist; or it may be lifting a heavy object.
2. The worker reports that "something happened to my back" (often described as a kink or hitch) during some kind of movement of the lumbar spine. The symptoms are so minor that they are usually disregarded. However, after a day or two, the symptoms intensify and become just as severe as the sudden attack described above.
3. The worker describes a smooth gradual transition from the less severe symptoms of lumbar insufficiency into the intense pain of lumbago. There may be no connection between the onset of pain and particular spinal movement.

Sciatica is the pain that radiates into either leg, usually down the posterior or lateral aspect of the thigh and lower leg, and frequently is associated with numbness or tingling in the foot and toes. The symptoms may be mild and transitory or more pronounced and incapacitating. It is important to note that buttock and thigh pain alone do not constitute sciatica since pain can be referred from the back to these areas, as mediated by the posterior primary ramus.

Muscle spasms are frequently present with low back pain and may prevent the worker from standing fully erect. When present, muscle spasms are often regarded as a cause of low back pain and lead to a diagnosis of muscle strain. However, as indicated earlier, there is no definite proof that low back pain is associated with the muscles. Therefore, muscle spasms should be regarded as a physical sign of low back pain and not as a cause.

Most authorities report that women are afflicted with low back pain as often as men. The average age of compensatable low back pain is 34 for males and 35 for females. However, the greatest incidence of compensatable low back pain (number of compensation claims per 100 workers per year) occurs in the twenties [6]. Although the incidence of low back pain is greater with younger workers, the severity of the disorder is not as great as with older workers. In the twenties, low back pain is usually mild, diffuse, and of short duration, followed by a return to full activity. In the thirties, there are more frequent attacks of localized and lateralized pain, relieved by rest, and followed by pain-free periods. In the forties, low back pain may be accompanied by episodes of sciatica, with residual pain between attacks. In the fifties, the pain often becomes less severe and more arthritic in nature, with stiffness in the morning that is usually relieved by physical activity. Finally, in the sixties, many individuals will find substantial relief from pain, although range of spinal motion is also decreased.

DIAGNOSIS

In arriving at a diagnosis for low back pain, the physician must first determine whether the disorder is regional or systemic. The use of x-rays and extensive laboratory tests are of little value except in confirming systemic disease.

A thorough history provides important clues in determining whether the disorder is regional or systemic. The onset of regional low back pain is acute and can occur at any working age; the pain is aggravated by exercise and relieved by lying down (unloading the spine). The back pain of ankylosing spondylitis, on the other hand, is characterized by insidious onset gradually at an age of less than 40 years, duration of at least 3 months, stiffness in the morning, and improvement with exercise. The bone pain of metastasis or myeloma tends to be more continuous, progressive, and prominent when recumbent. Referred pain from pelvic or abdominal viscera is unrelated to spinal movement or posture and may be associated with indigestion, renal colic or dysuria, or phases of the menstrual cycle. Back pain from infection may be accompanied by fever.

If the low back disorder is considered regional, the physician must then determine whether a surgical emergency exists. A surgical emergency exists only when there are signs and symptoms suggesting the *cauda equina* syndrome, caused by central or midline herniation of a disc or a tumor in the spinal canal. Symptoms of cauda equina syndrome include bladder and bowel dysfunction, saddle anesthesia, and reduced rectal sphincter tone and cremasteric reflexes. Measurements of spinal motion contribute little to the diagnosis of this syndrome.

If there are indications of sciatica or nerve root irritation, a diagnosis of discogenic low back pain can be made. Pain during straight-leg raising (SLR) suggests root irritation and is suggestive, but not diagnostic, of discal herniation. A positive SLR result occurs when back pain (not merely posterior leg pain) is reproduced at less than 70°; pain occurring beyond 70° is nonspecific. Other neurologic tests involving motor, sensory, and reflex changes will also indicate nerve root irritation. However, most cases of regional low back pain will not have these indications and must be diagnosed as nonspecific low back pain.

Nonspecific low back pain has no pathologic connotations and represents an honest appraisal of our current state of knowledge. The diagnosis of nonspecific low back pain is preferred over diagnoses such as lumbosacral strain, sacroiliac strain, or apophyseal joint subluxation, for which there are no demonstrated pathologic changes. Persons diagnosed as suffering nonspecific low back pain should be reevaluated at regular intervals to determine if any specific pathology develops.

HIGH-RISK JOBS

The risk of developing low back pain is high in the construction, mining, transportation, and manufacturing industries, especially with jobs requiring heavy physical demands, awkward postures, or postures that must be sustained for prolonged periods of time. The jobs with the highest incidence of compensatable low back pain are (in descending order): miscellaneous laborers, garbage collectors, warehouse workers, miscellaneous mechanics, nursing aides, nonspecific laborers, material handlers, lumber workers, practical nurses, and construction laborers [6]. Epidemiologic studies estimate that truck drivers are almost 5 times more likely to develop an acute herniated lumbar disc than others [7]. Truck drivers, of course, often load and unload trucks; these tasks contribute to the high risks they face for this and other musculoskeletal disorders. Measurements of intradiscal pressure are higher when sitting (especially without adequate lumbar support) than when standing [3]. The adverse effect of vehicular vibration is also considered as a risk factor.

Insurance company data indicate that a worker is 3 times more susceptible to compensatable low back pain if exposed to excessive manual handling tasks [8]. Studies of physically heavy jobs in the electronic, steel, rubber, and aluminum industries have reported similar findings [9]. In this context, the worker's perception of the job is important. Several investigators have found that when workers were asked to rate subjectively the degree of physical effort or strain in their jobs, low back pain appeared significantly more often in those who believed their work to be harder. It is also important to realize that low back pain in a sedentary worker is not nearly as incapacitating as the same problem in a material handler.

The work of nurses and nursing aides—especially the moving of patients (see Fig. 31-3)—is similar to that of material handlers who move heavy objects in industry. Some data indicate much low back pain among nurses, but other data show little difference between nurses and more sedentary workers in the overall prevalence of low back pain [10]. However, the onset of low back pain in nurses comes at an earlier age and is largely precipitated by factors at work; in sedentary workers, low back pain increases gradually with age and is generally nonoccupational.

Awkward postures are common in many nursing and industrial tasks, particularly bending forward and reaching out. When handling heavy objects, intradiscal pressure, myoelectric activity, and intra-abdominal pressure increase substantially as the distance between the object and the body increases [11]. Postures that must be sustained for long periods have also been associated with low back pain. For example, a high incidence of low back pain has been shown in workers who sit for prolonged periods and in those who stand for prolonged periods; a much smaller incidence of low back pain is shown in workers who can vary their posture by sitting for short, repeated periods of time [12].

MANAGEMENT

Most authorities now agree that safe, inexpensive conservative treatment is indicated for at least the first 3 months of nonspecific and discogenic low back pain. Surgery should not be considered during this period except under the emergency conditions described earlier. Approximately half of all sciatica patients will be greatly improved after 6 weeks. If surgery is indicated by good objective criteria, the best results are achieved when surgery is performed at approximately 3 months [13] (see also Nachemson in bibliography).

Bed rest is necessary for those who are highly incapacitated. However, too much bed rest can be counterproductive. The length of bed rest needs to be tempered by clinical judgment. One study concluded that for patients without neurologic deficits, 2 days of bed rest was just as good as 7 days [14]. Almost every patient will benefit from modest doses of aspirin. Controlled studies have demonstrated the benefits of isometric abdominal exercises. Rotational manipulation has been shown to reduce pain for short periods. The effectiveness of traction, corsets, and braces has not yet been demonstrated. Objective studies are also lacking for other treatments, such as ultrasound, shortwave diathermy, heat, and cold.

Almost every low back pain patient suffers from anxieties about chronic pain and long-term functional impairment. The physician must address these issues in a supportive and honest manner. The concepts of managing back pain must be explained in whatever detail is comprehensible to the patient, including mechanical advice regarding the avoidance of lifting, bending, and prolonged sitting during the acute phase. The patient should be encouraged to participate and be a partner in the management of the disorder and to attend a back school or rehabilitation program.

Physicians must remember that they are not treating backs, but human beings who happen to have painful backs. Assessment of the patient's personality and an understanding of its relationship to the back condition, job, and status in life are prerequisites to the effective management of low back pain. True malingering at the onset of low back pain is rare. Accusations of malingering, whether direct or indirect, will lead to an adversary situation that interferes with recovery. It is important to establish an emotionally satisfactory relationship between the patient and the physician, and the physician should coordinate management of the case with the patient's family and job supervisor. Systematic follow-up is necessary to provide the physician with progress information and the patient with reassurance.

PROGNOSIS

Nonspecific low back pain is a self-limiting disorder that resolves itself in over 90 percent of cases.

Approximately 40 percent of the patients will recover within 1 week, 80 percent within 3 weeks, and 90 percent within 6 weeks, regardless of treatment. The rate of recurrence, however, is very high—estimates range up to 90 percent. A British study indicates that the probability of low back pain is almost 4 times greater in individuals who have had previous episodes of low back pain [15].

At the onset of low back pain, it is very difficult to predict the cases that will require longer than 6 weeks to recover. A specific diagnosis, prior injury, and psychologic impairment have all been correlated with long recovery times. If workers have been off the job for longer than 6 months, it is estimated that there is only a 50 percent possibility of ever returning to productive employment; over 1 year, only 25 percent; and over 2 years, almost none [16].

Early return to work is now considered an important part of the therapy. However, there are many reasons why patients do not go back to work. Patients may suffer from illness behavior, especially if they have been disabled longer than 3 months. The obstacles to early return to work are several. These include: (1) the problem of identifying and providing modified work; (2) the unwillingness to accept workers back unless they are 100 percent recovered (despite evidence that accepting a partially recovered worker may be less costly and more effective in promoting recovery than continued disability); (3) difficulties imposed by rigid work rules; (4) inappropriate treatment by practitioners, or prolonged use of ineffective treatment; and (5) legal advice to accept a lump sum settlement instead of a rehabilitation program designed to return the person to work. The physician should be aware of these situations and recognize their relative importance in each case of low back pain.

CONTROL

There is no simple control for the complex problem of low back pain. It is impossible to prevent low back pain completely in industry, especially since the pathophysiology is not clearly understood. However, it does appear possible to control low back pain by reducing the probability of the initial episode, reducing the severity of the symptoms, reducing the length of disability, and reducing the chance of recurrence. Low back pain prevention is accomplished by a combination of measures that are listed in Table 22-1. No single measure by itself will control low back pain; it must be a combination of all the measures. Nevertheless, some measures are more effective than others, and these should be implemented first.

Table 22-1. Prevention of low back pain

Job design (ergonomics)
    Mechanical aids
    Optimum work level
    Good workplace layout
    Sit/stand work stations
    Appropriate packaging
Job placement (selection)
    Careful history
    Thorough physical examination
    No routine x-rays
    Strength testing
    Job-rating programs
Training and education
    Training workers
        Biomechanics of body movement (safe lifting)
        Strength and fitness
        Back schools
    Training managers
        Response to low back pain
        Early return to work
        Ergonomic principles of job design
    Training labor union representatives
        Early return to work
        Flexible work rules
        Reasonable referrals
    Training practitioners
        Appropriate medication
        Prudent use of x-rays
        Limited bed rest
        Early return to work (with restrictions, if
          necessary)

For example, it is estimated that good ergonomic design of the job can reduce up to one-third of compensatable low back pain in industry. Not only can good job design reduce the probability of initial and recurring episodes, it will also allow the worker with moderate symptoms to stay on the job longer and permit the disabled worker to return to the job sooner. Good ergonomic design reduces the worker's exposure to the risk factors of low back pain through the following:

1. Mechanical aids (powered or manual) to assist with heavy weights and forces (Figs. 22-2 and 22-3).
2. Optimum work level to reduce unnecessary bending (Fig. 22-4).
3. Good workplace layout to reduce unnecessary twisting and reaching (Fig. 22-5).
4. Sit/stand work stations to reduce prolonged sitting and standing.
5. Appropriate packaging to match object weights with human capabilities.

The National Institute for Occupational Safety and Health (NIOSH) has provided guidelines for evaluating and designing manual lifting tasks [17] (see Chap. 9). Guidelines for other manual-handling tasks, (such as pushing, pulling, or carrying) have been developed [18].

Although job design may be applicable to many manufacturing operations, there are other jobs that are difficult to design and control, such as fire fighting, police work, and certain construction and delivery operations. These jobs require greater dependence on preplacement testing and selection of workers. The preplacement medical examination has been used in many industries, especially since the enactment of workers' compensation laws. It has been estimated that, with careful history taking and a thorough examination, about 7 or 8 percent of young individuals prone to future back problems might be identified. The identification rate would be substantially higher with applicants in older age groups, where the findings of disease are more frequent and more obvious.

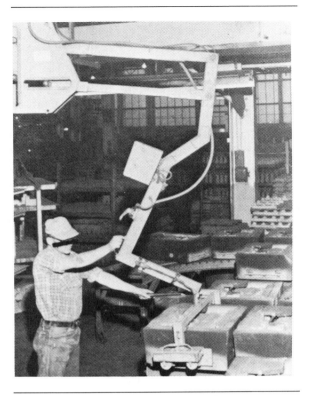

Fig. 22-2. Load positioners offer the ability to counterbalance the weight of a load, enabling the operator to position it accurately. They are particularly applicable to loading and unloading heavy pieces into machines. They use air pressure to balance the weight but still require the operator to move the piece in the direction needed, giving the operator more actual control and greater speed than with an electric chain hoist. (From Liberty Mutual Insurance Company.)

Many authorities feel that the medical history is the most important part of the medical examination in identifying workers who are susceptible to future low back pain. Knowing that the worker has had previous low back pain is significant, because after an initial episode of back pain, the probability of additional episodes of low back pain is 4 times greater [15].

Routine x-rays of the lumbar spine have often been part of the preplacement medical examination, although much evidence indicates that the small yield does not justify the radiation exposure or increased cost. According to guidelines issued by the American Occupational Medical Association, lumbar spine x-ray examinations should not be used as a risk-assessment procedure for back problems, but only as a special diagnostic procedure used by the physician when there are appropriate indications. Such indications include recurrent episodes of back pain and suspicion of an underlying congenital defect, or rheumatologic, neoplastic, or infectious etiology. Recent advances have been made in measuring the size of the spinal canal by ultrasound [19]. This noninvasive technique has been used to show that patients with symptomatic disc lesions have lumbar spinal canals that are significantly more narrow than asymptomatic subjects [20]. Other investigators, however, have not been able to reproduce these results.

Several studies have demonstrated the relationship between strength/fitness and the incidence of low back pain. Studies of isometric strength testing have shown that the probability of a musculoskeletal disorder is up to 3 times greater when job-lifting requirements approach or exceed the worker's isometric strength capability [9]. A recent study revealed that men who experience low back pain for the first time had lower isometric endurance of the back muscles when measured up to 1 year before the episode [21]. The results for women, however, were not the same. Although isometric strength testing may be an effective selection technique, it should only be used for jobs that are difficult to design or control and for which a careful ergonomic evaluation has been made. Strength testing should never be used as a substitute for good job design. Several attempts have been made to develop dynamic lifting tests, since dynamic lifting represents a better simulation of the actual lifting task. Unfortunately, there have been no studies showing the effectiveness of dy-

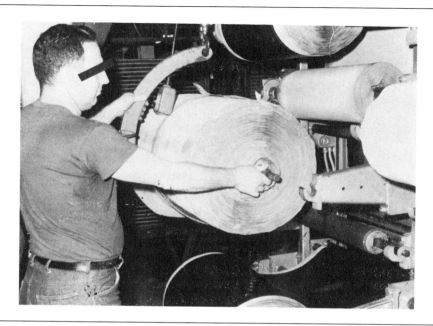

Fig. 22-3. Overhead hoists/lifting attachments. Overhead hoists with specially designed lifting attachments to fit the objects being handled eliminate the awkward manual handling tasks. This C-shaped attachment allows quick and easy placement of heavy rolls on a tire building machine. (From Liberty Mutual Insurance Company.)

namic strength testing as a preplacement technique for reducing the incidence and severity of musculoskeletal disorders.

Job-rating programs are structured attempts to evaluate the job as well as the worker, and then to obtain a good match between the two. These programs not only screen out inappropriate applicants, but also find suitable work for people of varying abilities. However, these programs have not been proven to reduce the occurrence of low back pain.

Training and education are the oldest and most commonly used approaches for reducing low back pain in industry. Safety and personnel departments have typically used education and training to instruct employees in proper methods and work procedures. For example, training the worker in the biomechanics of safe lifting has been a part of safety programs in industry for over 50 years. However, according to NIOSH, the value of training programs in safe lifting is open to question because there have been no controlled studies showing consequent decreases in rates of manual-handling accidents or back injuries [17]. A major problem is compliance; even after training, most workers do not lift correctly because it is a more difficult way to lift. Greater training compliance results from workers who have (or have had) low back pain. It appears that this type of training would be more effective if concentrated on workers with a history of low back pain. Exercises to increase strength and fitness have been a part of

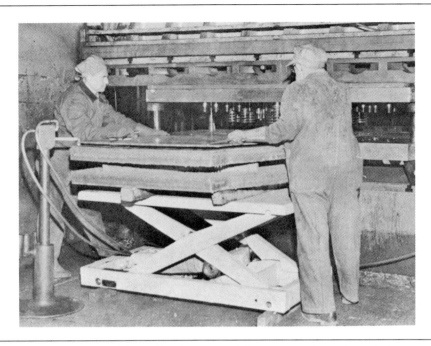

Fig. 22-4. Scissors lift. Hydraulic scissors lifts have a variety of uses in industry to position the workpiece so that a minimum of effort must be used to perform the operation. They can place the workpiece at the proper height to convert lifting and lowering tasks to carries or pushes. (From Liberty Mutual Insurance Company.)

low back pain treatment programs for many years, but only recently have strength and fitness programs been advocated in industry to reduce or prevent the onset of low back pain.

The back school is an attempt to educate the worker in all aspects of back care; it represents a much more comprehensive approach to back care that includes the previous topics of safe lifting, strength, and physical fitness. The original concept of the back school was to educate patients who were already suffering (or had recently suffered) from low back pain—that is, it was a form of treatment. A more recent use of the back school is to educate workers in industry on how to prevent low back pain. Controlled studies have demonstrated the effectiveness of a low back school when

used as treatment for patients [22]. However, no controlled study has been reported showing the effectiveness of a low back school as a preventive technique for workers.

Training managers is as important as training workers. Although low back pain cannot be totally prevented at the present time, managers can help prevent long-term disability from low back pain that does occur. Long-term disability is associated with adversary situations, litigation, hospitalization, and lack of follow-up and concern. Many of these situations can be alleviated by training foremen, supervisors, and upper-level managers in appropriate responses to low back pain. Also important is providing modified, alternative, or part-time work as a means of re-

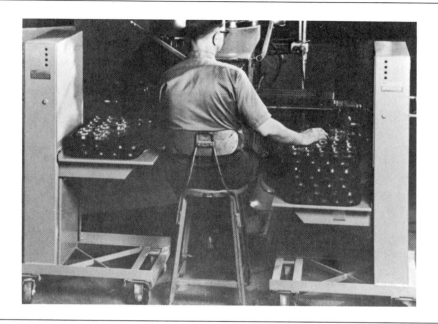

Fig. 22-5. Work dispensers are self-leveling devices designed to keep parts at a particular height eliminating the need to bend over to pick up or release an item. Models are available to utilize trays or pans, as well as for bulk-dispensing of small parts. The dispensers are portable and may be wheeled from station to station, eliminating the need to lift, carry, and lower trays as well as individual parts. (From Liberty Mutual Insurance Company.)

turning the worker to the job as quickly as possible.

A program in which management was trained in the positive acceptance of low back pain has been described [23, 24]. An atmosphere was created in which workers were encouraged to report all episodes of low back pain—even minor episodes—to the company clinic. Immediate and conservative in-house treatment, including worker education, was provided by the company nurse. Attempts were made to keep the worker on the job—often with modified duties or redesigned job. If necessary, referrals were made to the company physician, who closely monitored treatment and progress. Over a 3-year period, annual workers' compensation costs for low back pain claims were reduced from over $200,000 to less than $20,000. Although this was not a controlled study, the results are certainly impressive.

Unions must also be instructed in appropriate responses to their members with low back pain. Early return to work should be encouraged, especially where management is willing to provide modified, alternative, or part-time work. Union-management cooperation is, of course, necessary to achieve this goal. Early return to work is an important part of the treatment of low back pain. Unions can often assist in the recovery of their members by allowing early return to work through flexible work rules and referrals to clinicians and lawyers who will not unnecessarily prolong the disability.

Company medical personnel should be trained in the benefits of early intervention, conservative treatment, patient follow-up, and job placement techniques. Both physicians and nurses should be familiar with recent literature that objectively evaluates various types of treatment for low back pain. Medical personnel should also be familiar with the physical demands of jobs performed in the company in order to adequately place injured workers—and new employees.

The effectiveness of a standardized approach to the diagnosis and treatment of low back pain in industry has been demonstrated (see Wiesel in bibliography). This approach was used to monitor the course and treatment for employees with low back pain. If there was any disagreement between the investigators (who were orthopedic surgeons) and the treating physician, they discussed the case together in detail. Usually, they reached an agreement; if they did not, another physician was consulted for an independent opinion. This program dramatically decreased the number of low back patients, the number of days lost, and the number of cases sent to surgery.

Although knowledge of low back pain is limited, it is quite clear that enough is already known to adequately control the problem in industry. Instead of waiting for a major medical breakthrough to occur, emphasis should be placed on applying the knowledge that is already available. Low back pain control requires the combined efforts of workers, managers, unions, nurses, physicians, and others.

Work-Related Disorders of the Neck and Upper Extremity

Lawrence J. Fine and Barbara A. Silverstein

A 31-year-old, right-handed man had been employed in a variety of automobile-manufacturing jobs for 13 years. Two years ago he switched to a new plant and was assigned to a job requiring him to move a spotwelding machine beneath cars moving overhead. He had a minute to complete four welds on each car. The spot welder, which had metal handles, required substantial force to position it appropriately, and it had to be repositioned 4 times for each car. The worker's wrists were in complete extension for a substantial portion of the job cycle.

When the worker started on this job, the weekday work shift was 9 hours long and Saturday work was required in most weeks. After 3 weeks on the job, he noted that he had pain in both wrists. He also noted numbness and tingling in the first four fingers of his left hand, first only at night, a few nights each week, after he had fallen asleep. When he awoke at night with the numbness, he would get up and walk around shaking his hands; in about 10 minutes, he would be able to go back to sleep. Gradually over the next several months, the numbness and pain worsened both in frequency and intensity. His left hand would feel numb by the end of the work shift, and any time he was driving, his hands would become numb. Since he liked his job and did not want to be placed on restriction, which would mean he could not work overtime, he decided to visit his private physician rather than the company physician. He also was not sure that the company physician would be very sympathetic to his complaints.

His physician found on physical examination that he had decreased sensitivity to light touch in the left index and middle fingers and a positive Phalen's test of the left hand (see appendix to this chapter). She suspected carpal tunnel syndrome (CTS) and suspected that the disorder might be work-related because the patient was young, male, and had no other risk factors, such as diabetes, past history of wrist fracture, or recent trauma to the wrist. The physician discussed job changes with the patient. She also prescribed wrist splints to be used only at night.

The splints relieved some of the nighttime numbness for a period. However, over the next 6 months, the patient's symptoms began to be present all of the time, and he thought that his left hand was becoming weaker. He also developed similar symptoms in his right hand.

The patient felt he could no longer do his job and returned to his physician. She noted that the Phalen's test was now positive bilaterally. She referred him to a hand surgeon. Nerve conduction tests showed slowing of sensory nerve impulse conduction in the median nerve in the region of the carpal tunnel.

One year after the problem was first noted, he had

surgery, first on the left hand and then on the right hand. Following surgery, he was placed in a transitional work center by the company for a 3-month period where he worked at his own pace and had no symptoms. He then returned to the assembly line with the restriction that he not use welding guns or air-powered hand tools. While he worked on the line, he occasionally had symptoms, but they were substantially less intense and less frequent than before.

Now, he has transferred to a warehouse, because he felt that he would have a better chance of avoiding long layoffs there. He was placed on a job that required use of a stapling gun to seal packages. Three weeks after being placed on this job, his symptoms began to return with their former intensity. Through ordinary channels, he immediately sought and was given a transfer to a position driving a forklift truck. This change reduced, but did not eliminate, his symptoms. He has numbness, tingling, and pain in the fingers of both hands about twice a month. Playing volleyball usually triggers a severe attack. With the use of nighttime splints, he can sleep through most nights without awakening. While he feels that his hands are weaker than before he developed his symptoms, he still is able to perform his job. He decided that as long as his symptoms remain at this level, he will continue working.

This case illustrates the intermittent and progressive nature of the common work-related disorders of the upper extremity. These disorders, in contrast to low back pain, which is often not clinically easy to relate to a disorder of a specific tendon, joint, or compressed nerve, can be more easily related to a specific anatomic site. Common examples of disorders of the neck and upper extremity that may be related to work include CTS [25], DeQuervain's disease [26], trigger finger [27], lateral epicondylitis (tennis elbow) [28], rotator (or rotor) cuff tendinitis (mainly supraspinatus) [29], and tension neck syndrome (costalscapular syndrome) [30]. This family of disorders may involve muscles (tension neck syndrome), tendons (DeQuervain's disease), joints (degenerative joint disease [31]), skin (callouses), nerves (CTS), or blood vessels (vibration white-finger disease, or Raynaud's phenomenon of occupational origin [32]).

In addition to these disorders with specific physical findings on physical examination, workers in certain occupations (for example, musicians, meat packers, and keypunch operators) often have an elevated rate of complaints of pain in the upper extremity or neck. These symptoms are similar to low back pain because a specific anatomic source of this pain cannot be identified on clinical evaluation. As with low back pain, these pains are common, often intermittent in nature, and lead to disability and impairment, although they do so less frequently than back pain does.

Few of the specific disorders, and none of the nonspecific disorders have been adequately studied epidemiologically in working populations. Specific jobs in many manufacturing and nonmanufacturing industries have been associated with elevated rates of work-related disorders of the neck and upper extremity, including meat cutters, grinders, welders, sewer workers, and numerous other workers.

Conceptually these disorders have some of the characteristics of both occupational diseases and work-related diseases as defined by the World Health Organization (WHO) (see box in Chap. 3), depending on the specific disorder and occupation under study.

The WHO concept of "work-relatedness" is not only useful in understanding differences between different diseases or disorders, but is also useful in understanding the association between different types of work and the etiology of a single disorder. Some occupational factors, such as highly forceful and repetitive flexion and extension of the wrist, will cause CTS in a large enough fraction of the exposed population, regardless of age or gender, to conform to most characteristics of occupational disease in these highly exposed populations. In some situations, the relationship between work factors and disorders of the upper extremity will be at the other end of the spectrum (such as with ganglions and thoracic outlet syndrome) with an unclear, weak, or inconsistent relationship.

SIGNS AND SYMPTOMS

This broad group of work-related disorders of the neck and upper extremity has a very diverse set of symptoms and physical findings. However, a history and physical examination of the upper limb and neck can tentatively diagnose many of these disorders [33] (see appendix to this chapter).

PATHOPHYSIOLOGY

Clinical, laboratory, and epidemiologic studies all have contributed to the current understanding of the pathophysiology of work-related musculoskeletal disorders of the upper extremity and neck. While the current level of knowledge is incomplete, it nevertheless guides both treatment and preventive strategies. Five occupational factors are important in the etiology of these disorders: repetitive motions, forceful motions, mechanical stresses, static or awkward postures, and local vibration (Fig. 22-6).

Repetitive motions of the hands, wrists, shoulders, and neck commonly occur in the workplace. A data entry operator may perform 20,000 keystrokes per hour, a worker in a meat-processing plant may perform 12,000 cuts with a knife per day, and a worker on an assembly line may elevate the right shoulder above the level of the acromion 7,500 times per day. These repetitive motions in an individual may eventually exceed the ability to recover from this stress, especially if forceful contractions of muscles are involved in the repetitive motions.

The failure to recover usually implies the persistence of inflammation ("condition into which tissues enter as a reaction to injury"). In musculoskeletal work-related disorders the sites of inflammation most commonly involve tendons, tendon sheaths, and tendon attachments to bones, bursae, and joints. This persistent inflammation can lead to nerve compression (CTS), chronic fibrous reaction in the tendon, tendon rupture, calcium deposits, or fibrous nodule formations in a tendon, leading to trigger finger [34].

Abrupt increases in the number of repetitive motions performed by the worker each day is clinically well recognized as a cause of tendinitis. Too many forceful contractions of muscles can cause their corresponding tendons to stretch, compressing the microstructures of the tendons, leading to

Fig. 22-6. Schematic representation of pathophysiology of work-related disorders of the upper extremity and neck.

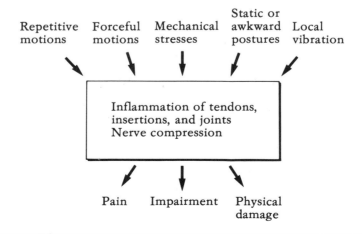

ischemia, microscopic tears in tendons, progressive lengthening, and sliding of tendon fibers through the ground substance matrix. All these vents can cause inflammation of tendons.

An important, but inadequately investigated, question is whether the repetitive stresses to the joints of upper limbs that occur in some occupations lead to the accelerated development of localized osteoarthrosis (LOA). Since LOA is not a specific disease but the final common pathway of biomechanical and pathologic changes in cartilage, subchondral bone, and bone-surrounding joints, it is reasonable to assume that repetitive stresses can accelerate its development [31, 34]. The pathophysiology of the nonspecific localized pain that is not clearly related to a specific episode of tendinitis, LOA, or nerve compression, is not clear.

In addition to repetitive and forceful motions, three other exposure variables that influence the development of work-related musculoskeletal disorders are mechanical stress, work performed in awkward or static postures, and segmental (localized) vibration.

Mechanical stress in tendons results from muscle contractions or when a tendon or other tissues is compressed because of contact between the body and another object. One of the major determinants of the level of the mechanical stress is the force of the muscle contractions. For example, a pinch that is very forceful will be more stressful than one that is not very forceful. Mechanical stress is often produced by hand-held tools with hard sharp edges or short handles. The tool exerts just as much force on the hand as the hand does on the tool.

Work performed in awkward or static postures is another important influence on the development of work-related musculoskeletal disorders. The level of mechanical stress produced by a muscle contraction varies with the posture of a joint. For example, it is believed that contraction of the finger flexors is more stressful if the wrist is flexed. Work with the arm elevated more than 60 degrees from the trunk is more stressful for the rotator cuff

tendons than work performed with the arm at the trunk. Work performed in static postures that requires prolonged low-level muscle contractions of the upper limb or neck may also trigger chronic localized pain by an unknown mechanism.

Mechanical stress to nerve or other soft tissues can occur when they come into contact with structures harder than themselves, particularly external hard or sharp objects. These stresses can lead to nerve compression. Examples include (1) a digital neuritis associated with the edge of scissors handles or bowling ball holes coming into forceful contact with the sides of the fingers or thumb; and (2) cubital tunnel syndrome in a microscopist who must position the elbow on a hard surface for long periods. Short-handled tools that dig into the base of the palm exert as much force on the hand, particularly the superficial branches of the median nerve, as the hand does on the hand.

Gloves will protect the hands from cold exposures, but gloves will also decrease grip strength (requiring more forceful exertion), decrease tactile sensitivity, decrease manipulative ability, increase space requirements, and increase the risk of becoming caught in moving parts.

Segmental vibration is transmitted to the upper extremity from impact tools, power tools, and bench-mounted buffers and grinders. The mechanism by which localized vibration from power tools contribute to the development of work-related Raynaud's phenomenon is not clear. Nevertheless, it has been associated with several types of power tools, such as chain saws, rock drillers, chipping hammers, and grinding tools.

In summary, excessive repetitive or forceful motions, high levels of mechanical stress, work in static or awkward postures, and the use of vibrating power tools singularly—or more frequently in combination—can cause inflammation and chronic localized pain in the upper limb and neck. Precise dose-response relationships have not been developed for these risk factors. In addition to these occupational factors, the risk associated with any exposure depends on nonoccupational factors. Personal risk factors, such as age, gender, peak muscle strength, or the size of the carpal tunnel, have not been adequately studied with rigorous scientific methods to demonstrate that these are powerful predictors of susceptibility.

TREATMENT

Since inflammation or nerve compression are the most common underlying causes of the symptoms of work-related musculoskeletal disorders, treatment is usually directed at two goals: to reduce inflammation or nerve compression, and to assist in the repair of any tissue damage. Symptomatic relief is provided by (1) the use of anti-inflammatory medications, (2) rest (often facilitated by splints), and (3) application of heat or cold. Physical therapy techniques are used to assist in symptom relief, to ensure normal joint motion, and to recondition muscles after periods of rest or reduced use. Surgery, even in CTS, may be ineffective if the worker is returned to the job without an effort to reduce occupational causes that are present. Few scientifically valid studies evaluate the treatment of the work-related musculoskeletal disorders of the upper limb and neck.

PREVENTIVE STRATEGY

Preventive strategy, largely experience-based, has not been comprehensively evaluated by scientific studies. The principles outlined below must be adapted to fit the specific characteristics of each working environment. They should be viewed as only a guide, requiring ongoing scientific evaluation rather than a detailed blueprint [35].

Three standard preventive strategies might be considered: (1) a reduction of the exposure to suspected occupational risk factors such as vibrating hand tools; (2) a conditioning process that increases the tolerance of workers to the suspected occupational risk factors; or (3) development of a preplacement process that is highly predictive and reliable to identify those persons at unusually high risk of developing an upper extremity disorder.

The remainder of this chapter discusses the first strategy in detail. Before this discussion, however, brief comment is in order for the other strategies.

Development of a preplacement process is the least desirable of these strategies because (1) there are no scientifically valid screening procedures to identify those persons at high risk of developing CTS; and (2) this shifts the cost of reducing the incidence of symptoms to the workers, who are denied employment or placement, and increases the cost of the hiring and preplacement processes.

For those persons in forceful action or repetitive-action jobs, the second approach, creating a period of time during which workers can gradually adapt their muscles and tendons to the new demands on them, could be useful. Training of new workers in the most efficient and least stressful way of performing their jobs may be useful, provided that the work tasks can be done in alternate ways, which are *both* less stressful and at least as fast. Similarly, workers with symptoms may, with training, be able to adapt an equally efficient, but less stressful, work method. Training activities have not been evaluated specifically. Several employers, perceiving long-term benefits in the "phasing-in period," have established transitional or training areas where employees may work at a reduced pace for a limited time.

The standard preventive approach, which is directed at control of occupational factors, has the most promise. This approach often requires changes in the work station, work process, or use of tools. Sometimes administrative changes, such as work restrictions, the use of personal protective equipment (for example, palm pads), or job rotation are useful alternatives. Job rotation of work requiring different types of motions of the upper extremity, however, may simply expose a larger number of workers to a considerable degree of risk.

The first step required for instituting changes in work stations or work processes in order to reduce exposure is to analyze the specific characteristics of suspected high-risk jobs. While the job review may be conducted by an industrial engineer or occupational health professional with training in ergonomics, the involvement of those persons most knowledgeable about the job is important. Experience has shown that not only can operators and supervisors with limited training successfully identify many of the hazardous aspects of a specific job, but also specific solutions may not be effective or accepted without their involvement in the job review and the development of solutions.

REDUCING EXPOSURE TO RISK FACTORS

A job analysis performed on the patient with the spot-welding job in the earlier case would have identified several exposure factors. The job was repetitive and required forceful gripping of the handles of the welding gun. The wrists were extended through most of the job cycle.

After a job analysis has identified the potentially hazardous exposures associated with a specific job, specific solutions should be solicited from individuals who have the greatest knowledge about the job. With limited training in the control principles (discussed in the next section), engineers, production employees, and frontline supervisors often propose the most useful methods for eliminating hazardous risk factors. If several factors are present, it can be difficult to determine which factor is the most detrimental one.

Control of repetitiveness, forcefulness, awkward posture, mechanical stress, vibration, gloves, and cold is often possible as illustrated below:

Control of Repetitiveness

1. Use mechanical assists and other types of automation. For example, in packing operations, a device can be used for transferring parts rather than using the hands.
2. Rotate workers between jobs requiring different types of motions. Rotation must be viewed as a temporary administrative control, one used until a more permanent solution can be found.
3. Implement horizontal work enlargement by adding different elements or steps to a job, particularly steps that do not require the same motions as the current work cycle.
4. Increase work allowances or decrease production standards. This control strategy is rarely looked on favorably by industry.
5. Design a tool for use in either hand and also so that fingers are not used for triggering motions.

Control of Forcefulness

1. Decrease the weight held in the hand by providing adjustable fixtures to hold parts being worked on. Many conventional balancers are available to neutralize tool weight. Articulating arms are being used in many plants to hold and manipulate heavy tools into awkward positions.
2. Control torque reaction force in power hand tools by using torque reaction bars, torque-absorbing overhead balancers, and mounted nutholding devices. Control the time that a worker is exposed to torque reaction by using shutoff rather than stall power tools. Avoid jerky motions by hand-held tools.
3. Design jobs so that a power grip rather than a pinch can be used whenever possible. (Maximum voluntary contraction in a power grip is approximately 3 times greater than in a pinch.)
4. Increase the coefficient of friction on hand tools to reduce slipperiness—for example, by plastic sleeves that can be slipped over metal handles of tools.

Control of Awkward Posture

The primary method for reducing awkward postures is to design adjustability of position into the job. Wrist, elbow, and shoulder postures required on a job are often determined by the height of the work surface with respect to the location of the worker. A tall worker may use less wrist flexion or ulnar deviation than a shorter worker. Additionally, awkward postures can be reduced by doing the following:

1. Altering the location or method of the work. For example, in automotive assembly opera-

tions, changing the line location where a part is installed may result in easier access.

2. Redesigning tools or changing the type of tool used. For example, when wrist flexion occurs with a pistol-shaped tool that is used on a horizontal surface, correction may involve using an in-line type tool or lowering the work station.

3. Altering the orientation of the work.

4. Avoiding job tasks that require shoulder abduction or forward flexion greater than 30 to 45 degrees, elbow flexion greater than 110 degrees, wrist flexion or extension greater than 30 to 45 degrees, and neck flexion greater than 20 degrees or frequent neck rotation.

Control of Vibration

1. Do not use impact wrenches and piercing hammers.

2. Use balancers, isolators, and damping materials.

3. Use handle coatings that attenuate vibrations and increase the coefficiency of friction to reduce strength requirements.

Control of Mechanical Stress

1. Round or flare the edges of sharp objects, such as guards and container edges.

2. Use different types of palm button guards, which allow room for the operator to use the button without contact with the guard.

3. Use palm pads, which may provide some protection until tools can be developed to eliminate hand hammering.

4. Use compliant cushioning material on handles or increase the length of the handles to cause the force to dissipate over a greater surface of the hand.

5. Use different-sized tools for different-sized hands.

6. Avoid narrow tool handles that concentrate large forces onto small areas of the hand.

Control of Gloves and Cold

1. Properly maintain power tool air hoses to eliminate cold exhaust air leaks onto the workers' hands or arms.

2. Provide a variety of styles and sizes of gloves to ensure proper fit of gloves.

3. Cover only that part of the hand that is necessary for protection. Examples include using safety tape for the finger tips with fingerless gloves and palm pads for the palm.

REFERENCES

1. Holbrook TL, Grazier K, Kelsey JL, Stauffer RN. The frequency of occurrence, impact and cost of selected musculoskeletal conditions in the United States. Chicago: American Academy of Orthopaedic Surgeons, 1984.

2. Jayson MIV. Back pain: some new approaches. Med J Aust 1979; 1:513–6.

3. Nachemson AL. The lumbar spine: an orthopaedic challenge. Spine 1976; 1:59–71.

4. Lipson, SJ. Adult low back pain. Current Concepts. Kalamazoo, MI: Upjohn, 1982.

5. Hult L. Cervical, dorsal and lumbar spine syndromes. Acta Orthop Scand [Suppl] 1954; no. 17.

6. Klein BP, Jensen RC, Sanderson LM. Assessment of workers' compensation claims for back strains/sprains. J Occup Med 1984; 26:443–8.

7. Kelsey JL. An epidemiological study of acute herniated lumbar intervertebral discs. Rheumatol Rehab 1975; 14:144–59.

8. Snook SH, Campanelli RA, Hart JW. A study of three preventive approaches to low back injury. J Occup Med 1978; 20:478–81.

9. Chaffin DB, Herrin GD, Keyserling WM. Preemployment strength testing: an updated position. J Occup Med 1978; 20:403–8.

10. Cust G, Pearson JCG, Mair A. The prevalence of low back pain in nurses. Int Nurs Rev 1972; 19:169–78.

11. Andersson GBJ, Ortengren R, Nachemson A. Quantitative studies of back loads in lifting. Spine 1976; 1:178–85.

12. Magora A. Investigation of the relation between low back pain and occupation. Indust Med Surg 1972; 41:5–9.

13. Weber H. Lumbar disk herniation: a controlled, perspective study with ten years of observation. Spine 1983; 8:131–40.

14. Deyo RA, Diehl AK, Rosenthal M. How many days

of bed rest for acute low back pain? A randomized clinical trial. N Engl J Med 1986; 315:1064–70.

15. Dillane JB, Fry J, Kalton G. Acute back syndrome: a study from general practice. B Med J 1966; 2:82–4.

16. McGill CM. Industrial back problems: a control program. J Occup Med 1968; 10:174–8.

17. U.S. Department of Health and Human Services. Work practices guide for manual lifting. Washington, DC.; DHHS, 1981. (NIOSH) publication no. 81-122.

18. Snook SH. The design of manual handling tasks. Ergonomics 1978; 21:963–85.

19. Porter RW, Wicks M, Ottewell D. Measurement of the spinal canal by diagnostic ultrasound. J Bone Joint Surg [Br] 1978; 60B:481–4.

20. Macdonald EB, Porter R, Hibbert C, Hart J. The relationship between spinal canal diameter and back pain in coal miners. J Occup Med 1984; 26:23–8.

21. Biering-Sorensen F. Physical measurements as risk indicators for low-back trouble over a one-year period. Spine 1984; 9:106–19.

22. Bergquist-Ullman M, Larsson U. Acute low back pain in industry. Acta Orthop Scand [Suppl] 1977; no. 170.

23. Fitzler SL, Berger RA. Attitudinal change: the Chelsea back program. Occup Health Saf Feb. 1982, pp. 24–26.

24. Fitzler SL, Berger RA. Chelsea back program: one year later. Occup Health Saf July 1983, pp. 52–54.

25. Phalen G. The carpal tunnel syndrome. Clinical evaluation of 598 hands. Clin Orthop 1972; 83:29.

26. Finkelstein H. Stenosing tendovaginitis at the radial styloid process. J Bone Joint Surg [AM] 1930; 12:509–40.

27. Cailliet R. Hand pain and impairment. 2nd ed. Philadelphia: Davis, 1981.

28. Steiner C. Tennis elbow. J Am Osteopath Assoc 1976; 75(1–6):575–81.

29. Bland D et al. The painful shoulder. Semin Arthritis Rheum 1977; 7:1, 21–47.

30. Waris P et al. Epidemiologic screening of occupational neck and upper limb disorders. Scand J Work Environ Health [Suppl 3] 1979; 5:25.

31. Halder N, Gillings DB, Imbus HR, et al. Hand structure and function in an industrial setting. Arthritis Rheum 1978; 21:210–20.

32. Cargile CH. Raynaud's disease in stonecutters using pneumatic tools. JAMA 1915; 64:582.

33. Silverstein BA, Fine LJ. Evaluation of upper extremity and low back cumulative trauma disorders: A screening manual. Ann Arbor: University of Michigan, 1984.

34. Kelly WN, Harris ED, Ruddy S, Sledge CG. Textbook of rheumatology. Philadelphia: Saunders, 1981. Vol. 2.

35. Silverstein B, Fine LJ, Armstrong TJ. Carpal tunnel syndrome: causes and a preventive strategy. Semin Occup Med 1986; 1:213–21.

BIBLIOGRAPHY

Cailliet R. Hand pain and impairment. 2nd ed. Philadelphia: Davis, 1981.
A good introductory text with excellent illustrations.

Deyo RA. Conservative therapy for low back pain: distinguishing useful from useless therapy. JAMA 1983; 250:1057.
Reviews the evidence supporting commonly used conservative therapies for low back pain. Methodologic criteria for validity and applicability were applied to 57 original articles describing trials of exercise, traction, use of corsets, bed rest, spinal manipulation, transcutaneous nerve stimulation, and drug therapy. The better studies are summarized with an indication of their design features and limitations.

Armstrong TJ, Silverstein BA. Upper-extremity pain in the workplace, role of usage in causality. In MM Hadler, ed. Clinical concepts in regional musculoskeletal illness. New York: Grune & Stratton, 1987. Ch. 19.
This chapter provides the clearest delineation of the association of upper extremity disorders with work exposures.

Nachemson A. Advances in low back pain. Clin Ortho 1985; 200:266.
An objective and thorough review of current knowledge about low back pain. Topics include epidemiology, etiology, biomechanics, and treatment. Emphasis is placed on the benefits of patient education and motion, and the disadvantages of prolonged bed rest (inactivity) and repeat surgery.

Quinet RJ, Hadler NM. Diagnosis and treatment of backache. Semin Arthritis Rheum 1979; 8:261.
A very comprehensive, objective, and well-written review of the etiology, diagnosis, and treatment of low back pain. The authors discuss traction, drugs, diathermy, heat, cold, manipulation, corsets, braces, injection therapy, exercises, chemonucleolysis, and surgery.

Rowe ML. Backache at work. Fairport, NY: Perinton, 1983.
Describes the results of a 20-year clinical study of low back pain at a large company. Included in the study are 1500 cases. The effectiveness of current selection techniques in preventing low back pain is discussed.

Emphasis is also placed on preventing the disability.
Wiesel SW, Feffer HL, Rothman RH. Industrial low-back pain: a prospective evaluation of a standardized diagnostic and treatment protocol. Spine 1984; 9:199.
Describes a standardized approach to the diagnosis and treatment of low back pain in employees at a

large company. Two orthopedic surgeons monitored the course and treatment of employee low back pain and intervened when they felt it necessary. The program dramatically decreased the number of patients, the number of days lost, and the number of cases sent to surgery.

Appendix
Symptoms and Physical Signs of Work-Related Disorders of the Upper Limb and Neck

Disorder	History	Physical examination
WRIST		
Carpal tunnel syndrome	Pain, tingling, or numbness in medial sensory distribution of the hand. Nocturnal exacerbation. Problems with dropping things.	Positive Phalen's test (Fig. 22-7). Positive Tinel's test (Fig. 22-7). Thenar atrophy in severe cases. Rule out pronator teres syndrome, cervical root syndrome.
DeQuervain's disease	Pain in anatomic snuffbox. May radiate up forearm. No history of radial fracture or wrist fracture.	Rule out radial nerve entrapment. Positive Finkelstein test (Fig. 22-7) with sharp pain rather than just pulling sensation.
Trigger finger	Finger locks in extension or flexion. Requires assistance in unlocking. Nodule on tendon.	Nodule at base of digit palpable. Locking in flexion or extension of digits.
Ulnar nerve compression (Guyon canal syndrome)	Burning, tingling or numbness in fourth and fifth digits. Clumsiness in fine movements.	Rule out cervical root disorder, rule out thoracic outlet syndrome. Rule out cubital tunnel syndrome. Decreased pinch strength. Weakness on resisted abduction and adduction of digits. Positive Tinel's sign at Guyon canal. Positive Phalen's test in ulnar distribution.
Tendinitis, tenosynovitis	Localized pain and swelling over muscle-tendon structure.	Pain exacerbated by resisted motions. Possibly fine crepitus on passive range-of-motion (ROM). No pain on passive ROM. Pronounced asymmetric grip strength.
ELBOW/FOREARM		
Lateral epicondylitis (tennis elbow)	Pain at lateral epicondyle during rest or active motion of wrists and fingers.	Pain on resisted extension of wrist with fingers flexed. No pain or limitation on full passive ROM. Pain at epicondyle on palpation. Pain on resisted radial deviation. Rule out radial nerve entrapment.

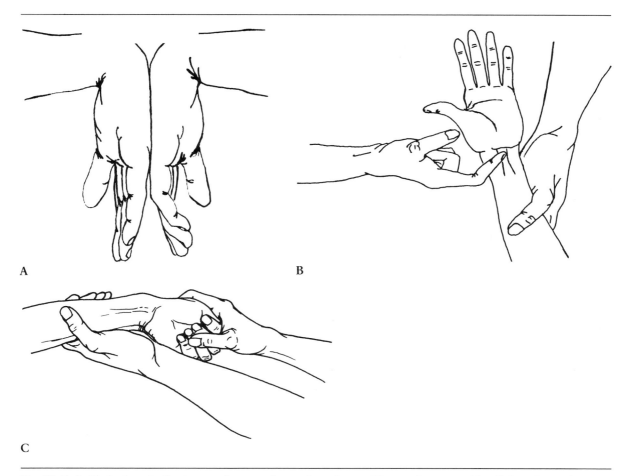

Fig. 22-7. A. Phalen's wrist flexion test for carpal tunnel syndrome. The results are positive if there is numbness and/or tingling in the fingers within 1 minute. B. Tinel's sign for carpal tunnel syndrome. A light tapping elicits numbness and/or tingling in the fingers. C. Finkelstein's test for DeQuervain's disease. Sharp pain around radial styloid and forearm, not just a pulling sensation.

Disorder	History	Physical examination
Medial epicondylitis (golfer's elbow)	Pain at medial epicondyle during rest or active motion of wrist and fingers.	No pain on passive ROM. Pain on resisted wrist flexion and resisted forearm pronation. Pain at medial epicondyle on palpation.

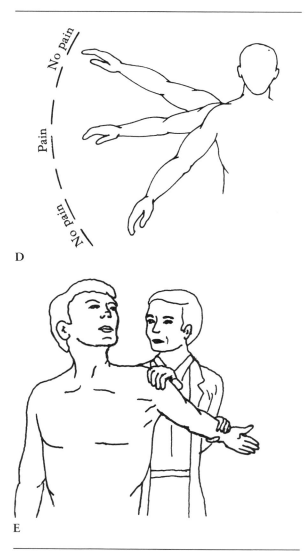

D

E

Fig. 22-7 (continued). D. A painful arc is often seen with rotator tendinitis, particularly of the supraspinatus tendon. E. Adson's test for thoracic outlet syndrome. Obtain a radial pulse and have the patient cock the head and take a deep breath. A positive test is a diminished pulse and symptoms in the fingers. (Drawings by Mary Weed, Audiovisual Department, School of Public Health, University of Michigan, Ann Arbor, MI. 48109-2029.)

Disorder	History	Physical Examination
Olecranon bursitis	Pain and swelling at olecranon.	No pain on passive or resisted ROM. Swelling around olecranon on palpation (rule out rheumatoid arthritis).
Pronator teres syndrome	Burning pain in first three digits of hand and forearm.	Increased pain in forearm by resisted pronation with clenched fist and flexed wrist (Mills's test). Sensory impairment of thenar eminence. Rule out carpal tunnel syndrome.
SHOULDER		
Rotator cuff tendinitis (mainly supraspinatus)	Dull ache generally localized to the deltoid area without neck or arm radiation. There are no symptoms of distal paresthesia. There is nocturnal exacerbation. The subject may note a "catch" on movement.	Diffuse tenderness over the shoulder, especially over the humeral head and lateral to the acromion. If tenderness is localized, it is most often over the supraspinatus insertion. Weakness is uncommon. *Supraspinatus:* Shrugs shoulder on abduction, painful arc at 70–90 degrees. Passive ROM normal. Pain on resisted abduction. *Infraspinatus:* Pain on resisted external rotation. Painful arc (Fig. 22-7). *Subscapularis:* Pain on resisted internal rotation. Painful arc. Rule out rheumatoid arthritis (other joints affected bilaterally, diffusely full and swollen; decreased ROM in all directions, especially rotation and abduction).
Bicipital tenosynovitis	Pain localized to the bicipital groove area. It may radiate to anterior aspect of the arm. There is no distal paresthesia. There is nocturnal exacerbation. The subject is able to use the forearm when the upper arm is held against the chest. The subject notes pain on abduction and rotation.	Normal passive and active ROM. Positive Yergason's test (resisted supination), or positive Speed's test (resisted wrist flexion).
Degenerative joint disease— Acromioclavicular joint	Generalized aching shoulder pain exacerbated by motion. Least difficulty in the morning but worse as the day progresses.	Limitation is similar on active and passive ROM. Most discomfort is with mild abduction. Crepitus is common. Tenderness on palpation directly over acromioclavicular articulation. Pain is reproduced as arm is abducted more than 90 degrees. Pain on shoulder shrug.

Disorder	History	Physical examination
Degenerative joint disease—Glenohumeral joint	Pain is very diffuse and nocturnal.	Tenderness to palpation along joint line. No deltoid or supraspinatus pain. Passive ROM is full but painful. Active ROM is retarded on flexion and extension. (Normal is 240 degrees in youth, 190 degrees at age 70. Normal abduction in youth is 166 degrees, 116 degrees at age 70.)
Thoracic outlet syndrome	Paresthesia usually in the ulnar distribution of hand and arm. Pain and sensation of "weakness." Deep dull ache in arm and hand. Problem holding small objects. Nocturnal exacerbation common.	Positive Adson's test (Fig. 22-7). Hyperabduction or costoclavicular test. Decreased grip strength.
NECK/SCAPULA		
Tension neck syndrome (costalscapular syndrome)	Neck pain or stiffness. No history of herniated cervical disk, injury, or ankylosing spondylitis.	Muscle tightness, palpable hardening and tender spots. Pain on resisted neck lateral flexion and rotation.
Cervical root syndrome	Pain radiating from the neck to one or both arms with numbness in the hand(s). Exacerbated by cough.	Limited passive and active ROM. Radiating pain on passive motions. Positive foraminal test. Decreased pinprick in dermatome. Absence of joint findings.

23
Skin Disorders

Kenneth A. Arndt and Michael Bigby

Any cutaneous abnormality or inflammation caused directly or indirectly by the work environment is an occupational skin disorder. Work-related cutaneous reactions and clinical syndromes are as varied as the environments in which people work. Skin disorders are the most frequently reported occupational diseases. A basic understanding of occupational skin disorders is therefore essential for everyone involved in occupational health.

An occupational skin injury is defined as an immediate adverse effect on the skin that results from instantaneous trauma or brief exposure to toxic agents involving a single incident in the work environment [1]. Occupational skin injuries account for 23 to 35 percent of all occupational injuries. Based on data collected in 1983 by the Bureau of Labor Statistics, it was estimated that the annual incidence of occupational skin injuries was 1.4 to 2.2 per 100 full-time workers. Lacerations and punctures are the most common skin injuries and in 1983 accounted for 82 percent of recorded occupational skin injuries. Thermal and chemical burns (14%), abrasions (3.4%), cold injuries (0.2%) and radiation injuries (.04%) also occur [1].

Occupational skin diseases or illnesses also result from exposure to toxic agents or environmental factors at work. In contrast to occupational skin injuries, occupational skin diseases require prolonged exposures and involve longer intervals between exposure and occurrence of disease [1]. Skin diseases account for 34 to 50 percent of all reported occupational diseases in the United States. In California, where physicians are required to report work-related disability lasting more than 1 day or requiring medical service other than first aid, skin diseases lead the list of occupational diseases. In 1985, 37 percent of the reported occupational diseases in California were skin conditions or chemical burns of the skin [2]. In 1984, skin diseases accounted for 34 percent of occupational illnesses recorded by the Bureau of Labor Statistics Annual Survey of Occupational Injuries and Illnesses [1]. However, in comparison with other occupational health problems, skin disorders are often more easily diagnosed and recognized as work-related.

The average annual reported incidence of occupational skin disease in the United States in 1976 was 1.5 cases per 1,000 workers. The average annual reported incidence had declined to 0.7 cases per 1,000 workers by 1982. Much of the decline, however, may be attributed to changes in federal rules regarding reporting rather than a true fall in the actual incidence of occupational skin diseases [3]. It is estimated that the actual incidence is 10 to 50 times higher than the reported incidence [3, 4].

Occupational skin disease is also a leading cause of time lost from work. From 20 to 25 percent of all reported occupational skin disease cases lose an average of 11 workdays annually. However, at least one-third of skin disorders in workers may not be directly related to their jobs.

The annual cost of occupational skin disease in the United States is great: at least 200,000 lost workdays, an estimated direct economic cost (lost wages or productivity) of $9.6 million, and a total cost (adding the costs of replacement workers, indemnity, medical costs, and insurance) of $20 to $30 million. If this estimate is multiplied 10 to 50 times to compensate for underreporting, the actual annual cost may be $250 million to $1.25 billion [3, 4].

Occupational skin disorders are unevenly distributed among industries. A worker in agriculture, forestry, fishing, or manufacturing has 3 times the risk of developing a work-related skin disease than workers in other industries. The incidence of occupational dermatologic conditions in the major industrial divisions in the United States is shown in Table 23-1.

SKIN: STRUCTURE AND FUNCTION
To understand skin disorders, a basic review of skin structure and function is helpful. Skin is the boundary between humans and their environment and is therefore very often the first site exposed to

environmental insults. Skin is the largest organ of the body. It weighs 3 to 4 kilograms, constitutes 6 percent of body weight, and covers about 20 square feet (about 2 m²) of the average adult. It consists of three principal layers.

The *epidermis* is the most superficial layer (Fig. 23-1). Its outermost compartment, the anucleate stratum corneum or horny layer, is very thin but supple and resilient. The stratum corneum acts as the principal barrier that retains water and interferes with the entrance of microorganisms and toxic substances. This barrier is quite impermeable to aqueous substances. Percutaneous absorption is greater with lipophilic compounds and through inflamed or abraded skin (see Chap. 14). Melanocytes of neural crest origin lie within the epidermis and synthesize the pigment melanin, which protects against ultraviolet radiation. Langerhans cells, which are dendritic antigen-presenting* cells important in the development of allergic contact dermatitis, also reside within the lower layers of the epidermis.

The *dermis* consists primarily of the fibrous protein collagen in a glycosaminoglycan† ground substance, both of which protect against trauma and envelop the body in a strong and flexible wrap. Also within the dermis are blood vessels, lymphatics, nerves, and the epidermal appendages: eccrine and apocrine sweat glands, sebaceous glands, and hair follicles. The epidermal appendages, especially the pilosebaceous unit (hair follicle and sebaceous gland), are important portals of entry for chemical irritants and allergens.

The third layer is the *subcutaneous tissue*. The thick, fatty subcutaneous tissue helps conserve the body heat and serves as an additional shock-absorbing buffer.

Certain aspects of normal or altered skin are particularly important for workers in an industrial

Table 23-1. Cases and incidence rate of occupational dermatologic conditions, in a segment of workers, by major industrial divisions—United States, 1984

Industrial division	Number	Incidence rate*
Agriculture/forestry/ fishing	2,233	28.5
Manufacturing	23,017	12.3
Construction	2,456	6.6
Services	7,973	5.0
Transportation/utilities	2,114	4.3
Mining	393	4.0
Wholesale/retail trade	3,770	2.1
Finance/insurance/real estate	563	1.1

*Per 10,000 full-time workers (2,000 employment hours/ full-time worker/year).
Source: Occupational Injuries and Illnesses in the United States by Industry, 1984. U.S. Department of Labor Bureau of Labor Statistics. Bulletin 2259, 1986.

*Dendritic cell that has the capacity to process (engulf, partially metabolize, and display on its surface) antigens and present antigens to lymphocytes.
†Polysaccharide (glycan) structure containing hexosamines (glycosamino) (hyaluronic acid, deymatin sulfate, and chondroitin sulfates).

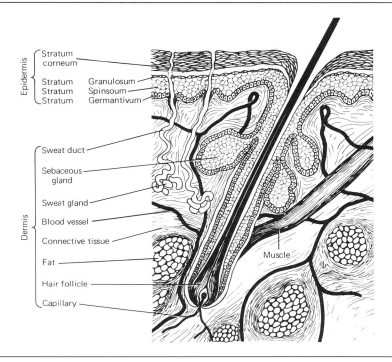

Fig. 23-1. Cross-section of human skin. The outermost stratum cor- neum is the principal barrier to chemical absorption. (From J Doull, CD Klaasen, MO Amdur, eds. *Casarett and Doull's Toxicology* 2nd ed. New York: Macmillan, 1980:18. © 1980 by Macmillan Publish- ing Co.)

environment. Induced or inherent alterations of barrier-layer function increase susceptibility to the effects of workplace exposures and open the skin to further damage. This phenomenon occurs in contact dermatitis, psoriasis, and atopic dermati- tis. Workers with atopic dermatitis are estimated to have a thirteen-fold higher prevalence of occu- pational irritant dermatitis [5]. Patients with pso- riasis may develop psoriasis in areas exposed to trauma or irritation (Koebner's phenomenon). These two common skin diseases, if noted on pre- placement examination, may be sufficient reason to place a worker where exposure to irritating or

sensitizing chemicals or to physical trauma does not occur.

Poorly pigmented skin is far more susceptible to ultraviolet light damage. Workers who tan poorly or not at all and who develop sunburns easily are more likely to develop basal cell and squamous cell skin cancers as a result of chronic exposure to sun- light. Such fair-skinned workers should protect their skin from ultraviolet damage by using sun- screens and wearing hats and long sleeves, espe- cially if they work in outdoor occupations, such as agriculture, fishing, forestry, and construction.

Excessive eccrine (sweat) gland function results

in hyperhidrosis (excessive perspiration), which may make it difficult to grasp objects. In the metal industry, malfunction of metal components occurs because of the problem of "rusters"—workers whose palmar sweat has a tendency to cause corrosion of metal objects. Another problem exacerbated by sweating results when otherwise harmless dusts, such as soda ash, may become hazardous by going into a solution after being deposited on wet (but otherwise normal) skin.

Disorders affecting the pilosebaceous follicles, such as acne, are worsened after exposure to heavy oils, greases, and hot and humid working conditions.

CAUSES OF OCCUPATIONAL DERMATOSES

Those workplace agents that may induce skin disorders can be arbitrarily divided in categories as described in Table 23-2. Chemical agents produce the great majority of occupational dermatoses by inducing either irritant or allergic contact sensitivity reactions. Poison oak (Rhus oleoresin) was the most common cause of occupational skin disease in California in 1985, accounting for 28 percent of total cases and 21 percent of lost workday cases. The other most common offenders include acids, soaps, detergents, and solvents.

Plant and wood substances may induce contact dermatitis or a light-activated photocontact dermatitis, which occurs when contact with the photosensitizing substance is followed by exposure to sunlight [6]. Dermatoses caused by vegetation are most commonly found among outdoor workers, especially farmers, construction laborers, lumber workers, and fire fighters.

Among the physical agents, ultraviolet radiation can cause both acute and chronic skin disorders. Acute exposures to ultraviolet radiation can result in sunburn that may vary from erythema to severe blistering accompanied by fever, chills, and malaise. Shortwave ultraviolet radiation (UVB) damages epidermal cells. The subsequent release of prostaglandins and leukotrienes causes vascular

dilatation in the dermis. Longer-wave ultraviolet light (UVA) can penetrate into the dermis and directly damage vessels. Acute ultraviolet exposure also causes increased production and dispersion of melanin, which causes darkening of the skin (tanning).

Chronic exposure to ultraviolet radiation causes solar elastosis, actinic keratoses, basal cell carcinomas, and squamous cell carcinomas. Solar elastosis is characterized by dryness and cracking of the stratum corneum, hyperpigmentation, decreased elasticity of the skin, and telangiectasia. Actinic keratoses are premalignant, erythematous, rough, scaly plaques that may develop into squamous cell carcinomas if left untreated. Solar ultraviolet radiation is responsible for the great majority of new skin cancers each year. All of the chronic effects of ultraviolet radiation occur most commonly and are most severe in lightly pigmented individuals who tan poorly and sunburn easily.

Ionizing radiation can also induce basal cell and squamous cell skin cancers. Chronic exposure to x-irradiation can cause a peculiar abnormality of the skin known as poikiloderma (areas of atrophy, telangiectasia, hyperpigmentation, and hypopigmentation) (see Chap. 16).

Exposure to cold temperatures may precipitate pernio (chilblains),* Raynaud's phenomenon, or may cause frostbite. Working in hot and humid environments predisposes one to the development of intertrigo and miliaria (heat rash) (see Chap. 18).

Biologic agents are said to be the second most common cause of occupational skin diseases. Skin diseases caused by biologic agents are often difficult to diagnose. In contrast to most occupational skin disorders, it is often difficult to recognize that the skin disease is work-related. Making the correct diagnosis requires insight and thoroughness. Examples of occupational skin diseases caused by biologic agents include herpetic infections of the

---

*Tender purple papules and nodules that develop on the hands and feet after exposure to cold weather.

Table 23-2. Examples of workplace agents that induce skin disorders

Chemical agents
  Rhus oleoresin (poison ivy and oak)
  Acids
  Alkalis
  Solvents
  Oils
  Soaps and detergents
  Plastics
  Resins
  Paraphenylenediamine
  Chromates
  Acrylates
  Nickel compounds
  Rubber chemicals
  Petroleum products not used as solvents
  Glass dust
Plant and wood substances
  Pink rot celery
  Citrus fruit
Physical agents
  Ionizing and nonionizing radiation
  Wind
  Sunlight
  Temperature extremes
  Humidity
Viruses
  Orf (sheep)*
  Milker's nodule (cows)
  Herpes simplex (patients)
Rickettsiae
  Rocky Mountain spotted fever (ticks)
  Murine typhus (fleas)
  Tick typhus (ticks)
  Rickettsialpox (mites)
  Scrub typhus (mites)

Bacteria
  Secondary superinfection
  Impetigo
  Furuncles
  Anthrax (infected hides)
  Brucellosis (animals)
  Erysipeloid (fish and poultry)
  Mycobacteria infection (animals and fish tanks)
  Tularemia (rodents)
  Cat-scratch disease (cats)
  Lyme disease (tick bites)
Fungi
  Candida infection (moist conditions)
  Dermatophytosis (animals, soil, and humans)
  Sporotrichosis (soil)
  Blastomycosis (inhalation)
  Coccidiodomycosis (inhalation)
Ectoparasites
  Cutaneous larva migrans
  Scabies
  Grain itch (mites)
  Bites (ticks, fleas, mites, and spiders)
  Swimmers' itch (schistosomes)
Biting animals
Mechanical factors
  Pressure
  Friction
  Vibration

*Agents of transmission or most common sources appear in parentheses.

hands, as seen in dentists and respiratory therapists, and orf in sheep handlers (see Table 23-2).

Mechanical factors may cause callouses and fissures. Fibers that are too small to see with the naked eye, such as those of fibrous glass, may become embedded in the skin and cause pruritus and excoriation. The use of pneumatic devices, such as jackhammers and chain saws, is an often forgotten cause of occupational Raynaud's phenomenon.

REACTION PATTERNS IN OCCUPATIONAL DERMATOLOGY

Occupational skin diseases may be classified into several clinical patterns, including contact dermatitis, infections, pilosebaceous unit abnormalities, pigment disorders, and neoplasms. (Inflammation in the skin is called "dermatitis.") This system of classification can serve as a tool for remembering a wide variety of work-related clinical syndromes and can also serve as a reminder of etiologies of occupational skin diseases.

Contact Dermatitis

The most common skin reaction seen in the industrial setting, contact dermatitis, accounts for approximately 90 percent of all occupational dermatoses. Contact dermatitis may be produced either by irritants or by allergic sensitizers. It occurs at the site of contact with the irritant or sensitizer, usually on exposed surfaces, especially the hands. It may take the form of acute changes of redness, swelling, blister formation, and exudation, leading to crusting and scaling, or more chronic changes may occur—thickening (lichenification), excoriations, and often hypo- or hyperpigmentation.

Primary irritant contact dermatitis is a nonallergic reaction of the skin caused by exposure to irritating substances (Fig. 23-2). Any substance can act as an irritant, provided the concentration and duration of contact are sufficient. Most irritants are chemical substances, although physical and biologic agents may produce the same clinical picture. Approximately 80 percent of occupational contact reactions are of an irritant type.

Irritants may be classified as mild, relative, or marginal irritants that require repeated or prolonged contact to produce inflammation (including soaps, detergents, and most solvents), and as strong or absolute irritants that will injure skin immediately on contact (including strong acids and alkalis). Exposure to strong acids and alkalis constitutes a medical emergency that should be treated by washing the area with copious amounts of cool water to limit tissue damage. Hydrofluoric (HF) acid is particularly damaging to the skin and may cause rapid, deep, and extensive tissue necrosis. Therapy for hydrofluoric acid burns may require

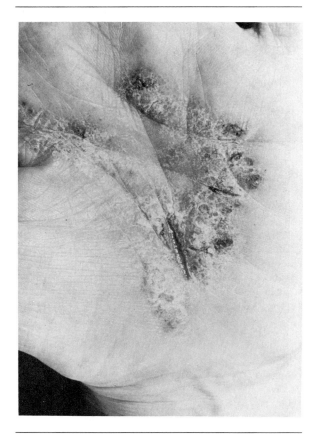

Fig. 23-2. Chronic irritant hand dermatitis. Skin is thickened, scaling, and inelastic to touch, and shows a deep fissure.

injection of 5 percent calcium gluconate solution or application of a calcium gluconate gel or ointment after washing [7]. Follow-up care to prevent superinfection is essential for all chemical burns.

If exposure to mild irritants is constant, normal skin in some workers may become "hardened" or tolerant of this trauma, and contact may be continued without further evidence of inflammation. Irritants may act as sensitizers but pure sensitizers are not primary irritants.

Allergic contact dermatitis is a manifestation of

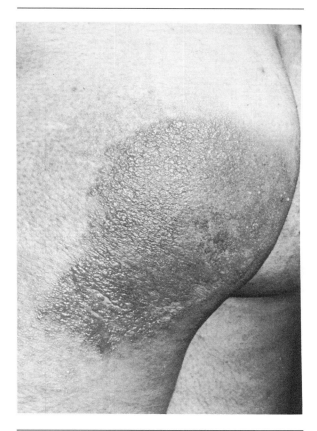

Fig. 23-3. Allergic contact dermatitis to MACE. This tear gas, methylchloroform chloracetophone, is a potent sensitizer. The patient was a security guard who sat down on a MACE spray can, whose nozzle was pointed toward his buttocks.

delayed-type hypersensitivity and results from the exposure of sensitized individuals to contact allergens (Fig. 23-3). Most contact allergens produce sensitization in only a small percentage of those exposed. *Rhus* antigens, which induce sensitization in more than 70 percent of those exposed to poison ivy, oak, or sumac, are marked exceptions to this rule. The incubation period after initial sensitization to an antigen is 5 to 21 days, but the

reaction time after subsequent reexposure is 6 to 72 hours. The normal reaction of a sensitized person after exposure to a moderate amount of poison oak or ivy is the appearance of a rash in 2 to 3 days and clearing within 1 to 2 weeks; with massive exposure, lesions appear more quickly (6–12 hours) and heal more slowly (2–3 weeks).

Irritants and allergens cause itching as the primary symptom of contact dermatitis. Irritants also can cause an inelastic skin, discomfort due to dryness, and pain related to fissures, blisters, and ulcers (Fig. 23-4). Strong irritants can cause blistering and erosions; mild irritants or allergens may cause dermatitis with microvesicles, erythema, and oozing. Allergens most typically cause grouped or linear tense vesicles or blisters. Edema can occur and may be severe particularly on the face and the genital areas. Most often contact dermatitis can be distinguished from other types of eczema/dermatitis not by the specific morphology of lesions but by their distribution and configuration—that is,

Fig. 23-4. Ulcer caused by contact with arsenic trioxide dust. This dust affected the whole community surrounding a gold smelting plant (From DJ Birmingham et al. An outbreak of arsenical dermatoses in a mining community. *Arch Dermatol* 91:457, 1965. Copyright 1965, American Medical Association.)

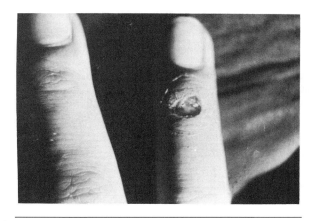

the rash occurs in exposed or contact areas, often with a bizarre or artificial pattern of sharp margins, acute angles, and straight lines.

Infections

Pyodermas induced by streptococci or staphylococci are the most common bacterial skin infections. These infections may occur as a result of trauma or as a complication of other occupational dermatoses. Barbers and cosmeticians who have contact in their work with customers suffering from contagious skin diseases are particularly at risk for bacterial and fungal infections. Lesions range from the superficial, such as impetigo, to the deep, such as folliculitis, carbuncles, cellulitis, and secondary lymphangitis. Diagnosis is made by clinical appearance, Gram's stain, and culture. A less common infection is erysipeloid among meat and fish handlers; even rarer is anthrax among sheep handlers and animal hide and wool workers (see Chap. 19).

Fungal infections with dermatophytes (ringworm) or the yeast-like fungus *Candida albicans* are often found in a local environment of moisture, warmth, and maceration; they therefore occur frequently in body folds and during warm seasons. The lesions of ringworm are annular, red, and scaling at the periphery with clearing in the center, whereas those of *Candida* are erythematous follicular papules or pustules outside skinfold areas. Both organisms may involve the nail, but the paronychial area is most often affected by *Candida,* particularly in workers whose hands are often exposed to water such as dishwashers, hairdressers, and canning industry workers who handle fruit. Demonstrating septate hyphae or budding yeasts and pseudohyphae on potassium hydroxide (KOH) examination will confirm the presence of fungal or yeast infection, and culture will delineate the type of organism.

Herpes simplex is the most frequently identified work-related viral skin infection in the United States. Health care workers, especially those who are exposed to oral secretions such as dental technicians, nurses, and anesthetists, may develop painful infections in their fingertips and around their nails (herpetic whitlow). These are often confused with felons or bacterial paronychial infections. Diagnoses is confirmed by finding viral giant cells on microscopic examination of scrapings from the vesicle floor (Tzanck preparation).

Pilosebaceous Follicle Abnormalities

Acne vulgaris, a multifactorial disorder involving the pilosebaceous follicles, is usually first noted in teenage years and subsides by early adulthood. Heavy oils such as insoluble cutting oils and greases used by machine-tool operators (or machinists) may aggravate idiopathic acne or cause comedo-like follicular plugging and folliculitis (Fig. 23-5). Skin under saturated clothing is most at risk, but lesions are also found on the dorsal surfaces of the hands and on extensor surfaces of the forearms. "Oil boils" may develop as the result of entrapment of surface bacteria.

Some halogenated aromatic hydrocarbons will induce chloracne, an acneiform eruption consisting of comedones, hyperpigmentation, and the pathognomonic oil cysts on exposed skin sites.

Fig. 23-5. Oil folliculitis. These acne-like lesions were induced by insoluble cutting oils which had saturated work pants. (From American Academy of Dermatology set of teaching slides on occupational dermatitis.)

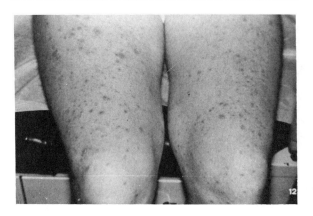

These disfiguring lesions can last for as many as 15 years. Though chloracne is not itself a disabling illness, it is important evidence of percutaneous absorption of chloracnegens. These chlorinated hydrocarbons have been associated with hepatic damage and malignancies in animals. Workers at risk include herbicide manufacturers and cable splicers and others exposed to polychlorinated biphenyls (PCBs) in dielectric applications (electrical insulation). Chloracne has been a side effect of recent massive environmental contamination by herbicides such as occurred in Seveso, Italy, in 1976, where an explosion in a nearby chemical plant sent a toxic cloud containing dioxin into the air. Dioxin, a trace contaminant of the chlorinated hydrocarbon 2,4,5-trichlorophenoxyacetic acid (2,4,5-T), is one of the most toxic substances known, second only to the neurotoxin botulin, and certain nerve gas and chemical warfare components. The dioxin-containing cloud settled on Seveso, a rural community of 5,000 people. There were 187 confirmed cases of chloracne, many in children; the long-term effects of this accident remain to be seen. Another exposure to dioxin occurred among inhabitants of and military personnel in Vietnam between 1962 and 1971, when Agent Orange, which contains 2,4,5-T, was used as a defoliant.

Pigment Disorders

Occupational exposures can produce many pigments on the skin. Some are stains adhering to the stratum corneum, some are a result of systemic absorption or inoculation (tattoo) of heavy metals, but most are due to altered melanin pigmentation.

Postinflammatory hyper- and hypopigmentation are the most common pigment disorders (Fig. 23-6). Any dermatitis or other trauma to the skin, such as thermal or chemical burns, may lead to temporary increase or decrease in melanin pigmen-

Fig. 23-6. Depigmentation caused by monobenzylether of hydroquinone. This chemical was used as an antioxidant in workers' gloves. (From EA Oliver, L Schwartz, LN Warren. Occupational leukoderma: Preliminary report. *JAMA* 1939; 113:927. Copyright 1939, American Medical Association.)

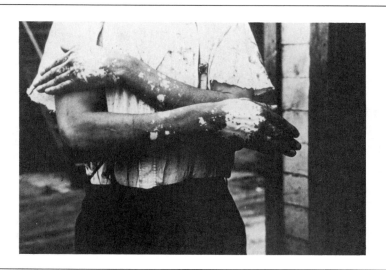

tation in that area. More heavily pigmented individuals show these findings most notably and with slower reversibility. If damage has been severe, melanocytes may have been destroyed and permanent depigmentation may occur, sometimes with scarring. Exposure to sun or other sources of ultraviolet light in the presence of photosensitizers such as tar, pitch, and psoralens will lead to enhanced erythema and, later, tanning.

An antioxidant used in rubber manufacturing, monobenzyl ether of hydroquinone, is the chemical most notorious for inducing permanent work-related loss of pigment (leukoderma). Metastatic lesions of hypopigmentation not in sites of direct contact may also be found. In the recent past other phenolic compounds used as antioxidants or germicidal disinfectants have been found to produce pigment loss.

Neoplasms
Occupational neoplasms may be benign, premalignant, or cancerous (Fig. 23-7). Foreign-body granulomas or granulomatous inflammatory nodules due to beryllium or silica are important examples of benign lesions. Keratoses produced by exposure to shale oils or to ultraviolet light are examples of premalignant lesions. Examples of cancerous lesions include squamous cell carcinoma and basal cell carcinoma from chronic exposure to ultraviolet light; scrotal cancer from occupational exposure to hydrocarbons such as those in soot; and squamous cell carcinoma, often on the scrotum, historically among cotton spinners and currently among metal machinists exposed to carcinogens in lubricating oils. Oncogenic agents include: ionizing radiation; ultraviolet light; some insoluble oils and greases, especially shale oils; and degradation products of the incomplete combustion of woods, oils, and tar. A diagnostic skin biopsy is always necessary when a skin cancer is suspected.

DIAGNOSIS OF OCCUPATIONAL SKIN DISORDERS
Occupational skin disorders are diagnosed by an accurate, detailed, and discerning history; a careful physical examination; laboratory tests; and tests for allergic contact dermatitis.

The history is of utmost importance in making a diagnosis of occupational skin disorders. The history should include a detailed description of the patient's job and a complete list of chemical, physical, and biological agents and mechanical factors to which the patient is exposed. The onset of the skin disorder in relation to starting or changing job duties is important. Occupational skin disorders often improve on weekends and during vacations. Up to one-third of skin disorders seen in workers are unrelated to their jobs, since exposure to irritants and allergens often occurs in the patient's home. Finally, all patients with contact dermatitis should be questioned about a past history of atopic dermatitis.

In the physical examination, emphasis should be placed on recognizing the patterns of occupational skin disorders. These disorders predominantly affect the hands, wrists, and forearms. The face, eye-

Fig. 23-7. Squamous cell carcinoma. This roofer had years of exposure to tars and sunlight. (From American Academy of Dermatology set of teaching slides on occupational dermatitis.)

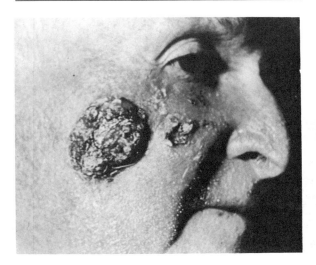

lids, and ears may also be involved. Examination of the entire cutaneous surface is recommended. Attention to spared areas as well as involved areas may provide clues to the etiology of the skin disorder. For example, phototoxic eruptions tend to spare areas covered by clothing, the upper eyelids, under the chin, and behind the ears.

Laboratory tests may include smears and cultures for viruses, bacteria, and fungi. A skin biopsy may be useful. A description of the laboratory tests used to help establish a diagnosis of skin disorders may be found in several references in the Bibliography.

Patch testing is used to document and validate a diagnosis of allergic contact sensitization and identify the causative agent (Fig. 23-8). It may also be of value as a screening procedure in patients with chronic or unexplained dermatitis to assess whether or not contact allergy is playing a causative role. The patch test is a unique means of in vivo reproduction of disease on a small scale since sensitization affects the whole body and may therefore be elicited at any cutaneous site; it is easier and safer than the "use" test because test items

can be applied in low concentrations on small areas of skin for short periods of time. Patch testing is of no value in diagnosing irritant dermatitis except to exclude allergic contact dermatitis as a primary or contributing cause. Proper performance and interpretation of patch tests require considerable experience. Possible side effects include a severe local reaction, possible secondary autosensitization reaction, or actually sensitizing someone to the testing compound. Patch-test allergens are often available commercially; sometimes they must be prepared from the occupational agent suspected. These substances must be nonirritating and nontoxic. Patch-testing procedures and techniques of proper dilution of reagents may be found in several references in the Bibliography.

MANAGEMENT OF SKIN DISEASES

The treatment of occupational skin disease generally depends on accurate diagnosis of the clinical reaction pattern. While it may be possible to treat some disorders successfully without having an exact etiologic diagnosis, an exact diagnosis should always be made for purposes of workers' compensation and prevention of the disorder in other workers. There are no differences between the management of skin diseases caused by occupational and nonoccupational factors. The following is a brief summary of the more commonly used therapies; for detailed management strategies, texts on dermatologic therapy should be consulted.

Contact Dermatitis

Acute exudative and vesicular contact dermatitis should be treated with compresses or dressings such as Burow's solution and topical anti-inflammatory agents. Topical corticosteroids are the anti-inflammatory agents of choice; they usually hasten resolution of the dermatitis and reduce itching. If the eruption is severe and accompanied by marked edema, a short course of oral corticosteroids may be necessary. Antihistamine drugs may reduce itching, and oral antibiotics are effective in eliminating

Fig. 23-8. Patch testing. Chemicals are applied to a Finn chamber made of aluminum, which is then taped to the patient's skin for 48 hours.

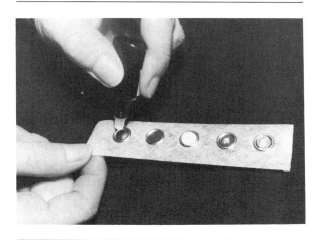

secondary infection. Chronic contact dermatitis requires adequate lubrication and the skillful use of topical corticosteroids.

Infections

Systemic antibiotics are usually warranted for cutaneous pyodermas. With fungal infections the topical imidazole drugs miconazole and clotrimazole are almost always effective in eliminating ringworm (dermatophyte) or yeast (C. *albicans*) infection. Oral and intravenous acyclovir are available for the treatment of selected patients with herpes simplex infection. (Acyclovir is the only antiviral drug available to treat skin disorders.)

Pilosebaceous Follicle Abnormalities

Acne and chloracne respond to topical and systemic treatment, but chloracne is far more recalcitrant and responds less completely. In most instances topical creams and gels containing tretinoin or benzoyl peroxide are the agents of choice. Lesions of chloracne often last months to years in spite of therapy.

Pigment Disorders

Postinflammatory pigment changes slowly resolve with time. That part of postinflammatory hyperpigmentation reflective of increased epidermal melanocyte activity may be treated with hydroquinone-containing creams. Usually, however, "bleaching" creams are of limited value. The leukoderma caused by monobenzyl ether of hydroquinone or phenolic disinfectants is not amenable to treatment.

Neoplasms

Premalignant keratoses may be treated with topical 5-fluorouracil (5-FU) or with liquid nitrogen cryosurgery, electrosurgery, or curettage. Cryotherapy, scalpel excision, and radiation therapy are appropriate for basal or squamous cell carcinomas. The best therapy in any instance depends on factors such as the size and site of the lesion and the patient's age and history of cutaneous carcinomas.

PROGNOSIS

The prognosis of occupational skin disorders depends on several variables including type of cutaneous reaction pattern, its exact cause (if determined), duration of eruption prior to diagnosis, type and effectiveness of treatment, patient compliance, and adequacy of preventive measures. Those workers with a specific allergic contact sensitivity may do well if they can avoid the allergen in work and home environments; in industrial settings it is almost always necessary to transfer such workers to another area of the plant. Workers with irritant contact reactions may be able to continue at work if the duration and intensity of exposure to contactants is decreased by environmental or protective measures. Those with atopy or a long history of dermatitis have a particularly dismal prognosis.

Persistence of what is presumed to be a work-related eruption even after the worker has been removed from the putative cause is not uncommon and may occur in the majority of cases [8,9]. However, persistence of a work-related skin disorder should raise several potential questions: Was the correct diagnosis made and the best treatment prescribed? Has the patient conscientiously carried out the treatment plan? Has work exposure been eliminated, and are there other possible sources of contact in second jobs or at home? Are psychologic factors playing a role, and is there any evidence of malingering? These questions are often difficult to answer definitely, just as it is often difficult to delineate the specific cause of an occupational dermatosis.

In 1970 the American Medical Association published guidelines on evaluating the degree of impairment and disability induced by occupational skin disorders; its criteria are shown in Table 23-3. As opposed to permanent skin impairment, functional loss is best evaluated by assessing the degree of itching, scarring, and disfigurement.

Table 23-3. Criteria for evaluating
permanent skin impairment

Category	Impairment	Comments
Class 1	0–5%	With treatment there is no or minimal limitation in the performance of the activities of daily living, although certain physical and chemical agents might temporarily increase the extent of limitation.
Class 2	10–20%	Intermittent treatment is required, *and* there is limitation in the performance of some of the activities of daily living.
Class 3	25–50%	Continuous treatment is required, *and* there is limitation in the performance of many of the activities of daily living.
Class 4	55–80%	Continuous treatment is required, which may include periodic confinement at home or other domicile, *and* there is limitation in the performance of many of the activities of daily living.
Class 5	85–95%	Continuous treatment is required that necessitates confinement at home or other domicile, *and* there is severe limitation in the performance of the activities of daily living.

Source: AMA Subcommittee on the Skin. Guides to evaluation of permanent impairment—the skin. JAMA 1970; 211:106. Copyright 1970, American Medical Association.

PREVENTION

Occupational skin diseases are almost always preventable by a combination of environmental, personal, and medical measures.

Environmental Measures

Environmental cleanliness is paramount in preventing occupational dermatoses. Maintaining a clean workplace involves the frequent cleaning of floors, walls, windows, and machinery; recognizing hazardous materials and either providing substitutes or altering or eliminating them from the workplace; ensuring proper ventilation; and the use of exhaust hoods, splash guards, and other protective devices and systems.

Personal Measures

Personal cleanliness is a key element in preventing occupational skin disease. Washing facilities with hot and cold running water, towels, and proper cleansing agents must be easily accessible and strategically placed. The *mildest* soap that will clean the skin should always be used. Appropriate cleansing agents might include waterless hand cleaners for oils, greases, or adherent soils. Safety showers must be available if highly corrosive chemicals are being handled. If strong irritants are in the work environment, it is necessary for workers to shower at the end of each shift, or possibly more often. In some industries it is appropriate to supply clothing and laundering to ensure both the use of proper types of material as well as daily clothes changes. If water is not easily accessible for washing, waterless hand cleansers can be used. Solvents such as kerosene, gasoline, and turpentine should *never* be used for skin cleansing; they are quite damaging to the skin since they "dissolve" the cutaneous barrier and can either induce an irritant contact dermatitis or predispose to a cumulative insult contact dermatitis. A skin moisturizer should be used after hand washing, especially if frequent washing is necessary.

Protective clothing is often all that is needed to

prevent a dermatitis by blocking contact of chemicals with the skin. The clothing should be chosen based on the skin site needing protection and the type of chemical involved (some solvents will dissolve certain fabrics or materials). Natural rubber gloves are impervious to aqueous compounds but deteriorate after exposure to strong acids and bases. Synthetic rubbers are more resistant to alkalis and solvents; however, some are altered by chlorinated hydrocarbon solvents. It is always useful to wear absorbent, replaceable soft cotton liners inside protective gloves to make them more comfortable. Commercially available gear includes gloves of different lengths, sleeves, safety shoes and boots, aprons, and coveralls composed of materials such as plastic, rubber, glass fiber, metal, and combinations of these materials. Clothing that might become caught in machines must be avoided for safety reasons.

Protective creams, referred to as "barrier" creams, afford much less protection than does clothing. However, these creams can be valuable when gloves would interfere with the sense of touch required to perform the job or when use of a face shield might be awkward. Barrier creams should be applied to clean skin, removed when the skin becomes excessively soiled or at the end of each work period, and then reapplied. Proper use of a barrier cream not only provides some degree of protection but induces the worker to wash at least twice during the work shift.

There are four types of protective creams. *Vanishing creams* contain soap, which remains on the skin and facilitates removal of soil when washing. *Water-repellent* creams leave a film of water-repellent substances such as lanolin, petrolatum, or silicone on the skin to help prevent direct contact with water-soluble irritants like acids and alkalis. *Solvent-repellent* creams repel oils and solvents and may leave either an ointment film or a dry, oil-repellent film on the skin surface. *Special creams* include sun shades, sunscreens absorbent of UVA, UVB, or both spectra of ultraviolet light, and insect repellents.

Medical Measures

Careful screening of new workers in preplacement examinations will decrease the incidence of job-related dermatoses. Individuals with a history of atopic dermatitis should not work in occupations involving frequent exposure to harsh chemicals or water, such as certain machining, cooking, bottle-washing, and operating-room jobs. Those with psoriasis of the hands would do poorly in the same situation and furthermore may respond with a Koebner reaction in which psoriatic lesions develop in sites of heavy trauma. Such trauma includes scratches, abrasions, and cuts that disrupt the epidermis as well as rough handwork or continual kneeling.

Workers with dermatographism*, at high risk for annoying pruritic responses to trauma or to foreign bodies such as fibrous glass, should avoid these occupational exposures; workers with acne should not be employed in hot and humid workplaces or where they would be exposed to oil mists, heavy oils, or greases; and fair-skinned or sunlight-sensitive individuals should not work in intense ultraviolet light (see Chap. 18) or around potentially photosensitizing chemicals such as tar, pitch, and psoralens. Job applicants should be questioned concerning previous skin diseases, including childhood eczema and atopic diseases, contact dermatitis, psoriasis, fungal infections, and allergic reactions to drugs or other agents.

Preplacement patch testing is generally not advised; although it may occasionally identify a previously allergic person, the yield is very low and it has the greater risk of inducing contact sensitization. Chemical agents used in the workplace should undergo toxicologic testing to detect irritancy, allergenicity, acnegenicity, carcinogenicity, and other properties. When potentially hazardous substances are detected, they should be properly

---

*Urticaria due to physical factors, in which moderately firm stroking or scratching of the skin with a dull instrument produces a persistent, pale, raised wheal, with a red flare on each side.

labelled, and workers should be educated about these hazards and how to avoid them.

Workers with severe, chronic, or unremitting allergic dermatoses should be transferred to other plant areas, if possible. By definition, allergy implies sensitivity to very low levels of an antigen, and it is usually not possible to continue working in the same site even though careful precautions are taken. Those with irritant dermatoses are often, but not always, able to continue working by decreasing the duration and intensity of exposure to irritants. Relocation of workers is more easily accomplished within large industries; however, only one-third of the workforce is employed in such industries. Most cases of occupational dermatitis occur in small plants with poorly developed preventive services and less sophisticated or no supervisory and medical personnel.

REFERENCES

1. Centers for Disease Control. Leading work-related diseases and injuries. Morbidity and Mortality Weekly Report 1986; 35:561–3.
2. Division of Labor and Statistics. Occupational disease in California, 1985. San Francisco: California Department of Industrial Relations, 1987.
3. Mathias CGT. The cost of occupational skin disease. Arch Dermatol 1985; 121:332–4.
4. National Institute for Occupational Safety and Health. Pilot Study for Development of an Occupational Disease Surveillance Method. Cincinnati: NIOSH, 1975. (Publication no. 75–162).
5. Shmunes E, Keil JE. Occupational dermatoses in South Carolina: a descriptive analysis of cost variables. J Am Acad Dermatol 1983; 9:861–6.
6. Berkley SF, Hightower AW, Beier RC et al. Dermatitis in grocery workers associated with high natural concentrations of furocoumarins in celery. Ann Intern Med 1986; 105:351–5.
7. Trevino MA, Herrman GH, Sproue WL. Treatment of severe hydrofluoric acid exposures. J Occup Med 1983; 25:861–3.
8. Keczkes K, Bhate SM, Wyatt EH. The outcome of primary irritant hand dermatitis. Br J Dermatol 1983; 109:665–8.
9. Burrows D. Prognosis and factors influencing prognosis in industrial dermatitis. Br J Dermatol [105 Suppl] 1981; 21:65–70.

BIBLIOGRAPHY

Adams RM. Occupational skin disease. New York: Grune & Stratton, 1983.
A thorough and comprehensive general reference book. An essential book for the serious student of occupational skin disorders.

Adams RM, ed. Occupational medicine: state of the art reviews. Occupational skin disease. Philadelphia: Hanley & Belfus, 1986.
A concise, well-written and up-to-date treatise on this subject, which covers the basics of occupational skin diseases. The role of atopy in occupational skin disease, vibration syndromes, and AIDS in the workplace are among the interesting topics covered.

AMA Subcommittee on the Skin. Guides to evaluation of permanent impairment—the skin. JAMA 1970; 211:106.
This material was also published in the AMA volume Guides to the evaluation of permanent impairment. Chicago: American Medical Association, :143–8. Ch. 12.

Arndt KA. Manual of dermatologic therapeutics: With essentials of diagnosis. 4th ed. Boston: Little, Brown, 1988.
A practical manual. Discusses the pathophysiology, diagnosis, and treatment of common skin disorders seen in ambulatory patients. Patch testing is described.

Fisher AA. Contact Dermatitis. 3rd ed. Philadelphia: Lea & Febiger, 1986.
Essential, detailed reference on contact dermatitis. Contains a glossary that describes the proper patch-test concentrations of many common antigens.

de Groot AC. Patch testing. Amsterdam: Elsevier, 1986.
This book provides recommendations for test concentrations and vehicles for 2800 allergens.

Maibach, HI. Occupational and industrial dermatology. 2nd ed. Chicago: Year Book, 1986.
A comprehensive, well-written book that includes the basics of occupational and industrial dermatology, dermatotoxicology, and specific industrial problems.

24
Eye Disorders

Paul F. Vinger and David H. Sliney

A 52-year-old metal worker was polishing a brass fixture on a buffing wheel. The fixture was torn from his grasp by the wheel and struck his left eye. In addition to a full-thickness laceration of the left upper eyelid, a severe laceration of the globe of the eye was apparent when he was evaluated at a hospital soon afterward. It was discovered then that the patient had a best-corrected vision in the uninjured right eye enabling him only to count fingers because of dense amblyopia ("lazy eye" secondary to unilateral uncorrected high myopia, or nearsightedness). Despite extensive surgical procedures, vision was lost in the injured left eye. Attempts to improve the vision in the uninjured right eye by optical means were not successful. He is now legally blind with no hope of recovery of useful vision. He can no longer drive or perform his usual work.

An 18-year-old arc-welding student stared at an electric welding arc while a piece of aluminum was being welded by another welder. He was outside a protective curtain and about 200 cm (about 6.5 ft) from the arc, yet was able to stare at the arc with his right eye for approximately 10 minutes. He sustained a retinal injury that initially resulted in marked visual loss. This loss slowly resolved over 16 months, leaving him with normal visual acuity and a residual, partially pigmented foveal lesion (*foveal* meaning in the central portion of the retina, which is required for normal reading and driving visual acuity and accurate color vision).

A scientist was working with a relatively weak neodymium-yag (neodymium-yttrium-*a*luminum-garnet) laser without safety goggles. He was not looking directly at the beam but heard a popping sound inside his eye accompanied by almost immediate obscuring of his vision. The laser burn, between the fovea and the optic nerve of his left eye, resulted in a large, permanent blind area in his visual field.

Every working day, there are over 2,000 preventable job-related eye injuries to workers in the United States. Occupational vision programs, including preplacement examinations and requirements for appropriate eye protectors in certain occupations, can prevent many of these injuries. Such programs could have prevented the loss of vision in the above situations.

CAUSES OF OCCUPATIONAL EYE INJURIES

Direct Trauma
Direct trauma is the most frequent cause of occupational eye injuries. Jobs in which there is the risk of high-speed flying particulate material as well as the tradition of working without eye protectors, such as automobile mechanics, present the highest risk (Table 24-1). Eye injuries from direct trauma are almost totally preventable with protective eyewear. Symptoms and signs of serious eye injury are shown in the box on p. 388.

Chemicals
Many different types of chemicals are commonly involved in industrial eye injuries (see box). These include alkalis, acids, esters, ketones, and other selected chemicals (see box on p. 395).

Light, Laser, Heat, and Ionizing Radiation
Eye injuries can occur from essentially all portions of the electromagnetic spectrum; however, some sources of electromagnetic energy are far more

Table 24-1. Emergency room visits, Massachusetts Eye and Ear Infirmary March 15 to September 15, 1985

3185 eye trauma patients:
  48% at work—highest rate in auto repair
  5% of injuries deemed serious
  $2 million in hospital bills
  30 person-years of work lost
  9% involved in litigation

Source: OD Schein, PL Hibbard, BJ Shingelton et al. The spectrum and burden of ocular injury. Ophthalmology 1988; 95:300–305.

SYMPTOMS AND SIGNS OF SERIOUS EYE INJURY

Symptoms of serious eye injury indicating immediate referral are the following:

1. Blurred vision that does not clear with blinking
2. Loss of all or part of the visual field of an eye
3. Sharp stabbing or deep throbbing pain
4. Double vision

Signs of eye injury that require ophthalmologic evaluation are the following:

1. Black eye
2. Red eye
3. An object on the cornea
4. One eye that does not move as completely as the other
5. One eye protruding forward more than the other
6. One eye with an abnormal pupil size, shape, or reaction to light, as compared to the other eye
7. A layer of blood between the cornea and the iris (hyphema)
8. Laceration of the eyelid, especially if it involves the lid margin
9. Laceration or perforation of the eye

hazardous to the eye because (1) the eye is more sensitive to the particular wavelengths, (2) the energy dose can be very high, or (3) the energy is delivered in a very brief interval (see Chap. 18).

Ionizing radiation is rarely a cause of industrial eye injury because standard precautions from exposure to ionizing radiation give adequate eye protection.

Exposure to excess heat can cause thermal burns to the lids and eye. Cataracts occur in unprotected glass blowers and furnace workers. Heat-absorbing or heat-reflecting protective eyewear is available. Other protective clothing or head or face shields may be indicated, depending on the severity of heat exposure.

Optical radiation is considered nonionizing radiation because photon energies for ultraviolet (UV) wavelengths greater than approximately 180 nm are insufficient to individually ionize atoms found in important biologic molecules (see Chap. 18). Unlike the nonthreshold biologic effects of ionizing radiation, such as x-rays, a threshold appears to exist for each biologic effect of optical radiation. In the UV and visible regions of the spectrum, photochemical damage mechanisms are demonstrable. Thermal injury mechanisms dominate for most pulsed laser exposures and infrared (IR) radiation exposures.

The optical spectrum includes the UV, visible (light), and IR regions of the electromagnetic spectrum. Lasers, which can emit wavelengths in all parts of the spectrum, are unique sources of optical radiation, with extremely high brightness.

Although most workers are aware of the potential for lasers to cause eye injury, it must be stressed that more conventional light sources, especially with high output in the UV portion of the spectrum, such as welding arcs and sun lamps, can also be extremely hazardous. Figure 24-1 correlates the potential for retinal injury with the absorbed retinal irradiance of various light sources.

There are at least five separate types of hazards to the eye and skin from lasers and other more conventional optical sources:

1. UV photochemical injury to the skin (erythema and carcinogenic effects) and to the cornea (photokeratitis) and lens (cataract) of the eye (180–400 nm).

2. Thermal injury to the retina of the eye (400–1,400 nm).
3. Blue-light photochemical injury to the retina of the eye (principally 400–550 nm).
4. Near-infrared thermal hazards to the lens (approximately 800–3,000 nm).
5. Thermal injury (burns) of the skin (approximately 340 nm–1 mm) and of the cornea of the eye (approximately 1,400 nm–1 mm).

Fig. 24-1. Retinal irradiances (exposure dose rates) from representative light sources. Levels above 10^{-4} W/cm² may cause photochemical blue-light injury from fixating the source. Above 10 W/cm² (depending on image size), thermal burns may result from brief exposures. (From D Sliney and M Wolbarsht. Safety with lasers and other optical sources. New York: Plenum, 1980.)

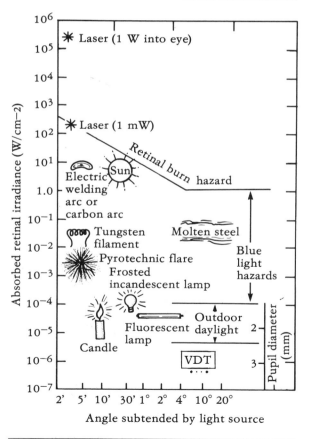

Company-Organized Sports and Exercise Programs
Many companies have physical fitness and sports programs that are important to the well-being, happiness, and ultimate on-the-job productivity of employees. However, many sports have an eye injury potential that can exceed the on-the-job eye injury risk. Hockey and the racket sports have very high eye-injury risk. Eye protection that meets American Society of Testing Materials (ASTM) standards should be mandated for these sports. Baseball, softball, basketball, and soccer have relatively high eye-injury risk. Safety glasses with polycarbonate lenses are indicated for these sports.

PREPLACEMENT EXAMINATION AND SAFETY EDUCATION
The purpose of preplacement examinations is to: (1) check for preexisting eye disorders, (2) identify individuals who are functionally one-eyed, (3) prescribe appropriate protective eyewear, and (4) ascertain that workers such as truck drivers meet standards for visual performance. The examination must be accompanied by education to teach the employee the potential for ocular injuries on the job, the importance of protection, and workplace rules regarding eye safety.

Checking for Preexisting Disorders
In any work setting where there is eye injury risk, it is important that the employer document basic visual skills and rule out significant preexisting eye disease. In addition to guiding decisions about job

placement and eye protection, this documentation protects both the employee and the company by providing baseline data that can be compared with results of subsequent screenings after any apparent eye injury and when the employee leaves the company.

For most occupations, satisfactory visual screening includes: central visual acuity (both for distant and near vision), muscle balance and eye coordination, depth and color discrimination, and horizontal peripheral fields. These screening tests can be measured by a nurse or a physician's assistant in 7 minutes or less on one of a variety of available binocular test instruments. These instruments are simple to operate, easy to transport, and relatively inexpensive, and they rarely require maintenance. For occupations that have a higher risk of eye injury, such as some work with high-powered lasers, screening by an ophthalmologist is preferable. Additional test procedures may be desirable, such as Amsler grid, fundus photos, peripheral visual fields, refraction, or a comprehensive eye examination; the value of particular test procedures can be discussed with the consulting ophthalmologist. Standardized reporting forms have been developed for these screening tests.

Discovering the Functionally One-Eyed

A person is functionally one-eyed when loss of the better eye would result in a significant change in life-style due to poorer vision in the remaining eye. There is no question that a person with 20/200 or poorer best corrected vision in one eye is functionally one-eyed since loss of the good eye would result in legal or total blindness and a burden both to the individual and society. On the other hand, most of us would function quite well with 20/40 or better vision in one eye. More difficult is advising employees with best-corrected vision in the poorer eye between 20/40 and 20/200. The loss of the ability to drive legally in most states would be a significant handicap to most persons and would significantly interfere with many present and potential future work and commuting situations.

Therefore, we could safely conclude that an employee is effectively one-eyed if the best-correctable vision in the poorer eye is less than 20/40.

Every employee who tests less than 20/40 (with glasses, if worn) on the preplacement examination *must* be evaluated by an optometrist or an ophthalmologist to determine if the subnormal vision is simply due to a change in refraction. If the best-corrected vision in either eye is less than 20/40 after refraction, ophthalmologic evaluation to obtain a definitive diagnosis of the visual deficit and an accurate preplacement ocular evaluation is indicated.

If the employee is functionally one-eyed, the potential serious, long-term consequences of injury to the better eye should be discussed in detail prior to assigning work with intrinsic ocular risk. This discussion is essential even if the employee feels that life would not be changed if vision in the better eye were lost.

Effective eye protection is possible only when the employee understands the risks and is willing to cooperate with protective measures. Having the unconvinced employee wear an occluder over the better eye for several days will allow a better evaluation of the ability to function with the poorer eye. Usually, with an honest appraisal by the employee it is fairly easy to reach an agreement between the employer, the employee, and the ophthalmologist as to whether the employee is functionally one-eyed and the level of extra protection needed to decrease the risk of eye injury to the lowest possible level.

Most jobs that pose a high risk to unprotected eyes can be made quite safe with the use of appropriate protective devices. The employee deserves a careful explanation of the eye injury risk in the proposed job category, both with and without various types of eye protectors.

In addition to on-the-job protective eyewear, it is prudent for functionally one-eyed people to protect the good eye when they are not at work by wearing glasses made of polycarbonate lenses mounted in a sturdy frame. This is especially true of active people who are subject to eye injury in leisure activities. *The important role of glasses as a protective device cannot be overemphasized.*

Prescribing Appropriate Protective Eyewear

Prescribing appropriate protective eyewear requires knowledge of the potential on-the-job risks and the best available means of protection. The nonexpert can get advice from an ophthalmologist, optometrist, or safety consultant who is experienced in eye hazards and protective eyewear.

All safety eyewear must meet the American National Standards Institute (ANSI) Z87.1 standard requirements. Again, polycarbonate plastic is best suited for use in a protective device unless special filtration or optical considerations make it impossible.

Since the total protection is decreased by up to 25 percent when side shields are removed (Fig.

24-2), dispensing safety eyewear without side shields cannot be justified for any work situation with a potential risk of flying particles or a significant risk of class 3 or class 4 laser exposure. Side shields are *always* indicated on safety eyewear (Fig. 24-3) unless the eyewear is to be used *only* in an office environment.

Goggles are indicated for (1) work where there is a higher potential for many fine flying particles, (2) use with certain lasers, (3) use over streetwear spectacles, (4) use with chemicals, and (5) welding that does not require a full-face shield (Figs. 24-4 and 24-5).

Face shields are required for arc welding (Fig. 24-6) or for use with tools that can project particles that pose an injury potential to the face, including the eyes. Protective eyeglasses or goggles should *always* be worn under face shields, since workers frequently raise the shield to chip slag, ex-

Fig. 24-2. View of the area of coverage of safety glasses without side shields. Note 90 degrees of unprotected eyes exposed to penetration by a fragment.

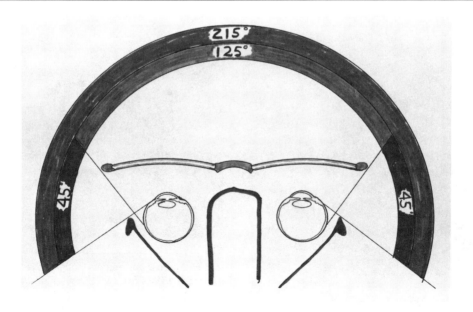

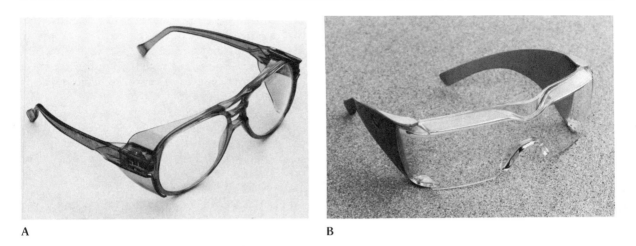

Fig. 24-3. Safety wear with side shields, for use (A) by workers who require a prescription lens or (B) by workers who require eye protection, but do not need a spectacle lens for better vision.

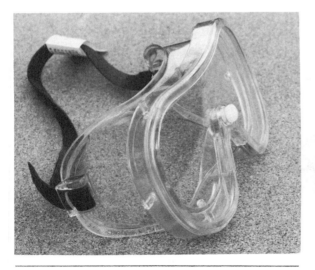

Fig. 24-4. Goggles, designed to protect eyes from chemical splash, suitable for use alone or over other spectacles.

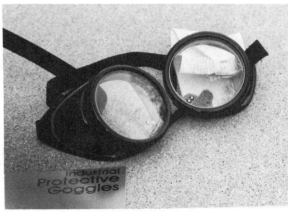

Fig. 24-5. Dust and impact goggles that could support protective lenses for impact, welding, or laser use.

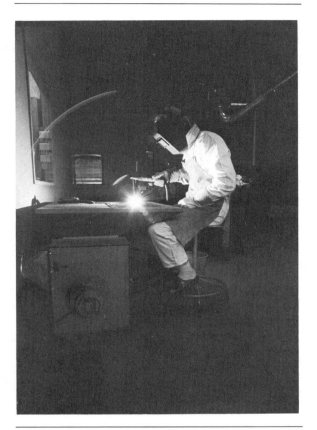

Fig. 24-6. Welder wearing protection against ultraviolet light. (Photograph by Denny Lorentzen from *Newsletter,* National Swedish Board of Occupational Safety and Health, January 1981.)

amine a work piece, or breathe more easily—thus temporarily exposing the eyes to risk of injury.

Laser eye protection is designed to provide the greatest visual transmission along with an adequate optical density at the laser wavelengths. Most laser hazard controls are common-sense procedures designed to limit personnel from the beam path and to limit the primary and reflected beams from occupied areas. The degree of control must be correlated with the injury potential of the laser in use (Table 24-2).

Table 24-2. Laser hazard categories

Class 4: high power, can produce hazardous diffuse reflections and may also present a fire hazard or significant skin hazard.

Class 3: medium power, cannot produce hazardous diffuse reflections but does present a hazard when the beam is viewed directly.

Class 2: low power, (<1 mW) are visible lasers safe for momentary (<0.25 sec) viewing; the eye's aversion response to bright light would normally preclude a person from staring into the light.

Class 1: nonhazardous, emit less than the recommended limits for intrabeam viewing for the maximal reasonable viewing duration.

Selecting appropriate protective eyewear for laser use requires knowing (1) at least three output parameters of the laser—maximum exposure duration, wavelength, and output power (or energy); (2) applicable safe corneal radiant exposure; and (3) environmental factors, such as ambient lighting and the nature of the laser operation.

The laser wavelength(s) for which the type of eye shields were designed should be specified. Commercial protective eyewear is designed to greatly reduce or essentially prevent particular wavelength(s) from reaching the eye. Although most lasers emit only one wavelength, many lasers emit more, in which case each wavelength must be considered. It is seldom adequate to merely mark on the goggle that it will protect against radiation from a particular laser or it will protect against only the wavelength corresponding to the greatest output power. For example, a helium-neon laser may emit 100 mW at 632 nm and only 10 mW at 1,150 nm; however, safety goggles that absorb at the 632 nm wavelength may absorb little or nothing at the 1,150 nm wavelength. Hence, the wavelength range of use must be specified.

Eye protection filters for glass workers, steel and foundry workers, and welders are specified by *shades* (logarithmic representations of visual transmission). Typical shade values are the following:

Acetylene flames	Shade 3 or 4
Electric welding arcs	Shade 10 to 13
Viewing the sun or plasma cutting/spraying	Shade 13 or higher

These densities greatly exceed those necessary to prevent retinal burns but are required to reduce the luminance (brightness) to comfortable viewing levels. The user of the eye protection should therefore be permitted to choose the shade most personally desirable for the particular operation. Actinic UV radiation from welding arcs is effectively eliminated in all standard welding filters. Few people use welding goggles for arc welding because a welding helmet or shield is necessary to protect the face as well as the eyes from radiant energy.

Contact lenses give no eye protection and are contraindicated when the employee is exposed to chemicals, especially alkalis. The contact lens can be very difficult to remove when the employee has a chemical corneal burn that involves extreme uncontrolled eyelid closure. The contact lens then will make irrigation far less effective since chemicals or caustic particles may be trapped beneath the lens, away from the flushing stream. Contact lenses are relatively contraindicated in areas where there is a large amount of dust, since particles trapped beneath the lens may increase the chance of corneal injury.

Contact lenses give no protection from UV keratitis (flash burn). Despite cases in the media reporting the "welding" of contact lenses to the cornea, a contact lens cannot be welded to the eye. All cases investigated have proven to be false reports. The pain that resulted was, in all investigated cases, due to UV keratitis because proper protection was not used over the contact lenses.

Developing Occupational Group Standards for Visual Performance

Various job categories require different visual skills. A receptionist could be totally blind, whereas a precision machine worker might require better-than-average skills for near vision. However, some highly motivated but visually impaired employees may, with the help of low vision aids, function quite well in jobs that usually require good visual skills; they may do so as long as their placement on the job will not cause undue hazard to themselves or other employees. Thus, while visual guidelines are important, there may be exceptions.

Basic guidelines for visual skills associated with successful performance of various job tasks are noted in the Purdue Vision Standards*. However, these standards must be combined with information gathered at the work station. This information includes observation of the employee's performance on the job so as not to discriminate against the visually handicapped but highly motivated employee who may be performing the job in a more satisfactory manner than a less-motivated, "hawk-eyed" coworker.

Teaching Employees Company Rules on Eye Safety

Every company that has jobs with risk of eye injury *must* have written, enforced rules concerning eye safety. The employee must know both the rules and the consequences for not obeying them. A laissez-faire attitude on the part of the safety officer will result in noncompliance with the eye safety program, leading to eye injuries, disability, and litigation.

FIRST AID AND REFERRAL PROGRAM FOR OCCUPATIONAL EYE INJURIES

Chemicals must be copiously and thoroughly irrigated from the eye. All employees who might receive ocular chemical burns through their work must be taught the principle and methodology of prompt irrigation for any chemical that comes in

---

*Source: American Academy of Ophthalmology. Interprofessional Education Committee. *The Worker's Eye.* San Francisco: American Academy of Ophthalmology, 1981.

CHEMICALS COMMONLY INVOLVED IN EYE INJURIES

Alkalis are especially dangerous because of their ability to rapidly penetrate into the interior of the eye with severe consequences. (Ammonia penetrates into the interior of the eye within seconds and sodium hydroxide within minutes.) The severity of ocular injury is proportional to alkalinity and not to a specific cation. Many workers do not realize that wet plaster containing lime is sufficiently alkaline to result in blindness if not immediately and thoroughly removed from the eye.

Acids can burn the eye. Acid burns are usually less severe than alkali burns since acids do not penetrate into the eye as readily. However, since sulfuric acid is one of the most frequently used compounds in industry, permanent corneal scarring from acids is not rare.

Carbon dioxide poisoning may result in retinal degeneration, photophobia, abnormalities of eye movements, constriction of peripheral visual fields, enlargement of the blind spots, and deficient dark adaptation.

Alkyl esters of sulfuric acid are intensely irritating to the conjunctiva, cornea, and eyelid. Many esters are irritating to the conjunctiva.

Hydrogen sulfide causes a keratoconjunctivitis that is responsible for colored rings around lights and increased photophobia—a possible warning sign of early poisoning.

Quinone vapor and hydroxyquinone dust cause corneal and conjunctival pigmentation that can result in significant visual loss.

Ketones can be irritating to the eyes and mucous membranes.

Methanol can cause total blindness from optic atrophy.

Concentrated *nitric acid,* when splashed into the eye, produces immediate opacification of the cornea. Severe nitric acid burns cause blindness, symblepharon (adhesion of the eyelids to the globe of the eye), and phthisis (blind, soft eye).

Although *silver* results in argyrosis—the dramatic staining of the conjunctiva, cornea, and rarely the lens—significant associated visual loss has not been reported.

Organic *tin* compounds can cause intense chemical conjunctivitis associated with severe itching.

---

contact with the eye. Emergency eyewash fountains must be located conveniently in chemical laboratories and in industrial chemical facilities. Eyewash fountains need to be tested regularly to make sure that they function properly.

Occupational health nursing personnel must be taught the symptoms and signs of serious eye injury (see box on p. 388), treatment of which consists of: (1) application of a dry, sterile eye pad to the injured eye; (2) the use of a protective shield if laceration of the globe of the eye is suspected; and (3) prompt referral to an ophthalmologist. The nurses must have constant access to immediate ophthalmologic consultation by a prearranged agreement with a hospital emergency department that has ophthalmologic coverage *or* an independent ophthalmologist (or group of ophthalmologists) who agrees to give full-time coverage for serious eye injuries.

MANAGEMENT OF EYE INJURIES

1. *Immediate emergency action followed by a referral to an ophthalmologist* is indicated for all chemical injuries. Any chemical splashed into the eye(s) must be considered a vision-threatening emergency. Forcibly keep the patient's eyelids open while irrigating with water from any source for at least 5 minutes, *then* refer the patient to an

ophthalmologist. Inform the ophthalmologist of the nature of the chemical contaminant.

2. *Injuries that require prompt referral* include all injuries with signs or symptoms of serious eye injury (see box on p. 388). Patch the injured eye lightly with a dry, sterile eye pad. If laceration of the eye is suspected, add a protective shield over the sterile eye pad. Instruct the patient not to tightly squeeze the eye shut because it greatly elevates the intraocular pressure. Calmly transport the patient to the ophthalmologist.

3. *Injuries that are treatable at the site* include conjunctival foreign body, dislodged contact lens, and spontaneous nontraumatic asymptomatic subconjunctival hemorrhage. Conjunctivitis, with normal vision and a clear cornea, may be treated with an antibiotic eye ointment for several days. If there is no improvement, referral to the ophthalmologist is indicated.

Never put eye ointment in an eye about to be seen by the ophthalmologist. The ointment makes clear visualization of the retina very difficult.

Never give a patient a topical anesthetic to relieve pain, such as from a flash burn. The prolonged use of topical anesthetics can result in blindness from corneal breakdown.

Never treat a patient with a topical steroid unless directed by the ophthalmologist. Topical steroids can make several conditions much worse, such as herpes simplex keratitis, fungal infections, and some bacterial infections.

If in doubt as to how severe an ocular symptom or sign is, *always err on the side of caution* and refer the employee to the ophthalmologist for diagnosis and treatment.

OTHER REQUIREMENTS FOR EYE SAFETY PROGRAMS

Site evaluation and effective preventive eye care in the workplace needs a great deal of improvement. Full-site evaluation and determination of visual and safety needs require input from an occupational health team including occupational and primary care physicians, ophthalmologists, nurses, optometrists, opticians, industrial hygienists, laser safety officers, and other safety personnel.

The occupational health team evaluates and preserves vision and ocular health by assessing:

the visual requirements needed to adequately and safely perform the job
the worker's visual skills
the safety of various job tasks
the illumination and visual/ergonomic conditions of the worksite
the intrinsic safety of the worksite
the availability and suitability of protective eye wear
medical access and a system for first aid and definitive care in the event of injury
obviously stated safety rules easily seen by all workers at the site
a definite statement concerning enforced company penalties for violations of safety rules.

SAFETY AT THE WORKPLACE
Direct Trauma

Prevention of eye injury from direct trauma requires a combination of: making equipment safer with proper shields; positioning workers so that flying particles from one worker's area do not enter the space of a nearby worker; prescribing, dispensing, and maintaining protective eye wear; and ensuring that safety eye wear is worn at all times.

Light and Laser Hazards

Three factors enter into any analysis of light and laser hazards (1) the type of laser or light source and the potential hazards of associated equipment, (2) the environment, and (3) potentially exposed individuals. Since many combinations are possible, numerous, rigid laser safety regulations should be avoided.

Since bright, continuous visible sources elicit a normal aversion or pain response that can protect the eye from injury, visual comfort can often be used as an approximate hazard index for the design of goggles and other hazard controls. Almost all conceivable accident situations require a hazardous exposure to be delivered within the period of the blink reflex. Few arc sources are sufficiently large and bright enough to be a retinal burn hazard under normal viewing conditions, but if the arc or tungsten filament is greatly magnified by an optical projection system, it is possible for hazardous irradiances to be imaged on a sufficiently large area of the retina to cause a burn. If an arc were initiated at a close viewing range (a few meters for all but the most powerful xenon searchlights, or a few inches from a welding arc, most movie projection equipment, or movie lamps) a retinal burn could result. Several hazard-reduction options are available to prevent individuals from viewing the source at close range.

The probability of hazardous *laser* retinal exposure is almost always remote. The pencil beam from most lasers is so small that direct entry into the 2 to 7 mm pupil of the eye is unlikely unless deliberate exposure occurs or unless an extremely careless atmosphere exists in the laser work area. However, the perception of a low likelihood of injury is probably the greatest single problem that exists with laser safety programs. When workers who do not follow precautions or who do not wear eye protectors are not injured, overconfidence, a lack of trust in the health and safety professionals, and a continued disregard for safety programs results. The only solution is a sound program of education, coupled with strict enforcement of company safety regulations. If workers understand that the laser hazard is somewhat similar to Russian roulette, they are more likely to take precautions. Better-educated workers may also be less likely to attribute all eye irritation or vision changes they experience to work with the lasers.

Safety Enforcement Policies

It is not possible to overstate the importance of eye injury prevention in terms of worker pain and suffering, the medical costs to society, and the direct and indirect costs to industry. Safety is as much a concern of management as it is of the occupational health team. Management must ensure that safety rules are followed, that overall planning includes safety, and that safety activities are promoted—through newsletters or membership in the Wise Owl Club, which is sponsored by the National Society to Prevent Blindness.

BIBLIOGRAPHY

American Academy of Ophthalmology, Interprofessional Education Committee. The Worker's Eye. San Francisco: American Academy of Ophthalmology, 1981.
   Text and slides on workers' eye safety programs.
American National Standards Institute (New York). Standards:
ANSI Z87.1—1979 practice for occupational and educational eye and face protection.
ANSI Z136.1—1986 safe use of lasers
ANSI Z49.1 welding and cutting
Duke-Elder S, MacFaul PA. System of Ophthalmology Injuries. St. Louis: Mosby, 1972. Vol. 14.
   A complete description of injuries with an excellent bibliography.
Sliney D, Wolbarsht M. Safety with lasers and other optical sources. New York: Plenum, 1980.
   A detailed text with multiple references.
Vinger PF. The eye and sports medicine. In: Duane TD, ed. Clinical Ophthalmology. Philadelphia: Harper & Row, 1985. Vol. 5 Ch. 45.
   Charts on polycarbonate included. Safety in sports programs featured.

25
Neurologic and Behavioral Disorders

Edward L. Baker, Jr.

A 29-year-old man was seen following 8 years of employment in a chlor-alkali plant where he was primarily employed in maintenance and operation of the electrolytic cells. Four years after beginning work in the plant he began to notice increased nervousness and irritability. His nervousness continued for 2 years; he then began to experience episodes of severe depression. At that time he also experienced a tremor of the hands, bleeding gums, easy fatiguability, increased salivation, and loss of appetite. He sustained an injury to his left Achilles tendon and was away from work for 7 months, during which time most of his symptoms improved. Tremulousness, nervousness, and depression, however, remained.

This man and his wife reported that prior to his employment at the plant he was outgoing, calm, and patient. He had been a military policeman in the Marines and did not experience emotional upsets during his tour of duty despite significant stress.

Urine mercury monitoring, which had been performed by his employer during his entire period of employment, had demonstrated numerous values over 500 μg per liter, the highest of which was 736 μg per liter in his fifth year of employment (normal range in general population 5–30 μg per liter).

Physical examination performed at the end of his 7-month removal from work showed no evidence of tremor, a mild loss of pinprick sensation on the dorsal aspect of his arms, and an otherwise normal neurologic exam. Lines of increased pigmentation were observed at the gingival margins of several teeth.

Neuropsychologic testing showed normal levels of intellectual functioning. He showed mild defects in his ability to perform mental calculations and in his immediate verbal and visual memory. Written spelling was particularly impaired with an inability to copy simple sentences. He could not concentrate on various tasks and, as a result, his performance was erratic with incorrect answers to simple questions and correct answers to more difficult ones. He was emotionally labile in the test situation, appearing anxious and depressed. He displayed average performance on tests of manual dexterity.

This patient's illness was manifest primarily by emotional disturbances that had secondary effects on standardized tasks of psychologic performance. He showed no particular deficits in memory, psychomotor performance, learning ability, or recall of current events. His most striking deficit was one of impaired concentration, which resulted in erratic performance on various tests. These effects were still detected months after he was removed from mercury exposure.

During recent years increasing concern has developed over the occurrence of neurobehavioral disorders among workers in various occupations. In many instances, as in this case study, specific chemical substances have been identified that are responsible for characteristic pathologic processes within the nervous system. In other cases groups of substances such as solvents have been associated epidemiologically with manifestations of nervous system disease. Although exposure to industrial toxins has been known for hundreds of years to affect behavior, recent studies have applied quantitative methods to the study of behavioral aberrations following toxin exposure and have demonstrated a wide range of clinical and subclinical effects for numerous substances. It has been shown that many neurotoxic agents produce a dose-related spectrum of impairment, ranging from mild slowing of nerve conduction velocity or prolongation in reaction time to neuropathy and frank encephalopathy.

Disorders with predominantly psychiatric manifestations have been described in some workers, ranging from acute psychosis and "mass psychogenic illness" to chronic neurasthenia (a condition characterized by mildly impaired responses to behavioral tests and symptoms of persistent fatigue). Although specific chemical substances have been identified that may be associated with certain of these psychiatric syndromes, etiologic mechanisms are unclear.

In view of the increasing diversity of industrial hazards, neurologic disorders are likely to follow the introduction of some new substances into the workplace. This happened in the 1970s when an industrial catalyst, dimethylaminopropionitrile (DMAPN), was found to be associated with bladder neuropathy in workers producing polyurethane foam; it also recently occurred when peripheral neuropathy in employees in a coated-fabrics plant was traced to the introduction of a neurotoxic solvent, methyl *n*-butyl ketone (MBK).

NEUROLOGIC DISORDERS

Pathophysiology

Peripheral Nervous System Effects. Two basic forms of damage to peripheral nerves have been identified as responsible for the peripheral neuropathies associated with occupational exposure to neurotoxins. *Segmental demyelination* results from primary destruction of the neuronal myelin sheath, with relative sparing of the axons. This process begins at the nodes of Ranvier and results in slowing of nerve conduction. There is characteristically no evidence of muscle denervation, although disuse atrophy may occur if paralysis is prolonged. As remyelination begins during the recovery phase, recovery is rapid and usually complete in mild to moderate neuropathies.

Axonal degeneration is associated with metabolic derangement of the entire neuron and is manifest by degeneration of the distal portion of

the nerve fiber. Myelin sheath degeneration may occur secondarily. Nerve conduction rates are usually normal until the condition is relatively far advanced. Distal muscles show changes of denervation. Recovery may occur by axonal regeneration but is very slow and incomplete.

In many instances, axonal degeneration and segmental demyelination may coexist, presumably due to secondary effects derived from damage to each system. Therefore, although the above descriptions of classic manifestations of these syndromes hold in experimental models, the clinical manifestations of neuropathy in exposed individuals may represent a combination of both pathologic processes.

Central Nervous System Effects. Recent studies, including investigations of lead, chlordecone (Kepone), and carbon monoxide, have shown significant disruption of neurotransmitter metabolism, affecting dopamine, norepinephrine, gammaaminobutyric acid (GABA), and serotonin, which correlates with behavioral aberrations in experimental animals. Furthermore, many industrial solvents cause acute depression of central nervous system (CNS) synaptic transmission resulting in drowsiness and weakness. Such mechanisms are undoubtedly responsible for the poorly understood manifestations of CNS toxicity induced by workplace substances.

Combined Peripheral and Central Nervous System Effects. Certain industrial neurotoxins cause distal degeneration of axons in both the central and peripheral nervous systems. This form of axonal degeneration was originally described as "dying back" neuropathy. In view of the association of central and peripheral nervous system degeneration, it has been recently suggested that this process be referred to as central-peripheral distal axonopathy. Substances associated with this effect include acrylamide, *n*-hexane, MBK, carbon disulfide, and organophosphorus compounds, the most notable of which is tri-ortho-cresyl phosphate (TOCP).

Characteristically, distal degeneration occurs within the long nerve fiber tracts of both the peripheral and central nervous systems. Once degeneration begins peripherally, it becomes more severe in the initially affected nerve segments while progressing centrally to involve more proximal segments of nerve fibers. Within the spinal cord the long ascending and descending tracts (the spinocerebellar and corticospinal tracts) appear to be the most severely affected. Involved fiber tracts demonstrate axonal swellings, which are often focal and are associated with neurofilament accumulation within the axon. Although the length of the axon is a key determinant of fiber susceptibility, fiber diameter may also be important: Large-diameter, myelinated fibers are more frequently affected.

The precise locus of the metabolic derangement that is responsible for these manifestations of axonal damage in unknown. Chemical substances may bind to the inactivate intra-axonal enzyme systems required for maintenance of normal axonal transport mechanisms.

Manifestations

Peripheral Nervous System. Virtually all of the industrial toxins that affect the peripheral nervous system cause a mixed sensorimotor peripheral neuropathy. The initial manifestations of this disorder consist of intermittent numbness and tingling in the hands and feet; motor weakness in the feet or hands may develop somewhat later and progress to the development of an ataxic gait or an inability to grasp heavy objects. Although the distal portion of the extremities is involved initially and to a greater degree, severe cases may also manifest proximal muscle weakness and muscle atrophy. Nerve biopsies in affected individuals have shown axonal swellings and paranodal myelin retraction. Extensor muscle groups usually manifest weakness before flexors.

Although the manifestations are fairly consistent from one toxin to another, certain specific characteristics are unique to individual agents (Table 25-1). Painful limbs and increased sensitivity of the feet to touch are particularly characteristic of arsenical neuropathy. Sensory involvement predominates in the relatively rare neuropathy seen with alkyl mercury poisoning. Both motor and sensory disorders are observed in the neuropathies associated with exposure to n-hexane, MBK, and acrylamide.

The peripheral neuropathy associated with lead exposure is unusual because only the motor system is involved. The most characteristic early manifestation of lead neuropathy is wrist extensor weakness. Reports of involvement of the lower extremities resulting in ankle drop were made during the 1930s, when cabaret dancers consumed lead-contaminated illicit whiskey and developed lead neuropathy in the muscles that they used most actively. Overt wrist drop, which was a characteristic manifestation of lead neuropathy in reports of many years ago, is quite rare today.

The development of these syndromes is usually insidious. Very slow development of numbness and tingling of the fingers and toes occurs over several weeks and may then be followed by motor weakness. Of particular interest is the case of several toxins, including acrylamide, n-hexane, and MBK, in which the neuropathy may progress even after workers are removed from exposure. This deterioration persists for 3 to 4 weeks after removal from exposure; at that point recovery may begin. The duration of the recovery process is proportional to the degree of severity of neuropathy: Less severely affected cases may totally resolve over a 3-to-6 month period, whereas individuals with advanced disease may show persistent signs and symptoms 1 to 2 years later.

Physical examination of affected individuals shows a characteristic distribution of sensory loss, particularly to pain and temperature discrimination (Fig. 25-1). Frequently vibration sensation is impaired and touch perception, particularly with acrylamide poisoning, is lost. Tremor of the hands is particularly common in several types of chemical intoxication. In most instances the tremor is a

Table 25-1. Peripheral nervous system effects of occupational toxins*

Effect	Toxin	Comments
Motor neuropathy	Lead	Primarily wrist extensors
		Wrist drop and ankle drop rare
Mixed sensorimotor neuropathy	Acrylamide	Ataxia common
		Desquamation of hands and soles
		Sweating of palms
	Arsenic	Distal paresthesias earliest symptom
		Painful limbs, especially in calves
		Hyperpathia of feet
		Weakness prominent in legs
	Carbon disulfide	Peripheral neuropathy rather mild
		CNS effects more important
	Carbon monoxide	Seen only after severe intoxication
	DDT	Only seen with ingestions
	n-hexane and methyl n-butyl ketone (MBK)	Distal paresthesias and motor weakness
		Weight loss, fatigue, and muscle cramps common
	Mercury	Predominantly distal sensory involvement
		More common with alkyl mercury exposure

*This table and subsequent tables include most but not all of the neurotoxic substances associated with listed conditions.

resting tremor that is not increased with movement. The tremor seen with chlordecone (Kepone) poisoning is a frequent manifestation of the disease and has characteristic features: irregular, non-purposive, and most severe when the limb is static but unsupported against gravity. In contrast the tremor seen with mercury poisoning is fine and affects the eyelids, tongue, and outstretched hands. Motor weakness in toxic neuropathies is characteristically found in distal muscles of the arms and legs (Fig. 25-1). Intrinsic muscles of the hands and feet are particularly affected in neuropathies caused by n-hexane, MBK, and acrylamide. Extensor weakness of the forearms is characteristic of lead neuropathy. Impaired coordination is often seen in individuals with motor weakness in the extremities; cerebellar pathology need not be present for these manifestations to occur. In summary, distal sensory and motor impairment characterized by numbness and weakness of the hands and feet is followed by more proximal involvement as the toxic neuropathy develops.

Other Neurological Manifestations. A wide variety of additional manifestations may be seen that are specific to individual toxins (Table 25-2). Movement disorders that resemble Parkinson's disease have been reported in individuals exposed to carbon disulfide, carbon monoxide, and manganese; hypotonia, dystonia, and other disorders of locomotion occur in individuals with excessive exposure to these substances. In the case of manganese toxicity, significant improvement following drug therapy was seen in the characteristic mask-like facies of a patient with occupational exposure to this toxin (Fig. 25-2).

A characteristic abnormality of eye movements called opsoclonus can be caused by chlordecone (Kepone) exposure. It consists of irregular bursts of involuntary, abrupt, rapid jerks of both eyes simultaneously, usually horizontal, but multi-directional in severely affected individuals.

Seizures are often seen in individuals with acute excessive exposure to industrial toxins. Organochlorine insecticides such as DDT and chlordane

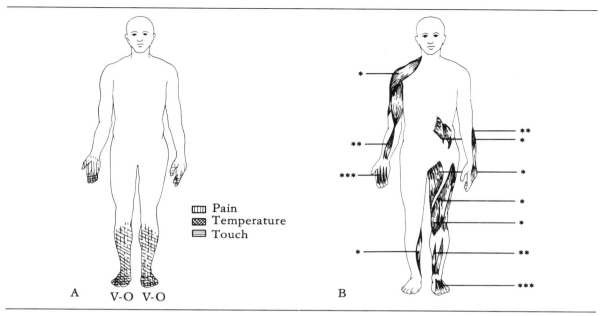

Fig. 25-1. A. Pattern of sensory loss in a severe case of MBK neuropathy. B. Distribution of muscle weakness in MBK neuropathy with degree of weakness proportional to number of asterisks. (From N Allen. Solvents and other industrial organic compounds. In PJ Vinken and GW Bruyn, eds., Intoxications of the nervous system. Part I [Volume 36] in Handbook of Clinical Neurology. Amsterdam: Elsevier/North-Holland Biomedical Press, 1979.)

have been associated with seizures following acute ingestion of large doses. Seizures are a rare manifestation of lead encephalopathy in adults.

Cranial nerve involvement is uncommon with the peripheral neurotoxins mentioned above. However, trichloroethylene has a predilection for the trigeminal facial nerves and has been associated with facial numbness and weakness. Carbon disulfide exposure is also associated with cranial neuropathies.

Excesses of CNS tumors have been reported among workers in the petrochemical industry; studies are currently being performed to determine if these are work-related.

An unusual manifestation of neurotoxicity was seen several years ago in a group of workers exposed to an industrial catalyst, dimethylamino-propionitrile (DMAPN). This substance caused a neuropathy in the bladder, resulting in urinary retention, urinary hesitancy, and sexual dysfunction. Although the symptoms improved after removal of the affected individuals from exposure to this substance, symptoms and signs persisted in some individuals for at least 2 years.

Diagnosis

Electrophysiologic tests that assess peripheral nerve function, including electromyograms (EMGs) and nerve conduction measurements, are important tools in assessing the extent and severity of neurologic disorders in workers exposed to industrial toxins. These techniques are useful often in the evaluation of individual patients. Recently, noninvasive techniques that measure sensory thresholds for vibration and temperature have been developed to monitor diabetic patients for the occurrence of sensory neuropa-

Table 25-2. Other neurologic manifestations of occupational toxins

Manifestation	Agent
Ataxic gait	Acrylamide
	Chlordane
	Chlordecone (Kepone)
	DDT
	n-hexane
	Manganese
	Mercury (especially methyl mercury)
	Methyl *n*-butyl ketone (MBK)
	Methyl chloride
	Toluene
Bladder neuropathy	Dimethylaminopropionitrile (DMAPN)
Constricted visual fields	Mercury
Cranial neuropathy	Carbon disulfide
	Trichloroethylene
Headache	Lead
	Nickel
Impaired visual acuity	*n*-hexane
	Mercury
	Methanol
Increased intracranial pressure	Lead
	Organotin compounds
Myoclonus	Benzene hexachloride
	Mercury
Nystagmus	Mercury
Opsoclonus	Chlordecone (Kepone)
Paraplegia	Organotin compounds
Parkinsonism	Carbon disulfide
	Carbon monoxide
	Manganese
Seizures	Lead
	Organic mercurials
	Organochlorine insecticides
	Organotin compounds
Tremor	Carbon disulfide
	Chlordecone (Kepone)
	DDT
	Manganese
	Mercury

thy. These techniques are also efficient tools for reliable screening of workers with significant exposure to neurotoxic agents or with early sensory symptoms. In addition to detection of toxic neuropathy, these instruments may also be useful in detection of compression neuropathies, such as carpal tunnel syndrome.

Electroencephalograms (EEGs) have also been used in the evaluation of workers exposed to neurotoxins. However, these have not usually been as useful as nerve conduction tests. EEGs may be of value as an adjunct to the assessment of altered states of consciousness of unknown etiology. A more promising extension of EEG use is the measurement of cortical-evoked potentials following auditory or visual stimuli; for example, prolonged latency of visually evoked responses has been reported in individuals chronically exposed to *n*-hexane.

BEHAVIORAL DISORDERS
Manifestations
Excessive exposure to industrial toxins may result in behavioral effects, ranging from mild symptoms of fatigue to overt psychosis. In view of the vagueness of many behavioral manifestations of neurotoxin exposure, standardized psychometric testing has greatly facilitated the evaluation of these disorders. In general, neurotoxins particularly affect psychomotor performance by causing slowness in response time, impaired eye-hand coordination, and diminished concentration ability. Emotional effects are also seen and consist of irritability and, at times, emotional lability. Recent memory may be disrupted, manifest in testing situations as an inability to learn new material. Aspects of cognitive functioning that are usually not affected by toxins include remote memory and fund of general information.

Although few toxins have unique behavioral effects, several substances deserve particular attention (Table 25-3). Carbon disulfide affects all levels of the CNS and may result in bizarre clinical

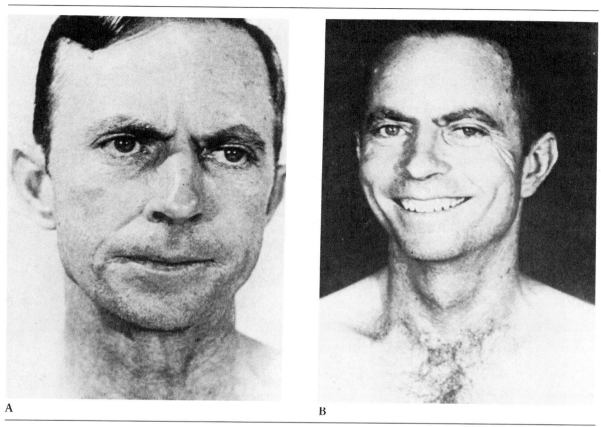

A   B

Fig. 25-2. A. Mask-like facies of patient with manganese toxicity prior to therapeutic trial with L-dopa. B. Full facial expression of same patient being maintained on L-dopa. (From HA Rosenstock, DG Simons, JS Meyer. Chronic manganism: neurologic and laboratory studies during treatment with levodopa. JAMA, 1971; 217:1355. Copyright 1971, American Medical Association.)

syndromes including acute psychosis. Heavy over-exposure has been associated with suicide in at least one worker. Although neurotoxins may cause both behavioral effects and peripheral neuropathy in the same individual, one effect usually predominates.

Most chlorinated hydrocarbon solvents in current use in industry cause a relatively brief "high" following exposure to significantly elevated concentrations in air. Intentional abuse of industrial solvents by individuals desiring these intoxicating effects has been reported to cause permanent damage to the peripheral and central nervous systems. Such use should obviously be proscribed in view of the potentially severe consequences.

Diagnosis
Standardized psychometric testing using measures of memory, intelligence, attention, dexterity, reaction time, personality, and general psychomotor function are very useful in evaluating exposed individuals as well as groups of workers. Recently

Table 25-3. Behavioral effects of occupational toxins

Manifestation	Agent
Acute psychosis or marked emotional instability	Carbon disulfide Manganese Toluene (rare)
Impaired psychomotor function	Carbon disulfide Lead Mercury Organophosphate insecticides Perchloroethylene and other solvents Styrene
Memory impairment	Arsenic Carbon disulfide Lead Manganese
Neurasthenia, irritability, and other mild systemic symptoms	Acrylamide Arsenic Lead Manganese Mercury Methyl *n*-butyl ketone (MBK) Organotin compounds Solvents Styrene

neurobehavioral tests have been adapted for computer administration to facilitate reproducibility in testing groups and to improve data-handling efficiency. In the future, computerized testing will be used in epidemiologic and clinical research to evaluate health effects of new agents or previously recognized toxins. Periodic monitoring of exposed workers will also become common. Interpretation of test results must take into account confounding factors such as age, education, alcohol consumption, and preexisting neurologic disease in order to evaluate correctly the etiologic role of toxin exposure. The most important feature of the diagnostic process is a carefully obtained occupational history that identifies specific neurotoxins and assesses the magnitude and duration of exposure to

each. The work history is particularly important in evaluating behavioral disorders since these conditions are often attributed to factors unrelated to work.

MANAGEMENT AND CONTROL

Management of occupationally induced neurologic problems consists primarily of identification of the offending agent and removal of the worker from continued exposure. In some episodes—for example, that of DMAPN exposure—removal of the offending agent from the workplace may result in cessation of the development of new cases. Some workers with known exposure may develop mild, early symptoms of neurotoxicity; objective demonstration of functional impairment using standardized tests is essential in the management of individual cases. Workers with evidence of toxin-related symptoms or functional impairment should be removed from exposure until these deficits resolve and exposure in the workplace is terminated.

Prevention of occupationally induced neurologic disorders can be accomplished through workplace medical and environmental control programs. The goal of environmental control is to reduce concentrations of neurotoxic substances in the worker's environment by various manipulations. Medical strategies designed to reduce neurologic morbidity include preemployment or preplacement evaluation and periodic medical monitoring. The goal of preemployment or preplacement evaluation as it relates to neurologic disorders is to avoid placement of individuals with preexisting disease (such as peripheral neuropathies) in jobs with exposures that might exacerbate these conditions. Furthermore, conditions that might impair workers' ability to perform their jobs, such as uncontrolled epilepsy in persons operating hazardous machinery, would be grounds for medical exclusion of such individuals from these jobs.

Periodic medical monitoring programs are becoming more common in industries where neurotoxins are used. An important element of such monitoring programs is the measurement of the neurotoxic agent in biologic fluids. The most common such application occurs in industries where lead and mercury are used.

Periodic monitoring of lead-exposed workers should include a work and medical history; physical examination, with special attention to the nervous system; blood and urine studies to evaluate hematologic and renal effects of lead exposure; and, most importantly, determination of blood concentration of lead and zinc protoporphyrin (ZPP). The content of such exams is mandated by the recent Occupational Safety and Health Administration (OSHA) standard on occupational exposure to lead, in which specific guidelines are given for job transfer of workers with excessive concentrations of lead in their blood. The OSHA standard for inorganic lead requires that employers make routine blood lead monitoring available to all employees exposed to lead above the action level of 30 μg per cubic meter, regardless of whether respirators are worn. The standard requires that testing be repeated every 6 months when the most recent blood lead level is less than 40 μg per dl. If the employee's blood lead level is greater than 50 μg per dl and this level is confirmed by a second blood lead level (which must be obtained within 2 weeks of the employer's receipt of the first level), the employee is to be removed from any job in which exposure is above the action level of 30 μg per cubic meter. Such workers must be retested monthly and not returned to an exposed job until their blood lead is below 40 μg per dl on two analyses. If a worker's blood lead is greater than or equal to 40 μg per dl but less than or equal to 60 μg per dl the worker must be retested every 2 months. If the average of the last 3 blood lead measurements taken within the last 6 months is greater than 50 μg per dl a worker must also be removed from exposure and retested monthly until the blood lead is less than 40 μg per dl. Any worker removed from a job because of elevated blood lead is protected by the medical removal protection (MRP) provision of

the OSHA lead standard. This provision requires an employer to "maintain the worker's earnings, seniority, and other employment rights and benefits (as though the worker had not been removed) for a period of up to 18 months."

The evaluation of mercury-exposed workers is similar with three exceptions. Urine mercury determinations are used rather than blood measurements; there is no enzymatic test such as the ZPP test that measures the metabolic toxicity of mercury exposure; and finally, there is no comprehensive OSHA standard for occupational mercury exposure that prescribes the content of periodic medical evaluations and medical action levels for job transfer. Workers exposed to cadmium and arsenic should be monitored periodically with urinary determinations of these two metals in addition to standard medical evaluations.

Workers chronically exposed to solvents should have periodic medical histories and physical examinations with attention to the nervous system. Standardized behavioral tests show promise as periodic monitoring tools, and measurement of urinary metabolites of solvents is sometimes helpful as an adjunct to other medical monitoring techniques.

Pesticide-exposed workers, particularly those using organophosphate insecticides, should be periodically evaluated with red blood cell cholinesterase levels to assess their degree of pesticide exposure. Although some recommendations have been made that periodic nerve conduction testing should be performed in addition to standard medical history and physical examination, this test is not suitable for routine monitoring of asymptomatic workers.

Treatment of occupational neurologic disease beyond removal of the worker from continued toxic exposure may consist of the administration of drugs designed to remove the offending agent or counteract its effects. Chelating drugs, such as ethylene diamine tetraacetic acid (EDTA) and penicillamine, are given as treatment for symptomatic poisoning by lead and other heavy metals. These drugs should only be given as treatment for symptomatic disease and not prophylactically to lower blood levels of the metal; they have known toxicity, which may add to the toxic effects of the metals and may also increase gastrointestinal absorption of the metal. Workers should be removed from exposure to the offending agent prior to initiation of drug therapy.

Treatment of organophosphate insecticide poisoning is accomplished primarily by giving atropine, a pharmacologic antagonist of the pesticide. If patients are seen very soon after exposure, other drugs (oximes) may be given to regenerate inhibited cholinesterase enzyme.

Ultimately, prevention of occupational diseases of the nervous system rests on adequate testing of chemicals prior to their introduction into the workplace and in environmental measures designed to reduce exposure. The Toxic Substances Control ACT (TSCA) addresses the issue of premarket testing, and the Environmental Protection Agency (EPA) has specified criteria for neurologic evaluation of chemical substances. Biologic assays of organophosphate compounds have successfully predicted those substances that will be neurotoxic to humans. Substances such as n-hexane and MBK, which produce an axonal neuropathy in exposed humans, have been shown to produce similar effects in animals, and the neurologic disorder associated with Kepone toxicity was seen in experimental animals several years before it was reported in exposed humans. Therefore, testing of industrial substances by administration of toxins to experimental animals is essential in the identification of substances with neurotoxic potential.

In rare instances structural similarity alone has proved useful in predicting toxicity. N-hexane and MBK are metabolized to 2,5-hexanedione, which is thought to be responsible for the neurotoxic manifestations of these two industrial chemicals. Thus, investigation of structure-activity relationships may be of value in identifying substances with potential neurotoxicity. In those instances where neurotoxicity is suspected because of the chemical structure of the compound, animal tests are still required.

As standardized tests of neurologic function become increasingly available, field studies of industrial toxins using these techniques will be used to determine the appropriate levels of industrial exposure. These levels, referred to as threshold limit values (TLVs) or permissible exposure limits (PELs), have in the past been based on informed opinion of experts. In the future, as epidemiologic studies become more precise in assessing the neurotoxic hazard of these substances, control measures and specific exposure standards will be based on much more objective information.

EFFECTS OF SELECTED NEUROTOXINS

Lead

The most commonly encountered workplace substance with clearly recognized neurotoxic effects is lead (see also Chaps. 14, 26, 28, and 30). The National Institute for Occupational Safety and Health (NIOSH) has estimated that over 1 million U.S. workers are daily exposed to lead (Fig. 25-3). The manifestations of lead neurotoxicity as currently encountered differ significantly from those seen in reports from the earlier part of this century when more overt disorders were observed. The most common neurologic finding in workers exposed to lead is impaired CNS function manifested by symptoms of fatigue, irritability, difficulty in concentrating, and inability to perform tasks requiring sustained concentration. These symptoms are associated with abnormalities on standardized neuropsychologic testing showing impairment of verbal intelligence, memory, and perceptual speed. Symptoms of arm weakness characteristically affecting extensor muscle groups are also seen in the early phases of lead toxicity. Often, weakness occurs before abnormalities are seen on nerve conduction testing. Such abnormalities tend to develop in individuals with blood lead levels in the range of 60 μg per deciliter and become more apparent as the blood lead level rises. After removal from exposure, these symptoms and abnormalities resolve slowly over weeks to months, the duration

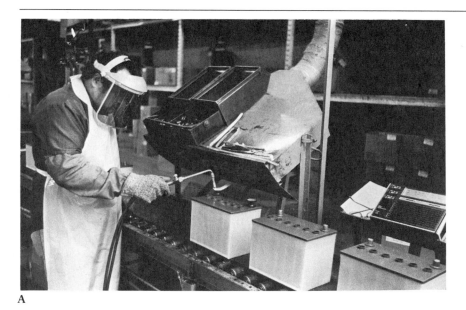

A

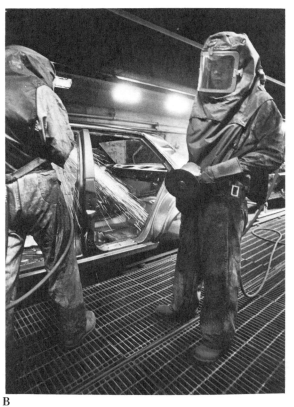

B

Fig. 25-3. Current work practice rules require significant personal and environmental protection in lead exposures. A. Lead battery worker is protected mainly by local exhaust ventilation. B. Automobile lead grinder is protected by air-supplied hood and floor exhaust ventilation.
(Photographs by Earl Dotter.)

depending on their initial intensity and other factors.

Neurologic abnormalities following lead exposure usually occur after hematologic toxicity as manifested by elevated ZPP level and reduction in blood hemoglobin concentration. Permanent renal damage occurs much later than neurologic dysfunction and characteristically develops only after at least 5 years of lead exposure. In contrast, neurologic abnormalities may develop within 2 to 3 months of the onset of work in a lead environment, particularly in those places where exposure is relatively poorly controlled. Abnormalities of nerve conduction tend not to occur before at least 6 to 8 months of chronic exposure to lead.

Mercury

Although disease as striking as that experienced by Lewis Carroll's Mad Hatter no longer occurs in plants in the United States, behavioral effects of exposure to elemental mercury are seen. Erethism, a set of behavioral symptoms classically associated with mercury toxicity, is characterized by unusual shyness, anxiety, inability to concentrate, and irritability. Standardized memory tests have been shown to be affected in individuals with urine mercury concentrations of 200 μg per liter or above. A fine tremor of the hands is associated with mercury poisoning, and computer-assisted analysis of EMGs has shown a shift in the frequency of normal forearm tremor as an early manifestation of mercury toxicity. Peripheral neuropathy is not a recognized feature of elemental mercury poisoning. Measurement of mercury in urine and blood is a useful tool in the assessment of workplace exposure. Urine mercury levels above 300 μg per liter are considered excessive.

Organic mercurials, particularly alkyl mercury compounds such as methyl mercury, have a strong affinity for the CNS, and severe neurologic effects have been associated with excessive exposure (see also Chap. 26). The best described episode of organic mercury poisoning occurred in Minamata, Japan, where early symptoms of poisoning consisted of distal paresthesias, cerebellar disorders, visual impairment, deafness, and mental disturbances. Sensory deficits were seen with loss of position sense, impaired two-point discrimination, astereognosis, and mild hypalgesia. Visual impairment characteristically consisted of constriction of visual fields. Mental disturbances were characterized by agitation alternating with periods of stupor and mutism. The more severe cases exhibited dystonic flexion postures. Peripheral neuropathies were not seen in this group of individuals.

The devastating and usually irreversible effects on the nervous system of organic mercury poisoning should be prevented through restriction of the use of these substances. To that end, the practice of treating seed grain with organic mercurial fungicides has been curtailed by the EPA following outbreaks of neurologic disease in the United States and Iraq among persons ingesting food inadvertently contaminated with these substances.

Organophosphate Insecticides

Acute organophosphate insecticide poisoning is characterized by the inhibition of acetylcholinesterase with resulting overactivity of cholinergic components of the autonomic nervous system, inhibition of conduction across myoneural junctions in skeletal muscle, and interference of CNS synaptic transmission. Manifestations of acute toxicity include meiosis, blurring of vision, chest tightness, increased bronchial secretion, and wheezing. Gastrointestinal effects are also seen, including abdominal cramps, nausea, and vomiting. Increased sweating, salivation, and lacrimation are also characteristic features.

Atropine is the drug of choice for treating the acute manifestations of organophosphate insecticide poisoning. Repeated doses are given to the point of atropinization, and subsequent doses of the drug may be required since the duration of action of atropine is less than that of organophosphate insecticides. Since organophosphate compounds bind irreversibly to cholinesterase, reactivation of the enzyme system occurs only through synthesis of additional cholinesterase molecules. Therefore, recovery of normal cholinesterase concentrations in red blood cells is slow, and repeated exposure may result in cumulative depression of cholinesterase stores. Recovery following an acute episode of poisoning is usually complete within 7 days unless anoxia has occurred during the acute phase of the episode. Measurement of red blood cell cholinesterase concentrations is valuable during the acute intoxication episode and is also used for surveillance of occupationally exposed workers. Plasma cholinesterase concentrations are of less value in occupational settings since many factors may alter them.

A syndrome of delayed neurotoxicity has been reported with certain organophosphate compounds (although not with organophosphate pesticides currently used in the United States). This syndrome develops 8 to 35 days after exposure to the organophosphorus compounds. Progressive weakness begins in the distal lower extremities, and toe and foot drop often develop; finger weakness and wrist drop follow lower extremity manifestations. Sensory loss is minimal. Deep tendon reflexes are frequently depressed. The disease may progress for 1 to 3 months following onset, and recovery is very slow.

Recent studies of workers occupationally exposed to organophosphates have revealed some evidence of psychomotor impairment and abnormal EEG. Further studies are required to assess the extent and nature of these disorders. Evaluation of patients exposed to organophosphate insecticides should include, in addition to work history, a neurologic exam with attention to manifestations of autonomic nervous system dysfunction. Measurement of red blood cell cholinesterase concentration is valuable; cholinesterase levels correlate reasonably well with manifestations of clinical toxicity.

Organic Solvents
Exposure to organic solvents occurs daily for over one million U.S. workers. The most frequently used include toluene, xylene, trichloroethylene, ethanol, methylene chloride, and methyl chloroform. Although chemically heterogeneous, these compounds are often discussed as a group because of toxicologically similar effects and the high frequency of exposure to various combinations of these substances.

Acute narcosis follows exposure to high concentrations of solvent vapors, and lower levels may produce a transient intoxication syndrome similar to that seen with ethanol consumption.

To facilitate the characterization of persistent health effects of solvent exposure, a nomenclature has been developed by a World Health Organization (WHO) working group and by a workshop of invited experts held in the United States. The mildest form of effect, organic affective syndrome (or type 1 solvent health effect), is characterized by symptoms of irritability, fatiguability, difficulty in concentrating, and loss of interest in daily events. This type of effect is typically reversible. The second, a more severe form of effect, mild chronic toxic encephalopathy, is characterized by objective abnormalities on neurobehavioral testing and by symptoms that are similar to organic affective syndrome (type 1 effect) but are more pronounced. Sustained personality or mood change (type 2a effect) or impairment in intellectual function (type 2b) may be seen at this level of effect, singly or in combination. Severe chronic toxic encephalopathy (type 3 effect) is characterized clinically as a type of dementia with global deterioration of memory and other cognitive functions; reversibility is unlikely. Workers exposed to solvents may exhibit any of these three syndromes depending on the intensity and duration of their exposure. Epidemiologic studies have frequently shown a decrease in reaction time, dexterity, speed, and memory among workers with prolonged solvent exposure. Relatively few abnormalities have been demonstrated in peripheral nervous system function; nerve conduction abnormalities have been reported in one study of mixed solvent exposure. Measurement of urinary metabolites such as hippuric acid in toluene exposure may be of value in monitoring exposed populations. Further research is needed to develop a more complete approach to prevention of solvent-induced disease.

MASS PSYCHOGENIC ILLNESS
Mass psychogenic illness (MPI) may be defined as the collective occurrence of physical symptoms and beliefs about the origin of these symptoms among a group of persons in the absence of a plausible biologic explanation. Reports of MPI have described workers employed at repetitive, boring tasks in workplaces having physical as well as emotional stressors. Symptoms are vague (often headache, dizziness, nausea, and weakness) and not consistent among outbreaks. The onset of an MPI outbreak has been described as precipitous, with many cases occurring over a few hours; it has been reported to follow a "trigger stimulus," which is often a noxious odor. Recurrences of similar symptoms in those initially affected are also common. Studies using psychometric testing have purported to identify "susceptible individuals" who are at risk for MPI. The poorly described nature of this entity increases the likelihood that attention will be focused on the worker when no obvious environmental agent is readily found. For this reason investigation of suspected outbreaks of MPI should focus intently on excluding environmental toxins as etiologic agents.

Diagnosis and Management
In practice the determination that an outbreak of acute illness is due to psychogenic factors is often impossible. Exclusion of toxic agents as etiologically responsible is often very difficult in view of the paucity of understanding of the effects of workplace toxins and the complexity of exposures in the work environment. Since efforts to identify susceptible workers shift the focus away from improving the work environment, this approach is not in keeping with accepted public health practice. Many descriptions of MPI have stressed that women are more frequently affected than men; this difference in attack rates may well relate to traditional hiring practices in which women are assigned to more repetitive, boring jobs than men. Chronic stress-related complaints have often been described in plants in which MPI has occurred,

suggesting that workplace factors may play an important role in the genesis of MPI. Primary attention should be directed to alleviation of chronic sources of stress in the workplace (see Chap. 20). Investigations that merely identify so-called susceptible individuals as a means of controlling this problem will fail to achieve satisfactory results and will often infringe on workers' rights.

BIBLIOGRAPHY
Allen N et al. Toxic polyneuropathy due to methyl *n*-butyl ketone. Arch Neurol 1975; 32:209.
A careful description of a classic outbreak of neurotoxicity.
Baker EL, Fine LJ. Solvent neurotoxicity: the current evidence. J Occup Med 1986; 28:126–9.
A review of current concepts on solvent neurotoxicity.
Bove F et al. Quantitative sensory testing in occupational medicine. Semin Occup Med 1986; 1:185.
A description of the theoretical and practical issues concerning the use of quantitative sensory testing.
Cranmer JM, Goldberg L, eds. Proceedings of the Workshop on Neurobehavioral Effects of Solvents. Neurotoxicology 1987; 7:1–95.
A comprehensive review of solvent-related health effects developed by a workshop of international experts.
Editorial. Hexacarbon neuropathy. Lancet 1979; 2:942.
A brief review of relevant literature on hexane and MBK.
Elofsson S-A et al. Exposure to organic solvents. Scand J Work Environ Health 1980: 6:239–73.
An extensive study of diverse neurologic effects of solvents with discussion of previous relevant research.
Feldman RG, Ricks NL, Baker EL. Neuropsychological effects of industrial toxins; a review. Am J Ind Med 1980; 1:211.
An overview of behavioral toxicology of workplace substances.
Heyman A et al. Peripheral neuropathy caused by arsenical intoxication. N Engl J Med 1956; 254:401.
Largest series of cases of arsenical neuropathy. Careful discussion of prognosis and treatment.
Kurland LT et al. Minamata disease. World Neurol 1960; 1:370.
Extensive discussion of historic outbreak of methyl mercury poisoning.
Letz RE, Baker EL. Computer-administered neurobe-

havioral testing in occupational health. Semin Occup Med 1986; 1:197.
A description of the development of a computerized neurobehavioral testing system for monitoring workplace exposures.

Namba T et al. Poisoning due to organophosphate insecticides—acute and chronic manifestations. Am J Med 1971; 50:475.
A clinical review with excellent discussion of treatment.

Spencer PS, Schaumberg HH, eds. Experimental and clinical neurotoxicology. Baltimore: Williams & Wilkins, 1980.
In-depth discussion of the pathophysiology of neurotoxin-induced disease.

Taylor JR et al. Chlordecone intoxication in man. Neurology 1978; 28:626.
A complete description of a severe outbreak of occupational neurologic disease.

Vinken PJ, Bruyn GW, eds. Handbook of clinical neurology. Intoxications of the nervous system, parts I and II. Amsterdam: Elsevier, 1979. Vols. 36 and 37.
A collection of comprehensive monographs on various neurotoxins. An excellent reference work.

World Health Organization, Nordic Council of Ministers. Chronic effects of organic solvents on the central nervous system and diagnostic criteria. Copenhagen: WHO Regional Office for Europe, 1985.
An important summary of a consensus WHO workshop on the nature of organic solvent neurotoxicity.

26
Reproductive Disorders

Maureen C. Hatch and Zena A. Stein

In this chapter, work-related experiences in men and women that might affect their reproductive function are discussed. Although the National Institute for Occupational Safety and Health (NIOSH) includes reproductive disorders in its list of 10 leading work-related disorders, there are few firmly based associations with occupation, in spite of the potential for physical, chemical, biologic or stress-related exposures to affect the reproductive system adversely. Hence, any strategy for *preventing* reproductive problems must necessarily emphasize research.

Most current knowledge about reproductive toxicity comes from laboratory studies of rodents, whose anatomy, physiology, rate of development, pharmacokinetics, and metabolism differ from those of humans. Population studies have been uncommon, and many that have been reported are of poor quality. In part, the reason is that reproductive hazards research is a relatively new field and appropriate study methods are still being developed. Not only is the field new, but it is also quite complex: researchers have to contend with multiple targets for exposure (male, female, and conceptus) and a wide range of possible effects. The recent advances in bioassay technology—for example, in imaging, immunology, and genetics—have the potential to provide sophisticated tools for measuring dose or assessing function that will greatly extend existing methodologies. As increasingly sensitive strategies are used, it is possible that new associations will be demonstrated. It is also possible that the reproductive processes, because of their crucial evolutionary significance, are, in fact, well protected against a wide range of environmental stimuli.

REPRODUCTIVE BIOLOGY IN BRIEF

Reproduction in humans is a complex, dynamic, interdependent system involving the brain, pituitary, and gonads. The following features of normal reproductive biology may be important in the context of toxic exposures (Table 26-1).

In males, germ cell production is continuous from the time of puberty and dependent on a pool of constantly dividing stem cells. Mature sperm develop through a staged process that takes approximately 80 to 90 days. Thus, damaged sperm cells are lost within one cycle of spermatogenesis, unless the damage occurs to the long-lived stem cells. In this case, all subsequent generations of cells could be affected; fortunately, the stem cells appear to be relatively resistant to injury, although they can be affected by antimitotic agents. The more susceptible maturing cells are enclosed by a blood-testis barrier that blocks the passage of some agents from the general circulation; penetration appears to follow simple diffusion kinetics so that small, lipid-soluble molecules are most likely to gain entry.

A number of compounds, many of them pharmaceuticals, are known to affect spermatogenesis. Using sperm cells and seminal fluid obtained from the ejaculate, it is possible to examine several parameters of semen quality. As a result of computer-based automation, methods and definitions of the normal range have become reasonably well estab-

Table 26-1. Salient features of human reproduction

Male	Female
Continuous, cyclic generation of germ cells from puberty onward	Fixed store of germ cells, in meiosis at birth
Blood-testis barrier	Reproductive cycle with marked endocrinologic fluctuations
Germ cells accessible for study	Shorter, more circumscribed reproductive lifespan
	Potential for transplacental and transmammary influence on the offspring

lished for sperm concentration and motility. However, a standardized scoring method for sperm morphology is currently lacking. Newer assays requiring sperm DNA are under development, and they may ultimately provide a direct measure of genetic damage.

In females, gametogenesis has a different chronology from that in the male. Production of germ cells begins and ends prior to birth, at which point the entire supply of egg cells has already entered meiosis. The first meiotic division is then suspended and the maturation process only resumes years later when a particular oocyte is recruited for ovulation. The sparse evidence available on the integrity of human germ cells suggests that the rate of chromosome anomalies is far greater in oocytes than in sperm; on the other hand, oocytes appear to be less vulnerable to gene mutation than sperm cells (perhaps because sperm cells undergo many more divisions). In our species and others, there is a geometric decline in oocyte number with age, largely due to a process of atresia. Eventually, the ovarian stock of oocytes is sufficiently depleted to induce menopause. Like menarche and ovulation, onset of menopause can be affected by exposure to xenobiotics.

Once a couple conceives, it is the woman who provides the environment for implantation of the fertilized egg and subsequent embryonic development. It has been suggested that the pregnant state might alter maternal susceptibility to toxic exposures. For example, pregnancy-related increases in plasma lipids and adipose tissue may lead to an increased body burden of lipophilic compounds. In turn, toxins in the maternal milieu can impinge on the developing conceptus via the fetoplacental unit, and later, on the newborn through contaminated breast milk.

REPRODUCTIVE EFFECTS OF EXPOSURES TO WOMEN

Reproductive processes in women include (1) hormonal function (age at menarche and at menopause, regularity of menstrual cycle and of ovulation); (2) fecundability (capacity for fertilization and implantation, as well as ovulation); (3) fertility (capacity to conceive and to carry a viable offspring); (4) the delivery of normal progeny; and (5) lactation. Although several of these functions have been studied at least once in the workplace, the results in many cases remain uncertain. Recent technical advances promise more sophisticated approaches in the future. The following sections summarize what has been learned about the effects of exposures on hormonal function, fecundability and fertility, miscarriage, malformation, and prematurity and birth weight. (See also Chap. 31.)

Hormonal Function

The menstrual cycle, as a measure of reproductive capacity in females, has not been fully exploited in the way that semen analysis has been in males, but some human observations warn against complacency regarding exposure to women. For example, anovular cycles have been observed in women athletes and dancers [1] and in other women who engage in sustained and heavy exercise [2]. Although this degree of physical activity would be unusual in the workplace, the association should still be noted and may apply to working women in developing countries. In India, for example, women are often employed as stone breakers on the streets or in quarries, although we have no evidence on their reproductive function. In the United States, women miners who work at the rock face or women working as fire fighters might be observed for this association.

There are a few observations that directly relate workplace exposures to menstrual function. Studies to date have relied on reports of cycle characteristics, which are not a direct measure of ovarian function and will fail to detect anovulation or other such problems in the presence of regular menses. Despite such limitations, menstrual disorders have been observed in a cohort of women occupationally exposed to synthetic hormones [3]. In Eastern Europe, studies have associated solvent exposure with menstrual dysfunction, although a recent U.S. study of women working with styrene found no increase in reported menstrual disorders [4]. Cycle length has been examined in women exposed to inorganic mercury vapor, with some indication that higher levels of exposure increase the risk of oligomenorrhea [5]. It is not surprising to find that hormones or central nervous system toxins, such as metals, can disturb menstrual function, which depends on a timely sequence of events involving the brain, pituitary, and ovaries.

Women who smoke cigarettes experience menopause at a somewhat younger age than do nonsmokers [6]. This association may reflect oocyte killing by cigarette smoke constituents. However, it could also relate to hormonal effects on ovulation, as smoking is known to be antiestrogenic. Several studies have found that for couples planning a pregnancy, the interval between attempting and achieving a conception is longer on average for women who smoke than for those who do not [7]. This observation might relate to anovular cycles. It is possible that prolonged exposure to passive smoking in the workplace could act similarly, although surely the delay in conception would be less.

Fecundability and Fertility

Fecundability and fertility are measured by the success or failure of couples to reproduce, hence the term *couple infertility* [8]. A woman could have hormonal insufficiency so that ovulation does not occur, occurs infrequently, or occurs in some anomalous fashion; without ovulation, a woman is clearly not fecund. Experimental animals have been rendered anovular through in utero exposure to ionizing radiation, the presumed cause being destruction of oocytes, which undergo development very early in prenatal life. In humans, there may be another later period of female germ cell vulnerability prior to ovulation, when the oocyte resumes the meiotic division that has been suspended since birth. Although purely speculative, the suggestion of susceptibility in the preovulatory period is certainly reasonable.

Germ cell mutations could simulate infecundability by causing very early loss of the zygote. As with the loss of ova, germ cell mutations might arise from stimuli in the prenatal period, during embryonal development, or they could occur at later stages from exposures in the cycle immediately before the index conception. Effects might be from single or cumulative doses. If such mutations did indeed occur, there might be (1) no pregnancy at all (the egg failed to mature and burst through the follicle, or the extruded egg proved impermeable to the sperm), or (2) a pregnancy might occur but fail before, around, or immediately after implantation. We do know that the latter phenomena can be induced in the laboratory. Observations of pre- and postimplantation loss have been made on rats and mice following exposure of the female to, for example, cyclophosphamide and ionizing radiation. No human examples can be cited, but the means to identify early postimplantation loss using sensitive hormonal assays is now being field-tested [9]. A method based on subject reports of time-to-pregnancy (that is, the number of cycles required for a noncontracepting couple to conceive) has also been proposed as a way of monitoring fecundity [10]. As yet the method has not been applied to occupational exposures. It also cannot distinguish delayed conception from very early loss.

Relatively few human observations on *couple infertility* among workers have attempted to separate male from female causes. One common method of studying couple infertility is to note the number of offspring born to workers compared to an expected number based on some standard population; this approach is unlikely to be sensitive to less dramatic influences affecting women than, say, DBCP has proved to be among men (see box). Quite recently, couples seeking help at infertility clinics have served as "cases" in case-control studies to advance epidemiologic understanding of human infertility. Despite the obvious difficulties in generalizing from self-selected couples using infertility clinics to the population as a whole, some useful material is beginning to emerge, which

should in time help to focus study of hazards in the workplace. Many of the positive findings for couple infertility noted in the appendix to this chapter relate to female exposure (for example, noise, dyes, lead, mercury, and cadmium) and were identified through the case-control approach (see reference 8 for a review).

Pregnancy Outcome

The next sections deal with effects of exposures around the time of conception and after to pregnant workers and women contemplating pregnancy, or at least "at risk" (that is, sexually active and not using contraception).

Regarding *miscarriage*, there have been conflicting findings about risks to pregnant laboratory workers in different industrial settings, and currently, anecdotal reports about increased risk among video display terminal operators are being pursued in systematic studies. Apart from this, women working in hospitals and health care facilities have furnished most of the available information. In spite of several large studies of exposure to anesthetic gases [12], the evidence for an association with miscarriage is unsubstantiated at present. There are, however, two work exposures to women (also to hospital workers) that are tentatively accepted as valid: (1) ethylene oxide, used as a sterilant, and (2) antineoplastic agents, medications dispensed to cancer patients. These associations were identified in separate investigations in Finland: the first, a retrospective cohort study of hospital sterilizing staff [13] and the second, a case-control study of fetal loss among nurses preparing drug doses at major cancer chemotherapy centers [14]. Both studies used existing national registries of health care personnel and obstetric events. In the study of the sterilizing staff, the risk of miscarriage was increased 60 percent or more among nurses exposed during pregnancy to ethylene oxide (and perhaps also glutaraldehyde). The case-control study reported a risk ratio of 2.3 for exposure to antineoplastic agents but was not able to separate the effects of particular drugs. Anti-

---

DBCP: A POTENT
REPRODUCTIVE TOXIN

In 1977, a small group of men in a northern California chemical plant noticed that few of them had recently fathered children. Investigation of the full cohort of production workers subsequently found a strong association between decreased sperm count and exposure to DBCP, a brominated organochlorine used as a nematocide since the mid-1950s. The spermatotoxic effects in some of the exposed men were sufficient to render them sterile. Testicular biopsies showed the seminiferous tubules to be the site of action and spermatogonia to be the target cell. The relationship between reduced sperm count and exposure to DBCP, both in its manufacture and use, has been confirmed in studies of other plants in the United States and abroad. Follow-up of workers after cessation of exposure shows that spermatogenic function is eventually recovered in those less severely affected. However, many of the azoospermic men have remained azoospermic [11].

cancer drugs commonly used include alkylating agents, antimitotics, antimetabolites, and antibiotics.

A distinction should be made between (1) germ cell toxins, which affect the egg or its contents, and (2) teratogens or abortifacients, which affect the developing embryo or fetus. Given their toxicologic properties, ethylene oxide and the various antineoplastic agents have the potential to act in either way. For the antineoplastic agents, the fact that fetal loss was linked to first trimester exposure, and *not* to exposure accumulated prior to conception, in this case, suggests that the exposure was not operating as a germ cell toxin. From the perspective of the woman worker, the distinction is very important because if an exposure is an abortifacient or a teratogen, then work before conception would not be harmful and there would be no rationale for limiting exposure in this period. Preventive strategies could be focused on the time when a pregnancy is being planned or has already begun.

Unfortunately, recognized miscarriage, a relatively common outcome, is, like death, an event that may follow different types of disorders, some of which originate before conception and some after. Direct cytogenetic examination of the fresh abortus specimen may reveal whether the zygote was chromosomally abnormal. In this case, if a maternal occupational exposure was responsible, it would almost certainly have been preconceptional. If the zygote were chromosomally normal, a postconceptional exposure remains a possibility. No occupational exposures to women have yet been characterized in such specific terms. However, since both maternal fever and cigarette smoking have been associated with chromosomally normal miscarriage, a model exists for adverse postconceptional influences on pregnancy that can lead to miscarriage. These adverse influences may also include other exposures: There is one report of increased fetal loss in relation to heavy lifting [15], and the effect of shift work is now a topic of study.

Malformations

Malformations, either at miscarriage or at birth, have not been convincingly shown to be related to occupational exposures in women. The observation of affected offspring among nurses exposed to cytostatic drugs [16] is worth noting, given the strength of the observed association and the mechanism of action of the agent. There are also conflicting reports for laboratory workers exposed to solvents. Alcohol, polychlorinated biphenyls (PCBs), organic mercury, and ionizing radiation are proven human teratogens, but none have actually been studied for women in the workplace. A type of cerebral palsy, first recognized in Minamata Bay, Japan, has resulted from contamination of the pregnant woman's diet with methyl mercury [17]. In the Minamata Bay episode, the pollution was a byproduct of industry, and similar episodes have occurred in other places. Lead, certainly hazardous to the infant and child, may also be hazardous to the embryo and fetus, but more evidence is needed on possible teratogenic levels.

It would not be entirely surprising if *prematurity* (delivery before 36 weeks) and *low birth weight* (< 2,500 gm) were related to particular occupational exposures, because both have been associated with maternal smoking. In fact, maternal exposure to PCBs, both occupationally at a capacitor-manufacturing facility [18] and environmentally through consumption of contaminated fish [19], has been associated with reduced birth weight and earlier delivery of offspring. Suspicion has fallen on hard exercise [20] in relation to prematurity and on prolonged standing in relation to low birth weight, but the evidence for both these possible associations is insufficient. One study examined the type of work done by women during pregnancy and inferred that stressful occupations, shift work, and a high level of fatigue were associated with prematurity [21]. Much research is now being focused on the role of psychosocial strain in prematurity and such factors as enforced time keeping, scarcity of breaks, and very long hours or shifts. There is also interest in whether pregnancy is affected by long periods of standing and by working into the third trimester.

Is it in the interests of a woman as well as of her offspring if she continues to work outside the home during pregnancy? A definitive answer to this question is not possible now, largely because the working woman, as the working man, is by definition a relatively healthy person when compared to the nonworker. Not surprisingly, no studies have shown the nonworking woman to be at any advantage in terms of pregnancy or childbirth. For the pregnant woman, "working" might be considered both for the type of work and for the stage of gestation. Thus, some believe that in France, because benefits are given to those who stop work in the third trimester, there is a reduction in prematurity and improved survival of infants at birth. In the United States, there is some evidence suggesting that among women living in poverty and poor psychosocial circumstances, those who work until term have more adverse experiences in childbearing than do those who give up work sooner; however, these experiences need not be attributable to the nature and duration of the work as much as to the social circumstances of women workers.

REPRODUCTIVE DISORDERS AMONG MALE WORKERS

Reproductive system disorders in men can be considered in terms of fecundity (sexuality and semen quality), fertility, and effects on progeny, including childhood cancers.

Fecundity

Normal sexual function is a prerequisite for fertility and is most likely to be affected by agents that interfere with hormonal balance or that act directly on the nervous system. Thus, while parameters of sexual behavior (libido and potency) are obviously difficult to measure, the effects on sexuality reported among workers exposed to estrogens and to heavy metals, such as lead and manganese, are at least plausible. Decreased libido and

impotence have also been observed among workers exposed to phenoxy herbicides [22], which appear to alter hormone metabolism.

The finding in 1977 that the nematocide dibromochloropropane (DBCP) affects spermatogenesis [23] stimulated a decade of research on potential alterations in semen quality from various workplace agents. Early on, interpretation of study findings was made difficult by methodologic problems in recruiting sufficient study subjects (particularly unexposed controls) and in standardizing procedures for collecting and analyzing seminal fluid. However, with time and field experience, protocols have improved substantially and appear to have gained acceptance among worker populations (excepting certain religious and cultural groups). Many of the more recent studies of semen quality also include some measure of gonadotropic hormones, although these appear to be less sensitive indices of testicular toxicity than semen parameters.

Besides DBCP and ionizing radiation, which has long been recognized as a spermatotoxic factor, only lead, chlordecone (Kepone), and carbon disulfide (at high doses) have shown adverse effects on spermatogenesis among exposed workers [24]; microwave exposure has also been implicated. Several other associations have been examined but with less clear-cut results because of shortcomings in the research design and analysis. Experience suggests that the conventional approach of collecting a single sample from exposed and unexposed workers and then comparing the mean values in the two groups is unlikely to yield a significant finding unless a large proportion of men at risk are quite seriously affected (for example, azoospermic).

Fertility

Thus far, two methods have been used to examine fertility in couples where the male partner is exposed to a suspected reproductive toxin. The first is based on comparing the live birth rate in the exposed cohort with that in a "standard" population. This approach (which assumes that contraceptive use is independent of work exposure) has suggested that manganese [25] and perhaps ethylene dibromide (EDB) [26], contribute to male infertility. The second method, involving case-control studies of infertile couples, implicates exposure to excessive heat [27] as a male factor. (Hyperthermia has long been thought to be spermatotoxic.)

Effects on Progeny

Increases in fetal loss have been observed among couples where the male partner was exposed (and the woman presumably unexposed). Such associations have been reported for several agents (vinyl chloride and its structural analog chloroprene, DBCP, anesthetic gases—especially those used in dental anesthesia), and some work settings (a waste water treatment plant and a smelter) [24]. However, most of these associations derive from a single study and require replication before being accepted. Moreover, in most of these investigations, the obstetric history was obtained from the male worker rather than his wife and therefore may be inaccurate, particularly with regard to the number of miscarriages.

Childhood cancer is another reproductive outcome that has been linked to paternal occupation. A careful review of this literature [28] concludes that no large general effect is present. For the moment, greatest credence is given to the association between childhood brain cancer and paternal work exposure to paints and solvents; in this case, sizable risks (twofold or more) have been found in studies with reasonable exposure data and adjustment for potentially confounding variables.

The possible mechanisms for male-mediated effects on pregnancy outcome are genetic (fertilization by a mutant sperm) or epigenetic (transport of toxin into the home environment, or transport of toxin into the female genital tract via sperm or seminal fluid). Concerning a genetic mechanism, several agents implicated in male-mediated effects, such as vinyl chloride, DBCP, and nitrous oxide, are mutagenic in in vitro tests. In the future, it will be possible to look directly for associations between exposure and human sperm chromosome lesions using the hamster egg system (human sperm are placed in contact with hamster ova from which the species-specific outer membrane has been removed; the sperm enter the ova and begin to divide, at which time the chromosomes may be visualized); with this approach, a dose-response relation has recently been reported for ionizing radiation [29]. Concerning an epigenetic mechanism, one can imagine a male worker carrying some toxins home on his clothes or person, but it is difficult to see how there could be transmission of volatile substances such as anesthetic gases. In theory, semen and sperm are routes of exposure and, in fact, several toxins, including PCBs and lead, have been identified in seminal fluid. There are even documented instances of vaginal absorption of substances in semen. What seems more speculative is that uterine concentrations would be sufficient to affect the developing organism. Thus, a genetic mechanism appears to be more likely than an epigenetic one for male-mediated effects on offspring.

PREVENTION AND CONTROL

Although specific instances of work-related exposures affecting reproduction have been rare, each positive report has had grave repercussions. There is wide agreement that workers should be protected from potential hazards to the reproductive process. This protection should ensure that the fertility of both men and women remains unaffected by the demands of their jobs and that no harm is done to the growing embryo or fetus. The best safeguard is vigilance, and the surveillance of workers is strongly advocated.

In the Workplace

Either employers or unions, or both, may institute programs of reproductive health surveillance. Such programs, which track reproductive function in a cohort of workers, can be based on histories, physician examinations, or analyses of biologic samples. The components of the program and the end-

Fig. 26-1. Sample annual questionnaire for workplace reproductive surveillance. (From M Hatch, V Scott, Z Stein. Surveillance of reproductive health in the U.S. A survey of activity within and outside industry. Washington, DC: American Petroleum Institute, 1983.)

Please do not write your name on the form, because the system must be kept anonymous. Instead, think up your own five-letter code, using letters or numbers or both, and write your code in the five boxes provided. Choose something that you will be able to remember next year, when we ask you to fill out another form like this.

Employee Code ☐☐☐☐☐   **Year of Birth: 19** ☐☐   **Sex** ___ F   ___ M

Please answer the following questions by filling in the square next to the appropriate answer. After completing the form, drop it into the ballot box provided. Thank you for your cooperation.

A. If you are single or have taken no steps toward adding to your family this past year, mark this box ☐. Go no further and drop the form into the ballot box. Otherwise continue.

B. In the past year, have you and your spouse had:

	Yes	No
1. Any problems with fertility or with becoming pregnant (trying for at least one year)?	☐	☐
2. Any miscarriages?	☐	☐
3. A premature baby (born weighing less than 5 lbs. or before the eighth month)?	☐	☐
4. A live birth?	☐	☐
5. A loss of an infant around the time of birth (stillbirth or death up to one month of age)?	☐	☐
6. Any problems with a child (birth defect, serious illness, loss)? If yes, please explain here:	☐	☐

points to be monitored will be influenced by (1) the nature of the exposures, (2) the size and sex distribution of the workforce, and (3) institutional resources and constraints. In a review of reproductive surveillance activities in industry [30], existing programs tended to incorporate this information into the employee health system by adding a lengthy reproductive questionnaire to the medical history. As an alternative, we have proposed that a brief annual questionnaire, independent of the periodic health examination may be a more effective vehicle for workplace monitoring (Fig. 26-1). Vital records are another potential data source on reproductive outcomes and might be used to supplement subject reports. In some states, however, difficulties or delays in gaining access to such records have been experienced by researchers.

In addition to reproductive health surveillance, employers obviously should be concerned with exposure surveillance. Environmental and biologic monitoring can be used as means to ensure that exposure of workers to known or suspected reproductive toxins is kept to acceptable levels.

In the Clinical Setting

When evaluating a reproductive disorder or enrolling an obstetric patient, clinicians should routinely obtain occupational histories from both parents. Patients may ask their health care providers' advice about exposures that they or their partners have sustained and whether work during pregnancy should continue. (Various services exist to help in responding to such inquiries; some of these are listed in Table 26-2.) The degree of risk associated with the job and the need to continue working both have to be taken into consideration. Usually, information is limited on the potential hazard to reproductive health of a workplace exposure. In the end, judgments need to be made by the woman, her partner, and the clinician together. The American College of Obstetricians and Gynecologists has developed a set of guidelines for

Table 26-2. Selected listing of teratogen information services

UNITED STATES

Connecticut* (serves only Connecticut)	Connecticut Pregnancy Exposure Information Service University of Connecticut Health Sciences Center Farmington, CT (800) 325-5391 (in CT only) or (203) 679-2676
Massachusetts	Teratogen Information Service National Birth Defects Center, Kennedy Memorial Hospital Brighton, MA (800) 322-5014 (in MA only) or (617) 787-4957
Utah* (serves only Utah and Montana)	Pregnancy Riskline University of Utah Medical Center Salt Lake City, UT (800) 822-BABY (in UT only) or (801) 583-2229
Washington	Washington State Poison Control Network University of Washington Seattle, WA (800) 732-6985 (in WA only), or (206) 526-2121 or (206) 543-3373

CANADA

Ontario	Motherisk Program Division of Pharmacology, Hospital for Sick Children Toronto, Ontario (416) 598-5781

*Will refer callers from other states to teratogen information services in their areas.

judging individual cases on the basis of information concerning the duties and exposures associated with a particular job [31]; the assumption is that a normal pregnancy is not, in itself, a contraindication to work (see Chap. 31).

By any standard, reproductive dysfunction is a significant health problem. Regardless of how large or how small the contribution of workplace exposures ultimately proves to be, they represent a potentially preventable portion. Precisely because such exposures are preventable, detection and control of reproductive hazards at work must be a priority.

REFERENCES

1. Feicht CB, Johnson TS, Martin BJ, et al. Secondary amenorrhea in athletics. Lancet 1987; 2:1145–6.
2. Green BB, Daling JR, Weiss NS, et al. Exercise as a risk factor for infertility with ovulatory dysfunction. Am J Public Health 1986; 76:1432–6.
3. Harrington JM, Stein GF, Rivera RO, et al. The occupational hazards of formulating oral contraceptives—a survey of plant employees. Arch Environ Health 1987; 33:12–5.
4. Lemasters GK, Hagen A, Samuels SJ. Reproductive outcomes in women exposed to solvents in 36 reinforced plastics companies. J Occup Med 1985; 27:490–4.
5. De Rosis F, Anastasio SP, Selvaggi L, et al. Female reproductive health in two lamp factories: effects of exposure to inorganic mercury vapour and stress factors. Br J Ind Med 1985; 42:488–94.
6. McKinlay SM, Bifano NL, McKinlay JB. Smoking and age at menopause in women. Ann Intern Med 1985; 103:350–6.
7. Baird DD, Wilcox AJ. Cigarette smoking associated with delayed conception. JAMA 1985; 253:2979–83.
8. Baird DD, Wilcox AJ. Effects of occupational exposures on the fertility of couples. Occup Med: State of the Art Reviews 1986; 1:361–74.
9. Wilcox AJ, Weinberg CR, Wehmann RE, et al. Measuring early pregnancy loss: laboratory and field methods. Fertil Steril 1985; 44:366–73.
10. Baird DD, Wilcox AJ, Weinberg CR. Use of time to pregnancy to study environmental exposures. Am J Epidemiol 1986; 124:470–80.
11. Whorton MD, Foliart DE. Mutagenicity, carcinogenicity and reproductive effects of dibromochloropropane (DBCP). Mutat Res 1983; 123:13–30.
12. Kline JK. Maternal occupation: Effects on spontaneous abortions and malformations. Occup Med: State of the Art Reviews 1986; 1:381–403.
13. Hemminki K, Mutanen P, Saloniemi I, et al. Spontaneous abortions in hospital staff engaged in sterilizing instruments with chemical agents. Br Med J 1982; 285:1461–3.
14. Selevan SG, Lindbohm M-L, Hornung RW, et al. A study of occupational exposure to antineoplastic drugs and fetal loss in nurses. N Engl J Med 1985; 313:1174–221.
15. Taskinen H, Lindbohm M-L, Hemminki K. Spontaneous abortions among women working in the pharmaceutical industry. Br J Ind Med 1986; 43:199–205.
16. Hemminki K, Kyyronen P, Lindbohm M-L. Spontaneous abortions and malformations in the offspring of nurses exposed to anaesthetic gases, cytostatic drugs, and other potential hazards in hospitals, based on registered information of outcome. J Epidemiol Community Health 1985; 39:141–7.
17. Koos, BJ, Longo LD. Mercury toxicity in the pregnant woman, fetus, and newborn infant. Am J Obstet Gynecol 1976; 126:390–409.
18. Taylor, PR, Lawrence CE, Hwang H-L, et al. Polychlorinated biphenyls: influence on birthweight and gestation. Am J Public Health 1984; 74:1153–4.
19. Fein GG, Jacobson JL, Jacobson SW, et al. Prenatal exposure to polychlorinated biphenyls: effects on birth size and gestational age. J Pediatr 1984; 105:315–20.
20. Stein ZA, Susser MW, Hatch MC. Working during pregnancy: physical and psychosocial strain. Occup Med: State of the Art Reviews 1986; 1:405–9.
21. Mamelle N, Laumon B, Lazar P. Prematurity and occupational activity during pregnancy. Am J Epidemiol 1984; 119:309–22.
22. Suskind RR, Hertzberg VS. Human health effects of 2,3,4-T and its toxic contaminants. JAMA 1984; 251:2372–80.
23. Whorton MD, Krauss RM, Marshall S, et al. Infertility in male pesticide workers. Lancet 1977; 7:1259–61.
24. Whorton MD. Male reproductive hazards. Occup Med: State of the Art Reviews 1986; 1:375–9.
25. Lauwerys R, Roels H, Genet P, et al. Fertility of male workers exposed to mercury vapor or to manganese dust: a questionnaire study. Am J Ind Med 1985; 7:171–6.

26. Wong O, Utidjian HM, Karten VS. Retrospective evaluation of reproductive performance of workers exposed to ethylene dibromide (EDB). J Occup Med 1979; 21:98–102.
27. Rachootin P, Olsen J. The risk of infertility and delayed conception associated with exposures in the Danish workplace. J Occup Med 1983; 25:394–402.
28. Savitz DA. Childhood cancer. Occup Med: State of the Art Reviews 1986; 1:415–29.
29. Martin RH, Hildebrand K, Yamamoto J, et al. An increased frequency of human sperm chromosomal abnormalities after radiotherapy. Mutat Res 1986; 174:219–25.
30. Hatch M, Scott V, Stein Z. Surveillance of reproductive health in the U.S.: a survey of activity within and outside industry. Washington, DC.: American Petroleum Institute, 1983.
31. American College of Obstetrics and Gynecologists. Guidelines on pregnancy and work. Rockville, Md.: NIOSH, 1977.

BIBLIOGRAPHY

American College of Obstetricians and Gynecologists. Guidelines on pregnancy and work. Rockville, Md.: NIOSH, 1977.
A guide for clinicians in counseling pregnant workers, including assessment of work tasks and exposures, and recommendations regarding modification or termination of work during pregnancy.
Barlow SM, Sullivan FM. Reproductive hazards of industrial chemicals: an evaluation of animal and human data. New York: Academic, 1982.
A useful synthesis of toxicologic and human data on environmental and occupational exposures. Extensive bibliography.
Bloom AD, ed. Guidelines for studies of human populations exposed to mutagenic and reproductive hazards. White Plains, NY: March of Dimes Birth Defects Foundation, 1982.
State-of-the-art research protocols for evaluating environmental hazards to reproduction. Contains useful background on the epidemiology of various reproductive disorders.
Hatch M, Scott V, Stein Z. Surveillance of reproductive health in the U.S.: a survey of activity within and outside industry. Washington, DC.: American Petroleum Institute, 1983.
A description of reproductive surveillance systems, existing and proposed, and of various national and local data sources on reproductive parameters. Includes recommendations regarding approaches to workplace surveillance.
Hunt VR. Work and the health of women. Boca Raton, Fl.: CRC, 1979.
A useful reference volume on the health effects of work.
Lockey JE, Lemasters GK, Keye WR, eds. Reproduction: the new frontier in occupational and environmental health research. New York: Liss, 1984.
The proceedings of a recent conference on occupation and reproduction. Useful papers on methodologic as well as substantive topics.
Office of Technology Assessment. Reproductive hazards in the workplace. Washington, DC.: U.S. Government Printing Office, 1985 (OTA-BA-266).
A comprehensive review of reproductive biology, reproductive hazards, and methods for assessing reproductive function.
Stein ZA, Hatch MC, eds. Reproductive problems in the workplace. Occup Med: state of the art reviews. Vol. 1, no. 2. Philadelphia: Hanley & Belfus, 1986.
A compilation of first-rate papers by experts in reproductive research. Includes chapters on the ethical, social, and legal aspects of work and reproduction.

APPENDIX

Review of Available Evidence on the Role of Workplace Agents in Reproductive Disorders

The workplace agents judged to be associated with reproductive disorders on the basis of available evidence are shown here.

If one compares results among columns, with each column representing a different end point, it becomes apparent that most of the findings relate to fecundity and fertility, which raises the possibility that these are susceptible processes that can usefully serve as focal end-points for monitoring reproductive toxicity in humans. It is difficult to know what inference to draw from the paucity of findings with respect to pregnancy outcome, but it certainly seems premature to conclude that these outcomes are refractory to exposure. Note that lactation represents a route of exposure for nursing offspring of women workers.

The rows list suspected reproductive toxins. Many of those cited, including solvents and metals such as lead and mercury, have not been comprehensively evaluated for effects of workplace exposure. As part of a preventive strategy, NIOSH has proposed that substances be ranked according to the "degree of evidence" that exists with regard to reproductive toxicity. This ranking should then be used to set priorities for further human or laboratory studies of those agents for which information is limited or inadequate. This follows the model developed by the International Agency for Research on Cancer, which has used the approach effectively to guide research and regulation in the cancer field.

Suspected reproductive effects

Agents	Couple fertility	Effects on male or female fecundity	Spontaneous abortion	Prematurity	Birth defects	Contaminated breast milk	Childhood cancer
HEAVY METALS							
Lead	M	M	?			x	
Mercury		?F			(methyl) x	x	
Cadmium	M					x	
Manganese	M	M					?
HALOGENATED HYDROCARBONS							?
Dibromochloro-propane (DBCP)	M	M					
Ethylene dibromide (EDB)	?M						
Chlordecone		M					
Polychlorinated biphenyls (PCBs)				x	x	x	
Paints							(brain) ?

Suspected reproductive effects (continued)

Agents	Couple fertility	Effects on male or female fecundity	Spontaneous abortion	Prematurity	Birth defects	Contaminated breast milk	Childhood cancer
SOLVENTS							
Carbon disulfide		M					
Organic solvents (for example, benzene)		?F			?	x	?
ESTROGENIC COMPOUNDS							
Oral contraceptives		M,F				x	
ANESTHETIC GASES							
Halogenated gases	?F						
Nitrous oxide			?				
PESTICIDES							
Organophosphates						x	
Organochlorine compounds (for example, 2,4,5-T)						x	

Suspected reproductive effects (continued)

Agents	Couple fertility	Effects on male or female fecundity	Spontaneous abortion	Prematurity	Birth defects	Contaminated breast milk	Childhood cancer
MISCELLANEOUS							
Heat	M	M					
Noise	M,F						
Textile dyes	F						
WORK ENVIRONMENT							
Stress				?			
Passive smoking				x			
STERILIZING AGENTS							
Ethylene oxide			x				

Suspected reproductive effects (continued)

Agents	Couple fertility	Effects on male or female fecundity	Spontaneous abortion	Prematurity	Birth defects	Contaminated breast milk	Childhood cancer
CYTOSTATIC AGENTS			x		x		
Alkylating agents			M				
Folate antagonists					x		
IONIZING RADIATION							
X-rays and gamma rays	M,F	M		x*	x*		x*

Key: x = positive findings; ? = contradictory findings; M = male; F = female.
*These effects of irradiation have not been explored in occupational settings but have been reported in connection with in utero exposures from medical x-rays or exposure to the atomic bomb. The pertinent literature is reviewed in Committee on the Biological Effects of Ionizing Radiation. The effects on populations of exposure to low levels of ionizing radiation, Washington, DC: National Academy of Sciences, 1980.
Source: Adapted from M Hatch and Z Stein. Agents in the workplace and effects on reproduction. Occup Med: State of the Art Reviews 1986; 1:531–534.

27
Cardiovascular Disorders

Gilles P. Thériault

A 37-year-old man, whose work consists of moving carts containing 180-kg rolls of wire from one side of a plant to the other, developed an acute myocardial infarction. One morning, at the end of his night shift, while trying to free his loaded cart that had become stuck in a hole in the floor, he felt an acute pain in his chest. On arrival at the hospital, an extensive myocardial infarction was diagnosed. Even though this man smoked a pack of cigarettes daily and had a father who had died from heart disease, the workers' compensation board awarded him a settlement for "an injury resulting from an accident at work."

A 55-year-old man with a past history of mild angina pectoris had been hired as a parking attendant in an underground parking garage. On a particularly cold winter day, when business had been heavier than usual, he developed severe chest pain and shortness of breath. When he arrived at the hospital, his carboxyhemoglobin (COHb) level was found to be 10 percent. He died during the night of myocardial infarction. Measurements of the garage air taken the following day showed levels of carbon monoxide (CO) of up to 100 ppm.

A 42-year-old lumberjack consulted his family doctor for severe loss of strength in both hands, so severe that he was unable to hold his chain saw. He reported a long history of episodic whitening of his fingers on exposure to vibration and damp weather. This phenomenon had started 3 years after he began work in forestry and had increased regularly in frequency and duration over time. He was a nonsmoker. Several fellow workers complained of similar problems.

Cardiovascular diseases, including hypertensive disease, ischemic heart disease (also designated as coronary heart disease [CHD]), other forms of heart disease, and cerebrovascular disease are re-

sponsible for more deaths in the United States each year than any other category of disease, even though the death rate from ischemic heart disease has declined markedly over the last 2 decades [1]. Because cardiovascular diseases cause so much mortality, preventing even a small increase in risk due to occupational exposures can involve large numbers of people and represent an important public health measure.

Personal risk factors that contribute to the development of CHD have been well studied, but the contribution of working conditions to this disease has been explored very little. In 1981, the American Heart Association recognized this gap in knowledge and recommended that occupational epidemiologic studies be performed [2].

RISK FACTORS FOR CORONARY HEART DISEASE

Risk factors associated with CHD can be divided into three categories: personal, hereditary, and environmental. As shown in Table 27-1, personal risk factors include sex, age, race, high serum cholesterol (most specifically low-density lipoprotein (LDL)/cholesterol ratio), high blood pressure, and cigarette smoking. The interaction between these factors is strong enough that a smoker with both high blood pressure and hypercholesterolemia is 8 times more at risk of developing CHD than a nonsmoker who has normal blood cholesterol and normal blood pressure [3].

Other personal risk factors, such as obesity, di-

Table 27-1. Personal risk factors associated with CHD

Risk factor	Feature
Sex	Mortality rates for women lag behind those of men by about 10 years
Age	Risk increases with age
Race	Prior to age 60, white males have lower death rates than non-white males; the inverse is true after 60
High serum cholesterol	Risk estimated at 1.7–3.5
High blood pressure	Risk estimated at 1.5–2.1
Cigarette smoking	Risk estimated at 1.5–2.9

abetes, and lack of physical exercise, have been associated with CHD, but their roles are considered minor compared with those cited above. In certain families, the risk of CHD is high and is correlated with the number of blood relatives who have developed the disease and the early age at which they developed it [4].

OCCUPATION AS A RISK FACTOR FOR CORONARY HEART DISEASE
While the association between personal risk factors and CHD is well documented, our knowledge of the role of occupational and environmental risk factors is still limited. Several chemical and physical agents have been suspected of causing CHD in workers chronically exposed to them. However, scientific evidence indicates a direct causal relationship for very few of them. For most of these agents, the evidence is based on isolated case reports or on a few unconfirmed studies. Table 27-2 lists some occupational hazards associated with cardiovascular disorders.

Carbon Monoxide
The potential for exposure to carbon monoxide (CO) in industry is high. This odorless and colorless gas is produced in most processes where there is fire, combustion, or oxidation. High exposures may occur in many workplaces, such as steel and iron foundries, petroleum refineries, pulp and paper mills, and plants where formaldehyde and coke are produced. One of the most common and insidious sources is the internal combustion engine; workers in garages and enclosed parking spaces may be chronically exposed to fairly high levels of CO. Fire fighters, apart from the usual hazards of their work, may be exposed to excessively high levels of CO in smoke.

Carbon monoxide causes a variety of signs and symptoms, dependent on concentration of expo-

Table 27-2. Some occupational hazards associated with cardiovascular disorders

Hazard	Effect	Strength of evidence
Carbon monoxide	Atherosclerosis	Weak
Carbon disulfide	Atherosclerosis	Satisfactory
Certain aliphatic nitrates	Coronary spasm	Strong
	Atherosclerosis	Weak
Arsenic	Coronary heart disease	Satisfactory
Lead, cadmium	Coronary heart disease secondary to nephrotoxicity	Satisfactory
Noise	Transient high blood pressure	Strong
	Long-term high blood pressure	Absent
Shift work	Coronary heart disease	Weak
Halogenated solvents	Arrhythmia	Satisfactory
Chronic hand-arm vibration	Vibration white finger	Strong

Table 27-3. Progressive effects of exposure to carbon monoxide[a]

8-hour average concentration (ppm)	Carboxyhemoglobin[b] concentration (%) after equilibrium	Main signs and symptoms
0	0.1–1.0	No signs or symptoms. Normal endogenous level.
25–50	2.5–5	No symptoms. Compensatory increase in blood flow to certain vital organs. Patients with severe cardiovascular disease may lack compensatory reserve.
50–100	5–10	Visual light threshold slightly increased.
100–250	10–20	Tightness across the forehead. Slight headache. Visual evoked response abnormal. Possibly slight breathlessness on exertion. May be lethal to fetus. May be lethal for patients with severe heart disease.
250–450	20–30	Slight or moderate headache and throbbing in the temples. Flushing. Nausea. Fine manual dexterity abnormal.
450–650	30–40	Severe headache, vertigo, nausea and vomiting. Weakness. Irritability and impaired judgment. Syncope on exertion.
650–1000	40–50	Same as above, but more severe with greater possibility of collapse and syncope.
1000–1500	50–60	Possibly coma with intermittent convulsions and Cheyne-Stokes respiration.
1500–2500	60–70	Coma with intermittent convulsions. Depressed respiration and heart action. Possibly death.
2500–4000	70–80	Weak pulse and slow respiration. Depression of respiratory center leading to death.

[a]Carboxyhemoglobin and carbon monoxide equivalents obtained from the formula developed by Gobbato and Mangiavacchi [5]. Main signs and symptoms extracted from Kurppa and Rantanen [6].
[b]Varies with pulmonary ventilation rate, endogenous carboxyhemoglobin production, blood volume, barometric pressure, and relative diffusion capability of the lungs.

sure (Table 27-3 and see case history in Chap. 14). Exposure to high concentrations of CO (> 1,500 ppm) can cause sudden death by anoxia. Exposure to low concentrations decreases myocardial oxygen consumption, concomitantly increases coronary flow and heart rate and lowers exercise tolerance of healthy persons. When a person already suffers from a certain degree of coronary insufficiency, such consequences may manifest by an increase of the S-T segment depression on electrocardiogram (ECG), the onset of angina pectoris [7], and occasionally by acute myocardial infarction.

However, the association between chronic exposure to low levels of CO and the development of coronary atherosclerosis leading to CHD has yet to be shown. Recent literature indicates that low exposure to CO accelerates the development of atherosclerosis in laboratory animals when combined with a diet rich in saturated fats, especially when exposure consists of intermittent peaks [8]. The few studies conducted so far among working groups have been unable to show a distinct relationship between chronic exposure to CO and the development of CHD. The known association of CHD with cigarette smoking, combined with recent observations that workers intermittently exposed to peaks of CO have higher risk of heart disease, keeps this question open to further research.

Carbon Disulfide

Of all the chemicals for which an association with heart disease has been studied, carbon disulfide (CS_2) shows the most convincing evidence. Although this chemical is used mostly as a solvent and in the production of organic chemicals, paints, fuels, and explosives, its use in the viscose rayon-producing industry revealed this association (Fig. 27-1). Mortality studies of viscose-rayon workers who were exposed to CS_2 have shown that they are at 2 to 5 times greater risk of dying from heart disease than unexposed workers. Reduction of exposures reduces the risk to workers [9]. In one study, the excess mortality declined from a relative risk of 4.7 to 1.0 over a 15-year period after implementation of exposure reduction measures [10].

The mechanism by which CS_2 causes heart dis-ease is not known, although it is hypothesized that it may be through changes in cholesterol metabolism with promotion of atherosclerosis of the coronary arteries.

Nitroglycerin and Other Aliphatic Nitrates

Some aliphatic nitrates are potent vasodilators of coronary vessels; this property has long been used for the treatment of angina pectoris. However, it has been reported that some workers exposed continually to nitroglycerin, and in particular to nitroglycol, during the manufacturing of explosives have suffered from angina pectoris on withdrawal from exposure (Fig. 27-2). This phenomenon, which occurs on weekends or on vacations, disappears on return to work. The mechanism involved is thought to be a coronary spasm. The reversal of this spasm by the administration of

Fig. 27-1. Worker tending machines that spool rayon thread from carbon disulfide. Worker exposure to carbon disulfide was high until this process was enclosed, which reduced worker exposure and, by recycling the carbon disulfide, saved the company a substantial amount of money [9]. (Photograph by Barry Levy.)

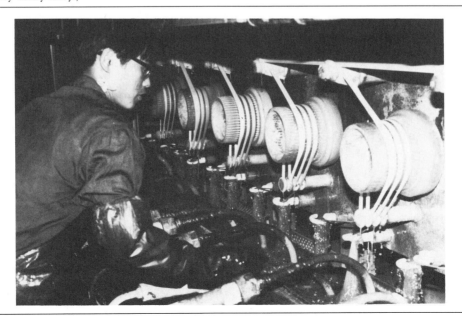

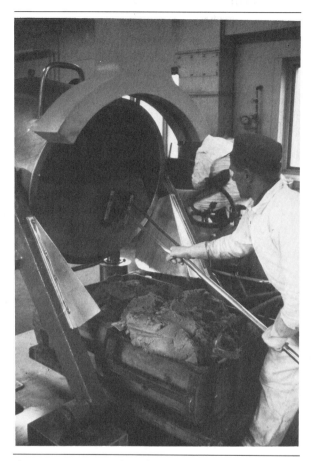

Fig. 27-2. Dynamite kneeding involves exposure to nitrates which, on days off, can result in rebound vasospasm of coronary arteries. Note local exhaust and protective clothing.
(Photograph courtesy of C. Högstedt.)

nitroglycerin has actually been observed with angiography during the withdrawal period.

Studies have reported elevated risk for CHD after some 20 years of exposure, which seems to indicate that nitro compounds are not only responsible for acute vasospastic reactions but may also increase the risk of CHD after long exposure by an increase in high blood pressure and atherosclerosis.

Metals

Poisoning by metals, such as lead, cadmium, and arsenic, is recognized as capable of causing CHD after long exposure to high levels. For lead and cadmium, this effect is a consequence of the renal damage caused by these metals. This effect is so remote from their actual toxicity that mention of it should be reserved for the description of their renal effects (see Chap. 30).

There are studies in the literature that seem to indicate that exposure to arsenic released during the smelting of copper may increase the rates of CHD, but this hypothesis remains unproven.

Noise

High levels of noise, exceeding 85 dBA, are common in the workplace. There are few factories, smelters, or mines where hazardous noise is never a problem. The association between chronic exposure to high noise levels and hearing loss is well documented (see Chap. 17).

Some researchers have proposed that noise can also damage the cardiovascular system indirectly by causing high blood pressure and, over a long period, may lead to atherosclerosis of the heart and blood vessels. Intermittent and impact noise would seem to be more harmful than continual noise in this respect. However, reports have been rather inconsistent on this issue and observations are frequently confounded by methodologic inadequacies.

Acute exposure to high levels of noise initiates cardiovascular responses that mimic the effects of acute stress: these include increases of blood pressure and heart rate; blood levels of catecholamines and lipids, such as low-density lipoproteins and fatty acids; and vascular tone of peripheral vessels. These changes are transitory, however, and disappear a short time after exposure ends [11]. Long-term effects of exposure to noise, such as chronic high blood pressure, coronary atherosclerosis, or ischemic heart problems, have yet to be demonstrated, if indeed they do exist.

Psychological Stress

Among other less well defined risks of CHD in the work environment is a wide array of psychologic stress factors. The most widely studied of these is the type A behavior pattern in "an individual who chronically struggles to obtain an unlimited number of goals in the shortest possible time, often in competition with other people or opposing forces in the environment" [12] (see Chap. 20).

An extensive review of the evidence on the association between CHD and type A behavior [13] concluded that population studies demonstrate type A behavior to be a risk factor for coronary heart disease among healthy working men, but not for recurrent events or for mortality in men having had a first heart attack or suffering from angina. Subsequent studies seem to point out that anger and hostility are associated both with type A behavior and coronary heart disease. These personality traits could well become the most meaningful risk factors to be considered in the future.

Contrary to previous beliefs, white-collar workers who are exposed to the more stressful psychologic environment of the decision-making process have shown lower mortality and incidence rates of CHD than blue-collar workers. This effect can be explained by the high socioeconomic status of white-collar workers and possibly also by their greater degree of control over their work environments; however, it could also indicate a risk associated with the physical stresses and exposures to pollutants of a blue-collar working environment [14].

Shift work and excessive overtime have recently been suspected of being associated with CHD [15]. More evidence is needed for such associations to be confirmed.

OCCUPATION AS A RISK FACTOR FOR CARDIOVASCULAR DISORDERS OTHER THAN CHD

Some cardiovascular disorders other than CHD have also been associated with exposure to chemical and physical agents at work. Among the most

noteworthy are myocarditis, congestive heart failure, cardiac arrhythmias, Raynaud's phenomenon, and skin telangiectasia.

An epidemic of fatal cardiomyopathies was reported among heavy beer drinkers after several breweries had added a foam-stabilizing, cobalt-containing substance to the beer. It has been suggested that the synergistic effects of alcohol, cobalt, and a protein-poor diet were at the root of the cobalt-induced cardiomyopathy, whose symptoms resemble thiamine deficiency [16]. Although reports on industrial exposures to cobalt suggest important consequences for the heart, the situation remains unclear.

In their advanced stages, silicosis, asbestosis, severe asthma following exposure to toluene diisocyanate (TDI), and other pulmonary diseases may develop into right-sided heart failure. This condition, called *chronic cor pulmonale,* can be regarded as the terminal stage of a long chronic evolution of the disease.

Acute exposures to some halogenated and non-halogenated industrial solvents, such as toluene, xylene, chloroform, and trichloroethylene, and to fluorocarbon aerosol propellants have been associated with sudden death. The mechanism underlying this effect is presumably a fatal cardiac arrhythmia. Case reports indicate that these sudden deaths are usually preceded by high levels of exposure to the solvents and concurrent stress, resulting in activation of the sympathetic nervous system.

Chronic exposure of the hands to vibration from vibrating tools, such as pneumatic drills, hammers, chisels, riveting tools, metal grinders, and chain saws has been associated with a vascular syndrome affecting the fingers. This syndrome, called Raynaud's phenomenon or vibration white finger (VWF), manifests by an episodic whitening of the fingers accompanied by numbness or complete loss of sensation. The toes can also be similarly affected. On recovery, there is reddening and tingling of the affected areas accompanied by pain. In forestry, the prevalence of this phenomenon has been estimated to be over 30 percent [17]. After several years of exposure, the syndrome becomes so disabling that the affected worker is forced to leave the job. Recovery takes place slowly once exposure is ceased (see Chap. 18).

Another vascular phenomenon that has been associated with a specific job is skin telangiectasias in aluminum workers. Primary aluminum reduction workers have developed numerous red spots on their chest, back, and upper limbs. These maculae are clusters of telangiectasias. Apart from their unaesthetic appearance, they do not seem to carry any other health significance. Neither the mechanism involved nor the causal chemical is known at this point, although it is proposed that a fluoride element bound to a hydrocarbon molecule excreted by the sweat may account for the phenomenon [18].

CARDIOVASCULAR DISORDERS AND CIGARETTE SMOKING

Although antitobacco campaigns have succeeded in decreasing the number of smokers, many workers still smoke cigarettes. It is therefore appropriate to stress the relationship between smoking and CHD.

Most studies have estimated the risk of CHD among smokers to be in the order of 2.5 as compared with nonsmokers. It seems that this risk is associated more closely with the number of cigarettes smoked per day than with the number of years of smoking. Recent investigations demonstrate that this risk is reversible after a person stops smoking: The risk decreases to the level of a nonsmoker after 10 years of abstention [19].

SCREENING FOR CORONARY ARTERY DISEASE IN ASYMPTOMATIC WORKERS

The use of exercise stress testing has been proposed as a means of screening out from strenuous jobs those persons who are at high risk of developing ischemic heart disease. This concept stemmed from the results of several studies show-ing that symptomatic persons undergoing exercise stress testing who present a lowering of the S-T segment on ECG develop 3 to 5 times more CHD after 5 years than those without this ECG change [20].

This type of screening may seem attractive, particularly in situations where persons are working under conditions that may represent a higher risk of CHD, such as regular exposure to low levels of CO or working in strenuous jobs. However, many sound arguments militate against this approach: (1) the low reliability of exercise stress testing in predicting the development of CHD; (2) discrimination in hiring of workers on unproven grounds; (3) the unavailability of preventive measures for those identified as being at higher risk; (4) the association of risk with numerous other factors; and, (5) the existence of risk associated with the testing itself.

After weighing all considerations, the benefits that can be gained from exercise stress testing to screen out persons potentially at risk of coronary artery disease appear to be substantially outweighed by the drawbacks. The procedure cannot be recommended for asymptomatic persons.

RETURN TO WORK AFTER MYOCARDIAL INFARCTION

There is no consensus on a policy for employment of workers returning to work after a heart attack, after heart surgery, or during active treatment for ischemic heart problems. Most cases are dealt with on an ad hoc basis.

The cardiologist is generally the physician who must decide when it is medically permissible for a worker who has suffered a recent myocardial infarction to return to work. The existing guidelines are meager. The healing period normally lasts from 6 to 8 weeks. The usual procedure is to advise the patient who has been moderately active outside the hospital during convalescence to resume work on a part-time basis—for example, 2 to 4 hours daily, while avoiding symptoms, fatigue, and emotional tension. The patient is cautioned to avoid public transportation and rush-hour traffic, as well as to limit after-hours social functions.

With the advent of specialists in exercise physiology and the development of cardiac rehabilitation centers, much has been done to quantitate job requirements, to assess the capacities of heart attack victims through performance testing, and to reassign workers to jobs tailored to their capacities.

Different methods have been developed to ensure sensible matching of the heart patient to the job. Assessment of caloric expenditure required by a job allows matching with the ability of the patient to attain that level of expenditure without symptoms. Job simulation in rehabilitation centers is another technique useful in assessing a heart patient's ability to accomplish a specific job. The use of telemetric ECGs for on-the-job monitoring allows direct evaluation of a subject's capacity. Many patients will not be able to avail themselves of this approach. In any case, occupational physicians should visit the workplace to assess hazards.

Modern technologic refinements and major developments in cardiology have succeeded in removing the stigma of frailty often associated with a heart attack victim: a more positive approach that benefits both the worker and the employer now prevails, although there are still good reasons for caution.

For ensuring protection and gaining personal confidence in the capability to return to work, the heart attack victim should return to work in a gradually progressive manner, based on a schedule prepared with the occupational physician. Part-time work, light work, and rest periods longer or more frequent than usual should be considered. Shift work should be avoided.

Victims of heart disease should not perform job tasks in which the safety of fellow workers or of the general public is directly concerned, such as driving public transit vehicles, piloting aircraft, and erecting scaffolding. Other than these types of work, there are no clear guidelines regarding what work such individuals are capable of performing.

A worker who has suffered a heart attack needs to resume work after recovery for economic as well as psychological reasons. With modern treatment, the risk of high absenteeism is much less than previously believed and is most likely negligible. The lack of motivation that can arise from remaining at home, coupled with long periods of inactivity and overprotection by a spouse, are factors that contribute most to a permanent handicap after a myocardial infarction.

CORONARY HEART DISEASE AND WORKERS' COMPENSATION

Even though CHD is considered to be a personal disease, it can, in certain circumstances, be recognized as work-related. Legal experts' opinions on the causal relationship between heart attack and work lie between two extremes: (1) an approach based on the lack of full understanding of the etiology of this disease, leading to an uncritical acceptance of exertion as the precipitating factor in its appearance in the workplace; and (2) a systematic rejection of any claim on the basis that CHD is essentially of personal origin and that no medical opinion on the existence of a causal relationship can be substantiated.

In most North American workers' compensation programs, CHD is considered to be an injury caused by accident rather than an occupational disease. The presence of an accident originally meant that some "unusual exertion" was a necessary precondition, but its definition has varied much with time and place [21].

It is reasonable to assume that most courts of law will accept cases when four conditions are met: (1) the asserted heart pathology is well demonstrated; (2) the CHD has followed an exertive activity, not encountered normally in the execution of the work (often this is in relation to an emergency situation); (3) the heart attack took place immediately or in a reasonable period of time after the effort; and (4) a physician states that the exertion, more probably than not, triggered the attack.

There seems to be general agreement that fire fighters and policemen are at high risk for CHD and, accordingly, several states have favorably considered compensation cases for these workers. The impetus for such an attitude has been a concern over the physical and emotional stresses of both occupations, and, in addition, the chemical hazards encountered in fighting fires.

REFERENCES

1. Levy RI. The decline in cardiovascular disease mortality. Annu Rev Public Health 1981; 2:49–70.
2. Harlan WR, Sharrett AR, Weill H, Turino GM, Borhani NO, Resnekob L. Impact of environment on cardiovascular disease. Report of the American Heart Association Task Force on Environment and the Cardiovascular System. Circulation 1981; 63(1):242A–71A.
3. Feinleib M. Risk assessment, environmental factors and coronary heart disease. J Am Coll Toxicol 1983; 2(1):91–104.
4. Barrett-Connor E, Khaw KT. Family history of heart attack as an independent predictor of death due to cardiovascular disease. Circulation 1986; 69:1065–9.
5. Gobbato F, Mangiavacchi D. Previsione del rischio di ossicarbonismo acuto. Nomogramma per il calcolo della carbossiemoglobina nel sangue in funzione della concentrazione del CO in aria, del tempo di esposizione e della ventilazione polmonare. (Prevision of the hazard of acute carbon monoxide poisoning. A nomogram for calculating blood COHb on the basis of the carbon monoxide concentration in air, the length of exposure and lung ventilation.) Lavoro Umano 1977; 29:129–40.
6. Kurppa K, Rantanen J. In: Parmeggiani L, ed. Encyclopedia of occupational health and safety. 3rd ed. Geneva: ILO, 1983: 395–9. Vol. 1.
7. Anderson EW, Andelman RJ, Strauch JM, Fortuin NJ, Knelson JH. Effect of low-level carbon monoxide exposure on onset and duration of angina pectoris. Ann Intern Med 1973; 79:46–50.
8. Weir FW, Fabiano VL. Re-evaluation of the role of carbon monoxide in production or aggravation of cardiovascular disease processes. J Occup Med 1982; 24(7):519–25.
9. Liang YX, Qu DZ. Cost benefit analysis of the recovery of carbon disulfide in the manufacturing of viscose rayon. Scand J Work Environ Health [Suppl. 4] 11:60–3.
10. Nurminen M, Hernberg S. Effects of intervention on the cardiovascular mortality of workers exposed to carbon disulphide: a 15 year follow-up. Br J Ind Med 1985; 42:32–5.
11. Delin CO. Noisy work and hypertension. Lancet 1984; 2:931.
12. Dorian B, Taylor CB. Stress factors in the development of coronary artery disease. J Occup Med 1984; 26(10):747–56.
13. Matthews KA, Haynes SG. Type A behavior pattern and coronary disease risk. Update and critical evaluation. Am J Epidemiol 1986; 123(6):923–60.
14. Kasarek R, Baker D, Marxer F, Ahlbom A, Theorell T. Job decision latitude, job demands and cardiovascular disease: a prospective study of Swedish men. Am J Public Health 1981; 71:694–705.
15. Knutsson A, Akerstedt T, Jonsson BG, Orth-Gomer K. Increased risk of ischaemic heart disease in shift workers. Lancet 1986; July 12:89–91.
16. Morin Y, Daniel P. Quebec beer drinkers cardiomyopathy: etiological considerations. Can Med Assoc J 1967; 97:925–8.
17. Thériault GP, De Guire L, Gingras S. Raynaud's phenomenon in forestry workers of the Province of Quebec. Can Med Assoc J 1982; 126(12):1404–8.
18. Thériault GP, Harvey R, Cordier S. Skin telangiectases in workers at an aluminum plant. N Engl J Med 1980; 303:1278–81.
19. Rosenberg L, Kaufman DW, Helmrich SP, Shapiro S. The risk of myocardial infarction after quitting smoking in men under 55 years of age. N Engl J Med 1985; 313(21):1511–14.
20. Hlatky MA. Exercise stress testing to screen for coronary artery disease in asymptomatic persons. J Occup Med 1986; 28(10):1020–5.
21. Barth PS, Hunt MA. Occupational disease in the law. In: Workers' compensation and work-related illnesses and diseases. Cambridge, MA: MIT Press, 1980:92–116.

BIBLIOGRAPHY

Epstein FP. The epidemiology of coronary heart disease. J Chronic Dis 1965; 18:735–74.
   A thorough review of the epidemiology of CHD including mortality, incidence and prevalence, and the importance and reduction of known risk factors. Old reference, but its findings are still applicable today.

Fine L. Occupational heart disease, In: Rom WN, ed. Environmental and occupational medicine. Boston: Little, Brown, 1983; 359–65.
   A review on the scientific evidence on the association

between CHD and chemical and nonchemical factors encountered at the workplace.

Kurppa K, Hietanen E, Klockars M et al. Chemical exposures at work and cardiovascular morbidity. Scand J Work Environ Health 1984; 10:381–8.
A review of the scientific evidence on the association between CHD and hazards encountered at the workplace.

Scott A. Employment of workers with cardiac disease. J Soc Occup Med 1985; 35:99–102.
Despite all the advances in management of the cardiac victims, it is still a sad fact that many patients do not return to gainful employment. The author discusses this issue in the socio-economic context of modern workplaces.

Stamler J, Wentworth D, Neaton JD. Is relationship between serum cholesterol and risk of premature death from coronary heart disease continuous and graded? JAMA 1986; 256(20):2823–8.
A very large study that illustrates remarkably well the risks associated with personal risk factors, age, serum cholesterol, high blood pressure, and smoking.

Turino GM. Effect of carbon monoxide on the cardiorespiratory system. Carbon monoxide toxicity: physiology and biochemistry. Circulation 1981; 63(1):253A–9A.
A critical review of the evidence of CO toxicity on the cardiorespiratory system.

28
Hematologic Disorders

Bernard D. Goldstein and Howard M. Kipen

The hematologic system is a primary end-point of effect for a variety of occupational health problems. It is also a conduit of unwanted material to other organ systems and often an early indicator of important effects in other tissues. In addition, a number of the most important hematologic problems in the workplace are due to chemical agents that may produce more than one hematologic effect [1, 2].

AGENTS THAT INTERFERE WITH BONE MARROW FUNCTION

Benzene: Aplastic Anemia and Acute Myelogenous Leukemia

The potent hematotoxicity of benzene was first described in workers in the nineteenth century. Life-threatening aplastic anemia appears to be an inevitable consequence of exposure to high levels of benzene. Acute myelogenous leukemia in association with benzene exposure was originally reported in 1927, and the causal relationship has since been established through epidemiologic research [3].

The control of benzene exposure in the workplace (Fig. 28-1) and in the general environment has been a subject of much interest and controversy during the past decade. A major reason for the controversy surrounding the regulatory control of benzene is that, among the organic chemicals that are known to be human carcinogens, it is produced in the highest volume (9.7 million tons in the United States in 1985) and has the greatest potential of exposure for workers and the general

public. The National Institute for Occupational Safety and Health (NIOSH) estimates that up to 2 million American workers may be exposed. Benzene is an integral component of petrochemical feed stocks and is present in gasoline in the United States in the range of 1.0 to 1.5 percent. It is a useful intermediate in organic synthesis and is frequently used in research and commercial laboratories. Benzene is also formed during coke oven operations. Although an excellent solvent, it can and should be largely replaced in this role by much less toxic solvents, such as toluene. Benzene, however, is likely to remain a ubiquitous component of our society for the near future.

The current U.S. occupational standard for benzene is 1 ppm TWA. In 1977, following discovery by NIOSH of a group of rubber workers with a very high incidence of acute myelogenous leukemia, the Occupational Safety and Health Administration (OSHA) attempted to lower the workplace standard for benzene to 1 ppm, first by an emergency temporary standard and then through a formal rule-making process. Both approaches were overturned by the courts, the latter in a 5-to-4 U.S. Supreme Court decision, which in part called on OSHA to calculate the benefits of its action. In 1987, using updated information on the rubber worker cohort, OSHA established the 1 ppm standard [4].

The mechanism by which benzene produces hematotoxicity has not been determined. Benzene does not produce bone marrow damage; one or more metabolites do. Approximately 50 percent of inhaled benzene is excreted by exhalation; the

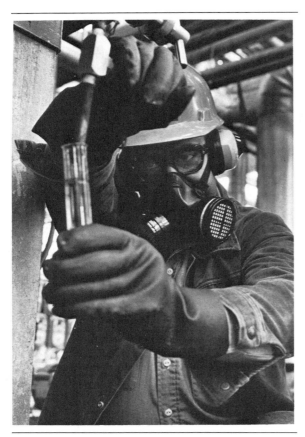

Fig. 28-1. Benzene worker with respiratory protection and impermeable gloves.
(Photograph by Earl Dotter.)

remainder is metabolized to a variety of products, particularly phenol. Measurement of urinary phenol has been used as a marker of benzene exposure. Although this is a useful technique to confirm relatively high-level exposure, the variation in background levels of urinary phenol, which are presumably from dietary sources, appears to preclude use of this assay as a technique to determine benzene exposure at levels present in a modern, well-regulated workplace. Benzene can also be measured in blood or in exhaled breath, both assays being in equilibrium with total body benzene.

While useful for determining instantaneous benzene body burden, the relatively steep slope of the disappearance curve of benzene following exposure makes such assays inappropriate as indicators of quantitative exposure. Studies in humans have determined that the half-life of benzene is relatively short, benzene being no longer detectable in the body approximately 1 week following exposure.

In laboratory animals, the metabolism of benzene has been reported to be inhibited by simultaneous exposure to toluene, resulting in protection against benzene-induced hematotoxicity. However, this protection does not occur at relatively low exposure levels in animals; in addition, toluene does not appear to inhibit benzene metabolism in humans exposed to usual workplace concentrations. In animal studies, benzene hematotoxicity has been shown to be potentiated by ethanol and by lead; however, the relevance of these findings to humans is yet to be determined. A potential interaction of note is the report that Japanese atom bomb survivors who developed leukemia were more likely to have also had an occupational exposure to benzene [5].

Studies of the toxicology of benzene in laboratory animals have clearly demonstrated benzene-induced aplastic anemia in a variety of species. However, only recently has it been possible to demonstrate tumorigenicity in laboratory animals, predominantly carcinomas and lymphatic tumors, in addition to a weak leukemic effect. While various lymphatic tumors have been associated with benzene exposure in humans, causality does not yet appear to be fully proven (Table 28-1) [6]. At present, the evidence that benzene is causally related to human nonhematologic neoplasms is minimal at best.

Benzene not only destroys the pluripotential stem cell responsible for red blood cells, platelets, and granulocytic white blood cells, it also causes a rapid loss in circulating lymphocytes in laboratory animals and humans. Based on studies in animals and the lymphocytopenic effects in humans, the potential for benzene effect on the immune system

Table 28-1. Relationship of benzene exposure to hematologic disorders

Causality proven
  Pancytopenia: aplastic anemia
  Acute myelogenous leukemia and variants (including
    acute myelomonocytic leukemia, acute
    promyelocytic leukemia, and erythroleukemia)
Causality reasonably likely
  Chronic myelogenous leukemia
  Chronic lymphocytic leukemia
  Hodgkin's disease
  Paroxysmal nocturnal hemoglobinuria (PNH)
Causality suggested but unproven
  Acute lymphoblastic leukemia
  Myelofibrosis and myeloid metaplasia
  Lymphoma: lymphocytic and histiocytic
  Thrombocythemia
  Multiple myeloma

in workers has been suggested but not demonstrated. There is evidence that benzene results not only in a decrease in number but also in structural and functional abnormalities in circulating blood cells. An increase in red cell mean corpuscular volume (MCV) and a decrease in lymphocyte count may be useful parameters for surveillance of potentially exposed workers. Cytogenetic abnormalities are common in significant benzene hematotoxicity and with advances in techniques may become useful in surveillance.

Aplastic anemia is frequently a fatal disorder, with death usually occurring due to (1) infection related to leukopenia or (2) hemorrhage due to thrombocytopenia. Studies of groups of workers with overt evidence of benzene hematotoxicity have often been initiated following the observation of a single individual with severe aplastic anemia. For the most part, those individuals who did not succumb relatively quickly to aplastic anemia demonstrated recovery following removal from benzene exposure. A follow-up study of a group of workers who previously had significant benzene-induced pancytopenia revealed minor residual hematologic abnormalities 10 years later [7]. An oc-

casional individual in these groups with initially relatively severe pancytopenia was observed to proceed from aplastic anemia through a preleukemic phase to the eventual development of acute myelogenous leukemia. This development is not unexpected since individuals with aplastic anemia from any cause appear to have a higher-than-expected likelihood of developing acute myelogenous leukemia. Accordingly, it has been suggested that acute myelogenous leukemia is not a direct consequence of a benzene effect on the genome, but rather that it occurs indirectly through the production of aplastic anemia, or at least significant pancytopenia. If true, this would imply that workplace control of benzene that prevented pancytopenia would be sufficient to also preclude a risk of myelogenous leukemia. However, based on currently available evidence, there is no reason to alter the present prudent public health approach of assuming that there is no threshold for the carcinogenic effect of benzene. In other words, we assume that every molecule of benzene to which an individual is exposed has some finite risk, albeit small, of producing a somatic mutation that may result in acute myelogenous leukemia.

Review of leukemia cases that have been reported to be associated with exposure to benzene reveals not only acute myelogenous leukemia but also a number of variants of this disorder, including acute myelomonocytic leukemia, promyelocytic leukemia, and erythroleukemia, the last of which is a relatively rare variant that has been disproportionately reported. Even in cases not specifically designated as erythroleukemia, evidence of erythroid dysplasia is relatively commonly noted in the bone marrow. Perhaps related is the observation of an increased MCV of erythrocytes as a fairly common and early manifestation of benzene hematotoxicity.

A typical case report of acute myelogenous leukemia in an individual heavily exposed to benzene is described below:

A 29-year-old white man went to his physician with complaints of nonspecific malaise and bleeding gums.

On physical examination, he was noted to be febrile and to have exquisite sternal tenderness. Laboratory findings included hematocrit, 32 percent; white blood count, 28,000 per cu mm; undifferentiated blast forms, 40 percent; and platelet count, 28,000 per cu mm. The bone marrow findings were diagnostic of acute myelogenous leukemia. Cytogenetic studies were not performed until following chemotherapy. Although abnormalities were observed, the findings could not clearly be related to the etiology of the acute leukemia.

The patient had been working in the chemical industry since age 20, when he received an associate degree in laboratory technology. Since that time, he has taken courses at two universities to earn a bachelor's degree in chemistry. Control of chemical exposure in the student laboratories of all three academic institutions was negligible to modest. Benzene was present in each. In only one laboratory course was there any specific instruction concerning the control of chemical hazards in the laboratory. His initial job was in the control room of a petrochemical plant, where he primarily checked dials. He rarely was outdoors or in the chemical area but did participate in the clean-up of occasional spills.

From 23 to 27 years of age, he worked as a technician in the quality control laboratory of a chemical company that produced chlorinated hydrocarbon pesticides. On about two-thirds of workdays, his job was to test the extent of chlorination of the product. The procedure included a solvent extraction in which 50 ml of benzene was added to each of 30 samples on a laboratory bench, and the samples were then placed into a hood containing a heating device. After a specified time, the 30 beakers were removed from the hood and, while still hot and bubbling, were placed on a laboratory bench. After titration and analysis, the residual material was dumped into a sink and the viscous residue was washed vigorously with hot water. He reported that the smell of benzene was particularly notable during the washing procedure, and on occasion he would become lightheaded. This feeling would clear in a few minutes if he left the room or stood by an open window.

During this period, his supervisor, who did much of the same procedures and had also been exposed to Lindane (gamma benzene hexachloride), developed fatal aplastic anemia. Benzene was used in the laboratory as a general solvent and kept in bottles out of the hood.

Two years before developing acute myelogenous leukemia, he began work in another chemical plant as a laboratory technician. In this laboratory he also performed chloride analysis, but acetone was used as the extractant and benzene was kept in the hood. In addition, the latter laboratory regularly received visits from industrial hygienists with monitoring equipment, and they presented lectures about laboratory safety.

Other Hematologic Disorders Due to Benzene

Benzene has also been associated with other myeloproliferative disorders including chronic myelogenous leukemia, myelofibrosis, and myeloid metaplasia; however, evidence is less convincing for a causal relationship with benzene exposure than it is for acute myelogenous leukemia. It is not surprising that cases of the relatively rare disorder paroxysmal nocturnal hemoglobinuria (PNH) have been reported in benzene-exposed workers. This paraneoplastic disorder is related both to aplastic anemia and to acute myelogenous leukemia. Lymphoproliferative disorders, including Hodgkin's and non-Hodgkin's lymphoma, acute and chronic lymphatic leukemia, and multiple myeloma, have also been reported in association with benzene exposure. Again the evidence of a causal relationship to benzene is suggestive but not conclusive.

Other Causes of Aplastic Anemia and Hematologic Neoplasia

Other agents in the workplace have been associated with aplastic anemia, the most notable being radiation. The effects of radiation on bone marrow stem cells have been employed in the therapy of leukemia. Similarly, a variety of chemotherapeutic alkylating agents produce aplasia and pose a risk to workers responsible for producing or administering these compounds. Radiation, benzene, and alkylating agents all appear to have a threshold concentration below which aplastic anemia will not occur. Protection of the production worker becomes more problematic when the agent has an idiosyncratic mode of action in which minuscule amounts may produce aplasia, such as chloramphenicol. A variety of other chemicals have been reported to be associated with aplastic anemia, but it is often difficult to determine causality. An example is the pesticide Lindane (gamma benzene hexachloride). Case reports have appeared, generally following relatively high levels of exposure, in which Lindane is associated with aplasia. This finding is far from being universal in humans, and there are no reports of Lindane-induced bone marrow toxicity in laboratory animals treated with large doses of this agent. Bone marrow hypoplasia has also been associated with exposure to ethylene glycol ethers, trinitrotoluene (TNT), and arsenic.

Hematologic neoplasms have been reported to occur in other occupational situations. There is some evidence that (1) farmers have a higher risk of lymphoma; (2) workers exposed to ethylene oxide, used primarily as a sterilant, have a great incidence of acute myelogenous leukemia; and (3) much more controversially, workers exposed to electromagnetic fields may possibly be at greater risk of leukemia [8, 9, 10]. Multiple myeloma has been associated with radiation and with solvent exposure. The reported association of toluene with aplastic anemia and leukemia almost certainly is incorrect, because this represents contamination of toluene with benzene.

AGENTS THAT AFFECT RED BLOOD CELLS

Agents that Interfere with Hemoglobin Oxygen Delivery

Certain toxins produce adverse effects by interfering with the orderly delivery of oxygen from red cell hemoglobin to tissues (see Chaps. 14 and 27).

Carbon Monoxide. Carbon monoxide (CO) binds relatively firmly with the oxygen-combining site of hemoglobin, thereby preventing the uptake of oxygen from the lungs. This effect is magnified because once one or more of the four oxygen-combining sites on a hemoglobin molecule is occupied by CO, it becomes more difficult for the oxygen on the molecule to be released at the tissue level. This "shift to the left" of the oxygen dissociation curve accounts for the potential lethality of carboxyhemoglobin (COHb) concentrations as low as 25 to 35 percent of total hemoglobin. The affinity of hemoglobin for CO is more than 200 times greater than it is for oxygen; that is, a gas mixture of 1,000 ppm CO and 20 percent oxygen (200,000 ppm) would result in about one-half oxyhemoglobin and one-half COHb at equilibrium. At the normal rate of respiration, equilibration occurs slowly, requiring approximately 8 to 12 hours. The rate of COHb level change depends on the rate of respiration, thereby putting active workers at greater risk.

There is a natural background level of approximately 0.5 percent COHb because of the formation of CO during metabolism. A pack-a-day cigarette smoker will achieve COHb levels of about 5 percent. The U.S. workplace standard for carbon monoxide is 50 ppm TWA, which will result in approximately 8 to 9 percent COHb at the end of an 8-hour workday. There is also a 400 ppm short-term exposure limit (STEL)—a 15-minute time-weighted average not to be exceeded at any time during a workday. There is roughly an additive effect of COHb levels from cigarette smoke and from ambient exposures.

In a workplace, CO poisoning is usually caused by incomplete combustion coupled with improper ventilation. Carbon monoxide is also formed through the metabolism of certain exogenous agents, most notably methylene chloride.

There is some evidence that COHb levels in the range of 5 percent are associated with a minimal decrement in psychomotor function, suggesting that at these or higher levels there may be an increased risk of performing tasks wrong, leading to industrial accidents [11]. Individuals with preexisting cardiovascular disease have been reported to have a decrease in exercise tolerance and earlier development of acute angina or intermittent claudication, with effects occurring at levels ranging down to perhaps 2.5 percent COHb.

Detection of CO poisoning depends primarily on clinical suspicion. Complaints include headache, weakness, lassitude, and mental obtundation. In severe cases, the blood has a characteristic cherry red color. Treatment includes removal from the contaminated air and ventilation with oxygen.

Methemoglobin-Producing Compounds. Methemoglobin is another form of hemoglobin that is incapable of delivering oxygen to the tissues. Hemoglobin iron must be in the reduced ferrous state in order to participate in the transport of oxygen. Under normal conditions, oxidation to methemoglobin, with iron in the ferric state, goes on continuously, resulting in approximately 0.5 percent of total hemoglobin in the form of methemoglobin in the steady state. Reduction to ferrous hemoglobin occurs through the activity of an NADH-dependent–methemoglobin reductase.

Clinically significant methemoglobinemia has been a not-uncommon event in industries using aniline dyes. Other chemicals frequently causing methemoglobinemia in the workplace have been nitrobenzenes, other organic and inorganic nitrites and nitrates, hydrazines, and a variety of quinones (Table 28-2) [12]. Cyanosis, confusion, and other signs of hypoxia are the usual symptoms. In chronically exposed individuals, blueness of the lips may be observed at levels of methemoglobinemia (approximately 10% or greater) that are without other overt consequences. The blood has a characteristic chocolate brown color. Treatment consists of avoiding further exposure. With significant symptoms, usually at methemoglobin levels

Table 28-2. Selected agents implicated in environmentally and occupationally acquired methemoglobinemia

Nitrate-contaminated well water
Nitrous gases (in welding and silos)
Aniline dyes
Food high in nitrates or nitrites
Moth balls (containing naphthalene)
Potassium chlorate
Nitrobenzenes
Phenylenediamine
Toluenediamine

greater than 40 percent, therapy with methylene blue or ascorbic acid can accelerate reduction of the methemoglobin level.

There are inherited disorders leading to persistent methemoglobinemia, either due to (1) heterozygosity for an abnormal hemoglobin, or (2) homozygosity for deficiency of red cell NADH-dependent methemoglobin reductase. Individuals who are heterozygous for this enzyme deficiency will not be able to decrease elevated methemoglobin levels caused by chemical exposures as rapidly as will individuals with normal enzyme levels.

In addition to oxidizing the iron component of hemoglobin, many of the chemicals causing methemoglobinemia, or their metabolites, are also relatively nonspecific oxidizing agents, which at high levels can cause a Heinz-body hemolytic anemia. This process is characterized by oxidative denaturation of hemoglobin, leading to the formation of punctate membrane-bound red cell inclusions known as Heinz bodies, which can be identified with special stains. Oxidative damage to the red cell membrane also occurs. While this may lead to significant hemolysis, the compounds listed in Table 28-2 primarily produce their adverse effects through the formation of methemoglobin, which may be life threatening, rather than through hemolysis, which is usually a limited process. In essence, two different red cell defense pathways are involved: (1) the NADH-dependent methemoglobin reductase required to reduce methemoglobin to normal hemoglobin, and (2) the NADPH-dependent process through the hexose monophosphate (HMP) shunt, leading to the maintenance of reduced glutathione as a means to defend against oxidizing species capable of producing Heinz-body hemolytic anemia (Fig. 28-2). Heinz-body hemolysis can be exacerbated by the treatment of methemoglobinemic patients with methylene blue because it requires NADPH for its methemoglobin-reducing effects. Hemolysis will also be a more prominent part of the clinical picture in individuals with (1) deficiencies in one of the enzymes of the NADPH oxidant defense pathway, or (2) an inherited unstable hemoglobin. Except for glucose

$$GSH + GSH + (0) \xrightarrow[\text{Peroxidase}]{\text{Glutathione}} GSSG + H_2O$$

$$GSSG + 2NADPH \xrightarrow[\text{Reductase}]{\text{Glutathione}} 2GSH + 2NADP$$

$$\text{Glucose-6-Phosphate} + NADP \xrightarrow{\text{G6PD}} \text{6-Phosphogluconate} + NADPH$$

$$Fe^{+++} \text{ Hemoglobin (Methemoglobin)} + NADH \xrightarrow[\text{Reductase}]{\text{Methemoglobin}} Fe^{++} \text{ Hemoglobin}$$

Fig. 28-2. Red blood cell enzymes of oxidant defense and related reactions.

6-phosphate dehydrogenase (G6PD) deficiency, described later in this chapter, these are relatively rare disorders.

Another form of hemoglobin alteration produced by oxidizing agents is a denatured species known as sulfhemoglobin. This irreversible product often can be detected in the blood of individuals with significant methemoglobinemia produced by oxidant chemicals. Sulfhemoglobin is the name also given, and more appropriately, to a specific product formed during hydrogen sulfide poisoning (see Chap. 14).

Hemolytic Agents: Arsine
The normal red blood cell survives in the circulation for 120 days. Shortening of this survival can lead to anemia if not compensated by an increase in red cell production within the bone marrow. There are essentially two types of hemolysis: (1) intravascular hemolysis, in which there is an immediate release of hemoglobin within the circulation; and (2) extravascular hemolysis, in which red cells are destroyed within the spleen or the liver.

One of the most potent intravascular hemolysins is arsine gas (AsH_3). Inhalation of a relatively small amount of this agent leads to swelling and eventual bursting of red blood cells within the cir-

culation. It may be difficult to detect the causal relation of workplace arsine exposure to an acute hemolytic episode. This is partly because the delay between exposure and onset of symptoms but primarily because the source of exposure is often not evident. Arsine gas is made and used commercially, often now in the electronics industry. However, most of the published reports of acute hemolytic episodes have been through the unexpected liberation of arsine gas as an unwanted byproduct of an industrial process—for example, if acid is added to a container made of arsenic-contaminated metal. (A characteristic untoward exposure is described below.) Any process that reduces arsenic, such as acidification, can lead to the liberation of arsine gas. As arsenic can be a contaminant of many metals and organic materials, such as coal, arsine exposure can often be unexpected. Stibine, the hydride of antimony, appears to produce a hemolytic effect similar to arsine.

NIOSH has recommended an immediate danger to life and health (IDLH) level of 6 to 30 ppm for 30 minutes and the National Academy of Sciences Committee on Toxicology has recommended an emergency exposure limit of 1 ppm for 1 hour. Death can occur directly due to complete loss of red blood cells. (A hematocrit of zero has been reported.) However, a major concern at arsine levels less than those producing complete hemolysis is acute renal failure due to the massive release of hemoglobin within the circulation (see Chap. 30). At much higher levels, arsine may produce acute pulmonary edema and possibly direct renal effects. Hypotension may accompany the acute episode. There is usually a delay of at least a few hours between inhalation of arsine and the onset of symptoms. In addition to red urine due to hemoglobinuria, the patient will frequently complain of abdominal pain and nausea, symptoms that occur concomitantly with acute intravascular hemolysis from a number of causes [13].

Treatment is aimed at maintenance of renal perfusion and transfusion of normal blood. As the circulating red cells affected by arsine appear to some extent to be doomed to intravascular hemolysis, an exchange transfusion in which arsine-exposed red cells are replaced by unexposed cells would appear to be optimal therapy. As in severe life-threatening hemorrhage, it is important that replacement red cells have adequate 2,3-diphosphoglyceric acid (DPG) levels so as to be able to deliver oxygen to the tissue.

Two maintenance workers were assigned to clean up a clogged drain with a mixture of sodium hydroxide, sodium nitrate, and aluminum chips, which together act to form hydrogen gas. Arsine was formed from the combination of hydrogen with arsenic, which was residual in the drain from a use 5 years before. Both men noted the development of a sewer-like odor during the 2 to 3 hours during which they worked on the drain. One man noted a headache, followed by numbness of tongue and cheeks, weakness, and nausea while at work. After being home for a few hours, he sought medical attention. The second patient first noted abdominal discomfort at the end of the workday and while at home experienced nausea, vomiting, and hematuria. He was treated at an emergency department that evening with "stomach medicine" and after being anuric all night was admitted the next morning to a local hospital. Both patients were treated for acute renal failure with partial recovery in one and a need for maintenance dialysis in the other patient [14].

There are a variety of other hemolytic agents in the workplace. As discussed before, for many the toxicity of concern is methemoglobinemia. Other hemolytic agents include naphthalene and its derivatives. In addition, certain metals, such as copper, and organometals, such as tributyl tin, will shorten red cell survival, at least in animal models. Mild hemolysis can also occur during traumatic physical exertion (march hemoglobinuria); a more modern observation is elevated white blood counts with prolonged exertion (jogger's leukocytosis). The most important of the metals that affects red cell formation and survival in workers is lead.

Hematologic Aspects of Lead Poisoning

Occupational exposure to dusts and fumes that contain lead compounds is a frequent concern of medical personnel who evaluate workers in a variety of occupational and environmental settings. In addition to occupations with well-recognized risks, such as battery makers, secondary lead smelter workers, and foundry workers, the list of potentially lead-exposed occupations includes more commonly encountered groups, such as firing range personnel, jewelry and pottery workers, iron workers, welders, and painters. The last three groups are at risk when sanding or burning through lead pigment-containing paints, particularly in a marine setting. Exposure usually is from inhalation of dust or lead oxide fumes. Skin absorption occurs readily only with organic lead compounds, such as tetraethyl lead (a gasoline antiknock additive being phased out in the United States); poor work habits and hygiene can predispose to ingestion and inhalation of lead on cigarettes. The finer the lead particle generated at work (as in lead fume from burning), the greater proportion of lead absorbed from the respiratory tract. An understanding of hematologic aspects of lead poisoning is important, in part, because the erythrocytic cells of the bone marrow and peripheral blood represent a major target for lead toxicity. (See also Chaps. 14, 25, 26, and 30.)

Pathophysiology of Lead Hematotoxicity

Although lead is known to inhibit most of the enzymes in the heme biosynthetic pathway, its most pronounced effect is inhibition of the final enzymatic reaction in heme formation, in which heme synthetase (ferrochelatase) catalyzes incorporation of ferrous iron into the heme ring (Fig. 28-3). The resultant decrease in intraerythroid levels of iron-containing heme releases earlier reactions in the biosynthetic pathway from feedback inhibition by the end product, particularly for the irreversible first reaction, the synthesis of Δ-aminolevulinic acid from succinyl-CoA and glycine, catalyzed by ALA synthetase. Increased production of Δ-ALA, and decreased incorporation of iron into protoporphyrin IX causes accumulation of abnormally high levels of all constituents of the pathway, particularly of the penultimate protoporphyrin IX. These high intracellular levels of erythrocyte protoporphyrin provide the biochemical basis for one group of valuable diagnostic tests in the evaluation of lead toxicity.

Interference with heme formation leads to a series of predictable abnormalities in red cell maturation. Bone marrow examination of the lead-intoxicated patient, while rarely clinically indicated, will reveal erythroid hyperplasia and sideroblastic changes in which the more mature cells display iron-staining granules in a perinuclear arc. Of greater clinical relevance are the peripheral red cell abnormalities. Due to a combination of decreased red blood cell production and reduced survival time (from membrane abnormalities), normochromic microcytic or normochromic normocytic anemia is the classic finding, although anemia is only expected with the combination of high blood levels and chronic exposures. Examination of the peripheral smear may demonstrate increased punctate basophilic stippling of red blood cells (stippled cells) and reticulocytosis. Decreased osmotic fragility may also be demonstrated in the laboratory.

It is of utmost importance that neither absence of the above hematologic changes nor absence of other signs and symptoms of clinical lead poison-

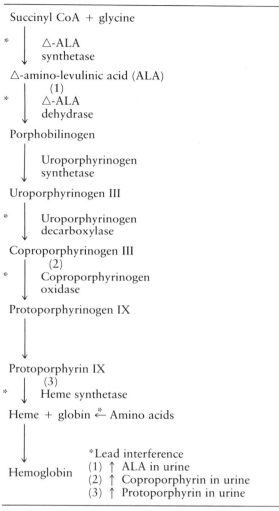

Fig. 28-3. Multiple sites of lead interference with hemoglobin synthesis. (From WN Rom. Environmental and occupational medicine. Boston: Little, Brown, 1982.)

ing (such as neurologic dysfunction) be used to rule out the presence of significantly high lead burdens in either individuals or populations. Development of overt hematologic disease from lead may be expected to result only after serious breaches of safety procedures and of recommended exposure limits, such as those of the 1978

OSHA lead standard. Air concentrations are limited to a TWA of of 50 ug per cubic meter, personal hygiene standards are set, and mandatory biologic monitoring of blood lead levels is now the law for those with significant exposures to lead [15]. Ideally, elevation of biologic indices, such as blood lead and zinc protoporphyrin (ZPP), the latter of which is not specified in the 1978 OSHA standard, will be recognized before overt hematologic disease supervenes.

In chronic lead intoxication, the marrow produces erythrocytes with a modestly decreased survival due to membrane abnormalities, and thus there is some hemolytic component to a resulting anemia. The unusual occurrence of acute lead intoxication due to massive inhalation of dust, as has occurred in some painters when sanding leaded paint from older homes, may result in acute hemolysis similar to that encountered following arsine exposure. The diagnosis is usually evident from the occupational history.

Hematologic Tests for Diagnosis of Lead Poisoning

The most commonly used test is direct measurement of the blood lead (PbB) concentration, routinely performed in clinical laboratories by atomic absorption. Only a few milliliters of whole venous blood is required. Since lead is a ubiquitous contaminant of industrialized societies, background levels in adults approximate 10 to 20 μg per dl although neurologic dysfunction has been suggested, especially in children, at the upper end of this "normal" range. Values greater than 35 μg per dl commonly indicate significant exposures. The OSHA lead standard is designed to control airborne exposures so that most workers' PbB will be less than 40 μg per dl, although it does not specify worker removal from exposure until blood lead reaches 50 μg per dl.

Blood lead levels best reflect recent exposure—that is, exposure within 2 to 3 weeks. Large amounts of lead are readily incorporated into bone and maintained in equilibrium with blood and soft tissue levels. Thus chronic or intermittent exposure may lead to relatively moderate elevations of PbB (30–60 $\mu g/dl$) in the face of a substantial total body burden. In situations with the opportunity for chronic or intermittent exposures, PbB may be an incomplete index of both body burden and toxicity, and the following two alternatives are indicated to supplement this evaluation.

As implied above, lead inhibition of heme synthetase results in large accumulations of various heme precursors within developing erythrocytes, the most prevalent of which is protoporphyrin IX. Increases in erythrocyte protoporphyrins (EPs) can be measured by extraction of the porphyrins from whole blood, followed by spectrophotometry or fluorometry. Additionally, they can be measured in urine, a common approach in the work-up of other abnormalities of porphyrin metabolism. A more recent and highly useful test is the fluorometric assay for intraerythrocytic zinc protoporphyrin (ZPP), which has been shown to correlate almost perfectly with free erythrocyte protoporphyrin (FEP) determinations [16]. Zinc is the most abundant intracellular heavy metal, apart from iron, and readily complexes with excess EP, forming a specific fluorescent product. During extraction, zinc is usually removed—hence the term *free* erythrocyte protoporphyrin. The direct assay of ZPP with a hematofluorometer can be performed in the field using only microcapillary amounts of whole blood. Rather than assaying a level of lead, it represents a sensitive indicator of biochemical dysfunction. Elevated protoporphyrin measurements are not specific for lead inhibition of heme synthesis; this parameter is commonly elevated in iron deficiency anemia. Thus, all abnormal values must be interpreted in the context of PbB and serum iron determinations.

It is important to recognize differences in the interpretation of PbB results, compared with those of ZPP [17]. ZPP measures intraerythrocytic abnormalities developed during bone marrow maturation; since the red cells of even a lead intoxicated individual circulate for over 100 days, ZPP reflects the cumulative average inhibition of heme synthesis over the preceding 3 to 4 months. It remains elevated for the life of an individual cell. However, PbB reflects more recent lead exposure. Thus, in an intermittently exposed worker, ZPP may be elevated from exposures of 1 to 2 months previously, whereas the blood lead initially rose, but subsequently fell due to redistribution to bone and slow renal excretion. Although no clear guideline has been established, in many laboratories a ZPP greater than 100 μg per dl is said to be beyond the usual range. Even lower levels may be of concern in protecting against lead-induced neurologic dysfunction, especially in children.

Finally, occult lead intoxication, especially if exposures have taken place more than 3 months before, may be demonstrated by a diagnostic challenge with calcium EDTA. This metal chelator will bind lead cations in bone and soft tissue. Excretion of greater than 600 μg of lead in a 24-hour urine specimen suggests previous significant exposure. In the presence of renal insufficiency, 72-hour urine collections may be required [18].

OTHER HEMATOLOGIC DISORDERS
White Blood Cells
There are a variety of drugs, such as propylthiourea (PTU), which are known to affect the production or survival of circulating polymorphonuclear leukocytes relatively selectively. In contrast, nonspecific bone marrow toxins affect the precursors of red cells and platelets as well. Workers engaged in the preparation or administration of such drugs should be considered at risk. There is one report of complete granulocytopenia in a worker poisoned with dinitrophenol. Alteration in lymphocyte number and function, and particularly of subtype distribution, is receiving more attention as a possible subtle mechanism of effects due to a variety of chemicals in the workplace or general environment, particularly chlorinated hydrocarbons, dioxins, and related compounds. Validation of the health implications of such changes is required.

Coagulation
Similar to leukopenia, there are many drugs that selectively decrease the production or survival of circulating platelets, which could be a problem in workers involved in the preparation or administration of such agents. Otherwise, there are only scattered reports of thrombocytopenia in workers. One study implicates toluene diisocyanate (TDI) as a cause of thrombocytopenic purpura. Abnormalities in the various blood factors involved in coagulation are not generally noted as a consequence of work. Individuals with preexisting coagulation abnormalities, such as hemophilia, often have difficulty entering the workforce. However, although a carefully considered exclusion from a few selected jobs is reasonable, such individuals are usually capable of normal functioning at work.

HEMATOLOGIC SCREENING AND SURVEILLANCE IN THE WORKPLACE
Markers of Susceptibility
Due in part to the ease in obtaining samples, more is known about inherited variations in human blood components than for those of any other organ. Extensive studies sparked by recognition of familial anemias have led to fundamental knowledge concerning the structural and functional implications of genetic alterations. Of pertinence to occupational health are those inherited variations that might lead to an increased susceptibility to workplace hazards. There are a number of such testable variations that have been considered or actually used for the screening of workers. The rapid increase in knowledge concerning human genetics makes it a certainty that we will have a better understanding of the inherited basis of variation in human response, and we will be more capable of predicting the extent of individual susceptibility through laboratory tests (see Chap. 6 and 32).

Before discussing the potential value of currently available susceptibility markers, the major ethical considerations in the use of such tests in workers should be emphasized. It has been questioned whether such tests favor exclusion of workers from a site rather than maintain a focus on improving the worksite for the benefit of the workers. Some distinction has been made between the use of susceptibility markers as a screening device at a preplacement examination and such use as part of an ongoing evaluation of employed workers. At the very least, before embarking on the use of a susceptibility marker at a workplace, the goals of the testing and consequences of the findings must be clear to all parties.

The two markers of hematologic susceptibility for which screening has taken place most frequently are sickle cell trait and glucose-6-phosphate dehydrogenase (G6PD) deficiency. The former is at most of marginal value in rare situations, and the latter is of no value whatsoever in most of the situations for which it has been advocated.

Sickle cell disease is a fairly common disorder in which the individual is homozygous for hemoglobin S (HbS). It is a relatively severe disease that often, but not always, precludes entering the workforce. The HbS gene may be inherited with other genes, such as HbC, which may reduce the severity of its effects. The basic defect in individuals with sickle cell disease is the polymerization of HbS, leading to microinfarction. Microinfarction can occur in episodes, known as sickle cell crises, and can be precipitated by external factors, particularly those leading to hypoxia and, to a lesser extent, dehydration. With a reasonably wide variation in the clinical course and well-being of those with sickle cell disease, employment evaluation should focus on the individual case history. Jobs that have the possibility of hypoxic exposures, such as those requiring frequent air travel, or those with a likelihood of significant dehydration, are not appropriate.

Much more common than sickle cell disease is sickle cell trait, the heterozygous condition in which there is inheritance of a gene for HbS and one gene for HbA. Individuals with this genetic pattern have been reported to undergo sickle cell crises under extreme conditions of hypoxia. Some consideration has been given to excluding individuals with sickle cell trait from jobs where hypoxia is a common risk, probably limited to the jobs on military aircraft or submarines, and perhaps on commercial aircraft. However, it must be emphasized that individuals with sickle cell trait do very well in almost every other situation. For example, athletes with sickle cell trait had no adverse effects from competing at the altitude of Mexico City (2,200 m, or 7,200 ft) during the 1968 Summer Olympics. Accordingly, with the few exceptions described above, there is no reason to consider exclusion or modification of work schedules for those with sickle cell trait.

Another common genetic variant of a red blood cell component is the A⁻ form of G6PD deficiency. It is inherited on the X chromosome as a sex-linked recessive gene and is present in approximately one in seven black males and one in 50 black females in the United States. As with sickle cell trait, G6PD deficiency provides a protective advantage against malaria. Under usual circumstances, individuals with this form of G6PD deficiency have red blood counts and indices within the normal range. However, due to the inability to regenerate reduced glutathione, their red blood cells are susceptible to hemolysis following ingestion of oxidant drugs and in certain disease states. This susceptibility to oxidizing agents has led to workplace screening on the erroneous assumption that individuals with the common A⁻ variant of G6PD deficiency will be at risk from the inhalation of oxidant gases. In fact, it would require exposure to many times higher than the levels at which such gases would cause fatal pulmonary edema before the red cells of G6PD-deficient individuals would receive oxidant stress sufficient to be of concern [19]. G6PD deficiency will increase the likelihood of overt Heinz-body hemolysis in individuals exposed to aniline dyes and other methemoglobin-provoking agents (Table 28-2), but in these cases the primary clinical problem remains the life-threatening methemoglobinemia. While knowledge of G6PD status might be useful in such cases, primarily to guide therapy, this knowledge should not be used to exclude workers from the workplace.

There are many other forms of familial G6PD deficiency, all far less common than the A⁻ variant. Certain of these variants, particularly in individuals from the Mediterranean basin and Central Asia, have much lower levels of G6PD activity in their red blood cells. Consequently the affected individual can be severely compromised by ongoing hemolytic anemia. Deficiencies in other enzymes active in defense against oxidants have also been reported as have unstable hemoglobins that render the red cell more susceptible to oxidant stress in the same manner as in G6PD deficiency.

Surveillance

One of the most difficult tasks in occupational medicine is to distinguish between statistical abnormality and clinical abnormality in the interpretation of laboratory tests obtained as part of surveillance. Surveillance differs substantially from clinical testing in both the evaluation of ill patients and the regular screening of presumably healthy individuals. In ill patients, a laboratory value just beyond normal limits is unlikely to explain the cause of the illness. Similarly, physicians evaluating apparently healthy individuals will tend to discount an unsupported finding of one laboratory test just beyond normal limits. In contrast the laboratory tests chosen for a surveillance program are in general those for which any abnormality is a matter of concern due to the nature of the job. These tests are not intended for diagnostic purposes, although they may be useful to supplement normal diagnostic testing. In an appropriately designed surveillance program, the aim is to prevent overt disease by picking up subtle early changes through the use of laboratory testing. Therefore, a slightly abnormal finding should automatically trigger a response—or at least a thorough review—by physicians.

To respond appropriately, the statistical basis of the "normal" laboratory value must be understood. For blood counts, it has been traditional to describe the "normal" range as including 95 percent of the distribution of blood counts in healthy people. This range implies that 1 of 20 clinically normal individuals will be statistically abnormal in any one blood count, 1 in 40 being higher than normal and 1 in 40 being lower than normal. This situation presents a problem when reviewing blood counts in that clinical information can be obtained by findings beyond either end of the normal range. For most hematotoxins, such as benzene, one is primarily concerned with the lower end of the range. The problem of making a distinction between statistical abnormality and clinical abnormality is further compounded by the number of tests in use and the relatively large number of workers who may be under surveillance. Consider that in a normal individual, blood counts for platelets, white cells, and red cells might each have a 1 in 40 chance of a count below the normal range. In a study of 100 healthy individuals with no known exposure to hematotoxins, it would not be surprising if perhaps 6 were found to have a statistically abnormal low count for one of these parameters. This finding would be the baseline of false-positives if a physician were evaluating 100 workers potentially exposed to benzene.

In the initial review of hematologic surveillance data in a workforce potentially exposed to a hematotoxin such as benzene, there are two major approaches that are particularly helpful in distinguishing false-positives. The first is the degree of the difference from normal. As the count gets further removed from the normal range, there is a rapid drop-off in the likelihood that it represents just a statistical anomaly. Second, one should take advantage of the totality of data for that individual, including normal values, keeping in mind the wide range of effects produced by benzene. For example, there is a much greater probability of a benzene effect if a slightly low platelet count is accompanied by a low-normal white blood cell count, a low-normal red cell count, and a high-normal MCV. Conversely, the relevance of this same platelet count to benzene hematotoxicity can be relatively discounted if the other blood counts are at the opposite end of the normal spectrum.

These same two considerations can be used in judging whether the individual should be removed from the workforce while awaiting further testing and whether the additional testing should consist only of a repeat complete blood count (CBC).

If there is any doubt as to the cause of the low count, the entire CBC should be repeated. If the low count is due to laboratory variability or some short-term biologic variability within the individual, it is less likely that the blood count will again be low. Comparison with preplacement or other available blood counts should help distinguish those individuals who have an inherent tendency to be on the lower end of the distribution. Detection of an individual worker with an effect due to a hematologic toxin should be considered a sentinel health event, prompting careful investigation of working conditions and of coworkers (see "Surveillance" in Chap. 3).

The wide range in normal laboratory values for blood counts can present an even greater challenge since there can be a substantial effect while counts are still within the normal range. For example, it is possible that a worker exposed to benzene or ionizing radiation may have a fall in hematocrit from 50 to 40 percent, a fall in the white blood cell count from 10,000 to 5,000 per cubic millimeter and a fall in the platelet count from 350,000 to 150,000 per cubic millimeter—that is, more than a 50 percent decrease in platelets; yet all these values are within the "normal" range of blood counts. Accordingly, a surveillance program that looks solely at "abnormal" blood counts may miss significant effects. Therefore, blood counts that decrease over time while staying in the normal range need particular attention.

Another challenging problem in workplace surveillance is the detection of a slight decrease in the mean blood count of an entire exposed population—for example, a decrease in mean white blood cell count from 7,500 to 7,000 per cubic millimeter because of a widespread exposure to benzene or ionizing radiation. Detection and appropriate evaluation of any such observation requires metic-ulous attention to standardization of laboratory test procedures, the availability of an appropriate control group, and careful statistical analysis.

REFERENCES

1. Wintrobe MM, Lee GR, Boggs DR et al. Clinical Hematology. Philadelphia: Lea & Febiger, 1981.
2. Williams WJ, Beutler E, Erslev AJ et al. Hematology. New York: McGraw-Hill, 1983.
3. Laskin S, Goldstein BD, eds. Benzene toxicity: a critical evaluation. J Toxicol Environ Health [Suppl 2], 1977.
4. Rinsky RA, Smith AB, Hornug R et al. Benzene and leukemia. An epidemiologic risk assessment. N Engl J Med 1987; 1044–50.
5. Ishimaru T, Okada H, Tomiyasu T et al. Occupational factors in the epidemiology of leukemia in Hiroshima and Nagasaki. Am J Epidemiol 1971; 93:157–65.
6. Goldstein BD. Clinical hematotoxicity of benzene. In: Carcinogenicity and toxicity of benzene. Princeton, NJ: Princeton Scientific, 1983: 51–61. Vol. 4.
7. Hernberg S, Savilahti M, Ahlman K et al. Prognostic aspects of benzene poisoning. Br J Ind Med 1966; 23:204.
8. Sheikh K. Exposure to electromagnetic fields and the risk of leukemia. Arch Environ Health 1986; 41:56–63.
9. Blair A, White DW. Leukemia cell types and agricultural practices in Nebraska. Arch Environ Health 1985; 40:211–4.
10. Hogstedt C, Aringer L, Gustavsson A. Epidemiologic support for ethylene oxide as a cancer-causing agent. JAMA 1986; 255:1575–8.
11. National Academy of Sciences, Committee on Medical and Biologic Effects of Environmental Pollutants. Carbon monoxide: effects on man and animals. Washington, DC.: NAS 1977: 68–167. Ch. 3.
12. Smith RP. Toxic responses of the blood. In: Casarett and Doull's Toxicology: the basic science of poisons, 3rd ed. New York: MacMillan, 1986.
13. Fowler BA, Wiessberg JB. Arsine poisoning. N Engl J Med 1974; 291:1171–4.
14. Parish GG, Glass R, Kimbrough R. Acute arsine poisoning in two workers cleaning a clogged drain. Arch Environ Health 1979; 34:224–7.
15. U.S. Department of Labor, Occupational Safety and Health Administration. Occupational exposure to lead: final standard. Federal Register

43(220):52952-53014 and 43(225):54353-54616, 1978; 46(238):60758-60776, 1981.

16. Lamola AA, Joselow M, Yamane T. Zinc proto-porphyrin (ZPP): a simple, sensitive, fluorometric screening test for lead poisoning. Clin Chem 1975; 21:93–7.

17. Fischbein A, Thornton JC, Lilis R et al. Zinc protoporphyrin, blood lead and clinical symptoms in two occupational groups with low-level exposure to lead. Am J Ind Med 1980; 1:391–399.

18. Lilis R, Fischbein A. Chelaton therapy in workers exposed to lead. JAMA 1976; 235:2823–4.

19. Amoruso MA, Ryer J, Easton D et al. Estimation of risk of glucose 6-phosphate dehydrogenase-deficient red cells to ozone and nitrogen dioxide. J Occup Med 1986; 28:473–9.

BIBLIOGRAPHY

Cullen MR, Robins JM, Eskenazi B. Adult inorganic lead intoxication: presentation of 31 new cases and a review of recent advances in the literature. Medicine 1983; 62:221–47.

A clinically oriented review with a good perspective on what is relevant.

Lilis R, Fischbein A, Eisinger J et al. Prevalence of lead disease among secondary lead smelter workers and biological indicators of lead exposure. Environ Res 1977; 14:255–85.

A complete clinical and laboratory evaluation of a cohort of highly exposed workers that clearly describes the relationship between ZPP, blood lead, and clinical findings.

Linet MS. The leukemias: epidemiological aspects. New York: Oxford University Press, 1985.

An excellent in-depth review of the epidemiology of leukemia. Contains valuable summary tables. The approach to the existing literature is both informative and critical.

Nielsen B. Arsine poisoning in a metal refining plant: fourteen simultaneous cases. Acta Med Scand [Suppl 496], 1969.

Contains five papers describing various aspects of an episode of arsine poisoning at a metal refining plant, including industrial hygiene studies, the clinical picture, and examination of the renal circulation in affected individuals.

29
Hepatic Disorders

Glenn S. Pransky

More than 100 chemicals are known to be toxic to the human liver, and many of these are frequently encountered in the workplace. Usually, hepatotoxicity of a particular substance has not been recognized until acute liver disease followed occupational exposure. Similar hepatotoxic effects can often be easily reproduced in laboratory animals. These investigations provide a method for predicting whether a new chemical is likely to cause acute hepatitis (but not chronic liver disease). As a result of substitution with less hepatotoxic alternatives and improved exposure control, the incidence of acute occupational hepatitis has decreased considerably.

In contrast to acute liver disease, causes of chronic liver diseases are much more difficult to determine. Animal models that allow prediction of effects after many years of low-level exposure do not exist. Although most cases are due to nonoccupational causes, such as alcohol, viral hepatitis, or autoimmune disease, epidemiologic studies have shown higher rates of hepatic carcinoma and cirrhosis in certain occupational groups, including rubber manufacturers and smelter workers. The specific etiologic chemical in these situations is often unknown.

Reports of industrial and experimental effects implicate haloalkanes (such as carbon tetrachloride), haloaromatics (such as polychlorinated biphenyls [PCBs]), azo dyes, nitrosamines, and nitroaromatics (such as dinitrobenzene) as types of organic compounds that are frequently hepatotoxic. Variation in toxicity exists within each class; for example, haloalkane toxicity increases as the number of atoms per molecule decreases, the number of halogen atoms increases, and the atomic weight of the halogen increases. Realization of these relationships has led to replacement, where possible, of the industrial solvents carbon tetrachloride (CCl_4) and tetrachloroethane ($C_2H_2Cl_4$) with methylene dichloride (CH_2Cl_2) and trichloroethylene (C_2HCl_3), which has substantially reduced the incidence of haloalkane-induced hepatotoxicity. Inorganic toxins include antimony, arsine, chromium, iodine, phosphorus, thallium, and thorium.

HIGH-RISK OCCUPATIONS

Occupations with exposure to hepatotoxins are found in many different industries including munitions, rubber, cosmetics, perfume, food processing, refrigeration, paint, insecticide and herbicide, pharmaceutical, plastics, and synthetic chemicals. Usually these workers are exposed by inhalation of fumes. Most hepatotoxins have pungent odors that warn of their presence, preventing accidental oral ingestion of large amounts; however, ingestion of imperceptible amounts of hepatotoxins over long periods of time may cause injury. Skin absorption has been a significant cause of disease only with TNT exposure in munitions workers and with methylenedianiline exposure in epoxy resin workers.

Table 29-1 indicates the effects and typical work exposures of several toxic chemicals; Table 29-2 lists some occupations with exposures to hepatotoxic chemicals.

457

Table 29-1. Some causes of occupational liver disease

Disease produced	Type of agent	Example	Types of workers exposed
ACUTE HEPATITIS			
Acute toxic hepatitis	Chlorinated hydrocarbons	Carbon tetrachloride Chloroform	Solvent workers, degreasers, cleaners, refrigeration workers
	Nitroaromatics	Dinitrophenol (DNP)	Chemical indicator workers
		Dinitrobenzene	Dye workers, explosives workers
	Ether	Dioxin	Herbicide workers, insecticide workers
	Halogenated aromatics	Polychlorinated biphenyls (PCBs)	Electrical component assemblers
		DDT	Insecticide workers, fumigators, disinfectant workers
		Chlordecone (Kepone)	
		Chlorobenzenes	Solvent workers, dye workers
		Halothane	Anesthesiologists
Acute cholestatic hepatitis	Epoxy resin	Methylenedianiline	Rubber workers, epoxy workers, synthetic fabric workers
	Inorganic element	Yellow phosphorus	Pyrotechnics workers
Acute viral hepatitis, type B	Virus	Hepatitis B	Health care workers (see Chap. 19)
Subacute hepatic necrosis	Nitroaromatic	TNT	Munitions workers
CHRONIC LIVER DISEASE			
Fibrosis/cirrhosis	Alcohol	Ethyl alcohol	Imbibing bartenders, wine producers, whiskey producers
	Virus	Hepatitis A, B, or non-A, non-B	Day-care workers, health care workers (see Chap. 19)
	Inorganic element	Arsenic	Vintners, smelter workers
	Haloalkene	Vinyl chloride	Vinyl chloride workers
Angiosarcoma	Haloalkene	Vinyl chloride	Vinyl chloride workers
Biliary tree carcinoma	Unknown agents	—	Rubber workers

PATHOPHYSIOLOGY

Most agents cause liver disease only after activation by hepatic enzymes. The liver performs two types of reactions on foreign compounds to enhance their removal from the body: *conjugations* (additions of side chains to increase water solubility) and *degradations* (oxidation, reduction, and hydration) (see Chap. 14). Degradation reactions may activate hepatotoxins into unstable intermediates capable of damaging hepatocytes; these reactions are chiefly responsible for toxic injury to the liver. In the metabolism of vinyl chloride (Fig. 29-1), for example, it is the unstable epoxide that is presumed to be responsible for the carcinogenicity of the chemical; another intermediate, the aldehyde, may cause acute hepatotoxicity. Some agents, such as halothane, affect only a small percentage of those exposed. These chemicals are probably metabolized to intermediates that may cause autoimmune hepatotoxicity in sensitized individuals.

Inducing agents are factors that increase levels

Table 29-2. Examples of occupations with exposure to hepatotoxic chemicals

Airplane hangar employees	Leather workers
Airplane pilots (insecticides)	Linoleum makers
Boat builders (styrene)	Nurses (chemotherapeutic drugs)
Cement (rubber, plastic) workers	Painters, paint makers
Chemical industry workers	Paint remover makers and users
Chemists	Paraffin workers
Cobblers	Perfume makers
Degreasers	Petroleum refiners
Dry cleaners	Pharmaceutical workers
Dye workers	Photographic material workers
Electrical transformer and condenser makers	Polish (metal) makers and users
Electroplaters	Printers
Enamel makers and enamelers	Pyroxylen-plastics workers
Extractors, oils and fats	Rayon makers
Fire extinguisher makers	Refrigerator workers
Galvanizers	Resin (synthetic) makers
Garage workers	Rubber workers
Gardeners (insecticides)	Scourers (metal)
Gas (illuminating) workers	Shoe factory workers
Glass (safety) makers	Soap makers
Glue workers	Straw hat makers
Ink makers	Thermometer makers
Insecticide makers	Varnish workers
Insulators (wire)	Waterproofers
Lacquer makers and lacquerers	

Source: HJ Zimmerman. Hepatotoxicity: the adverse effects of drugs and other chemicals on the liver. New York: Appleton-Century-Crofts, 1978. P. 307.

of degrading enzymes and thus enhance production of toxins. In small doses, most hepatotoxins are themselves inducing agents; other factors that induce enzymes are DDT and phenobarbital, high-protein diets, and fasting. Variations in thyroid and adrenal hormones may increase enzyme levels. Similar enzyme alterations from alcohol ingestion make heavy drinkers more susceptible than others to chlorinated hydrocarbon exposure. Also, hepatotoxin exposure may significantly alter drug and hormone metabolism

CLASSES OF OCCUPATIONAL LIVER DISEASE

Practically any type of liver disease can be caused by an occupational exposure. To the physician, these illnesses appear as either (1) acute hepatitis occurring soon after exposure, or (2) chronic liver disease becoming clinically evident after years of exposure.

Workplace exposures can cause liver disease in a variety of ways. Although true incidence is difficult to determine, the most common occupational liver disease in the United States is believed to be viral hepatitis, type B (see Chap. 19). Chemicals at work may contribute to liver disease by intensifying the effects of nonoccupational agents, such as viruses and alcohol. Several drugs, notably isoniazid (INH), phenobarbital, phenytoin, cytotoxic agents, androgens, and estrogens, may enhance the effects of workplace hepatotoxins by enzyme induction or by subclinical liver damage. Exposure to low levels of several different hepatotoxic agents in the workplace may cause much more toxicity than equivalent levels of a single agent. As clinical, laboratory, and pathologic features rarely implicate a specific chemical etiology, the relative importance of specific occupational and nonoccupational factors in an individual case can be difficult to determine.

Acute Hepatitis

The incidence of acute toxic hepatitis has declined as many compounds found to be responsible have been replaced with less hepatotoxic substitutes. The few cases still reported are usually caused by accidental inhalation of chemical fumes known to be hepatotoxic. The symptoms are similar to some of those of acute viral hepatitis (headache, dizziness, drowsiness, nausea, and vomiting), but they begin 12 to 48 hours after exposure, and patients

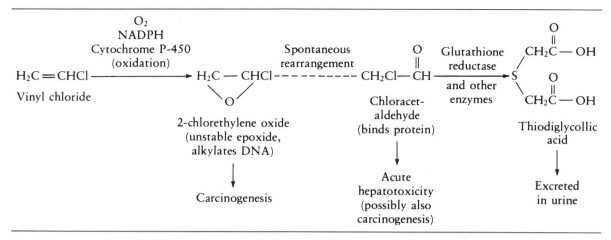

Fig. 29-1. Metabolism of vinyl chloride. (From T Green, DE Hathaway. The chemistry and biogenesis of S-containing metabolites of vinyl chloride interactions. Chem Biol Interact 1977; 17:137.)

remain afebrile. A history of exposure and appropriate liver function tests are sufficient to diagnose acute toxic hepatitis. Examination of liver tissue reveals zonal, massive, or submassive necrosis, often with fatty infiltration; jaundice and hepatomegaly are evident on physical exam. Patients usually recover within 4 to 6 weeks. Complications and death occur infrequently and are most often associated with extrahepatic diseases such as renal failure, which can result from the liver dysfunction or from direct toxicity of the substance to other organs.

The following case is typical of acute toxic hepatitis:

A 39-year-old man was exposed to high levels of carbon tetrachloride fumes when the ventilating system malfunctioned at the degreasing plant where he worked. Immediately after the exposure, he felt lightheaded and weak but was better several hours later. He noticed that his appetite was decreased the next day and presented to a physician complaining of increasing malaise.

Physical exam was normal, except for a tender liver edge palpable 4 fingerbreadths below the costal margin and minimal abdominal distension. Laboratory tests revealed a total serum bilirubin of 2.2 mg per deciliter, SGOT 1100, LDH 980, and a normal alkaline phosphatase.

The patient was unable to eat for the next 3 days at home and noticed dark urine for 5 days after this visit. He was able to slowly return to a normal diet over the next week but still felt generally weak 1 month later; follow-up exam then revealed a normal-sized liver and normal liver function tests.

Dinitrophenol and methylenedianiline cause acute cholestatic hepatitis, which begins with fever, chills, and pruritus, in addition to the usual symptoms of acute toxic hepatitis. If the initial injury to the liver is severe, it can be rapidly fatal. However, the liver damage associated with this disease is usually less extensive than that seen in acute toxic hepatitis, and most patients will recover within several days.

A variant of acute toxic hepatitis known as subacute hepatic necrosis is seen after months of exposure to TNT, PCBs, and tetrachloroethane. After weeks of skin, gastrointestinal, and neurologic complaints, symptoms of acute toxic hepatitis appear. Unlike acute toxic hepatitis, however, this variant may cause cirrhosis in survivors.

Chronic Liver Disease
Prolonged, often asymptomatic, exposure to toxic agents can lead to chronic liver disease, which is

usually manifest as cirrhosis or cancer. Because of the prolonged latency period (onset of symptoms 10–30 years after first exposure), the etiologic link to a specific agent is difficult to establish, and workers can be exposed for years before a compound is recognized to be toxic. For example, before the association between vinyl chloride exposure and liver angiosarcoma was recognized, an estimated 1 million workers were occupationally exposed to this chemical. Arsenic and thorium dioxide, as well as vinyl chloride, have been associated with hepatic angiosarcoma.

The following is a case history of angiosarcoma in a vinyl chloride worker. Three cases of this rare tumor occurred within 3 years at a plant that manufactured polyvinyl chloride (PVC). The physician and director of environmental health at the plant noticed this cluster of cases and discovered that they were associated with vinyl chloride exposure.

A 36-year-old white man was admitted to the hospital because of tarry stools. He worked for 15 years as a chemical helper and autoclave cleaner in the manufacture of polyvinyl chloride (Fig. 29-2) from vinyl chloride monomer. Past history was unremarkable. Physical examination was notable for pallor and black stools. Liver and spleen were not palpable. Although an upper GI series was interpreted as normal, a tentative diagnosis was made of a bleeding duodenal ulcer. Four months later, he was readmitted for persistently tarry stools. At this time his liver and spleen were palpable. Liver function tests were only slightly abnormal. A barium swallow test suggested esophageal varices. A liver scan was interpreted as being compatible with a large lesion of the left lobe, extending into the right lobe.

An exploratory laparotomy revealed marked enlargement of the liver and spleen, with the liver adherent to the anterior surface of the stomach. A biopsy of the liver revealed angiosarcoma.

The patient was treated with radiotherapy and chemotherapy. He was able to return to work for a short time. Twenty months after his first hospitalization he died [1].

This report, with several associated cases, was published in 1974 and immediately generated a

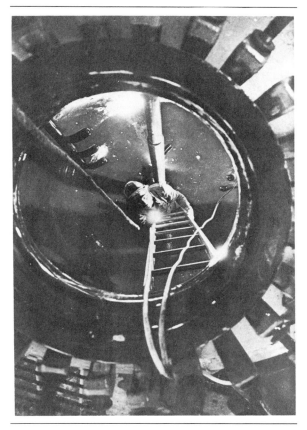

Fig. 29-2. Worker inspecting vinyl chloride polymerization chamber after cleaning. (From HF Mark, the Editors of Life. LIFE SCIENCE LIBRARY/Giant Molecules. Photograph by Gordon Tenney. Time-Life Books Inc. Publisher. © 1966 Time Inc.)

multinational epidemiologic investigation of cancer mortality in vinyl chloride plants. A high incidence of cancer, including angiosarcoma, was revealed.

Chronic exposures to most agents that cause acute hepatitis have not been associated with chronic liver disease, partly due to the lack of clinical features that would distinguish occupational from nonoccupational chronic liver disease and to the high incidence of chronic liver disease in the nonexposed population. Therefore, a causal relationship in any individual between work exposure and later development of cirrhosis or cancer is difficult to prove. Only by study of groups of exposed workers can it be proven that a substance causes chronic liver disease.

An abnormally high incidence of chronic liver disease has also been reported in refrigeration engineers, chemists, dry cleaners, rubber manufacturers, and workers exposed to tetrachloroethane and plutonium. Hepatocellular carcinoma (malignant hepatoma) in humans has not yet been clearly associated with occupational exposures.

Chronic liver disease is often first recognized when portal hypertension appears. Liver biopsy may show cirrhosis, but in the case of arsenic and vinyl chloride exposures, subcapsular or diffuse fibrosis and angiosarcoma may be found. In advanced cases severe hepatic dysfunction is typical. Prognosis is poor, with 75 percent mortality within 5 years. Even then the value of such medical monitoring is not proved.

TOOLS FOR DIAGNOSIS

Certain tests, developed for use in the diagnosis of patients with liver disease, have been used to screen workers with potentially hepatotoxic exposures. Most detect subtle liver damage by measuring serum liver enzymes or hepatic clearance of metabolites from blood and are good for confirming acute symptomatic liver disease. Unfortunately, these tests are not very sensitive for detection of early abnormalities in liver function (before symptoms appear) and are rarely specific for chemically-induced liver disease (see Chap 6). Typically, the occupational physician is faced with an asymptomatic worker who is exposed to a variety of potential hepatotoxins at work, drinks alcohol, and has abnormal liver enzymes on routine blood testing. A careful exposure history, review of alcohol intake, observations in coworkers, and follow-up after removal from exposure are necessary to distinguish between occupational and nonoccupational disease.

In subclinical chronic liver disease, abnormal values usually appear only after permanent damage has taken place. As the latency period of chronic liver disease may be several decades, periodic liver tests must be performed for many years after exposure has ceased to enable early detection of disease progression. Research has focused on the development of tests to enable detection of changes before they become irreversible. Unfortunately, no single test can sensitively detect change in the four major functional areas of the liver: detoxification/metabolic, reticuloendothelial/phagocytic, biliary excretion, and vascular.

Two screening tests for chronic liver disease show some promise. Levels of serum gammaglutamyl transpeptidase (GGTP), used to screen styrene workers, have shown good correlation with the extent of toxic exposure and the amount of hepatocellular damage. A group of vinyl chloride workers is being monitored by the indocyanine green excretion test, which measures the ability of the liver to take up and excrete this substance; the test has often detected vinyl chloride-induced liver disease when other tests were normal. Further development of such tests and proof of their effectiveness is necessary before advocating their widespread use for screening purposes.

A few tests are available that can help quantify the amount of previous exposure to a hepatotoxin. These include tests that can detect arsenic, vinyl chloride, and carbon tetrachloride metabolites in urine and can determine exposure levels to solvents in workplace air. Some tests are inexpensive, give reasonably quantitative results, and help assure that hepatotoxin exposure is within acceptable limits. However, the distinction between etiologies of liver disease is rarely clear, and it may become necessary to insist on removing the affected worker from all potentially hepatotoxic medications and exposures and to follow the individual with periodic tests of liver function.

MANAGEMENT AND PREVENTION

The management of occupational liver disease is identical to that of nonoccupational liver disease.

A multifaceted approach, with emphasis on recognition of hazards and use of environmental controls, is needed to prevent occupational liver disease. Work situations should be designed to minimize direct employee contact with hepatotoxins. Preplacement screening should focus on the identification of factors such as alcohol or barbiturate abuse that could make the worker particularly susceptible to the effects of hepatotoxic exposure. Those who work with potentially hepatotoxic substances should have periodic liver function tests. The appearance of confirmed abnormalities should initiate a careful investigation of the workplace, removing the affected worker from further exposure until the cause is identified and controlled. A worker with occupationally related liver disease should not return to the original job unless the substance is removed or adequate environmental control of it is established. Epidemiologic and laboratory studies to identify hepatotoxins should be given high priority. Substances capable of producing chronic hepatic disease can be identified by long-term epidemiologic studies only if age, alcohol intake, life-style, diet, and nonoccupational liver disease are carefully controlled.

REFERENCE

1. Creech JL, Johnson MN. Angiosarcoma of the liver in the manufacture of vinyl chloride. J Occup Med 1974; 16:150.

BIBLIOGRAPHY

Zimmerman HJ. Hepatotoxicity. New York: Appleton, 1978:597.

Schiff L. Diseases of the liver. 6th ed. Philadelphia: Lippincott, 1987.

Tamburro CH. Chemical hepatitis. Med Clin N Am 1979; 63:545.

Excellent general references. Zimmerman's book is listed first because it is a comprehensive source on hepatotoxicity due to chemicals and drugs (it includes chapters on occupational and environmental liver toxicity). Schiff's book is an exhaustive reference on liver disease, with detailed information on management, toxic hepatitis, and cirrhosis. Tamburro's article, an overview of hepatotoxic chemicals, contains examples of liver biopsies of each type of toxic liver injury, as well as a detailed description of the indocyanine green clearance test.

Dossing M, Skinhoj P. Occupational liver injury: present state of knowledge and future perspective. Int Arch Occup Environ Health 1985; 56:1.

An excellent review of the state-of-the-art and controversies in identification of occupational hepatotoxins.

Popper H et al. Environmental hepatic injury in man. In: Popper H, Schaffner F, eds. Progress in liver disease. New York: Grune & Stratton, 1979: 605–38.

A current and thorough overview of occupational and other environmental liver disease, with attention to mechanisms and experimental data. Good review of vinyl chloride problem.

Selikoff IJ, Hammond EC, eds. Toxicity of vinyl chloride-polyvinyl chloride. Ann N Y Acad Sci 1975; 246.

Several hundred pages by various authors on experimental, clinical, and epidemiologic data on vinyl chloride carcinogenesis.

Tamburro CH, Liss GM. Tests for hepatotoxicity: usefulness in screening workers. J Occup Med 1986; 28:1034.

A thorough review of various tests for screening exposed workers for early signs of hepatotoxicity.

30
Renal and Urinary Tract Disorders

Ruth Lilis and Philip J. Landrigan

Acute and chronic kidney failure are major causes of illness and death in the United States. Approximately 75,000 Americans suffer from end-stage renal disease (ESRD), and each year approximately 4,000 new cases are reported, for an annual incidence in the United States of about 50 cases per million [1]. The total cost of medical care of ESRD patients in 1982 was about $2.2 billion.

The proportion of ESRD that may be caused by occupational exposures is not known. However, a large number of known and suspected nephrotoxins are used in American industry (Table 30-1). The National Institute for Occupational Safety and Health (NIOSH) estimates that the number of workers with potential exposure to these compounds is 4 million.

For most cases of ESRD, no etiologic information is available. Several factors account for this absence of information. Exposures to nephrotoxins frequently go unnoticed. Few renal toxins produce easily recognizable acute syndromes; instead they produce chronic disease after many years of exposure [2, 3]. Because the kidneys have great reserve capacity and can function adequately despite progressive loss of nephrons, work-related kidney disease is typically not diagnosed until considerable dysfunction has occurred. By that time, the specific signatures of certain toxins, such as the intranuclear inclusion bodies of lead intoxication, have disappeared. On biopsy or postmortem examination, tissue specimens from most patients with ESRD look very much alike; regardless of etiology, they are characterized by nonspecific glo-

merulosclerosis, tubular dilation, and chronic interstitial inflammatory and fibrotic changes. Thus, histopathologic diagnosis of occupationally induced ESRD is seldom possible.

Societal and institutional factors also contribute to this failure of etiologic diagnosis. The Social Security Administration, to which ESRD cases are reported, has no requirement for collection of etiologic data. Furthermore, few physicians are trained adequately in occupational medicine or are competent to obtain a detailed history of past occupational exposures to nephrotoxins.

The kidney is a target organ for a number of toxic chemical compounds.

Renal excretion is the major route of elimination for many toxic compounds. The relatively high renal blood flow, about one-fourth of total cardiac output, exposes the renal structures to a relatively high toxic burden. Concentration of toxins in the glomerular ultrafiltrate through active reabsorption contributes further to the intensity of toxic exposures. The considerable endothelial surface represented by the extensive capillary network in the kidney, the presence in renal tubular cells of numerous important enzyme systems, the local synthesis of active peptides (for example, renin and prostaglandin), and the generally high metabolic rate of the organ are additional factors increasing the vulnerability of the kidneys to chemical toxins. These agents can adversely affect the delicate balance between blood flow, glomerular filtration, tubular reabsorption, and filtrate concentration.

465

Table 30-1. Estimated numbers of workers in the United States with potential occupational exposures* to proven or suspected nephrotoxins, 1971–1972

Substance	Nephrotoxicity	Estimated numbers of workers in the United States with potential exposure
Lead	Proven	615,000
Cadmium	Proven	52,000
Inorganic mercury	Proven	38,000
Uranium	Proven	1,000
Solvents	Suspected	3,373,000
Arsenic (including arsine)	Proven	6,000
Pesticides	Suspected	16,000
Beryllium	Suspected	11,000

*The phrase *potential occupational exposure* derives from the NIOSH National Occupational Hazard Survey, in which occupational groups are related to chemical exposures.

ACUTE AND CHRONIC RENAL EFFECTS OF OCCUPATIONAL AND ENVIRONMENTAL AGENTS

Acute nephropathies are the result of severe, usually short-term overexposures to toxic chemicals. These compounds can injure the kidney either directly, due to their intrinsic nephrotoxic effects, or indirectly as the result of systemic, prerenal toxic effects. Simultaneous toxicity to other organs, such as the liver, brain, and lungs, can occur, complicating clinical presentation and therapeutic management.

Pathogenic mechanisms in acute nephropathies are complex. Impaired glomerular filtration is frequently the prime abnormality and aberrant tubular reabsorption can be a secondary event. Tubular necrosis is often found and usually results in nonselective and almost complete reabsorption of glomerular filtrate. Increased renin production in the juxtaglomerular apparatus and disturbances in renal prostaglandin synthesis have also been documented. Reduction of renocortical blood flow and development of arterial and arteriolar vasoconstriction are thought to be major mechanisms in acute nephropathies of toxic etiology [4].

Sudden marked renal ischemia is an additional important causal mechanism resulting in acute nephropathies. It can occur as a result of systemic hypotension (due to dehydration, diarrhea, and shock) or massive hemolysis. Less frequently, physical agents, such as extreme heat (especially with concomitant extreme physical exercise), crush injuries, or high-voltage electrical injuries (resulting in muscle necrosis—rhabdomyolysis), can lead to acute post-traumatic renal failure.

Chronic nephrotoxicity due to occupational or environmental exposure has been associated with long-term exposure and absorption. The mechanisms of certain chemical compounds leading to chronic nephropathies have not been completely elucidated even for etiologic agents that have long been known to result in renal function impairment, such as lead. Functional tubular cell damage can remain subclinical for years; glomerular function impairment, either secondary to capillary lesions or due to direct toxic effects on glomerular cellular structures, can occur simultaneously with the slight and slowly progressing tubular injury; the result of this sequence of events is slow reduction in the number of functional nephrons, often with concomitant development of interstitial fibrotic changes. This process can continue and remain subclinical for years, until it reaches the critical level of nonfunctional nephrons, with resulting renal insufficiency, as expressed in significant reduction of glomerular filtration rate (creatinine clearance) and increase in blood urea nitrogen (BUN) and creatinine. In chronic cadmium nephropathy with proximal tubular dysfunction and proteinuria (distinguished by increased excretion of low molecular weight proteins), glomerular impairment may develop after long-lasting cadmium absorption.

More recently immunologic mechanisms have been found to be involved in the development of solvent-related glomerulopathies. Antibodies to solvent-altered basement membranes have been demonstrated and autoimmune glomerulonephritis has been found to occur more often in persons exposed to solvents. This area is being actively investigated.

Nephrotoxicity of Metals

Mercury. Mercury nephrotoxicity may follow accidental or intentional ingestion of mercuric salts; acute tubular injury and even tubular necrosis can result. Such severe nephrotoxicity is extremely unusual in occupational or environmental mercury poisoning.

Under present day circumstances of occupational or environmental exposure, the nephrotoxicity of mercury is usually limited to a moderate proximal tubular dysfunction; the clinical correlate is low-grade proteinuria. More sensitive tests have recently been introduced, such as measurements of urinary enzymes, including N-acetyl-beta-D-glucosaminidase (NAG), to assess early renal tubular dysfunction in mercury-exposed workers [5]. Another recently studied sensitive indicator of impaired renal function in mercury-exposed persons is urinary excretion of beta-galactosidase. Glomerular injury, due to toxic effects mediated by an autoimmune reaction, with formation of autoantibodies against glomerular structures has been reported in animal experiments [4]. Glomerular injury seldom has been described in humans. A few cases of nephrotic syndrome in mercury workers have been reported; recently case reports have documented glomerular lesions mediated by immunologic mechanisms [6].

Lead. The acute toxic effects of lead on the kidney are characterized by proximal tubular dysfunction and formation of intranuclear inclusion bodies composed of a lead-protein complex [7]. Mitochondrial abnormalities, related to impairment of cellular respiration and phosphorylation, are present in the proximal tubular cells. Aminoaciduria, glucosuria, and hyperphosphaturia (Fanconi's syndrome) [8] are characteristic clinical features of acute lead nephropathy. Renal tubular dysfunction is frequently present in acute episodes of childhood lead poisoning (mostly due to ingestion of lead-based paint). Acute lead poisoning in adults, due to occupational lead exposure, is exceedingly rare today in industrialized countries. The incidence in developing countries is not known.

Chronic lead nephropathy was well documented in the early decades of this century when heavy occupational lead exposure was widespread and severe lead poisoning was frequent. Progressive renal damage eventually resulting in renal failure (Bright's disease) was common in lead-exposed workers [9, 10].

With relatively less heavy lead exposure, there is a slow deterioration of renal function, with progressive reduction in renal blood flow and glomerular filtration rate. Increases in serum creatinine, BUN, and in some cases uric acid can occur [11, 12]. This chronic deterioration in function is more marked with higher lead exposure. Thus, a dose-response effect has been shown to exist [13].

A 61-year-old black man was examined during a clinical field survey of secondary lead smelter workers. He appeared to be chronically ill and complained of marked fatigue, weakness, muscle pain, loss of appetite, weight loss, frequent headache, and some deterioration of his memory. He had been employed at the same facility for 34 years. He had been repeatedly tested for blood lead levels; over the last several years of his employment, a blood lead test had been mandatory every 2 months. The patient's statement was that his blood lead level had been "always high." Also noteworthy was the fact that he had been treated with more than five courses of chelation therapy over the years. This fact confirmed that the blood lead levels had been significantly elevated. On repeated occasions, he had been removed from his work because of high blood lead levels. The last such episode was in 1970. The past medical history was negative for other diseases.

In February 1973, the patient had been examined by his physician whose help he sought because of tiredness, muscle pain, abdominal pain, constipation, and weight loss. Because of the intensity and persistence of these symptoms, he had to be admitted to a hospital. The blood lead level was found to be elevated, at 83 μg per dl. Slight anemia (hemoglobin 13.1 gm/dl), a finding not unusual for lead poisoning, was also present. Kidney impairment was indicated by an elevated BUN (25 mg/dl), coarse granular casts in the urine, and an elevated serum uric acid (8.3 mg/dl and 8.9 mg/dl). Chelation therapy with penicillamine 500 mg 4 times a day was started and relieved most of the symptoms. Ten months after this episode an elevated serum creatinine level (2.1 and 2.2 mg/dl) and uric acid (8.9 mg/dl) were again found. The creatinine clearance was markedly reduced to 43 ml per 1.73 square meters (normal is 80–140 ml). This marked reduction in the glomerular filtration rate indicated renal insufficiency. A repeated creatinine clearance test again showed a much depressed value of 35 ml. The blood lead level was 60 μg per dl, although the patient had discontinued his lead exposure for months.

The renal pathology in chronic lead nephropathy can affect all structures of the nephron. Glomerular obsolescence, periglomerular fibrosis, and diffuse damage to proximal tubules have been observed. With progressive renal insufficiency, interstitial fibrosis and loss of glomeruli are the most marked abnormalities, together with arteriolar endothelial proliferation [12].

Heavy environmental exposure of children to lead in Queensland, Australia, earlier in this century resulted in endemic childhood lead poisoning. Subsequently, endemic nephropathy with clinically overt renal failure was detected in numerous young and middle-aged adults in Queensland. A high lead body burden, demonstrated by positive EDTA chelation, (urinary lead excretion exceeding 600 μg per 24 hours after administration of 1 g EDTA) confirmed lead as the etiologic agent [14].

Other environmental lead exposure that has resulted in renal functional impairment has been chronic ingestion of drinking water with high lead content (in excess of 100 μg/liter). Chronic consumption of lead-contaminated "moonshine" whiskey has also been reported to produce severe lead poisoning including "saturnine gout."

Mortality studies of lead-exposed workers indicate excess death rates from chronic nephritis and from "other renal sclerosis," as well as "other hypertensive disease" (other than essential hypertension) [15, 16]. While this pattern of mortality reflects previous high lead exposure in certain industrial plants, the effects of recent lower-level occupational and environmental exposures are still not completely assessed. A no-effect level for lead with regard to renal function has not been established.

Cadmium. Acute high-dose overexposure to cadmium compounds, especially cadmium oxide fumes, has been reported to result from welding, soldering, and cutting cadmium metal and cadmium-containing alloys [17]. The major target organ under such circumstances is the lung, and severe, sometimes fatal chemical pneumonitis is the major clinical manifestation. In some of these cases, renal lesions, mainly affecting the tubular epithelium have been observed [8]. Marked proteinuria occurs. Bilateral renal cortical necrosis has been reported [18].

Chronic renal toxicity due to long-term exposure is the best-documented adverse health effect due to cadmium. It has been confirmed in numerous studies, in both humans and in experimental animals. It has been found under circumstances of both occupational and environmental exposure.

Increased urinary excretion of low molecular weight proteins is the most outstanding feature of chronic cadmium nephropathy [19]. Cadmium oxide fume or dust, cadmium sulfide, and cadmium stearate have all been found to be nephrotoxic and to produce proteinuria under conditions of long-term exposure. The low molecular weight protein-uria is characterized by increased excretion of beta-2 microglobulin (on which a sensitive test for biological monitoring is based), muramidase, ribonuclease, orosomucoid, transferrin, and retinol-binding protein. Recently, retinol-binding protein has also been used for biological monitoring; a sensitive and accurate radioimmunoassay has been developed.

Other features of proximal tubular dysfunction such as aminoaciduria and glycosuria have been found in some cases of cadmium nephropathy. Increased urinary levels of NAG, an enzyme abundant in renal tubular cells and released into the urine during tubular cell damage, have been reported.

Glomerular dysfunction, with significantly increased urinary albumin loss, decreased glomerular filtration rate (GFR) and increased serum creatinine levels has been documented in persons with longstanding cadmium nephrotoxicity [20]. Cadmium nephropathy, nevertheless, rarely results in chronic renal failure in humans.

The mechanism of cadmium nephrotoxicity is attributed to slow accumulation of cadmium in the kidney cortex. Cadmium in plasma is transported bound to the protein metallothionein. The cadmium-metallothionein complex is readily filtered through the glomerulus and then almost completely reabsorbed by the proximal tubular epithelium. Renal excretion of cadmium is slow and the half-life in the renal cortex is estimated to be several decades. When the concentration of cadmium in the renal cortex exceeds a certain "critical level," estimated to be in the range of 170 to 300 mg per kg, proteinuria can be detected, indicating disruption of proximal tubule reabsorption. The kidney cadmium concentration does not generally increase further after proteinuria has ensued; some of the proximal tubular cells with highest cadmium concentration are disrupted; their cadmium is lost in the urine. The critical urinary cadmium

level at which proteinuria is expected is 10 μg per gram of creatinine. When screening of cadmium-exposed workers reveals urinary excretion in excess of 10 μg per gram of creatinine, exposure must be discontinued to prevent overt clinical nephropathy.

Most studies in humans indicate that chronic cadmium nephropathy is not reversible and that proteinuria and slight decrements in glomerular function can persist and even progress for years after cessation of exposure [20].

Environmental cadmium contamination has occurred in Japan and has produced Itai-Itai (Ouch-ouch) disease in populations ingesting cadmium-contaminated rice and other foodstuffs [21]. Patterns of renal dysfunction similar to those described above have been found. In addition, osteomalacia, with pain in back and legs, especially in postmenopausal women is characteristic of this syndrome and thought to be due to the synergistic effects of dietary deficiencies and cadmium-induced disturbances in tubular reabsorption of calcium and phosphorus.

Uranium. Soluble uranium compounds are markedly nephrotoxic. Overt clinical nephropathy with proteinuria and increased BUN and serum creatinine has occurred after accidental occupational exposure to uranium hexafluoride and oxyfluoride. Restoration of function has generally occurred in such cases. Uranyl nitrate is a potent nephrotoxic agent that has been extensively used in experimental models for the study of renal tubular dysfunction [4].

Indirect Renal Effects of Potent Hemolytic Agents

Arsine. Acute arsine (AsH_3) poisoning is a severe and life-threatening occupational hazard. Arsine is a colorless gas, without irritant warning properties and is practically odorless when chemically pure. It usually is generated suddenly when metal ores or metals (such as lead, zinc, or cadmium) containing arsenic impurities come in contact with acid. Exposures also occur in the semiconductor industry, where arsine is used widely to "treat" crystals.

The major toxic effect of arsine is massive intravascular hemolysis; arsine is the most potent hemolytic agent encountered in industrial processes (see Chap. 28).

Acute nephropathy is a major manifestation of arsine poisoning. Although previously attributed to renal tubular obstruction by hemoglobin precipitates, the mechanisms of acute arsine-induced renal failure are presently thought to be due to ischemic tubular injury (secondary to sudden onset anemia and marked systemic hypotension) and also to a direct nephrotoxic effect of AsH_3 on the proximal tubular epithelium. Oliguria and anuria are the major manifestations of acute renal failure in arsine poisoning; hyperkalemia, metabolic acidosis, and increased BUN and creatinine can occur, especially in the most severe cases. Outcome is frequently fatal.

A 34-year-old chemical engineer had been working at the development of a method (pilot stage) for the extraction of cadmium from sludge. Analysis of the chemical reactions indicated that arsine could have been generated, since the mixture handled contained arsenic compounds. The patient was suddenly taken ill, with weakness, abdominal pain, unusual dizziness, and nausea. On admission, after several hours, she was markedly pale and jaundiced. Her red blood cell count fell rapidly and her bilirubin increased steadily for several days; oliguria was followed by anuria. All efforts to save this patient with acute arsine poisoning and renal failure (including dialysis), were unsuccessful; no recovery of her renal function occurred, indicating complete destruction of proximal tubular epithelium, including the basement membrane.

If a patient survives acute arsine nephropathy, urine flow returns to normal after an oliguric or anuric stage. Sometimes a polyuric stage ensues. Return of function may take many months, sometimes up to a year. Even in relatively mild cases of arsine poisoning, renal function tests indicate tubular dysfunction (due to direct nephrotoxicity of arsine) with markedly reduced concentrating capacity and reduced creatinine clearance.

Stibine and phosphine. Stibine (antimony hydride; SbH_3) and phosphine (phosphorus hydride; PH_3) produce clinical manifestations similar (although generally less severe) to those of arsine poisoning [22, 23].

SOLVENT NEPHROTOXICITY
Halogenated Aliphatic Hydrocarbons
Carbon tetrachloride (CCl_4) and chloroform ($CHCl_3$) are the best known nephrotoxic agents in this large group of chemical compounds. Dibromochloropropane (DBCP), ethylene dibromide, ethylene dichloride, hexachloro-1,3-butadiene, 1,1,2-trichloroethane, allyl chloride, trichloroethylene, and perchloroethylene are halogenated aliphatic hydrocarbons with high-volume production and numerous industrial and agricultural applications. Inadequate information on their nephrotoxicity is available, and it derives mainly from animal studies.

Acute overexposure to carbon tetrachloride or chloroform, such as with the use of carbon tetrachloride as a degreaser or in the chemical industry, can result in severe toxic nephropathy. Numerous such cases, due mostly to accidental inhalation or ingestion, have been documented. The proximal tubular epithelium is the principal target of aliphatic halogenated hydrocarbon renal injury; the severity of the lesion varies, but often includes tubular necrosis with acute oliguric or anuric renal failure. Concomitant hepatotoxicity may be a major complicating factor. Restoration of renal function generally occurs in 10 to 14 days as the tubular epithelium regenerates. In extreme cases, proximal tubular necrosis with disruption of the basement membrane precludes regeneration.

Release of halogenated aliphatic hydrocarbons into the general environment occurs through industrial effluents and emissions and also through pesticide application. Generation of low molecular weight chlorinated chemicals in surface waters, as a result of water chlorination, has also received increasing attention. Cumulative nephrotoxic effects of such long-term, low-level exposure are yet unknown [4]. Another issue of concern is the possible enhancement of halogenated hydrocarbon nephrotoxicity through concurrent absorption of chemical compounds, such as PCBs, which are inducers of mixed-function oxidases.

Diethylenedioxide (Dioxan)
Inhalation of the vapor of the pesticide dioxan can result in acute or subacute poisoning characterized by toxic effects on the central nervous system (CNS), hepatotoxicity, and nephrotoxicity [24].

Several chemically related compounds, such as ethylene glycol, diethylene glycol, ethyl diethylene glycol, and ethylene glycol diacetate, have nephrotoxic effects similar to those of dioxan. Their low vapor pressure at normal temperatures explains why no acute nephropathy from their inhalation has been reported. Accidental ingestion (particularly of ethylene glycol, a major component of antifreeze) has resulted in severe and sometimes fatal cases of neurotoxicity, toxic pulmonary edema, and nephrotoxicity.

Methanol (Methyl Alcohol)
Methyl alcohol, which has the chemical formula CH_3OH, is one of the most toxic organic solvents. Occupational exposure, with inhalation and skin contact, only rarely results in overt clinical poisoning since volatility is relatively low. Accidental ingestion, not unusual in industries where methyl alcohol is used, has resulted, however, in an important number of cases of severe poisoning, with a relatively high proportion of fatalities. Acute methyl alcohol poisoning is one of the most challenging medical emergencies; marked metabolic acidosis, neurotoxic effects with CNS depression and specific optic nerve injury, nephrotoxicity, hepatotoxicity, and injury of the pancreas can develop. In severe cases, toxic renal tubular injury can contribute significantly to fatal outcome. Correction of acidosis is important in management of such cases. Dialysis should be attempted in order to reduce methanol concentrations and allow return of renal function.

Solvent Nephropathy (Other Than Halogenated Aliphatic Hydrocarbons)
Numerous case reports have documented occurrence of glomerulonephritis with antibodies to glomerular basement membrane (anti-GM) after significant solvent exposure [25]. In case-control studies, it has been shown that a significantly higher prevalence of solvent exposure is found in patients with glomerulonephritis than in control groups. The pathophysiologic mechanism of this nephropathy is not yet clarified. It has, however, been suggested that inhaled vapors of hydrocarbon solvents may bind to the pulmonary alveolar basement membrane, resulting in the generation of an antigenic compound. Antibodies to this solvent-induced antigen may then be produced. The similar chemical structures of the alveolar and renal basement membrane makes the glomerular basement membrane vulnerable to these antibodies; thus, glomerulonephritis results. Cases of Goodpasture's syndrome as well as of acute autoimmune glomerulonephritis have been reported in persons exposed to solvents. An alternative possible pathophysiologic mechanism is that solvents may attach directly to the glomerular basement membrane, alter it, and thereby produce an antigenic compound that induces specific antibodies against the renal glomerular basement membrane. Chronic glomerulonephritis has been reported to develop following such a sequence of events. Several cohort mortality studies so far have not detected increased mortality from renal disease in solvent-exposed refinery, oil distribution, or paint and varnish workers [26].

In experimental animals, exposure to widely used mixtures of aliphatic hydrocarbons (alkanes and alkenes) has been found to result in nephrotoxic effects, primarily affecting the tubular epithelium, with clear dose-dependent severity of lesions. Reduction in urine concentrating ability and increase in urinary protein and glucose are the most frequent functional changes [27].

Carbon Disulfide. Long-term low-level exposure to carbon disulfide (CS_2) has been associated with an atherosclerosis-potentiating effect (see Chap. 27). Increased incidence of ischemic heart disease, cerebral atherosclerosis ("sulfocarbonic encephalopathy"), and vascular chronic nephropathy have been found in workers with long-term exposure. Reduced concentrating capacity is the most frequently described renal functional abnormality [28].

OCCUPATIONAL EXPOSURE AND CANCER OF THE KIDNEY AND URINARY TRACT
Renal Cancer
The possible work-relatedness of primary renal cancer has not been adequately explored. Increased numbers of deaths from primary renal tumors have been reported among workers in the petroleum industry as well as in steel workers exposed to coke oven emissions [29]. Two case reports of renal cancer in lead workers have been noted. Lead has been shown to produce renal tumors in three species of experimental animals [30].

Urinary Bladder and Urinary Tract Cancer
In the United States, the annual incidence of cancer of the bladder is 35,000 cases, and each year approximately 10,000 persons die of this neoplasm. The incidence of bladder cancer is increasing in both white and black men; mortality is stable in white men, but it is rising in black men [31].

Occupationally induced bladder cancer was first reported in 1895 among workers in Germany employed in the manufacture of synthetic aniline dyes. Subsequently, occupational bladder cancer spread worldwide following the international spread of the synthetic dyestuffs industry. The first cases of work-related bladder cancer in American chemical workers were reported in 1934.

The *aromatic amines* are the chemical compounds responsible for bladder cancer in dye workers. Carcinogenic amines in current use include benzidine, beta-napthylamine, and 4-aminobiphenyl. In some occupationally exposed groups, a very high total mortality from bladder cancer has been reported.

Exposure to aromatic amines occurs in textile, fur, and leather dyeing. Workers in those trades have been shown to absorb synthetic dyes such as Direct Black 38, Direct Brown 95, and Direct Blue 6. These dyes are metabolized to release benzidine and other aromatic amines. Benzidine is detectable in urine of workers exposed to synthetic dyes.

Aromatic amines are used also as antioxidants in rubber, and exposure to carcinogenic amines has been reported in rubber and cable manufacture. 4,4′-Methylene-bis-2-chloroaniline (MBOCA), an aromatic amine, is used as a stabilizer in plastics manufacture. MOCA is an animal carcinogen, and cases of bladder cancer have recently been reported among workers in Michigan occupationally exposed to MOCA.

The lag time between onset of occupational exposure to aromatic amines and bladder cancer ranges from 4 to over 40 years, with a mean of about 20 years. The minimum duration of exposure necessary to produce cancer is reported to be as short as 133 days.

Soots, tars, and *polycyclic aromatic hydrocarbons* including *benzo-a-pyrene,* have been shown to cause bladder cancer. Elevated risks of bladder cancer have been reported in creosote manufacture (creosote is a tar-based wood preservative) and in aluminum smelting; aluminum smelting involves heavy exposure to polycyclic aromatic hydrocarbons from carbon-graphite electrodes [31] (see Chap. 15).

Cigarette smoking has been shown to cause bladder cancer [31]. A multiplicative interaction may exist between occupational exposure to aromatic amines and cigarette smoking in the causation of bladder cancer [32].

Previously, bladder cancers resulting from occupational exposures were considered indistinguishable from nonoccupationally related bladder cancers [31]. However, it is now recognized that occupationally related bladder cancers differ in that they occur 15 years earlier on average than similar tumors in the general population. Also, occupationally induced malignancies appear more frequently to be preceded by carcinoma in situ.

Significant opportunities exist for early detection of work-related bladder cancer. Although the efficacy of early detection in curing and prolonging life of patients with bladder cancer has not yet fully been assessed, currently available data suggest that early detection may be life-saving [32]. Aggressive screening of workers at high risk for work-related bladder cancer is therefore strongly recommended. Early detection is most efficiently achieved by annual screening of workers at high risk for occult blood in urine. A positive finding of occult blood demands immediate cystoscopic examination. Evaluation of exfoliative urinary cytology (urine Papanicolaou's test) is another screening modality of promise.

OCCUPATIONAL URINARY TRACT DISEASE RESULTING FROM NEUROLOGIC IMPAIRMENT

Because the lower urinary tract is closely controlled by the autonomic nervous system, neurologic dysfunction may result in urinary tract disease. Urinary tract disease of neurologic origin is exemplified by the reported episodes of bladder paralysis in workers occupationally exposed to dimethylaminopropionitrile (DMAPN) (see Chap. 25).

DIAGNOSIS AND MANAGEMENT

A thorough exposure history is an essential prerequisite to early detection and correct diagnosis of adverse renal and urinary tract effects due to occupational or environmental hazards. It is very important that health providers be aware of a patient's occupational and environmental exposures (usual as well as accidental) and of the potentially toxic effects of those exposures, including nephrotoxic effects.

Acute nephropathy due either to direct toxicity or secondary to sudden renal ischemia always represents a serious medical emergency. It requires prompt diagnosis, intensive monitoring, and appropriate medical care. Hospital admission is an absolute necessity, since the possibility of rapidly developing acute renal failure exists. The most aggressive approach, including dialysis, might be necessary under such circumstances, and rapid intervention is crucial for a favorable outcome. In cases of severe overexposure to agents known to have potential for acute nephrotoxicity (such as metals, halogenated hydrocarbons, arsine, dioxane, ethylene glycol, or methyl alcohol), monitoring of urinary output is essential; proteinuria, and less often hematuria, are also significant alarm signals, as are rapid increases in serum creatinine, BUN, or potassium. The clinical picture is often complicated by simultaneous toxic effects on other organ systems, principally the CNS and the liver. Hemolysis is a major effect in arsine, stibine, or phosphine poisoning, and a sudden fall in the red blood cell count and hematocrit, together with increases in serum bilirubin and hemoglobin, are indicative of acute hemolysis.

Medical management of acute nephropathies caused by occupational or environmental agents is similar to that for acute severe nephropathies of other etiology. Discontinuing the hazardous exposure, and, when possible, reducing the body burden of chemical toxins are the only specific components in the management of such cases. Chelation therapy, which is effective in some metal poisonings,—for example, those due to lead, mercury, and arsenic—can rarely be used in the presence of nephrotoxicity, since most chelating agents can be nephrotoxic in large doses and could therefore compound the renal damage.

Documentation of increased urinary excretion or blood level of metals (lead, cadmium, mercury, and arsenic in the case of arsine) can significantly contribute to correct etiologic diagnosis. For acute nephropathies due to agents with a shorter half-life, identification of the etiologic agent can sometimes be made by exhaled breath analysis (for volatile solvents) soon after the accident or by detection of specific metabolites in blood or urine, or both, in the days following exposure. For example, oxalic acid is excreted in increased amounts in ethylene glycol poisoning; formic acid can be found in methyl alcohol poisoning.

Early Detection and Prevention

The recent development of sensitive tests of renal dysfunction permits earlier detection than previously was possible of nephrotoxic effects due to long-term exposure to chemical compounds. Increased excretion of high molecular weight proteins, mainly albumin, is an early indicator of glomerular dysfunction. Still under development are tests for the detection of glomerular basement membrane antigens in blood and urine or of circulating antibodies against glomerular basement membrane for monitoring of workers exposed to chemical compounds (for example, solvents) that may produce an immune-type glomerular dysfunction. Increased excretion of low molecular weight proteins, such as beta-2-microglobulin and retinol-binding protein, is a sensitive indicator for proximal tubular dysfunction. These tests have been particularly useful in the detection of chronic cadmium nephropathy.

Increased urinary enzyme excretion, due to proximal tubular cell injury, is a sensitive test for early detection of nephrotoxicity; an assay for NAG has been used in evaluation of renal injury following exposure to mercury, halogenated hydrocarbons, and cadmium. Tests for other urinary enzymes are still in the experimental stage. Decrease in concentrating capacity, reduction in glomerular filtration rate, and increase in serum creatinine and BUN are found in more advanced cases of chronic toxic nephropathies and may be used to assess the extent of functional loss.

Prevention of occupational nephropathy relies on maintaining exposure to potentially nephrotoxic agents at levels well below hazardous limits;

a safety margin is important, especially for agents for which information on a no-effect level is not yet available. Special caution is necessary for agents that have been shown to be nephrotoxic in animal studies but for which no human data are yet available.

REFERENCES

1. Sugimoto T, Rosansky SJ. The incidence of treated end stage renal disease in the eastern United States: 1973–1979. Am J Public Health. 1984; 74:14–7.
2. Landrigan PJ, Goyer RA, Clarkson TW et al. The work-relatedness of renal disease. Arch Environ Health 1984; 39:225–30.
3. Wedeen RP. Occupational renal disease: in-depth review. Am J Kidney Dis 1984; 3:241–57.
4. Hook JB, ed. Toxicology of the Kidney. New York: Raven, 1981.
5. Meyer BR, Fischbein A, Rosenman K, Lerman Y, Drayer DE, Reidenberg M. Increased urinary enzyme excretion in workers exposed to nephrotoxic chemicals. Am J Med 1984; 76(6):989–98.
6. Porter A, ed. Nephrotoxic mechanisms of drugs and environmental toxins. New York: Plenum, 1982.
7. Goyer RA, Leonard DL, Moore JF, Rhyne B, Krigman MR. Lead dosage and the role of the intranuclear inclusion body. Arch Environ Health 1970; 20:705–11.
8. Chisolm JJ. Aminoaciduria as a manifestation of renal tubular injury in lead intoxication and a comparison with patterns of aminoaciduria seen in other diseases. J Pediatr 1962; 60:1–17.
9. Lane RE. The care of the lead worker. Br J Ind Med 1949; 6:125–43.
10. Lilis R, Gavrilescu N, Nestorescu B, Dimitriu C, Roventa A. Nephropathy in chronic lead poisoning. Br J Ind Med 1968; 25:196–202.
11. Lilis R, Valciukas JA, Fischbein A, Andrews G, Selikoff IJ. Renal function impairment in secondary lead smelter workers: correlations with zinc protoporphyrin and blood lead levels. J Env Path Tox 1979; 2:1447–74.
12. Wedeen RP, Maesaka JK, Weines B et al. Occupational lead nephropathy. Am J Med 1975; 59:630–41.
13. Lilis R, Fischbein A, Valciukas JA, Blumberg W, Selikoff IJ. Kidney function and lead: relationships in several occupational groups with different levels of exposure. Am J Ind Med 1980; 1:405–12.
14. Henderson DA. The aetiology of chron-

ic nephritis in Queensland. Med J Aust 1958; 1:377–86.

15. Cooper WC, Gaffey WR. Mortality of lead workers. J Occup Med 1975; 17:100–7.

16. Selevan SG, Landrigan PJ, Stern FG, Jones JH. Mortality of lead smelter workers. Am J Epidemiol 1985; 122:673–83.

17. Lucas PA, Jarivalla AG, Jones JH, Gough J, Vale PT. Fatal cadmium fume inhalation. Lancet 1980; 26:205.

18. Beton DC, Andrews GS, Davies HJ, Howells L, Smith GF. Acute cadmium fume poisoning, five cases with one death from renal necrosis. Br J Ind Med 1966; 23:292–301.

19. Bernard A, Buchet JP, Roels H, Masson P, Lauwerys R. Renal excretion of protein and enzymes in workers exposed to cadmium. Eur J Clin Invest 1979; 9:11–22.

20. Roels H, Djubgang J, Buchet J-P, Bernard A, Lauwerys R. Evolution of cadmium-induced renal dysfunction in workers removed from exposure. Scand J Work Environ Health 1982; 8:191–200.

21. Friberg L, Piscator M, Nordberg GF, Kjellstrom T. Cadmium in the environment. 2nd ed. Boca Raton, Fl: CRC, 1974.

22. Casarett and Doull's Toxicology. 3rd ed. New York: MacMillan, 1986; 567–623.

23. Patty's industrial hygiene and toxicology. 3rd ed. Toxicology. New York: Wiley, 1981: 1511. Vol. 2A.

24. Encyclopedia of occupational health and safety. 3rd ed. Geneva: International Labour Office, 1983.

25. Klienknecht D, Morel-Maroger L, Callard P, Adhemar JP, Mahiev P. Antiglomerular basement membrane nephritis after solvent exposure. Arch Intern Med 1980; 140:230–2.

26. Morgan RW, Kaplan SD, Gaffey WR. A general mortality study of production workers in the paint and coatings manufacturing industry. J Occup Med 1981; 23:13–21.

27. Mehlman MA, Hemstreet GP III, Thorpe JJ, Weaver NK, eds. Renal effects of petroleum hydrocarbons. Princeton, NJ: Princeton Scientific, 1984.

28. World Health Organization. Environmental health criteria 10:carbon disulfide. Geneva: WHO, 1979.

29. Hanis NM, Holmes TM, Shallenberger LG, Jones KE. Epidemiologic study of refinery and chemical workers. J Occup Med 1982; 25:203–12.

30. Moore MR, Meredith PA. The carcinogenicity of lead. Review article. Arch Toxicol 1979; 42:87–94.

31. Matanowski GM, Elliot EA. Bladder cancer epidemiology. Epidemiol Rev 1981; 3:203–29.

32. Schulte PA, Ringen K, Hemstreet GP. Optimal management of asymptomatic workers at high risk of bladder cancer. J Occup Med 1986; 28:13–7.

BIBLIOGRAPHY

Fowler BA, ed. Biological and environmental effects of arsenic. Amsterdam: Elsevier, 1983.

This monograph is an excellent source of detailed information on the severe nephrotoxic effects of arsine.

Friberg L, Nordberg GF, Vouk VB, eds. Handbook on the toxicology of metals. 2nd edition. Amsterdam: Elsevier, 1986. Vols. 1 and 2.

Of particular interest is the chapter on cadmium, written by the world's most prominent experts on cadmium nephropathy who first described the condition in the 1950s. There is also valuable information on nephrotoxicity of mercury and uranium.

Hook JB, ed. Toxicology of the kidney. New York: Raven, 1981.

An excellent book on renal toxicology. The use of renal function tests in the evaluation of nephrotoxic effects, including renal clearance and use of enzymuria assessment are important for state-of-the-art evaluation of subclinical renal toxicity. A chapter on renal handling of environmental chemicals is very informative. The discussion of nephrotoxicity of low molecular weight alkane solvents, pesticides, and chemical intermediates includes valuable information on high volume chemicals such as ethylene dibromide, ethylene dichloride, perchloroethylene, trichloroethane, and others.

Landrigan PJ, Goyer RA, Clarkson TW et al. The work-relatedness of renal disease. Arch Environ Health 1984; 39(3):225–30.

A review addressing the important issue of the largely unknown etiology (in most cases) of chronic renal disease; the possibility that occupational factors might make a larger contribution than currently recognized is considered. Methods for diagnosis of subclinical nephrotoxicity, epidemiologic studies of populations exposed to compounds that have been shown to be nephrotoxic in animal experiments, as well as several other strategies are proposed for the more complete assessment of the contribution of occupational exposures to chronic renal disease.

Lauwerys RR, Bernard A. Early detection of nephrotoxic effects of industrial chemicals. State of the art and future prospects. Am J Ind Med 1987; 11:275–85.

This paper discusses several tests that may permit the early detection of renal changes induced by long-term exposure to nephrotoxic industrial chemicals and may possibly serve as advance warning of pending renal damage. Some tests mainly attempt to assess the integrity of the glomerulus: high molecular weight proteinuria, glomerular basement membrane (GBM) antigens in blood and in urine, circulating anti-GBM antibodies, glomerular filtration rate after an acute oral load of proteins, and estimation of membrane negative charges (that is, glomerular polyanion). Others mainly attempt to identify functional and morphologic changes at the tubular level: low molecular weight proteinuria, aminoaciduria, glucosuria, hyperphosphaturia, hypercalciuria, enzymuria, tubular antigen excretion, kallikrein, and prostaglandin excretion. Some of these tests are already routinely used, although controversy may still persist with regard to their clinical significance. Recently, new tests have been developed that may open new perspectives for assessing the significance of the early renal changes induced by chemicals.

Mehlman MA, Hemstreet GP III, Thorpe JJ, Weaver NK, eds. Renal effects of petroleum hydrocarbons. Princeton, NJ: Princeton Scientific, 1984.

This recent monograph provides much needed information on the problem of aliphatic hydrocarbon nephropathy. This is now a topic of intense interest, especially because of the large numbers of workers exposed. Human studies and experimental data are reviewed in detail.

Singhal RL, Thomas JA. Lead toxicity. Baltimore: Urban & Schwarzenberg, 1980.

An excellent chapter is dedicated to a thorough review of lead nephrotoxicity. Early effects are well described as are the results of chronic low-level exposure and absorption. Pathologic changes are presented in great detail. This is based on the personal experiences of the authors.

V
Selected Groups of Workers

31
Women and Work

Margaret M. Quinn and Susan R. Woskie

Women in the manufacturing industries, in the service sector, and in office work often report different health hazards and symptoms than men in these same jobs. The fact that many job assignments are gender-based can explain much of this difference [1] and is the result of a complex web of social and economic factors leading men and women into different occupations.

Since social and economic factors also determine many important aspects of an individual's work experience, such as income, the likelihood of being employed and remaining employed, opportunities for job advancement, and authority in workplace decisions, a woman who does the same job or a comparable job as a man is likely to have a different experience. For example, in 1986, women in the United States earned, on average, only 64 cents for every dollar earned by men. The median earnings of year-round workers in 1984 ranked, in order of highest to lowest: white men, Hispanic men, black men, white women, black women, and Hispanic women.

In addition, women who work outside of the home still do most of their household work as well. Added to the pressures of long working hours and the conflicting roles of family caretaker versus wage earner is the serious lack of social service supports for working women. Foremost among these is the lack of adequate child care, sick-child care, and elder care. Finally, there are stresses and hazards particular to women who find themselves in the great minority in industries that have traditionally hired only men.

There were almost 49 million working women in the United States in 1986, comprising 44 percent of the entire U.S. workforce and 55 percent of all women 16 years of age and older. The number of wage-earning women has been steadily increasing over this century and the increase is expected to continue. Women are moving into heavy industrial jobs (Fig. 31-1), the building trades, and professional fields in small, but increasing numbers. The number of families maintained by women grew almost 90 percent between 1970 and 1985. The growth of black female-headed families has been especially dramatic, more than doubling between 1970 and 1985. In 1985, 44 percent of all black families were headed by women compared with 23 percent of Hispanic families and 13 percent of white families. Almost 55 percent of children in families with a female head of household lived below the poverty level. Over two-thirds of black and Hispanic children whose mothers supported them lived in poverty, primarily because black and Hispanic women maintaining families had lower median earnings, lower median ages, and higher unemployment rates than white women maintaining families.

SOURCES OF OCCUPATIONAL STRESS

Stress can be defined as a physical or psychological stimulus that produces strain or disruption of the individual's normal physiologic equilibrium. Men and women may experience a wide range of stress

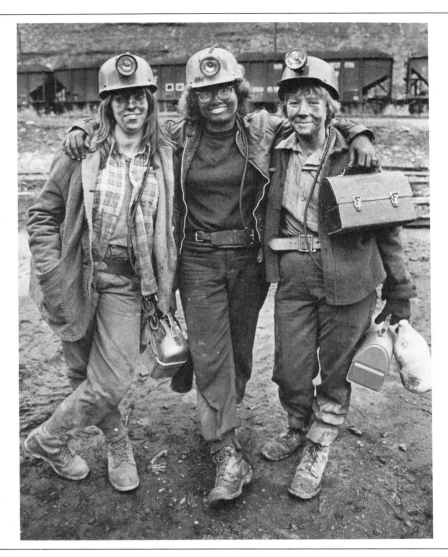

Fig. 31-1. Many women now work in jobs that were traditionally held only by men. (Photograph by Earl Dotter.)

reactions, including adverse health effects (see Chap. 20).

Problems of Multiple Roles

As the distinction fades between women who marry and have families and women who work, the enormous problem of managing both aspects of life at once emerges. Even if some of the domestic chores are assumed by men, the organization and care of the home, children, and elderly family members still largely remains the woman's responsibility. The average working woman puts in an estimated 80 hours a week in both job and household work. The extreme of this dual role exists for the full-time working mother, who has the sole responsibility for domestic family needs. She may work up to 105 hours per week, well past the maximum associated with worker efficiency [2]. This situation is compounded by the serious lack of social support services for dependents of working women. Working women frequently have to take their own sick leave to care for a sick child or elderly family member, which often means that they must work when they become ill.

Discrimination

Racial, sexual, and age discrimination all contribute to the stress experienced by working women. These types of discrimination take many forms and affect women in economic terms (lower pay than men who do comparable work), social terms (alienation from supervisors and coworkers), and personal terms (low self-esteem and reduced creative growth). Women who work in occupations where the majority of the workforce is male are often seen as unwelcome intruders and many experience widespread harassment for being female (gender harassment). They may also feel excessive pressure to perform faultlessly to prove that they are good enough. These experiences are likely to be even more extreme for women who represent a racial or ethnic minority, and they can have serious consequences for health and safety.

Sexual Harassment

In the workplace, sexual harassment continues to be a problem for many women. In a study of over 500 cases of sexual harassment on the job, 46 percent of the women said this behavior interfered with their work performance, despite expressions of pride at being able to do their jobs even with the harassment, and 36 percent reported physical ailments that they associated with the harassment. The most prevalent of these were nausea, vomiting, fatigue, depression, headaches, and drastic weight change. About one-fourth had sought medical or psychological help (see box) [3].

Job Control

When the Framingham Heart Study examined the relationship between employment status and the incidence of coronary heart disease, it found that 21 percent of women clerical workers develop coronary heart disease, a rate almost twice that of other nonclerical workers or housewives [3]. One study examined the widely held opinion that certain individuals are more prone to stress and bring their problems on themselves. It found that typical female jobs had much less control over decision-making than do typical male jobs. Clerical work ranked among the highest in this regard. The study concluded that it may be the concentration of women in these jobs that accounts for their higher prevalence of stress-related disorders rather than women's lack of ability to cope [3].

Recognizing the social, economic, and physical determinants of health effects related to occupational stressors instead of focusing solely on personal pathology is a first step in the complete and long-term management of stress-related problems. While many women may benefit from programs that provide individual coping and relaxation exercises, workplace stress management programs should also acknowledge the broader social and

SEXUAL HARASSMENT ON THE JOB—
Cathy Schwartz

What Is It?

Sexual harassment is any unwanted verbal or physical sexual advance, ranging from sexual comments and suggestions, to pressure for sexual favors accompanied by threats (outright or subtle) concerning one's job, to physical assault including rape.

How Widespread Is It?

Studies indicate that from 42 to 88 percent of working women report having been sexually harassed on the job.

*What are the Effects of
Sexual Harassment?*

Psychological trauma and stress-related physical symptoms are the effects of sexual harassment. Both types of effects are compounded if the woman's job is in jeopardy, if she is forced to resign, or if she is fired as a result of the harassment situation.

What Can Be Done?

Sexual harassment is illegal. It is a violation of rights under Title VII of the Civil Rights Act and of many state fair employment practice laws. A woman who is fired or resigns as a result of a harassment situation may be entitled to unemployment compensation. Organized protest against managers for sexual harassment is protected activity under the National Labor Relations Act.

Getting Help

A woman can seek help from her union, coworkers, and local women's organizations. Talking to other people and getting assistance can help the woman feel less isolated and frustrated and is probably necessary to effectively deal with the situation. It may be necessary to seek legal help and to go to a local or state agency that deals with fair employment practices or the closest office of the federal Equal Employment Opportunity Commission (EEOC).

---

economic constraints that provide the context for the daily lives of working women.

ERGONOMIC HAZARDS

Many workplaces are a haphazard layout of tools, machines, and work stations. Little thought is given to the fit of tools, the nature of the lifting tasks, or the fit of personal protective equipment (PPE) to the user. This lack of thought results in injuries that could be prevented if basic guidelines for lifting and for job and tool design were used. Although these issues are not particular to women, women often bear the brunt of poor workplace design because most tools, work stations, and PPE were manufactured for use by the "average" male.

Repetitive, sharply angular, and rotational motions have been associated with a number of occupational musculoskeletal disorders (see Chaps. 9 and 22). Neck, shoulder, and upper limb disorders (for example, cervicobrachial syndrome) have been identified among a number of jobs held largely by women including: keyboard operators of typewriters, telex, calculating machines, computers, and telephone exchangers; cash register operators; film roller and capper workers; cigarette rolling and packing workers; and scissors manufacture and assembly workers. Tenosynovitis has been reported among women assembly-line packers in a food production factory, women poultry-processing plant workers, and women scissors manufacture and assembly workers. Carpal tunnel syndrome (CTS) has been found among women garment workers, hotel cooks, maids, workers in the boning department of a poultry-processing plant, and cash register operators.

Carpal tunnel syndrome has been reported to be more common (1.4–16.0 times) in women than in men [4]. Hormonal changes following gynecologic surgery, especially hysterectomy with removal of the ovaries, has been related to increased risk of the disease [5]. Examination of CTS cases at one plant showed that workers in departments with repetitive-motion jobs had a very high risk of the disease while the risk attributed to gender, although elevated, was 20 times less than that attributed to having a job using repetitive motions [4]. Although women seem to be at a greater risk of developing CTS and related tendon disorders than men, gender is probably less important than work pattern, segmental vibration, and hand stress. Since women are concentrated in jobs that require repetitive motions, such as bench assembly and small parts manufacturing, it is difficult to determine whether there are aspects of this disease that are solely related to gender.

Reduction of musculoskeletal injuries can be accomplished through careful consideration of the ergonomics of the work process. Improvements of tool and work station design can contribute significantly to preventing musculoskeletal disorders.

One company made improvements in the working conditions of cash register operators, including shortened operating time, development of a work-rotation system, and change from mechanical to electronic registers with lighter key touches. The result was a decrease in the workload on the arms and hands and a significant drop in complaints of pain, dullness, stiffness, or numbness in the hands, fingers, and arms [6].

When visual display unit workers in an office were given an adjustable work station that they could adapt to their preferred settings for a number of factors, including keyboard and screen height, viewing angle, and screen distance, they reported significantly fewer complaints of these muscles or impairment in the neck, shoulder, back, and wrist [7].

Heavy physical work is associated with low back pain (LBP). For example, among nurses and nurse's aides, those in their twenties who spent more time lifting had higher prevalence of LBP than those whose jobs did not require heavy lifting. This pain may also be related to childbearing and child rearing, which increase the load on the back even more [8]. Whereas only 5 percent of the women in light industry report ever having LBP lasting more than 3 days, 35 percent of the women in heavy industry report LBP. Only 7 percent of women office and postal clerks report LBP compared to 17 percent of nurses. LBP is also common among working men (17% in nursing, 18% in light industry, and 19% in heavy industry), suggesting that much needs to be done to improve the ergonomic design of most jobs (see box on p. 484) [9].

PROBLEMS WITH PERSONAL PROTECTIVE EQUIPMENT

Personal protective equipment (PPE) should not be the primary method of controlling a worker's exposure to a workplace hazard, but it can be important in temporary situations, emergencies, or situations that cannot be controlled in other ways. However, for PPE to work, it must fit. In addition, PPE, such as gloves, that does not fit can increase the risk of accidents and increase the strength requirements for a task. For women, it is often hard to find manufacturers who make equipment in women's sizes. Often small, medium, and large sizes of equipment are available, but even the small size is designed for small men, not women. A survey of over 350 companies exhibiting at a National Safety Council annual meeting found that in women's sizes, only 14 percent provided ear protection, 58 percent hand protection, 18 percent respirators, 14 percent head and face protection, 50 percent body protection, and 59 percent foot protection [10]. Many women end up purchasing men's PPE and try to modify it to fit, or they purchase women's equipment that is not up to safety standards. Until PPE is available in a variety of sizes for women, it may actually be contributing to the risk of workplace injuries.

THE STRENGTH OF WOMEN—
Laura Punnett

How Do Women Compare To Men?
Women's total body strength is, on average, about two-thirds that of men. However, the static strength (ability to move a stationary weight) of men and women differs from 35 to 85 percent depending on the tasks and muscles involved. Women's average strength is closer to men's for static leg exertions and for certain dynamic lifting, pushing, and pulling activities.

Since muscle strength is greatest in the twenties and thirties, with a 20 percent decline by age 60, younger women and older men may have more similar strength capabilities.

Despite these average differences, there is also substantial overlap in the strength distribution between men and women, as much as 50 percent or more for certain muscle groups. In fact, the factors of gender, age, weight, and height only explain about one-third of the variability in human strength data.

Strength Testing
There is inconclusive evidence concerning the effectiveness of static strength testing to predict an individual's likelihood of injury. There is no evidence that worker selection based on medical or strength criteria has been effective in preventing musculoskeletal disorders. Although women are less strong than men on average, there is also no epidemiologic evidence that women suffer more work-related musculoskeletal injuries than men performing the same task.

Strength testing may provide an alternative to blanket discrimination based on sex. Since there is a large overlap between the population distributions of the static strength abilities of men and women, selection of individuals able to lift a given weight will not exclude all prospective women employees. However, using this criterion may unnecessarily exclude persons who would not suffer injury. In addition, these tests do not measure endurance (aerobic capacity) or flexibility, both of which on average, are greater in women than men, and which may be protective factors against the biomechanical stress of heavy lifting.

The best approach to eliminating musculoskeletal injuries from the workplace is the implementation of engineering controls. It has been estimated that the redesign of jobs to fit workers' capabilities could reduce injury rates by 6 percent.

Pregnancy and Strength
Studies suggest that a woman's aerobic capacity to do physical work does not change during pregnancy, except in the last few months. However, it may be difficult to maintain a particular work level if nausea or other health problems develop. Lifting capacity will be altered in later pregnancy as the center of gravity moves and as a woman's body size prevents an object from being lifted close to the body. In addition, the ligaments and muscles of the stomach and back are stretched and joints become more mobile, making lifting potentially more hazardous. There is evidence of increased risk of low back injury for pregnant women performing specific tasks, including heavy lifting, standing, and frequent climbing of stairs.

With regard to adverse pregnancy outcome, the epidemiologic evidence is still inconclusive. Heavy lifting, heavy industrial cleaning, and other strenuous exertions have been associated with both spontaneous abortions and premature birth. Long periods of standing at work appear to increase the risk of prematurity. These factors may also increase the rates of uterine contraction during pregnancy and low birth weight. The effect of ergonomic stressors on the pregnancies of women working in the home has not been evaluated.

REPRODUCTIVE HEALTH HAZARDS

Occupational reproductive hazards are often viewed as a "woman's problem." As a result, the individual woman is left to bear the burden of the social, economic, and health consequences of reproductive hazards while the hazards faced by men are ignored. In fact, almost all occupational crises with documented adverse reproductive effects, such as exposure to dibromochloropropane (DBCP), Kepone, exogenous estrogens, and dimethylaminopropionitrile (DMAPN), have involved men (see Chap. 26). In situations where men have been at risk, control of the hazard was achieved by elimination of the exposure. However, when even the potential for a reproductive health problem has existed for female workers, control of the "hazard" has been achieved often by eliminating women from the job, particularly if women are seeking a job in an industry that has not traditionally hired women. Both men and women will benefit if it is recognized that reproductive hazards may seriously compromise the health of all workers as well as the children they produce.

THE PREGNANT WORKER

Many organ system and musculoskeletal changes occur during pregnancy to accommodate the needs of the developing fetus. The most evident changes are modifications in cardiovascular, respiratory, and metabolic functions as well as shifts in the center of gravity associated with weight gain. These changes are normal and healthy and may or may not affect a woman's ability to work. Pregnant women can usually continue to perform the physical activities to which they have been accustomed; however, pregnancy may not be the time to change to a new or unfamiliar level of work activity unless the woman undertakes a carefully supervised program of physical conditioning. Some medical conditions can be compromised by pregnancy; others predispose the pregnant woman to an increased likelihood of complications during pregnancy. The American Medical Association has developed guidelines for the continuation of various levels of work during pregnancy [11].

As with pregnancy, data about postpartum readiness to resume work is lacking. In 1977, the American College of Obstetricians and Gynecologists stated the following in their *Guidelines on Pregnancy and Work:* "The normal woman with an uncomplicated pregnancy and a normal fetus in a job that presents no greater potential hazards than those encountered in normal daily life in the community may continue to work without interruption until the onset of labor and may resume working several weeks after an uncomplicated pregnancy" [12]. A woman's ability to work during pregnancy and return to work after pregnancy should be determined by the woman and her health care provider, considering the requirements of her job, her health status at the time she becomes pregnant, and her pregnancy experience.

The First Trimester

During the first trimester, many women experience nausea and vomiting as well as fatigue and breast swelling and tenderness. There is a large increase in total blood volume, which results in an increased heart and metabolic rate. The ventilation rate begins to increase (from a nonpregnant average of 7 liters/min to an average of 10 liters/min by term). Glomerular filtration increases about 50 percent above the nonpregnant level.

These physiologic changes may affect a working woman in several ways. The vomiting and fatigue may decrease her capacity for work. Some women are particularly sensitive to bad odors that may increase their nausea. The increased metabolic rate raises body temperature, increasing sensitivity to hot and humid environments. The increased blood volume decreases the total percentage of red blood cells in the circulating blood and leads to an anemia, which is normal for a pregnant woman. However, it is especially important that a pregnant woman does not already have anemia caused by work factors, such as lead or benzene. Since the percentage of hemoglobin-carrying red blood cells is decreased, she will also be more vulnerable to environmental agents that interfere with the blood's ability to carry oxygen, such as carbon monoxide. The increased ventilation rate can result in increased absorption of any toxic materials in the air. Increased kidney function results in increased urination, making access to suitable bathroom facilities particularly important [12].

The Second Trimester
While the body changes mentioned will persist throughout pregnancy, many of the symptoms will disappear and women often find they feel better during the second trimester. By the end of this period, there is a weight gain of approximately 7 kg (15 lb) and the uterus grows about 28 cm (11 in) above the pelvis. As the uterus enlarges, its bulk tilts the body forward and the lower spine curves inward. The pelvic joints also become increasingly mobile. In addition to aggravating any preexisting back problems, women often experience low back discomfort and stiffness. The change in the center of gravity may result in decreased ability to balance, and tolerance to physical exertion may vary widely. In general, women who are in good physical condition before pregnancy will have fewer problems and will be capable of greater exertion.

Along with these changes in body structure, there may be a greater tendency for the blood to pool in the legs. This can lead to dizziness and fainting with prolonged standing or working in hot environments, which increase the pooling. Varicose veins may also develop under these work conditions [12].

The Third Trimester
During the third trimester, the uterus continues to enlarge and total body weight gain increases to an average of 11 kg (24 lb). Peripheral edema is common because there may be a decrease in venous return from the legs due to the pressure of the uterus on the pelvic veins. As the third trimester progresses, many women also experience increasing fatigue, insomnia, and shortness of breath. These symptoms may be caused by the uterus pushing on the diaphragm, increased respiratory demands with a tendency toward an oxygen debt, and discomfort associated with weight gain. Near

delivery, the uterus pressing on the bladder may cause women to be incontinent or to urinate frequently [12]. Prolonged standing or jobs requiring balance, endurance, exertion, work in hot environments, or in locations remote from bathroom facilities may become increasingly difficult.

Breast-Feeding
Chemical exposures in the workplace may present a hazard to women and the infants they breast-feed. Toxic substances are passively transferred from plasma to breast milk if they are lipid soluble, polarized at body pH, and have a low molecular weight. These include many drugs, alcohol, some components of cigarette smoke, and many occupational and environmental toxins, such as lead, mercury, halogenated hydrocarbons, and organic solvents. The dose and duration of exposure to the infant also depends on how quickly the substance is metabolized or excreted by the mother. For chemicals such as dichloro-diphenyl-trichloroethane (DDT), polychlorinated biphenyls (PCBs), and related halogenated hydrocarbons, which are stored in body fat, breast milk can be a major route of excretion. The baby's dose may thus be as high as the mother's even after she has been removed from the exposure. However, solvents, though lipid soluble, are also metabolized or excreted through the liver, lung, and kidneys as well as breast milk, so maternal body burden rapidly decreases after removal from exposure [13].

What the Health Care Provider Can Do
Information on a pregnant woman's work activity and that of her partner (including wage-earning work and work done at home) and chemical and physical exposures should be an essential part of the comprehensive perinatal health history. This information should be obtained from her at the first prenatal visit and reconfirmed by inquiry at each subsequent visit. This inquiry can often best be done by means of a questionnaire [11]. In some instances, it may be important to augment the questionnaire information, with the woman's permission, from the physician, nurse, or industrial

hygienist in her employee health unit, from the plant safety director, or from the union representative. (See information on the occupational history in Chap. 3.)

Legal Rights of Pregnant Workers
When I told my new employer that I was pregnant, they lowered the amount of money they had offered to pay me, actually telling me I was worth less to them now. When my husband told his boss he was going to be a parent, he got a raise.

The 1978 Pregnancy Discrimination Act, an amendment to Title VII of the 1964 Civil Rights Act, requires that women affected by pregnancy and related conditions must be treated the same as other employees and applicants for employment when an employer determines their probable ability or inability to perform a job. This law protects a woman from being fired or refused a job or promotion merely because she is pregnant. A woman unable to work for pregnancy-related reasons is entitled to disability benefits, sick leave, and health insurance (except for abortions) just like employees disabled for other medical reasons. Under the law, pregnant workers temporarily unable to perform their jobs must be treated in the same manner as other disabled employees, such as by modifying the task, changing the work assignment, or granting disability leave or leave without pay. An employer who assigns a pregnant woman to another job because she cannot perform her regular work or because the job represents a hazard, however, can reduce her pay to that of the new job (Fig. 31-2).

The employer cannot enforce a rule prohibiting a return after childbirth for a set period of time. The woman's ability to return to work is the only test. Unless the employee on leave has informed the employer that she does not intend to return to work, her job must be held open on the same basis as jobs are held open for employees on sick or disability leave for other reasons. During her pregnancy-related leave, the employee must receive equal credit for seniority, vacations, or pay raises.

Pregnancy cannot have a role in the decision to

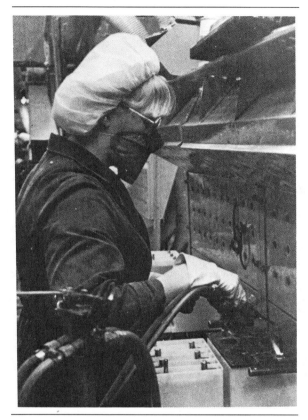

Fig. 31-2. There has been much controversy over whether women of childbearing age should work with lead, as this battery maker is doing. (See also Chap. 26.) (From C Zenz. Occupational medicine: principles and practical applications. Chicago: Year Book, 1975. Reproduced with permission.)

hire an employee. If the applicant can perform the major functions required by the position, pregnancy-related conditions cannot be considered. The employer cannot refuse to hire her because of any real or imagined preference of coworkers, customers, or suppliers. In addition, a woman's request for maternity leave must be honored if the employer grants employees the rights to leaves of absence for such purposes as travel or education.

If a woman believes she has been discriminated against because of childbirth or pregnancy-related conditions, she may sue the employer. The law requires filing a complaint first with the state agency dealing with discrimination. If this state agency does not proceed with informal mediation or legal action under state law after 60 days, then the woman can file a complaint with the federal Equal Employment Opportunity Commission (EEOC). The complaint must be filed within 6 months of the discriminatory event [14].

Despite the law, there are still at least three major stumbling blocks for working women and men who wish to become parents. First, although the law requires that pregnancy be treated as any other disability, many employers, including most branches of the federal government (the largest employer in the United States), have no established disability leave policy. Decisions affecting work and pregnancy-related issues are left to the discretion of the woman's supervisor. Second, the Pregnancy Discrimination Act applies only to workplaces employing 15 or more people, and many women work in smaller shops and offices. Third, there are no provisions for paternity leave, although some unions and employers are beginning to negotiate these provisions and the federal government may be beginning to develop legislation for paternity leave.

SPECIFIC OCCUPATIONS

Although women are found in nearly every job category, they continue to be concentrated in those that have been traditionally female. More than one-half of all women employed outside the home are in two broad occupational categories: clerical and service. Nontraditional jobs for women are defined by the Women's Bureau as those in which women make up 25 percent or less of the total number of workers. In this regard, one of the most important shifts in the employment of women has been the influx of women into the skilled trades. In 1981, there were over 800,000 women employed in these skilled trades in the United States, more than double the number in 1970 and almost 4 times the number in 1960. The number of women entering traditionally male occupations increased, at least in part, because of federal legislation and affirmative action programs. The appendix to this chapter summarizes many of the common hazards in industries that employ many women and some possible health effects of these hazards.

Household Work

The single largest type of work done by women in our society is that of unpaid household work. Despite the increasing number of women who work for wages, approximately one-third of married women in the United States are still full-time housewives, and most wage-earning women are responsible for work in their own households. In addition, there are over 1 million paid household workers who are employed as servants, nannies, housekeepers, janitors, or cleaners. The exact number of paid household workers is very difficult to determine, however, because much of this work is undocumented. The vast majority of these workers are female and more than one-third are of racial or ethnic minorities. Few household workers, paid or unpaid, get sick days and many have no health insurance, Social Security, or workers' compensation.

Household work is thought of as "women's work," and is often not regarded as work at all. This perception devalues the labor involved and implies that there are no health and safety concerns of importance. In fact, a wide range of industrial substances and equipment is used and stored in the home under relatively uncontrolled conditions. There is growing recognition that certain home environmental conditions may pose important health problems, and that homes are significant small-source generators of hazardous waste.

Among the products used routinely in the home are drain cleaners, chlorine bleaches, scouring powders, ammonia, oven cleaners containing lye, furniture polish, furniture or paint strippers containing organic solvents, glues, paints, epoxies, and pesticides. There is an aerosol product containing ammonia, chlorine, organic solvents, acids, or detergents for every surface of the bathroom. All of these products are potential hazards (see appendix to this chapter) and may become a problem, particularly when used in a confined space, such as an unventilated bathroom or attic, closet, crawl space, or the space beneath cabinets.

In well-insulated homes, potential health hazards may occur due to building, insulating, and decorating materials, such as formaldehyde emitted from particle board, plywood, carpeting, fabrics, and foam insulation; and asbestos in pipe lagging or furnace and boiler insulation. Toxic emissions from gas and wood stoves can accumulate in homes, as can radioactive radon.

In addition to hazardous chemical and physical agents in the home, some of the social factors that define the nature of housework can contribute to poor mental health. While many household workers enjoy their work and acquire a wide range of skills, their skills are largely unrecognized in the broader labor market, and they may have little long-term opportunity for job advancement or personal growth. For many, the work can be isolating and monotonous. In the industrial setting, it is recognized that such factors contribute to low job satisfaction. However, housewives are literally married to their jobs, and it can be difficult and threatening to grapple explicitly with low job satisfaction in this setting. The lack of support to directly address such dissatisfaction can lead to depression.

Sexual harassment and abuse are serious problems for women in the home. In fact, housework judged to be inadequate has been used as a pretext for wife battering. One police officer investigating an abuse case said, "If it had been my house, I would have beaten my wife for the condition it was in" [3].

An important step toward addressing the health and safety issues of women who work in the home is their recognition as legitimate workers with corresponding rights.

Electronics Manufacturing

Most workers involved in the assembly production processes of the electronics industry are female. Processes include precleaning and degreasing of fabrication materials with organic solvents, such as methylene chloride, 1,1,1-trichloroethane, trichloroethylene, perchloroethylene, xylene, or mineral spirits; etching with acids; electroplating; soldering; and packaging.

Many electronics assembly processes involve rapid, repetitive motions of the wrists, hands, and arms. Assemblers may have to maintain uncomfortable postures throughout the work shift. Thus, repetitive trauma and other musculoskeletal disorders are a serious problem in the electronics industry.

Health and safety concerns have been raised concerning a particular subgroup of electronics: the semiconductor industry. Although this industry was originally concentrated in California and Massachusetts, rapid technologic and economic growth has fostered production facilities in most industrialized areas in the United States and much of the world. It is now estimated that microelectronics production will be the fourth largest industry in the United States by the end of the century.

According to employment statistics for Santa Clara County, California, the site of "Silicon Valley," more than 75 percent of the semiconductor production workers there are female and at least 40 percent of them are minorities, primarily Hispanics and Asians. These workers are among the most poorly paid industrial workers in the United States today. This contrasts sharply with the large managerial and professional sector of this industry, which is nearly 90 percent white and male [3].

The major hazardous materials used in semiconductor manufacturing include hydrofluoric acid; solvents, such as freons and the glycol ethers (cellosolves); metals such as antimony and gallium; and toxic gases, such as arsine and phosphine. However, because the industry is relatively new, little is known about the chronic effects of the toxic materials used in this setting [15].

In 1980, the California Division of Labor Statistics and Research found that the rate of occupational illness among semiconductor workers was more than 3 times the rate among workers in the general manufacturing industry. The California Workers' Compensation statistics for 1980 through 1984 indicate that occupational illness in this industry accounted for 20 percent of all lost work-time injuries and illnesses, compared to 7 percent for the average of all manufacturing industries. These data also indicated that 47 percent of ill semiconductor workers experienced occupational illnesses attributable to exposure to toxic materials (called "systemic poisonings") as compared to 21 percent for all manufacturing industries [15].

Solutions for controlling hazards in the electronics industry include documentation of the nature and extent of materials used and integration of health and safety into the production process. The National Institute for Occupational Safety and Health (NIOSH) health hazard evaluations have repeatedly recommended installation of adequate local and general ventilation systems. The design of "clean rooms" should aim to minimize worker exposures as well as wafer contamination and, wherever possible, non-hazardous processes should be substituted for hazardous ones.

Hospital Work

Over 2.3 million women work in hospitals and another 4.5 million in other health services. Women make up over 80 percent of the total workforce of these industries but less than 24 percent in the health-diagnosing occupations (such as physician). In all health care occupations, women earn about 80 percent of what men earn, with the percentage dropping as the skill level of the occupation increases.

Stress is a major problem for health care workers, who are often overworked and yet have responsibility for human life. Six of the top 27 occupations showing mental health disorders are in the health care field [3]. Current cost-containment programs are expected to result in even more understaffing, as well as equipment maintenance problems and supply shortages. Rotating shifts, which are common among hospital workers, are another source of stress that can affect reproductive and cardiovascular health.

Nursing and personal care workers have an injury rate equal to that of agricultural workers. Hazards contributing to this high accident rate include electrical hazards from the extensive use of equipment to monitor and treat patients, needle sticks, slippery floors, and the movement of equipment and patients (Fig. 31-3).

Hospitals use a wide variety of chemicals for cleaning, sterilizing, lab analysis, and chemotherapy. A hospital worker can be exposed to chemicals or infectious agents through direct handling, cross-contamination of hospital areas due to poor ventilation design, the transport of waste, or the maintenance and cleaning of equipment or rooms.

Control methods have been developed for many of the hazardous substances to which hospital workers are exposed. For example, inexpensive scavenger systems are available to reduce exposures to anesthetic gases. Ventilation, substitution, and changes in work practices can minimize formaldehyde (formalin) exposures in autopsy, surgical pathology and histology labs, and renal dialysis units. The use of control procedures, such as complete evacuation of sterilizer units before opening, use of aeration cabinets and catalytic converters, and careful equipment maintenance, can reduce ethylene oxide exposures from sterilizers. Guidelines developed to minimize exposure to chemotherapeutic drugs include provisions for careful labeling of materials, use of biological safety cabinets in drug preparation, and use of gowns and gloves.

Radiation exposures can result from portable x-rays, other diagnostic tests or therapies using radiation, and patients emitting radiation after therapeutic implants or diagnostic tests. Shielding and distance from the radiation source are the best protection along with regular maintenance, personal monitoring, reductions in unnecessary procedures,

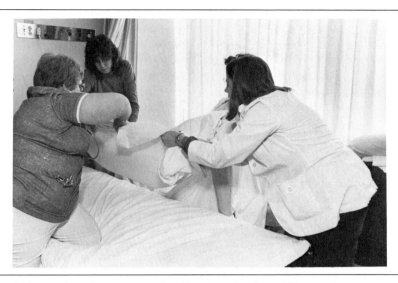

Fig. 31-3. Many female hospital workers are at risk of back strains from lifting patients. (Photograph by Marilee Caliendo.)

and careful labeling of materials, patients, and waste.

Hospital workers are exposed to a wide variety of infectious diseases, including hepatitis B, rubella, influenza, tuberculosis, meningitis, toxoplasmosis, cytomegalovirus disease, and AIDS. To prevent infections, all blood, excretions, and secretions should be treated as infectious, and personal hygiene should be strictly maintained [16] (see Chap. 19).

Office Work
"For a year-and-a-half, I worked 3 feet from a copier. . . . The fumes got so bad, I felt like I was being poisoned. . . . It's important that I have won a Workers' Compensation claim . . . but I cannot place an order for a new pair of lungs and I cannot wipe the worried look from the faces of the members of my family when I can't breathe, can't stop coughing, when I have to sit up to sleep. . . ."
—Former secretary before the House Subcommittee on Health

There are over 18 million clerical workers in the United States and nearly 80 percent of them are women. As illustrated by the above statement, despite its image of safe, clean white-collar work, there is a growing awareness of the hazards associated with office work. Among the more obvious safety hazards are slippery floors, open file cabinet drawers, electrical cords strung across the floor, swinging doors, and movement of bulky and heavy objects, such as cases of paper and office furniture.

The design of the office and its work stations are important in determining the extent to which noise, lighting, and ventilation are problems. The use of artificial fluorescent light can result in over-illumination and flicker. By using desk blotters and task lighting controlled by the worker, the shadows and glare that are often the source of eye strain can be reduced. Once the ventilation, copiers, typewriters, printers, and phones are operating in a modern, open office space occupied by many people, it is not uncommon for the noise level to exceed the 45 to 55 dBA recommended for easy office and phone conversation [17].

Many office buildings suffer from serious indoor air pollution. The combination of poor ventilation design, sealed buildings, the buildup of chemicals from building materials, office machines, and cigarette smoke has resulted in an office smog in many buildings. Photocopiers can produce ozone, nitropyrenes, and ultraviolet light (Fig. 31-4). Duplicating machines emit ethanol, methanol, and ammonia. Formaldehyde is found in carbonless paper, building materials, carpets, and draperies. Several solvents, including trichloroethane, tetrachloroethylene, and trichloroethylene, are used in liquid eraser products. Pesticides used in the building can remain in the air for extended periods [3, 17].

In buildings constructed primarily between 1930 and 1976, asbestos was used as insulation for ducts and pipes, as fire retardant on the structural steel of the building, and as a spray-on ceiling material. Office workers can be exposed to asbestos when it degrades from age, water damage, or disruption during renovations and when computer, phone, or electrical lines are installed between floors in a building. Motor vehicle exhaust is a frequent air contaminant in buildings that have air ducts near busy streets, parking garages, or loading docks. Buildings made of granite, bricks, or cement may accumulate surprisingly high levels of radon emitted from these materials. Offices in the basements of buildings may also have radon gas exposures from the soil. Microorganisms can flourish in the air-conditioning and humidifying systems, evaporative condensers, and cooling towers in many office buildings. The result may be allergies and respiratory infections, such as legionnaires' disease, that sometimes can reach epidemic proportions. Perhaps the most common office air pollutant is cigarette smoke, which can increase the level of respirable particles in the air by 5 times that of a nonsmoking office. Since research has linked the cigarette smoking of a spouse with the increased lung cancer risk of a nonsmoking

Fig. 31-4. In addition to the repetition and tedium of the job, office workers who operate duplicating machines may encounter hazardous chemicals.
(Photograph by Marilee Caliendo.)

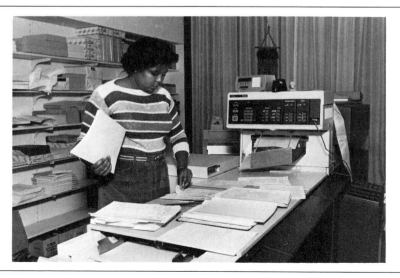

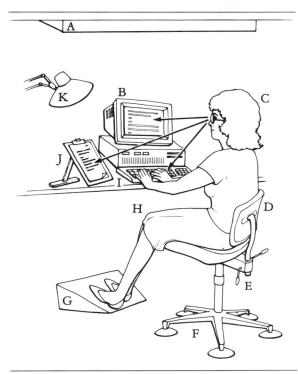

Fig. 31-5. A model video display terminal (VDT) work station. In addition to specific features, indicated below, it has adequate ventilation, no excess noise or crowding, adequate privacy, relaxing colors and nonglare surfaces, windows with blinds or curtains, and allows adequate social contact with coworkers. The terminal should be regularly serviced and cleaned, and records should be kept easily accessible. The printer should be in a separate area; if located near the work area, it should be equipped with a noise shield. The specific features, as shown on the figure, are (A) Indirect general lighting; moderate brightness (may be turned off if desired). (B) Screen about 1–2 feet away with midpoint slightly below eye level; characters are large and sharp enough to read easily; brightness and contrast controls present; adjustable height and tilt; glare-proof screen surface; no visible flicker of characters. (C) If necessary, special glasses for VDT viewing distance. (D) Adjustable backrest to support small of back. (E) Easily adjustable seat height and depth. (F) Swivel chair; safer with 5-point base and casters. (G) Feet firmly resting on the floor; footrest available. (H) Thighs approximately parallel to the floor. (I) Movable keyboard on surface with adjustable height; arms approximately parallel to the floor. (J) Copy holder at approximately same distance as screen; adjustable space for copy holder and other materials. (K) Direct, adjustable task lighting. (From Office Technology Education Project [OTEP]. Drawn by Beth Maynard.)

spouse, nonsmoking office workers may also be at risk.

Controlling the indoor air pollution of an office involves curtailing, alternating, or substituting some processes, isolating those sources of toxins that must be used, and improving the fresh-air ventilation of most buildings. For example, photocopiers should be kept in a separate room and vented, and substitutes should be used for carbonless copy paper containing sensitizing agents. Most office buildings have reduced fresh-air circulation to cut energy costs. The American Society of Heating, Refrigeration, and Air Conditioning Engineers recommends 20 cubic feet per minute (cfm) of fresh outdoor air per person where smoking is permitted (5 cfm where it is not) [18]. In addition, the relative humidity should be between 40 and 60 percent. By improving ventilation, the buildup of office smog can be avoided.

With the introduction of computers and video display terminals (VDTs) into the office, a series of health problems have surfaced. Among these problems are eye strain, headaches, neck and shoulder pain, carpal tunnel syndrome, and tenosynovitis.

Most VDTs in use today do not emit detectable levels of ionizing radiation (x-ray, gamma). Nonionizing radiation, in the form of very low frequency (VLF) and extremely low frequency (ELF) radiation, can be emitted from VDTs that are not shielded; however, there is much scientific debate about the health significance of exposure to this form of radiation (see Chap. 18). In the early 1980s, a series of miscarriage and birth defect clusters were reported among VDT users. There was some concern that they might be related to radiation leaks from VDT terminals. Since then, several studies have found inconsistent or inconclusive results regarding the association between VDT use and birth defects or miscarriage. However, these studies have been small and thus limited in their sensitivity. Several larger studies are currently being planned to examine this question.

Of the many recommendations made regarding VDTs, perhaps the most important is the need to provide workers with some control over their work patterns and environment. Many VDT data entry positions have been set up with required hourly key-stroke rates that are constantly monitored. The combination of this pressure, poor workplace design, and few, if any, breaks all contribute to the health problems experienced by these workers. NIOSH has recommended a 15-minute break for every 2 hours of VDT work or 15 minutes every hour if the workload or visual demands are high [19].

A review of the literature on VDT design suggests there is no consensus on the best ergonomic parameters for a VDT work station. Adjustable chairs and VDT tables, with separate and adjustable platforms for keyboard and screen, should be used so that each worker can find the best fit of viewing angle, distance, and keyboard height.

Supports for palm, hand, wrist, and arm may be desirable for prolonged typing. Chairs should provide a high seat back with proper support for both the lower and upper back. The VDT screen should have a glare reduction device, where necessary, and background lighting should be low with a separate light for the hard copy. The VDT unit should be positioned in the office to minimize glare on the screen. Each worker should be able to adjust the lighting and layout of the work station to his or her own comfort (Fig. 31-5).

Construction Trades Work

Women who work in "nontraditional" jobs, where the workforce is predominantly male, face different health and safety hazards, in part because the work is different from traditionally female occupations and in part because of the stress of being an unwelcome minority. In the past decade, women entered the skilled trades through special apprenticeship programs developed to respond to hiring goals set by many federal government contracts. Yet even now only 1.6 percent of the workers in the construction trades in the United States are women, and it is not uncommon for there to be a single woman on a job site employing hundreds of construction workers. Both the isolation and animosity that many men direct toward a woman in the trades is a source of significant stress on the job. Tradeswomen may end up working in isolated areas of a job site, where they might be harassed or assaulted. This hostility may pressure women to attempt work that is unsafe in order to prove they can make the grade.

The most common injuries in construction involve slips and falls from scaffolds, ladders, and roofs; falls on the ground; being struck by objects; overexertion during movement of building materials or equipment; and injuries from hand tools [20]. Although none of these is a hazard for women in particular, tradeswomen are often less likely to stop work and insist that conditions be improved because men, with more seniority, are willing to do the work or are critical of their "pampered" attitude. However, tradeswomen also report they may be more likely to notice potentially hazardous conditions because they are new in the field.

The health hazards encountered in construction depend in part on the trade of a worker. However, since most trades operate concurrently at the same site, there is much crossover of exposures. Trades workers doing renovation or demolition work often are exposed to asbestos. Some of the other health hazards encountered by construction workers include lime and silica in cement, fumes from welding, diesel exhaust, organic solvents, wood dust, and fibrous glass. In addition, in most construction, there are potentially hazardous exposures to poison oak and poison ivy, chemical wastes in the soil, noise, extremes of heat and cold, and vibration from tools or equipment [21]. A recent U.S. Department of Labor study reported that safety instructions for the work being done were never given to approximately one-half of construction laborers injured on the job. Over three-fourths of these workers were never provided with any information on asbestos or hazardous chemicals in their work, and over two-thirds wanted more information on safety and health risks found in their jobs [20].

Many construction jobs are repetitive and require stressful postures. Carpal tunnel syndrome, tenosynovitis, lower back injuries, and neck and shoulder pain are common problems for women as is the difficulty of finding tools and PPE that fits. Among tradeswomen, a common concern is the strength requirements for construction work. Tradeswomen are concerned about injuring themselves and at the same time they do not want to seek "special" treatment. In some cases, heavy lifting can be avoided by use of special tools or techniques, often used by older male workers, many of whom have been injured. In other cases, union agreements may define maximum lifting guides. Many tradeswomen lift weights or do other strength-conditioning exercises to prepare for work (see box on p. 484).

For pregnant construction workers, the heavy physical demands of nontraditional work may necessitate a transfer to a job where the needs for good balance and stamina are not as great. The worker, in conjunction with her health care provider, can determine if and when this is desirable. No research has been done to look at the reproductive outcomes of construction workers although some of the agents, such as noise, vibration, heat, cold, paints, and solvents, are thought to have potential adverse reproductive effects.

REFERENCES

1. Mergler D, Brabant C, Vezina N, Messing K. The weaker sex? Men in women's working conditions report similar health symptoms. J Occup Med 1987; 29:No. 5.
2. Warren-Gray B, Shapiro S. Hazards to women in the workplace. Department of Health, Education and Welfare, Health Resources Administration. Washington, DC.: DHEW, 1979. (HRA contract no. 232-78-0191).
3. Chavkin W, ed. Double exposure. New York: Monthly Review, 1984.
4. Armstrong TJ. Carpal tunnel syndrome and the female worker. Transactions of the 43rd Annual Meeting of the American Conference of Governmental Industrial Hygienists. Cincinnati, 1981:26–35.
5. Cannon LJ, Bernacki EJ, Walter SD. Personal and occupational factors associated with carpal tunnel syndrome. J Occup Med 1981; 23(4):255–8.
6. Ohara H, Aoyama H, Itani T. Health hazards among cash register operators and the effects of improved working conditions. J Hum Ergonomics 1976; 5:31–40.
7. Grandjean E, Hunting W, Nishiyama K. Preferred VDT workstation settings, body, posture and physical impairments. J Hum Ergonomics 1982; 11:45–53.
8. Videman T, Nurminen T, Tola S, Kuorinka I, Vanharauta H, Troup J. Low back pain in nurses and some loading factors of work, Spine 1984; 9(4):400–4.
9. Magora A. Investigation of the relation between low back pain and occupation. Industrial Medicine 1970; 39(11):465–71.
10. Murphy DC, Henifin MS, Stellman JM. Personal protective equipment for women: results of a manufacturers' and suppliers' survey. Transactions of the 43rd Annual Meeting of the American Conference of Governmental Industrial Hygienists. Cincinnati, 1981: 62–72.
11. Kipen H, Stellman J. Core curriculum: reproductive hazards in the workplace. White Plains, NY: March of Dimes, 1985.
12. National Institute for Occupational Safety and Health research report. Guidelines on pregnancy and work. The American College of Obstetricians and Gynecologists, U.S. Department of Health, Education, and Welfare. Rockville, MD.: NIOSH, 1977.
13. Welch LS. Decisionmaking about reproductive hazards. Semin Occup Med 1986; 1(2):97–106.
14. Goerth CG. Pregnant workers have discrimination protection. Occup Health Saf 1983:22–3.
15. Joseph LaDou, ed. The microelectronics industry. Occup Med: State of the Art Reviews. Vol. 1, No. 1, 1986.
16. Patterson WB, Craven DE, Schwartz DA, Nardell EA, Kasmer J, Noble J. Occupational hazards to hospital personnel. Ann Intern Med 1985; 102(5):658–90.

17. Stellman J, Henifen M. Office work can be dangerous to your health. New York: Pantheon, 1983.
18. American Society of Heating, Refrigeration and Air Conditioning Engineers. Standard: Ventilation for acceptable indoor air quality, Atlanta, GA: ASHRAE 1981. (ASHRAE publication no. 62-1981).
19. Murray WE, Moss CE, Parr WH. Potential health hazards of video display terminals. Rockland, MD.: National Institute for Occupational Safety and Health, 1981. (NIOSH publication no. 81–129).
20. U.S. Department of Labor, Bureau of Labor Statistics. Injuries to construction laborers. Washington, D.C.: 1986. Bulletin 2252.
21. Bertinuson J, Weinstein S. Occupational hazards of construction. Labor Occupational Health Program. Berkeley, CA: University of California, 1978.

BIBLIOGRAPHY

Chavkin W, ed. Double exposure: women's health hazards on the job and at home. New York: Monthly Review, 1984.
A thorough and well-documented selection of the social, economic, and scientific issues of women at work. Includes many important considerations that are often overlooked, including sections on household work, farm work, sexual harassment, and trade unions.

Clark E. Stopping sexual harassment, A handbook. Labor Education and Research Project, P. O. Box 2001, Detroit, MI 48220.
This handbook assists working women in identifying sexual harassment on the job and developing concrete strategies for change.

Davis L, Marbury M, Punnett L, Quinn M, Schwartz C, Woskie S. Our jobs, our health. Boston: Boston Women's Health Book Collective and Massachusetts Coalition for Occupational Safety on Health (MassCOSH), 625 Huntington Ave, Boston, MA 02115, 1983.
Written by the MassCOSH Women's Committee for women workers, this booklet is an overview of methods for recognition and control of workplace hazards. Chapters cover reproductive issues, stress, ergonomics, health and safety standards, toxic chemicals, legal rights, and accounts of women taking actions to correct workplace hazards.

Hunt VR. Work and the health of women. Boca Raton, FL.: CRC, 1979.
A comprehensive review of the physiologic, demographic, legal, and historical factors that affect the health and employment of women. Hazards of physical, chemical, and biologic environments are discussed including specific industries. Presents a concise summary of male reproductive hazards.

Stellman JM. Women's work, women's health. New York: Pantheon, 1977.
An overview of the history of working women, including stress, health hazards on the job, and policy issues concerning protective legislation and reproductive hazards.

U.S. Department of Labor. Facts of U.S. working women, 1986; Time of change: 1983 handbook on women workers Bulletin 298; Weekly earnings in 1985: a look at more than 200 occupations, September 1986; Occupational injuries and illnesses in the U.S. by industry. Bulletin 2259.
These publications were sources of the statistics on working women in this chapter. The Bureau of Labor Statistics publishes statistics on occupational safety, health, and wages; and the Women's Bureau has a wide variety of material on working women.

Appendix
Hazards in Industries That Employ Many Women

Marian Marbury

Type of work and estimated female employment*	Some common hazards	Some possible health effects
Household (1,100,000)	Cleaning substances (oven cleaners, bleach, detergents, aerosol sprays)	Dermatitis, mucous membrane and respiratory irritation
	Repetitive motions, lifting, slips, falls	Back strain, tendinitis, bursitis
	Sick children	Infectious diseases

Type of work and estimated female employment*	Some common hazards	Some possible health effects
Clerical (13,880,000)	Video display terminals	Eye, back, neck, and shoulder strain
	Poor office air quality and passive smoke exposure	Eye, mucous membrane, and respiratory irritation, headaches
	Poor lighting and chair design	Eye strain, musculoskeletal fatigue
	Stress	Headaches, fatigue, heart disease
Hospital (3,262,000)	Exposure to infectious patients and material	Infectious diseases including hepatitis
	Sterilizing and anesthetic gases, chemotherapeutic drugs	Skin and respiratory irritation, spontaneous abortions, birth defects (?), cancer, and central nervous system, liver, and kidney damage
	Radiation	Cancer, reproductive effects
	Lifting and falls	Low back strain, musculoskeletal fatigue, injuries to arms and legs
	Stress	Headaches, fatigue, heart disease
Retail sales (3,900,000)	Prolonged standing	Varicose veins, low back pain
	Safety hazards (blocked aisles and exits)	Injuries
	Poor indoor air quality and passive smoke exposure	Eye, mucous membrane and respiratory irritation, headaches
	Stress	Headaches, fatigue, heart disease
Textile (894,000)	Chemicals (fabric treatment, dyes, cleaning agents)	Dermatitis, respiratory irritation, liver and kidney damage
	Synthetic fiber and cotton dust	Asthma, chronic bronchitis, bysinnosis
	Noise	Irritability, hearing loss, high blood pressure
	Vibration	Raynaud's syndrome
	Extremes of temperature	Heat stress, dehydration, discomfort
	Unsafe equipment	Injuries
	Stress	Headaches, fatigue, heart disease
Art (100,000)	Solvents	Central nervous system depression, peripheral neuropathy, dermatitis
	Paints, soldering heavy metals	Damage to central nervous system, liver, kidneys
	Welding fumes	Chronic bronchitis, respiratory irritation
	Poor equipment maintenance	Injuries, burns

Type of work and estimated female employment*	Some common hazards	Some possible health effects
Laboratory (222,700)	Exposure to infectious biologic agents	Infectious diseases including hepatitis
	Solvents	Central nervous system depression, peripheral neuropathy, dermatitis
	Toxic chemicals, including mutagens and carcinogens; radioisotopes	Cancer and reproductive effects
Electronics (?)	Solvents	Central nervous system depression, peripheral neuropathy, dermatitis
	Acids	Skin burns, respiratory irritation
	Repetitive work	Tendinitis, carpal tunnel syndrome
	Fine work under microscopes	Eye and neck strain, headaches
	Solder fumes	Respiratory irritation
	Stress	Headaches, fatigue, heart disease
Cosmetology (635,800)	Prolonged standing	Varicose veins, low back pain
	Chemicals, including hair sprays, solvents	Dermatitis, respiratory and mucous membrane irritation, central nervous system depression
Laundry and dry cleaning (234,100)	Laundry: soaps, bleaches, acids	Dermatitis, respiratory irritation
	Dry cleaning: solvents	Central nervous system depression, peripheral neuropathy, dermatitis
	Lifting	Low back strain, musculoskeletal fatigue
	Heat	Heat stress, dehydration
Farm (231,400)	Awkward working positions	Low back strain, musculoskeletal disease
	Lack of field sanitation	Infectious diseases including urinary tract infection and parasitic infestation
	Pesticides	Pesticide poisoning
	Heat	Heat stress, dehydration
	Stress	Headaches, fatigue, heart disease

Type of work and estimated female employment*	Some common hazards	Some possible health effects
Construction (116,200)	Falling and flying objects, falls from scaffolding, electrocution	Injuries, death
	Lifting	Low back strain
	Noise	Irritability, hearing loss, high blood pressure
	Asbestos	Cancer, asbestosis
	Fibrous glass	Skin and respiratory system irritation
	Wood dust	Asthma, nasal cancer
	Carbon monoxide	Anoxia, heart disease, death
	Welding fumes	Chronic bronchitis, respiratory irritation
	Solvents	Central nervous system depression, peripheral neuropathy, dermatitis
Food preparation and service (3,184,000)	Repetitive motions	Tendinitis, carpal tunnel syndrome
	Slippery floors	Injuries
	Cold	Discomfort
	Lifting	Low back strain, musculoskeletal fatigue
	Unguarded machine saws	Laceration, amputation
	Plastic wrap fumes	Respiratory irritation
	Prolonged standing	Varicose veins, low back strain
	Unguarded heat sources	Burns

Source: Adapted from Our jobs, our health: a woman's guide to occupational health and safety. Boston: Massachusetts Coalition for Occupational Safety and Health and the Boston Women's Health Book Collective, 1983.
*U.S. Census Bureau, 1986.

32
Minority Workers

Bailus Walker, Jr.

The occupational health problems of minority workers* cannot be divorced from the nonoccupational health problems of the minority population, since many of the factors that influence the occurrence and progression of occupational disease are the same as those for nonoccupational disease. Moreover, occupational health according to the modern concept includes not only the prevention of occupational disease but also prevention of nonoccupational illness and the promotion of the health and welfare of the workforce.

The relationship of illness to occupation is complicated by occupations having two dimensions that affect health in different ways: (1) occupational status, which affects both the worker's health and that of the worker's family through the social and psychological environment of the society outside the workplace; and (2) the physical and, to a lesser extent, the social and psychological hazardous nature of the workplace, which affects only the worker's health.

MINORITY EMPLOYMENT

Before discussing aspects of occupational health problems of minorities, one should become familiar with the distribution of minority workers, since occupational health programs depend largely on this information.

*Although "minority workers" comprise many ethnic and racial groups, this chapter discusses mainly black workers because most of the limited information on minority workers concerns blacks. Their experience, however, likely represents the experiences of many other minority workers.

The United States, as other industrialized nations, has experienced a long-term shift from an agricultural to a goods-producing, then to a service-producing economic base. During the same period, nonwhites advanced both socially and economically, making notable strides in several areas, including educational attainment, voting rights, and earnings, as well as in employment.

Between 1972 and 1982, the number of employed nonwhites increased by 1.3 million (17%). The nonwhite proportion of the nation's employed workforce—9.4 percent—did not change, however, because the white employment level rose by 18 percent. While nonwhite advancement in several occupational categories was proportionately greater than that for whites, it was not sufficient to alter materially the overall nonwhite-to-white proportions of the previous decades. Nonwhites continue to represent a disproportionately small number of white-collar workers [1].

Nonwhite men increased their share of representation in a number of more highly skilled job categories, including electricians, painters, metal and printing craftsmen, and excavating and road-grading machine operators. The overall participation of nonwhite men in transport equipment operative positions held steady between 1972 and 1982, with nonwhites continuing to represent a disproportionately large number in these occupations. Nonwhites also made up about 20 percent or more of all men employed as clothing ironers and pressers, furnacemen, laundry and dry cleaning operators, sawyers, textile operators, bus drivers, forklift operators, and taxicab drivers. For the most part, participation by nonwhite men in these occupations increased or remained about the same between 1972 and 1982 because white men were moving out of these jobs.

Overall, shifts by nonwhites into the higher-salaried occupations were rather limited and were most apparent in central-city areas where most nonwhites live and where high concentrations of business activity exist. Many of the jobs created in urban centers—white-collar service positions requiring advanced skills—have been beyond the immediate reach of some urban minorities. Instead the jobs have gone to professionals who are returning to the central cities to take advantage of new employment opportunities.

OCCUPATIONAL MOBILITY

For certain purposes in occupational health, such as analysis of length of exposure to occupational stressors, it is appropriate to focus on workers' length of experience in their occupations. As would be expected, workers' length of tenure with their employers is strongly related to the age of the workers. For example, the vast majority of teenagers working in January 1985 held their jobs for 1 year or less. Workers aged 20 to 24 also had short tenures. In contrast, among workers aged 35 to 44, more than one-third had been employed at their jobs for at least 20 years.

On the average, men stay longer in the same occupation than women do. Black and Hispanic men all have longer occupational tenures than their female counterparts. As measured in 1985, the occupational mobility rate for Hispanic men was higher than that for white men and considerably higher than that for blacks. Black men had the lowest mobility rate in almost every age group. Thus, their duration of exposure to workplace hazards is much longer than more mobile workers, and they are more likely to be susceptible to specific work-related disease than workers with fewer years of exposure.

A number of factors are involved in occupational mobility. Among the positive factors, for ex-

ample, are better pay, increased postretirement benefits, and more appealing work. Negative factors include a forced change because of declining demand for one's preferred occupation. Because minority male workers predominated in industries sharply affected by the 1981 to 1982 recession, some of them may have been pushed, at least temporarily, into occupations with lower earnings, lower status, and higher risk of occupational disease and disability [1].

RISK IN MINORITY-INTENSIVE JOBS

Industry-specific epidemiologic studies can aid in establishing hypotheses of occupational disease causes. Minority workers, however, have often been underrepresented in such investigations. For example, a study of cancer mortality among members of a meat cutters' union examined only data for white males [2]; a study of leukemia risk among coal miners had no minorities in the sample [3]; the largest investigation of mortality patterns in aluminum reduction workers did not obtain data on race [4]; and a study of the health effects of automobile exhaust on tunnel and turnpike workers was limited to white male workers [5].

Even the most cursory consideration, however, leads to the empiric conclusion that minorities are more likely than nonminorities to work in occupations with a plethora of primary and secondary determinants of disease and disability. For minorities the probability of unhealthy employment is between 37 and 52 percent [6].

For most of its history, the United States has depended on minority workers to do much of the least desirable work. Since the turn of the century, the minority community has been the major source of labor for foundry work in the automobile industry, coke oven operations in the steel industry, construction jobs with the highest risk of exposure to hazardous dust and of physical injury, and public works jobs such as waste collection and disposal.

One of the earliest recorded examples of a minority occupational health problem was the so-called West Virginia Gauley Bridge tragedy that befell a large group of workers between 1930 and 1931. They were recruited from several southern states to construct a tunnel through a West Virginia mountain—a geological stratum composed mainly of sandstone with a high concentration of silica. Of the nearly 3,000 men who worked at least part of the time inside the tunnel, 75 percent were black. They drilled and removed the fragmented sandstones produced by drilling—the most dangerous of tunneling operations according to the most recent analysis of historical data on the disaster [7]. These workers experienced prolonged exposure to high concentrations of crystalline silica dust, which causes silicosis. Although the health effects of prolonged exposure to silica had been recognized for decades, the tunnel workers were not informed by management of the hazards associated with their jobs, nor did management take steps to reduce the risk of silica-induced disease through the application of appropriate industrial hygiene practices available at the time. These and other failures of management to implement a comprehensive occupational health program concerned both with prevention of silicosis and promotion of maximum health and welfare of the tunnel workers resulted in significant morbidity and mortality.

The death toll of the disaster at Gauley Bridge was immense when compared with any other outbreak of industrial disease in modern history. That toll was taken not by accident and a merciful, sudden death, but by prolonged illness and physical deterioration. And no statistical method has been devised to tally human suffering and despair [7].

Other examples that have attracted epidemiologic concerns can be summarized as follows:

1. A study of the mortality experience of coke oven workers revealed that nonwhites had a disproportionately high rate of lung cancer attribut-able to prolonged exposure to coke oven emissions [8, 9].

2. Some 85,000 black workers were employed in the textile mill industry between 1960 and 1979 (Fig. 32-1). Even though they had worked in the mills for a shorter period than whites, they were at a higher risk of developing byssinosis because the black workers were assigned to work areas with highest concentrations of dust of cotton, flax, or soft hemp [10].

3. Observations reveal that the incidence of bronchogenic carcinoma was significantly higher among black workers who comprised 41 percent of the laborers in the so-called dry end of the chromium-compound manufacturing process. In this section of the plant, workers were exposed to high concentrations of chromium dust [11, 12].

4. A report of five cases of pentachlorophenol (PCP) poisoning included two fatalities that occurred in two small wood preservative-manufacturing plants. All patients were black men less than 50 years of age. In one case, the worker's job involved crushing 2000-lb blocks of PCP with an electric jackhammer in a small, poorly ventilated room. The other cases were assigned jobs involving a dry-mixing process in which borax, kerosene, and sodium pentachlorophenate were emptied manually into a mixing tank. The process was dusty and the ventilation was poor. The workers often returned home from their jobs covered in dust [13].

5. A study of the mortality of workers in a construction equipment and diesel engine plant, where major exposures included solvents, cutting oils, and metal dust, found a significant excess among black males of deaths for all malignant neoplasms combined, for cancer of the pancreas, and for non-Hodgkin's lymphomas. These excess deaths occurred even though whites were more frequently employed earlier than blacks. Among white male workers, no significant deviations from expected deaths were recorded [14].

More recently, surveys of the U.S. occupational structure and of occupational illness indicate that

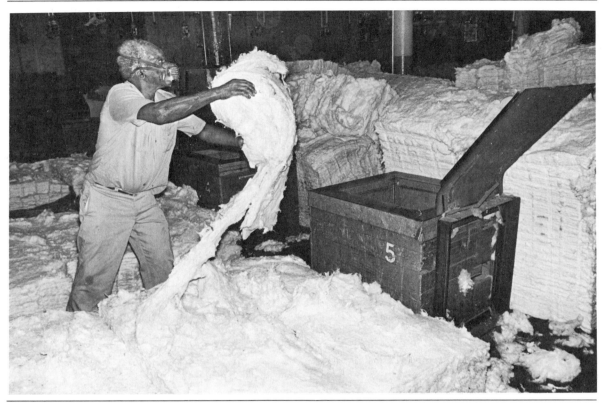

Fig. 32-1. Minority workers often are employed in the least desirable and most hazardous jobs, such as this worker opening bales of cotton—a job that has traditionally carried a high risk of byssinosis. (Photograph by Earl Dotter.)

minorities are still overrepresented in the high-risk sectors of the economy and in the more hazardous occupations within these industries. Table 32-1 shows the percentage of blacks in selected occupations and the lost work-day rate due to occupational illnesses and injuries per 100 full-time workers by occupation. It appears that blacks in general are overrepresented in the high-risk occupations. It is also evident that limited gains among blacks have been realized in the low-hazard occupations of banking, legal services, insurance, brokerage, underwriting. and accounting, which are among the fastest growing sectors of the U.S. economy.

Although the Occupational Safety and Health Act of 1970 increased the attention given to occupational health problems of minorities by health and safety professionals and employers, gains made in workplace risk reduction for all workers during the earlier phases of the act's implementation have been eroded. For example, during 1984, approximately 125,000 occupational illnesses were recorded, compared with approximately 106,000 illnesses in 1983—approximately 20 percent more. The largest proportion of illness cases was in agriculture (Fig. 32-2) and manufacturing (Fig. 32-3). The construction industry continued to have the highest injury incidence rate.

Table 32-1. Employed blacks as a percent of all employed men and women in selected occupations and the lost workday rate due to occupational illness and injuries (1984)

Occupation	Percent black		Lost workdays[a] (rate/100 full-time workers)
	Men	Women	
Meat cutters and butchers	9	19	181
Waste collectors	32	[b]	169
Construction workers	15	[b]	128
Furnace workers	25	[b]	109
Farm laborers	14	15	100
Garage workers and gas station attendants	8	[b]	47
Laundry and dry cleaners	28	21	43
Food service workers	11	10	34
Bank officials	3	5	11
Lawyers and judges	3	7	5
Insurance agents	4	8	4
Accountants	4	9	3

[a]Lost workdays include days away from work and days of restricted work activity because of occupational injury or illness.
[b]Data not shown where numerator is less than 4,000 or denominator is less than 35,000.
Sources: US Department of Labor, Bureau of Labor Statistics. Occupational injury and illness in the United States by industry, Washington, D.C.: U.S. Government Printing Office, 1984; and DN Westcott. Blacks in 1970s: did they scale the job ladder? Monthly Labor Review, 1982; 105:29–38.

The lowest rate was in wholesale and retail trades, where relatively few minority individuals work.

This upward trend in occupational injury and illness is due to a complex mix of economic, scientific, and regulatory issues, including intense competition among many economic sectors, weakened enforcement of health and safety regulations, and an overt conflict between health, safety, and job security.

Although the U.S. Bureau of Labor Statistics' surveys of work-related illness are comprehensive and well designed, there is a longstanding concern about the completeness of the recordkeeping on which the surveys are based. Such routinely published data may underestimate the true impact of the occupational environment on minority workers' health.

CORPORATE STRESSORS
Within the past two decades, the removal of several structural barriers to managerial jobs has en-

hanced minority employment in the corporate setting. There remain, however, cultural, attitudinal, and social barriers that often confront minorities who are newly introduced into these workplaces. Both real and perceived discrimination, which is often subtle and insidious, is a common stressor, as are a subjective sense of quantitative work overload, exacerbated by involvement in more than one job, and a sudden increase in job responsibility especially when there are conflicting demands and job dissatisfaction (see Chap. 20).

Although the links between socioenvironmental conditions and social support to disease and dysfunction require more thorough study, an increasing volume of literature is already suggesting a relationship between corporate stressors and stress-related disorders, such as hypertension, functional gastrointestinal disorders, general anxiety, and muscular tension.

Concepts and methodologies to measure precisely the health effects of subtle socioenvironmental stressors are only beginning to be devel-

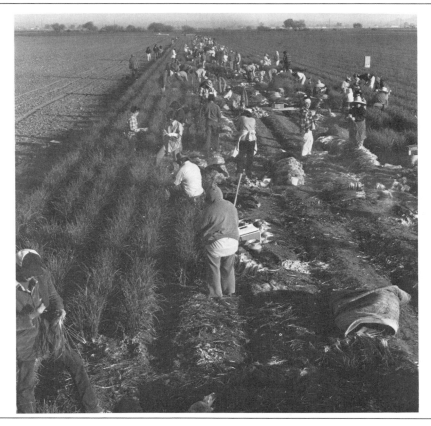

Fig. 32-2. Migrant farmworkers, often Hispanic, face many work-associated hazards, including physical stresses and exposure to pesticides.
(Photograph by Ken Light.)

oped. Nevertheless, occupational health specialists should be alert to emotional, health-related, cultural, and attitudinal barriers as possible sources of common physical and psychological symptoms in minority workers. Emotional health programs dedicated to the detection, prevention, education, treatment, referral, and follow-up of stressed employees should include systems for identifying pockets of stressor overload and systems for recommending to corporate management forms of early interventions.

GENETIC TESTING AND OCCUPATIONAL HEALTH

An increasing concern of minority workers and of health professionals concerned with minority health issues is the emphasis on genetic testing as a part of medical screening and monitoring in the workplace. Genetic testing is a collection of techniques used to examine workers for particular inherited genetic traits. It has been used by some major companies and utilities for medical evaluation and by others for research. Many more organiza-

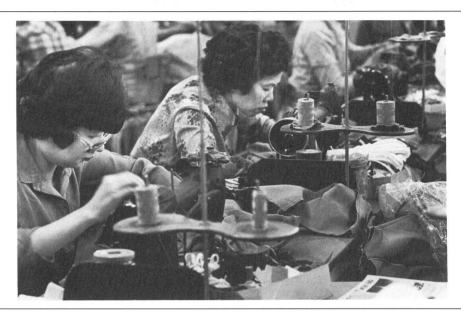

Fig. 32-3. Asian workers in the United States sometimes work in low-paying, monotonous jobs, such as in the garment industry, as shown here.
(Photograph by Earl Dotter.)

tions have expressed an interest in incorporating genetic testing into occupational health problems (see Chap. 28).

Since many of the genetic traits sought in screening are found disproportionately among some races and ethnic groups, there is a heightened awareness among these groups that test results could be used for discrimination on the basis of race, sex, or ethnicity. There is also concern that genetic testing may direct attention away from other ways to address risk of occupational disease.

In this context, occupational health specialists question whether an employee's risk of future illness is an appropriate factor for job selection, even if screening or monitoring are highly predictive. They argue that employees have no control over their genetic make-up and generally have no control over previous exposures to harmful agents. In addition, their increased risk would not affect their current ability to do the job.

The counterarguments to these assertions include: (1) society accepts immutable characteristics as possible proper criteria for employment selection; and (2) the autonomous interest of the individual should not be above the interest of society in reducing the economic and social cost of occupational illness.

But the role of genes in disease is still not fully understood, and the identification of genetic factors that may contribute to the occurrence of job-related illness is a science still in its infancy. Data are most lacking concerning the correlation of genetic traits to occupational disease susceptibility. Clearly genetic factors do not act in isolation from other biological variables, such as nutritional status and preexisting disease, which affect a worker's susceptibility to a broad spectrum of occupational stressors. Thus, the assessment of factors that may increase the risk of occupational disease should not stop at quantification of inherited genetic traits but should also incorporate many other biological variables.

A consequence of the public's concern and in some cases its opposition to genetic testing has been an attempt to address a number of issues within the broad scope of employee-employer relations, ranging from the nature of the physician-employee relationship through the proper use of the test results.

One frequently advocated approach includes the following: (1) prohibit job exclusion on the basis of genetic make-up; (2) prohibit job transfer because of genetic make-up or genetic damage, unless the transfer is to a comparable job at comparable pay and benefits; (3) require strict confidentiality of medical information; and (4) require that employees be told of the results of testing and be given counseling.

This approach would protect the interest of workers, preventing serious consequences to individuals who have no control over the misuse of test results. It would also be consistent with many established legal principles governing the rights and duties of employers, employees, and company medical personnel.

IMPLICATIONS FOR HEALTH PROFESSIONALS

As the service industry continues to grow and as manufacturing no longer provides adequate support for modern society, race and ethnicity, as labor market distinctions, will continue to erode. A different demographic profile will emerge. Within the next several decades, one in every three Americans will be nonwhite. Of those under 18, the proportion of nonwhites will be almost 45 percent, nearly 3 times what it was after World War II. Moreover, because black and Hispanic birth rates are above the national average, the percentage of minority children—and of potential minority entrants to the labor force—will continue to grow [15].

This changing demography, coupled with technologic pressure and expansion in the service industries, will create social, economic, and political demands for the training and employment of a much larger number of minorities than ever before in the U.S. economy.

In this setting, occupational health professionals must ensure that occupational health programs are consistently concerned not only with the prevention of disease and stress resulting from the occupation or the work environment, but also with the promotion of maximum health and welfare of the working population. For minorities, this aspect of occupational health involves a synthesis of (1) the philosophy, interest, resources, and efforts of many disciplines, and (2) the agencies and organizations, such as those concerned with public assistance, housing, education, social service, and health care, especially for the multiproblem worker. Occupational health personnel are not accustomed to advising a community to concentrate on better housing, equal education, and employment opportunities, but occasionally this advice would be sound in a comprehensive long-term effort to prevent the occurrence of occupational disease and dysfunction in minority workers.

Efficient use of occupational health professionals rests on the presence of other support services in the private and public sectors. Making this point clear may become a part of the occupational health education of the public and of policy-makers.

For example, the provision of appropriate nutrition counseling, adolescent health services, or adequate child care and housing assistance may be a high priority at a particular time and place in the occupational experience of minority workers. Fortunately, in most communities a wide variety of resources exist that may be called on by the occupational health professional. For some time, attempts have been made to provide some degree of joint service planning. Usually these attempts take the form of a council of health and social services agencies or a community health and welfare council in which there is membership by many of the agencies active in providing services to individuals and families.

Finally, comprehensive planning for occupational health services is only possible with a system that determines the incidence of illness and injuries among minorities. Health professionals have a responsibility to ensure that such systems operate and that the epidemiologic study of occupational disease includes minorities, whenever possible.

REFERENCES

1. Westcott DN. Blacks in 1970s: did they scale the job ladder? Monthly Labor Review 1982; 105:29–38.
2. Johnson E, Fischman HR, Matanoski GM, Diamond E. Cancer mortality among white males in the meat industry. J Occup Med 1986; 28:23–32.
3. Gilman PA, Ames RG, McCawley E. Leukemia risk among U.S. white male coal miners—a case control study. J Occup Med 1985; 27:669–71.
4. Gibbs GW. Mortality of aluminum reduction plant workers 1950 through 1977. J Occup Med 1985; 27:761–70.
5. Tollerud DJ, Weiss ST, Elting EH et al. The health effects of automobile exhaust. VI: relationship of respiratory symptoms and pulmonary function in tunnel and turnpike workers. Arch Environ Health 1983; 38:334–40.
6. Robinson JC. Racial inequality and the probability of occupation-related illness. Milbank Memorial Fund Quarterly/Health and Society 1984; 62:567–90.
7. Cherniack M. The Hawk's Nest incident: America's worst industrial disaster. New Haven, CT: Yale University Press, 1986.
8. Lloyd W. Long-term mortality study of steelworkers: V. respiratory cancer in coke plant workers. J Occup Med 1971; 13:53–68.
9. Redmond CK et al. Long-term mortality experience of steel workers. Cincinnati: NIOSH, 1981. (DHHS/NIOSH publication. no. 81–120).
10. Martin C, Higgins J. Byssinosis and other respiratory ailments: a survey of cotton textile employees. J Occup Med 1976; 18:455.
11. Gafafer W. Health of workers in the chromate producing industry: a study. Washington, DC.: U.S. Public Health Service, 1953.
12. Sunderman FW Jr. A review of the carcinogenicity of nickel, chromium and arsenic compounds in men and animals. Prev Med 1976; 5:279–90.
13. Wood S et al. Pentachlorophenol poisoning. J Occup Med 1983; 25:527–30.
14. Mallin K, Berkeley L, Young Q. A proportional mortality study of workers in a construction equipment and diesel engine manufacturing plant. Am J Ind Med 1986; 10:127–41.
15. Steen LA. Mathematics education: a predictor of scientific competitiveness. Science 1987; 237–52.

BIBLIOGRAPHY

Bell C. Occupational health hazards and the minority workers. Hazardous Material Management 1980; 2:37–41.
This article reviews research efforts needed to assess the impact of occupational exposures on morbidity and mortality rates of minority workers.

Canter EG. Employment discrimination of genetic screening in the workplace under Title VII and the Rehabilitation Act. Am J Law Med 1984; 10:323–47.
This report analyzes genetic screening cases with respect to currently available remedies contained in Title VII of the Civil Rights Act of 1964 and the Rehabilitation Act of 1973. The report concludes that Title VII claims will encounter enormous obstacles to relief. Additionally, the publication discusses some of the implications of the use of genetic screening in the workplace.

Davis ME. The impact of workplace safety and health on black workers: assessment and prognosis. Labor Law J 31:723, 1980.
An analysis of health problems among black workers. It also addresses policy issues and recommends strategies for solving these problems.

Sparacino J, Ronchi D et al. Blood pressure of male municipal employees: effects of job status and worksite. Percept Mot Skills 1982; 55:563–78.
A study of the resting blood pressure and heart rate of 441 municipal workers ranging widely in age, job level, and education. Higher rates were obtained for blue-collar as opposed to white-collar employees. Whites' and blacks' blood pressures deviated significantly from expected values. Social and psychologic mechanisms that may mediate these effects are discussed.

Walker B. The relevance of occupational medicine. J Nat Med Assoc 1982; 74:200–8.
A discussion of the relevance of occupational health services for minority populations. The author argues that workplace exposures are among the major determinants of health problems among minorities.

Wescott DN. Blacks in the 1970's: did they scale the job ladder? Monthly Labor Review 1982; 105:29–38.
An examination of occupational shifts of black workers between 1972 and 1980, using population survey data on employment by detailed occupation, race,

and sex. To further assess the extent of occupational mobility among blacks during this period, occupational data by area of residence and usual weekly earnings are also analyzed.

U.S. Department of Health and Human Services. Report of the Secretary's Task Force on Black and Minority Health. Washington, DC.: DHHS, 1985. Vol. 2.

A detailed analysis of social and economic determinants of the differential health experience of minorities and nonminorities. It contains a collection of papers on nutrition, socioeconomic position, and health services delivery to minorities.

33
Agricultural Workers

Molly Joel Coye and Richard Fenske

An 18-member work crew responsible for checking mushroom beds for blight entered one of the growing rooms in a mushroom plant. Their task was to inspect the beds for blight and to cut out the affected parts. The rooms were relatively dark, with no windows and only two doors. Several minutes after this crew began to work on the beds, an applicator crew, apparently unaware that the other crew was inside, sprayed the entrance of the growing room and the adjoining circulation vents with the organophosphate pesticide diazinon.

Within 15 to 20 minutes, all but one of the workers developed headache, dizziness, fatigue, and nausea. Four workers began to vomit and were taken to a local hospital, where they were admitted to the intensive care unit, decontaminated, and treated with atropine. All but one of the nonhospitalized workers were seen by the same physician who admitted the first four. Cholinesterase levels were drawn and the patients were followed on an outpatient basis. Workers were not allowed to return to work for varying periods of time; the four hospitalized patients were finally released for work 13 days after the incident with work restrictions, including an insecticide-free environment for the following month.

Red blood cell cholinesterase levels for the nine exposed workers who were seen by the local physician in the hospital and subsequently in his office were analyzed. All nine of workers' initial levels, in the 5 days after the incident, fell in the low-normal or below-normal range for the laboratory. Moreover, each of the workers had a marked increase in cholinesterase levels by 15 days after the incident, placing them well within the middle of the normal range. This information suggests an initial depression in cholinesterase levels with a subsequent return toward baseline, consistent with organophosphate poisoning and the severe symptoms that at least four of the workers initially had [1].

The total U.S. agricultural labor force is estimated at 4 to 5 million workers. Hired, nonfamily farm workers constitute between one-third and one-half of that total. Approximately one-half of all farm workers are seasonal. Seasonal workers are at greatest risk for occupational hazards in agriculture because they are concentrated in high-risk crops and activities: 80 percent of all pesticides used in agriculture are applied to 20 percent of the total crop acreage, where most seasonal field laborers work.

Farm workers are concentrated geographically in three migrant streams flowing (1) up the West Coast through California, (2) the Central plains from Texas to Wisconsin and Ohio, and (3), the East Coast from Florida to Maine. More than one-half of all hired farm workers on large farms are found in just two states, California and Florida, and 65 percent are employed in the production of vegetables, fruits, nuts, tobacco, or sugar [2].

Whereas farm workers migrate across states, farmers and agricultural service workers (pesticide applicators, equipment salespersons, repair workers, and others) commonly remain in the same community year-round. Where farms are small, the farmer may perform the full range of tasks from pesticide application to weeding and harvesting.

MORBIDITY AND MORTALITY IN AGRICULTURE

Agricultural work is one of the most dangerous and physically demanding occupations in America

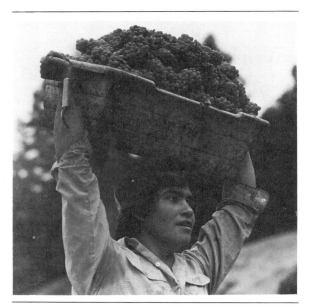

Fig. 33-1. Farmworkers, as illustrated by the work of this grape picker, face physically demanding jobs, which often predispose them to serious injury. (Photograph by Ken Light.)

(Fig. 33-1). Injury and death rates rank agriculture consistently among the three most hazardous industries in the United States. The death rate for agricultural workers is 54 per 100,000 workers in comparison with 57 and 63 per 1,000,000 workers for construction and mining, and the injury rate for agricultural workers is even greater than that for construction and mining [3].

As with injury rates, illness rates place agriculture among the most hazardous occupations. In California, occupational illnesses per 100 full-time workers in 1979 were 0.3 for all industries combined, 0.5 for manufacturing, 0.3 for mining, 0.3 for construction, 0.6 for agriculture [4]. While injury rates have been declining, occupational disease rates have not, and they represent a rising proportion of all morbidity among agricultural workers. In public health terms, this fact resembles the broader shift in developed industrial societies to predominant patterns of chronic disease.

Even in this industrial society, the living conditions of many migrant seasonal farm workers and of some poor family farmers more closely resemble those of families in developing nations (Fig. 33-2). Deficiencies in nutrition, housing, sanitation, education, and access to health care all constitute the general health status of these families and individuals and frequently exacerbate occupational health risks. Housing in or near fields exposes workers and their families to pesticide spray drift. Lack of adequate sanitation is associated with an increased prevalence of parasitic and infectious disease among migrant farm workers [5]. Lack of potable water in the fields and in some housing forces workers to drink irrigation water, which is frequently contaminated with pesticide run-off and is increasingly used as a direct method of pesticide application. Lack of education makes it difficult or impossible for workers to read pesticide labels and posted signs, a problem that is even more serious for the many agriculture workers in the United States who speak little or no English. Finally, the same economic and geographic factors that limit access to medical care for farm workers may also delay or prevent appropriate treatment for job-related injuries and illnesses.

Despite this pattern of morbidity and mortality, farm workers are specifically excluded from key labor laws, from almost all federal and state occupational safety and health laws and regulations, and, in one-half the states in the United States, from the workers' compensation system as well. As a result, injuries and illnesses are significantly underreported; although California is one of only two states to require notification regarding pesticide illnesses, the California Department of Health Services has estimated that an extremely small proportion of all pesticide-related illness among farm workers is reported [6].

Agriculture has been treated as a "special case" even in regard to basic workplace sanitation. All other workers—including those in similar outdoor and transient conditions of employment, such as construction and forestry—have been guaranteed rights to the provisions of basic sanitation since

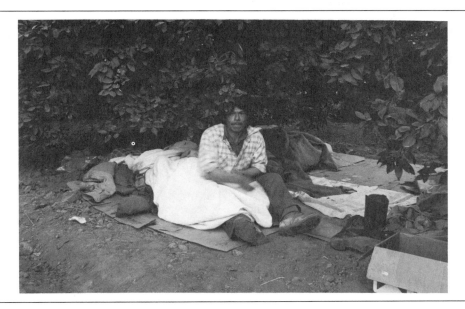

Fig. 33-2. Migrant farmworkers typically suffer from housing and other socioeconomic problems, as illustrated by these workers sleeping under orange trees because no housing was provided. (Photograph by Ken Light.)

1971: hand washing and potable water and portable toilets. The first farm worker petition to the Occupational Safety and Health Administration (OSHA) was filed in 1972; OSHA consistently denied such petitions and appealed multiple court orders to develop a field sanitation standard. Under threat of congressional action to legislate field sanitation protection, OSHA finally promulgated a field sanitation standard in 1987.

OCCUPATIONAL EXPOSURE AMONG FARM WORKERS

Pesticides

Pesticide exposure represents a major potential health hazard for farmers and agricultural field workers. As our knowledge of the toxicology of pesticides expands, it becomes increasingly important to characterize both the causes and the extent of chemical exposures. Exposure levels that were considered acceptable a decade ago are now being carefully evaluated for health risks.

Only recently have the principles of industrial hygiene been applied systematically to agriculture. The evaluation of pesticide use and exposure in agriculture is complex for several reasons. First, the physical nature of the chemical can vary greatly: Workers may be exposed to pesticides in their concentrated form, as a dilute aqueous spray, as granules or pellets, or as a residue on crops and foliage. Second, workers are exposed to a wide variety of chemicals over a single season: A potent and acutely toxic organophosphorus compound may be applied one day, a skin-irritating sulfur material the next day, and a mutagenic fungicide on the following day. Third, chemical exposures occur under totally uncontrolled environmental conditions: Factors such as wind, rain, and sunlight can dramatically alter exposure potential. Finally, unlike exposures in many industrial settings, the major route of exposure to pesticides in agriculture is dermal rather than respiratory. For this reason traditional industrial hygiene approaches, such as air sampling and adherence to threshold limit values (TLVs), have limited relevance. In considering the evaluation and control of agricultural pesticide exposures, it is useful to distinguish between workers who directly handle or those who are exposed to pesticides during application and field workers who are primarily exposed to crop residues.

Mixers and Applicators

As the organophosphate pesticides replaced organochlorines for many uses in the early 1950s, the U.S. Public Health Service recognized that pesticide applicators were at high risk for acute intoxication. Because agricultural exposure is primarily to the skin, investigators developed what has come to be known as the "patch technique," using gauze pads as collection devices on various parts of the body to determine levels of deposition. Hand exposure was measured by rinsing the hands with water or alcohol and concentrating the residue collected [7].

These methods provided enough information to draw several important conclusions. First, the highest exposures usually occur during mixing and handling of the concentrated material. Second, wind is the single most important factor determining dermal exposure during application. Third, in most cases, exposure to the hands constitutes a major fraction of the total exposure. Fourth, the use of protective clothing can substantially reduce total dermal exposure. More recently, fluorescent tracers have been employed to visualize patterns of pesticide deposition on the skin, allowing evaluation of protective clothing performance and effective worker education (Fig. 33-3) [8].

The primary method of preventing exposure during pesticide mixing is an engineering control: the closed system that transfers the pesticide from its container to the mixing tank without direct handling by the worker. When functioning properly, these systems can reduce exposure consider-

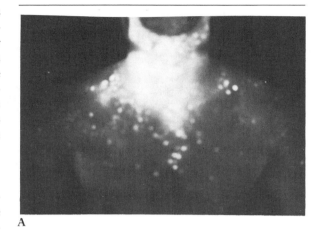

A

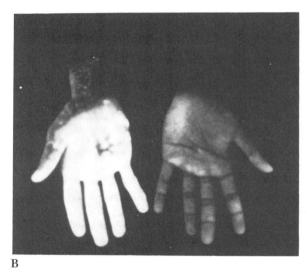

B

Fig. 33-3. A. Fluorescent tracer evaluation of a pesticide applicator reveals deposition on the neck and on the chest beneath coveralls. The area around the mouth was protected by a respirator. B. The use of gloves while handling pesticides can reduce exposure dramatically. The right hand, in this photograph done with a fluorescent tracer, was not protected by a glove, as the left one was.

ably. When a system failure occurs, however, potential exposure is very high.

The most common engineering control for exposure reduction during the actual application of pesticides is the closed cab tractor. The closed cab normally provides an effective barrier to dermal contact. However, the efficiency of the air filtration system is critical. If the cab is left partially open or if improper filters are employed, the utility of this approach is reduced drastically. Also, exposure may actually be higher inside the cab than outside if the worker enters the cab with boots and work clothes contaminated during mixing procedures.

A supplemental but very important preventive measure for mixers and applicators is training: Knowledge of the operation of closed systems, of the relative toxicity of compounds, of the proper handling and disposal of concentrated material, and of when to spray are all required. (Since windy conditions will increase exposures substantially during application, many agricultural regions prohibit pesticide spraying then.)

The final control strategy for mixers and applicators is protective clothing. Protective gear, such as gloves, face shields, aprons, and boots, can effectively reduce exposure. If mixing is only an intermittent and short-term activity, such a strategy may prove practical, but skin contamination can still occur in the removal of the gear or in cases where clothing is not properly cleaned before reuse [9].

Regulatory agencies, such as the U.S. Environmental Protection Agency (EPA), have recently turned to protective clothing as a primary strategy for exposure reduction in agriculture. This approach has always been considered a control of last resort by industrial hygienists for a number of important reasons. First, such a control strategy requires continual training of personnel in the proper use and maintenance of clothing. Second, the clothing must be inspected periodically and replaced when necessary. Third, use of chemical protective clothing often reduces the comfort, agility, and dexterity of the worker and may contribute to heat stress under agricultural conditions. Thus, an *effective* control program based on protective clothing may prove to be more costly and more difficult to monitor than equally effective engineering and administrative approaches.

Field Workers

The pesticide hazard that agricultural field workers confront takes the form of residues on fruit, foliage, or soil. This hazard is complicated by workers generally being unaware of their potential for exposure and the consequent health risks they face. Since many of these workers are migratory and are not involved with other farm operations, they may not know what pesticides have been used or when they were sprayed. Furthermore, a substantial number of studies have demonstrated that residue levels on foliage are difficult to predict. The arid regions of California and the southwestern United States are particularly problematic, as high residue levels can remain for many weeks. Under certain environmental conditions, a number of organophosphorus compounds can even be transformed into their more toxic "oxon" derivatives; for example, the oxon derivative of parathion, paraoxon, is 10 times more acutely toxic than parathion.

The thinning and harvesting operations that field workers perform require direct contact with foliage, and significant dermal exposure to any pesticide residues on the foliage is largely unavoidable. The hard physical labor and high temperatures typically encountered make protective clothing an even more unrealistic method for the prevention of exposure. Several decades of research point to the conclusion that the only practical means of minimizing exposure for field workers is to make certain that toxic levels of residues have degraded or dissipated before workers are allowed into the fields. To achieve this goal, *reentry intervals* are derived from repeated studies of pesticide residue decay on specific crops. The EPA has established a minimum reentry interval for all pesticide applications that requires waiting until the pesticide spray has dried and the pesticide dust (powder or granules) has settled. In addition, 24-hour and 48-hour reentry intervals are in effect nationwide for a number of acutely toxic compounds. In California, where "long-term" reentry is an issue because of the arid climate and persistent residues, the reentry interval may extend up to 60 days for particular pesticide and crop combinations.

Traditional engineering controls used in occupational health are usually not feasible as a means of reducing pesticide residue exposures in agriculture. However, several prevention strategies with engineering aspects are useful. One strategy is the provision of hand-washing facilities for the removal of pesticide residues before eating or using the bathroom and at the end of the workday. A second strategy is product substitution, in which a less toxic pesticide is used in place of a hazardous compound. A third approach is the development of alternative pest control technologies, such as biological control, that reduce pesticide use. A final engineering possibility is the application of alternative cultivation practices, such as crop rotation and the cultivation of mixed varieties, that reduce the need for heavy pesticide use.

Other Exposures
In addition to the occupational risks of pesticide exposure, agricultural work also entails risks associated with the use of equipment, exposure to animal-borne infectious diseases (see Chap. 19), geographic and social isolation, heat stress (see Chap. 18), and hearing loss (see Chap. 17) from the operation of heavy equipment such as tractors and combines. Traditional agricultural tools and labor practices exact a toll on the musculoskeletal system of life-long farmers. Modernization, in turn, has frequently brought more extensive use, and physiologically less adaptive uses, of traditional tools such as "el cortito," the short-handled hoe. The industrialization of agriculture has also introduced new equipment for harvesting and on-field packaging of many fruits and vegetables. This equipment has frequently been designed without the benefit of ergonomic analyses and produces new forms of musculoskeletal disease and risks of injury for farm workers and operators.

National health surveys find that farm workers have a higher prevalence of arthritis than white-collar, blue-collar, service, or all workers combined; musculoskeletal conditions are the most commonly reported ailments among farmers and farm managers, and farmers report over 50 percent more musculoskeletal disease than farm managers [10]. The significance of this evidence of widespread musculoskeletal disease must be emphasized because it is often ignored by clinicians, either because they look predominantly for signs of pesticide exposure or because they assume that musculoskeletal disease is an unavoidable result of farm labor. In fact, ergonomic strain associated with farm work can be minimized or entirely prevented with the appropriate redesign of equipment and labor practices. In forestry and construction occupations, related or similar to some in agriculture, such changes have significantly reduced the ergonomic problems of many tasks (see Chap. 9).

The mechanization of agriculture has had benefits. It has reduced the number of occupational injuries by replacing workers and lowered the rate of occupational injuries by mechanizing many hazardous hand-labor processes. However, it has also resulted in widespread unemployment within certain sectors of agriculture and has been accompanied by other changes with more adverse effects. No-till cultivation eliminates hand weeding and requires large quantities of herbicides instead to kill weeds. Reduced cultivation activities, such as weeding, encourages increased insect populations and thus greater use of pesticides. And subsequent development of resistance to the pesticides requires heavier chemical applications. Fortunately, these counterproductive cycles can now be interrupted in many crops with the aid of integrated pest management (IPM), which relies on the limited use of pesticides and more intensive use of other cultivation techniques and beneficial insects.

OCCUPATIONAL DISEASE AMONG FARMWORKERS

Dermatitis

As in much of industry, dermatitis is the most frequently reported occupational disease in agriculture. In California, the rate of occupational skin disease for all industries combined in 1977 was 2.1 cases per 1,000 workers; for manufacturing, construction, and mining, the rates were 4.1, 2.5, and 2.0, respectively, while for agriculture the rate was 8.6. Agriculture represented 3 percent of all jobs in the state but 13 percent of occupational dermatoses. Most agricultural dermatoses are due to plant exposures, although pesticide-related skin diseases often require extended periods of disability leave [11]. It is usually difficult to distinguish the clinical presentation of plant dermatoses from pesticide dermatoses, be they irritant contact dermatitis, allergic contact dermatitis, or a photosensitivity reaction.

The differential diagnosis of plant dermatosis versus pesticide dermatosis is accomplished primarily through the history of a temporal association between work in a certain field or crop, the agricultural cycle and chemical applications, and symptoms. For example, a recurrent rash in the early part of June may be related to a weed that flourishes then; a rash occurring in July may result from exposure to a herbicide used on the crop at that stage of the cycle each year. Distribution on the extremities may also provide a clue; pesticide residues dislodged from foliage often irritate the face and neck in addition to the forearms, hands, and ankles, whereas contact with plants may produce irritation on the forearms, hands, and ankles alone. Patch testing with plant extracts or pesticide samples will frequently permit a definitive diagnosis in cases of allergic contact dermatitis (see Chap. 23).

Diagnostic Approaches to Pesticide Illness

Moderate to Severe Acute Exposures. Acute pesticide exposures are frequently recognized in the initial presentation of the patient to the clinician, although the specific chemical may be unknown (Table 33-1). Most common among acute pesticide poisonings today are those caused by organophosphates with fairly typical symptoms, as illustrated in the case at the start of this chapter (Table 33-2). As emergency life-support procedures are instituted, samples of vomitus, urine, and blood should be taken, and the patient should be rapidly decontaminated. Also, care must be taken to protect health workers from exposure because exposures in handling bodily fluids or contaminated clothing may be substantial, and emergency room personnel have become very ill while assisting pesticide-poisoned patients.

Specific clinical treatment for acute and emergent pesticide exposure is comprehensively detailed in *Recognition and Management of Pesticide Poisonings* [12].

The clinical diagnosis of moderate or severe or-

Table 33-1. **Major chemical groups of pesticides**

Groups and examples	Action

Organophosphates
  Fensulfothion
  Mevinphos
  Parathion
	Cholinesterase
	  inhibition

Carbamates
  Aldicarb
  Methomyl
  Carbaryl
	Cholinesterase
	  inhibition

Organochlorines
  Endrin
  Chlordane
  DDT
	Central nervous system
	  stimulation

Anticoagulants
  Warfarin
  Coumarin
  Fumarin
	Slowed clotting

Nitro- and chlorophenols
  Dinitrophenol
  Dinitrocresol
  Pentachlorophenol
	Metabolic stimulation

Bipyridyls
  Paraquat
  Diquat
	Proliferative changes

Table 33-2. Symptoms of exposure to organophosphates and carbamates

Acute (mild)	Acute (moderate to severe)	Chronic
Fatigue	Weakness	Fatigue
Headache	Fasciculations	Headache
Dizziness	Dyspnea	Drowsiness
Blurred vision	Ataxia	Insomnia
Excessive sweating	Miosis	Disturbances of concentration and memory
Nausea/vomiting	Unconsciousness	Anxiety
Stomach cramps		
Diarrhea		

ganophosphate poisoning is confirmed when a test dose of atropine does not result in symptoms of atropinization, including flushing, rapid heart beat, large pupils, and dryness of the mouth. Biochemical tests for the presence of pesticide residues or their metabolites permit the subsequent identification of organophosphates and other compounds for medicolegal purposes, although usually not early enough to affect the course of clinical treatment. Because farm workers who become ill at work often must obtain medical assistance on their own, it is important to inquire whether other workers were potentially exposed, so that public health investigators can attempt to locate them both to investigate the incident and to offer medical care.

Chronic or Mild Acute Pesticide Exposures. Mild acute organophosphate exposure—not severe enough to require treatment with atropine—and chronic low-level exposures to field residues account for the most common forms of pesticide-related occupational disease among agricultural workers today. (See symptoms in Table 33-2.) Two decades ago, the majority of reported cases were "crew poisonings," in which entire crews of field workers (frequently harvesters in citrus orchards) became acutely ill after exposure to pesticide residues on foliage. The development of reentry periods for the most acutely toxic organophosphate compounds has largely eliminated such episodes in

routine field work. Reported cases of systemic illness in more recent years have predominantly been in individuals or small groups of workers encountering reentry violations or accidental exposures, as when a field about to be harvested is sprayed in error (see the case history at the beginning of this chapter).

Although chronic cases are rarely reported, they are now believed to represent most pesticide-related illness among field workers and perhaps also among applicators and other pesticide handlers. While the near-elimination of severe acute poisonings represents a major advance, current reentry schedules and enforcement do not provide farm workers with adequate protection from low-level residue exposure. Children under the age of 16 years are estimated to constitute as much as 16 percent of the agricultural work force, and their exposure is of particular concern. Although research in animal models suggests that their developing hormonal systems may be more susceptible to toxic effects of some compounds, the physiologic and clinical effects of pesticide exposure in children and adolescents are largely unevaluated.

A growing number of studies in California, New Jersey, Canada, Nebraska, and other agricultural areas have demonstrated that (1) continual or intermittent exposure to low levels of residues occurs regularly in field work; and (2) where the residues are of organophosphate compounds, there is a depression of cholinesterase activity levels in farm workers when pesticides are applied [13].

Low-level exposure to organophosphates, carbamates, and many other pesticides may produce a variety of nonspecific central nervous system symptoms that are easily mistaken for common nonoccupational diseases. Symptoms may include headache, fatigue, drowsiness, insomnia and other sleep disturbances, mental confusion, disturbances of concentration and memory, anxiety, and emotional lability. Unfortunately, it is extremely difficult to demonstrate a clinical association between residue exposure, symptoms, and the effect on cholinesterase activity levels because symptoms often occur at relatively slight levels of cholinesterase suppression.

Declines in plasma and red cell cholinesterase activity levels may reflect exposure to organophosphate and carbamate pesticides. Cholinesterase measurements have been used since the 1950s to evaluate acute poisonings and chronic exposure among pesticide applicators, and more recently to evaluate low-level exposure among farm workers. Although plasma cholinesterase measurements are more widely used, the red cell value—as an analog of the similar nervous system enzyme—is a more valid indicator of the physiologic effect of the pesticide on the nervous system. There is a significant degree of intraindividual and interindividual variation for both cholinesterases. Because of this variation, the reduction in cholinesterase activity required to diagnose pesticide-induced inhibition is relatively large even when a preexposure baseline value is available for comparison.

Without baseline values, plasma activity levels usually must be 30 percent or more below the laboratory normal range to achieve statistical significance. When a baseline value is available, a 20 percent decline in plasma and 15 percent decline in red cell activity is significant; even in a study that obtained 10 preexposure values, a 15 percent fall in plasma and an 11 percent fall in red cell activity was required for significance [14]. Unfortunately, mild, but persistent and disabling symptoms may occur at levels of inhibition far less impressive than these. In a large study of California lettuce harvesters exposed to mevinphos, for example, mod-

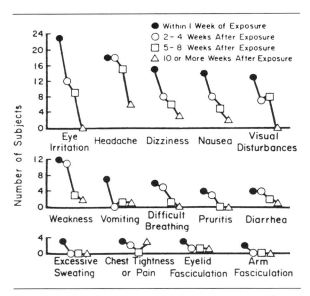

Fig. 33-4. The time course of symptoms reported by crew members exposed to organophosphates over the follow-up period (22–29 subjects examined at different times). (From MJ Coye, PG Barnett, JE Midtling, et al. Clinical confirmation of organophosphate poisoning of agricultural workers. Am J Ind Med 1986; 10:399–409.)

erately severe symptoms were reported despite plasma and red cell cholinesterase inhibition averages of 16 percent and 6 percent, respectively. The frequency and duration of their symptoms is suggested by results in Fig. 33-4 [15].

Because of intraindividual and laboratory-related variations, the upper limit of normal for cholinesterase determinations in a laboratory may be fully 225 percent of the lower-limit value. Workers suffering substantial and clinically significant declines from their own individual baselines may therefore have cholinesterase levels well within the laboratory normal range. Clinicians frequently fail to remember this fact and eliminate pesticide poisoning from their differential diagnoses, despite clear temporal relationships between exposure and symptoms.

Because most farm workers do not have baseline cholinesterase determinations and because their exposures and symptoms are often mild or moderate, it is particularly difficult to confirm pesticide poisoning in these cases. The use of sequential postexposure cholinesterase determinations to confirm cholinesterase inhibition and recovery appears to be a useful alternative to reliance on the laboratory normal range when individual baseline values are missing [16]. Plasma cholinesterase activity is frequently more markedly depressed on initial exposure and rebounds more rapidly than red cell activity. Plasma cholinesterase should increase at least 15 to 20 percent between the initial test at the time of exposure and retesting 2 to 3 days later if a significant organophosphate-induced inhibition has occurred.

Workers with probable pesticide-related symptoms or a cholinesterase inhibition of 30 percent or more, or both, should be withdrawn from work and retested; if the original test result is confirmed, the work situation and practices should be investigated. If the red cell or plasma declines from baseline are 40 percent or 50 percent, respectively, the clinician should not release the worker to any risk of further exposure until both cholinesterase levels return to baseline.

Release to work should depend on red cell cholinesterase activity, which more accurately reflects inhibition of the enzyme in the neurologic system. If a red cell value increases by more than 10 to 15 percent over the value 1 week earlier, the worker's normal baseline may not yet have been reached. Farm workers frequently return to work for economic reasons long before their red cell activity demonstrates complete recovery, however, or even before their symptoms have completely resolved.

MONITORING
Routine monitoring of cholinesterase levels is appropriate for workers handling organophosphate or carbamate pesticides on a regular basis, including applicators, mixers/loaders, flaggers, and equipment maintenance workers. Because carba-

mate-induced cholinesterase inhibition is rapidly reversed (often within 8–12 hours), both clinical diagnostic evaluations and routine monitoring should rely on such measurements with caution. In addition, there is some variation among organophosphates and carbamates in their relative inhibition of cholinesterase activity. While cholinesterase inhibition has not been characterized for all compounds, toxicologic texts should be consulted when the patterns of inhibition appear puzzling in the context of known exposures and reported symptoms.

Biological monitoring for compounds other than the organophosphates and carbamates has been limited to a few chemicals that can be reliably detected in blood or urine, are relatively rapidly eliminated from the body, and are potentially toxic enough to merit surveillance. These chemicals include pentachlorophenol, methyl bromide, and chlordimeform. Although analytical methods exist for the detection of many other compounds in biological samples, either intact or as metabolites, these tests are used primarily in research settings. In addition to research determining the absorption, metabolism, and excretion of pesticides, however, the tests are also useful in research establishing reentry periods or evaluating the effectiveness of engineering controls and protective clothing.

OPPORTUNITY AND RESPONSIBILITY FOR THE CLINICIAN
Agriculture has been treated as a "special case," resulting in the failure to adequately protect the health of many agricultural workers. The clinician serving agricultural workers therefore has a unique opportunity and responsibility to redress this inequity and to offer farm workers and agricultural service workers adequate information about these hazards and medical care appropriate to their consequences. Many farm workers in the United States are originally from Central America, Mexico, and the Caribbean. Agricultural practices

in these areas are characterized by the far-less-regulated use of pesticides; severe exposure of farm workers is fairly common, and agricultural communities are often heavily exposed through contamination of groundwater supplies, housing, clothing, and food products. This history leads many farm workers who have come to the United States—both immigrant and seasonal—to believe that they must accept pesticide exposures as a price of employment. Without a thorough review, the clinician is never justified in assuming that agricultural workers are adequately informed about the hazards of their work, or that they are adequately protected.

REFERENCES

1. NIOSH. West foods: HETA 81-366-1248. Washington, D.C.: U.S. Government Printing Office, January 1983.
2. Coye MJ. The health effects of agricultural production: I. the health of agricultural workers. J Public Health Policy 1985; 6(3):349–70.
3. Strigini P. On the political economy of risk: Farmworkers, pesticides, and dollars. Int J Health Serv 1982; 12:263–92.
4. Division of Labor Statistics and Research. Occupational injuries and illnesses survey: California, 1979. San Francisco, CA: California Department of Industrial Relations, May 1981.
5. Arbab DM, Weidner BL. Infectious diseases and field water supply and sanitation among migrant farmworkers. Am J Public Health 1986; 76(6): 694–5.
6. Kahn E. Pesticide related illness in California farm workers. J Occup Med 1976; 18:693–6.
7. Durham WF, Wolfe HR. Measurement of the exposure of workers to pesticides. WHO bulletin, 1962; 29:279–81.
8. Fenske RA, Long SM, Leffingwell JT, Spear RC. A video imaging technique for assessing dermal exposure. II. fluorescent tracer testing. Am Ind Hyg Assoc J 1986; 47(12):771–5.
9. Guidelines for the selection of chemical protective clothing. American Conference of Governmental Industrial Hygienists, Inc., 6500 Glenway Avenue, Bldg. D-5, Cincinnati, OH 45211.
10. NIOSH. Musculoskeletal disease in agricultural workers. Cincinnati: NIOSH, 1983. Internal Document. Information extracted for this chapter courtesy of Shiro Tanaka, M.D., Industry Wide Studies Branch, Division of Surveillance, Hazard Evaluations and Field Studies.
11. Division of Labor Statistics and Research. Occupational skin disease in California. San Francisco, CA: California Department of Industrial Relations, January 1982.
12. Morgan D. Recognition and management of pesticide poisonings. Washington, D.C.: Environmental Protection Agency, 1982. (EPA-540/9-80-005).
13. Coye MJ. The health effects of agricultural production: I. the health of agricultural workers. J Public Health Policy 1985; 6(3):349–70.
14. Coye MJ, Lowe JA, Maddy KJ. Biological monitoring of agriculture workers exposed to pesticides: I. cholinesterase activity determination; II. monitoring of intact pesticides and their metabolites. J Occup Med 1986; 28:8:619–27, 628–36.
15. Coye MJ, Barnett PG, Midtling JE. Clinical confirmation of organophosphate poisoning of agricultural workers. Am J Ind Med 1986; 10:399–409.
16. Midtling JE, Barnett PG, Coye MJ et al. Clinical management of field worker organophosphate poisoning: case report. West J Med 1985; 143:168–72.

VI
Approaches to Occupational Health

34
Occupational Health and Safety Programs in the Workplace

Duane L. Block

Workplace occupational health and safety programs have as their primary objective the prevention of work-related illnesses and injuries. Although these programs focus primarily on workers, they also affect the workers' families and those who live in the vicinity of the workplace since what affects one group may affect others. For example, a carcinogen produced in a factory might cause cancer in exposed workers if workplace controls are inadequate, in family members unless protected from workers' contaminated clothing, in individuals who live near the factory if environmental controls for the community are improper, and in consumers of the finished product unless proper preventive measures are taken. For these reasons and because of the interrelationships between work and health for all individuals, it is important for all health and safety professionals to understand these programs even though relatively few will work directly with them. Most such programs are operated by management, although there is some indication that this practice may change.

Descriptions of workplace health and safety programs are drawn from the author's experience as medical director of a multinational corporation with 370,000 employees engaged in diversified manufacturing and marketing operations. Note that whereas large employers frequently provide many of the services described, smaller employers usually provide few, if any, of them. The majority of employed persons in the United States work in plants that do not have formal workplace health and safety programs.

OBJECTIVES AND SCOPE OF OCCUPATIONAL HEALTH AND SAFETY PROGRAMS

The American Medical Association lists the following as the basic objectives of an occupational health and safety program:

1. To protect employees against health and safety hazards in their work situation.
2. Insofar as practical and feasible, to protect the general environment of the community.
3. To facilitate the placement of workers according to their physical, mental and emotional capacities in work they can perform with an acceptable degree of efficiency and without endangering their own health and safety or that of others.
4. To assure adequate medical care and rehabilitation of the occupationally ill or injured.
5. To encourage and assist in measures for personal health maintenance, including acquisition of a personal physician whenever possible [1].

These objectives are generally included in most workplace health and safety programs. However, workplace programs vary considerably in scope depending on the size of the workforce, the nature of workplace hazards, management attitudes and policies, demands from organized labor if the workforce is represented by a union, regulatory requirements, and various other factors.

A comprehensive workplace health and safety program should focus on the prevention of illness and injury and the effective use of human resources. To achieve this goal, the important program elements should include: (1) selective job placement, (2) ensuring a safe and healthful work environment, (3) treatment and rehabilitation of occupational illnesses and injuries, and (4) health maintenance or health promotion programs.

SELECTIVE JOB PLACEMENT

Selective job placement is a process by which the requirements of a given job are matched with the physical, mental, and emotional capacities of the worker. The process is operative not only at the time of initial employment but also at various other times during employment, such as following absence from work due to illness and at the time of periodic physical examinations—either of a routine nature or related to specific job assignments requiring special physical skills or proficiency.

For the process to be effective, the medical department staff must be thoroughly familiar with job requirements of the various activities and job classifications in the plant. Equally important is the accurate description of the worker's capacity for work in a manner that will be well understood by all of the interested parties. To achieve this goal, the plant medical staff must establish a physical examination protocol that will identify essential health information and also a means of collecting information from the worker's personal physician or specialists who may have evaluated the individual's health status.

Generally speaking, most employers can successfully place at suitable work most individuals with physical or mental impairments if the aforementioned process is followed. The key to the success of the effort is communication. The workplace medical staff must communicate effectively with the worker's physician, the worker, the worker's supervisor, and various personnel and union representatives. Some method should be devised for the resolution of professional differences of opinion when they arise.

The plant medical staff should also be thoroughly familiar with appropriate guidelines for the placement of handicapped individuals that are available from large companies or appropriate professional organizations, such as the American Medical Association or the American Occupational Medical Association (see Appendix C). It is also important that the medical staff be familiar with antidiscrimination and handicapped employment regulations, collective-bargaining agreements, and privacy considerations, as well as ethical and professional considerations related to the sharing of confidential information (see Chap. 13).

Selective job placement, if properly applied, will ensure that the worker can be most productively employed on a job that will not adversely affect the worker's health or jeopardize the health or safety of fellow employees.

ENSURING A SAFE AND HEALTHFUL WORK ENVIRONMENT

The cornerstones of an effective workplace occupational health and safety program are initiatives that ensure a safe and healthful work environment. Broadly speaking, this was the purpose of the Occupational Safety and Health Act of 1970 (see Chap. 10). It is a far-reaching and complex undertaking that requires the cooperation and collaboration of several groups and individuals in the workplace. It requires a commitment by management at all levels and labor officials as well, if the workers are represented by a union. It also requires participation and commitment by workers and technical and professional personnel from a number of activities within the workplace, including engineering, personnel, and health and safety professionals.

Great strides have been made in workplace accident prevention over the years. Between 1912 and 1984, accidental work deaths per 100,000 population were reduced 76 percent, from 21 to 5 per 100,000 population. In 1912, an estimated 18,000 to 21,000 workers' lives were lost. In 1984, in a workforce more than double in size and producing 10 times as much, there were 11,500 work-related deaths [2]. Although the reduction has not been as dramatic for work-related disabling injuries, these disabling injuries have been consistently fewer than off-the-job accidental disabling injuries. These advances have been due to workplace accident prevention programs, involving worker education, engineering controls that focus on equipment design and guarding, and the provision of personal protective equipment (PPE) for workers.

Although the primary responsibility for workplace accident prevention programs may rest with safety, management, or union personnel, the plant physician and nurse may play very important roles. They may contribute significantly in accident epidemiology, worker education, and the fitting and dispensing of PPE.

As important as worker safety education programs are programs designed to inform workers concerning other workplace hazards. The Occupational Safety and Health Administration (OSHA) Hazard Communication Standard, which became effective in 1986, has encouraged the development of these programs. Hazard communication programs have as their central theme the sharing of information concerning the potential health hazards related to materials used in manufacturing or maintenance processes in the workplace. They require the employer to collect information concerning potential adverse health consequences from exposure to materials used in the work environment. In addition, various means may be used to minimize employee exposure if there are potential adverse health consequences (see Chap. 7).

In order for PPE to be effective in hazard control, employees must be aware of the importance of their role in the proper fitting and wearing of it. Information-sharing programs are most effective if management, labor, and employees, as well as health and safety personnel, are involved in their development and implementation.

In the author's company, all materials to be used in manufacturing and maintenance processes are reviewed for their potential to cause adverse health effects by a staff of toxicologists. After the review, the conditions of usage are stipulated, including methods of controlling employee exposure, if necessary. All information known about the materials, including recommended methods of use, is included in a computerized data base. This information is available to employees at each plant so that questions regarding employee exposure to any material currently in use are easily answered. This data base was the focus for the development of the company hazard communication program. This program was developed jointly with the union and with assistance from two universities. During the summer of 1985, over 300 employees, who had been selected as workplace hazard communication coordinators, attended a 1-week training course. The course was conducted by the two universities and was designed to teach the coordinators how to use the information system and other training materials. These coordinators then returned to their respective workplaces to conduct hazard communication training programs for all employees. The program has been especially successful in building trust and in sharing information important in preventing work-related illness.

The plant physician and nurses were important contributors to the success of the workplace hazard communication program: They made certain that employees understood the potential adverse health consequences from hazardous workplace exposures and also emphasized the importance of proper fitting and wearing of PPE if it was indicated.

In addition to chemical hazards, other areas of workplace concern that involve the same principles are hearing conservation and ergonomics (see Chaps. 9, 17, and 22). There has been an excellent hearing conservation program in this multinational company for over 20 years with all of the essential elements, including employee education. A more recent program of interest relates to ergonomics. In 1984, two plants were to be rebuilt to accommodate a new product. Management decided that this change afforded an opportunity to redesign the workplace using ergonomic principles. In collaboration with the union and with assistance from a neighboring university, a program of workplace evaluation was undertaken. As a result, an extensive program involving workplace and tool design using ergonomic principles has evolved. The program also involves an extensive educational segment for management, supervisors, employees, and health and safety professionals on the role of ergonomics in the prevention of workplace-related illness and injury. There is also a significant research component to the program focused on methods of preventing the commonly encountered musculoskeletal conditions in the workplace. Although the program has not been operating long enough to produce documented results, early indications are that the engineering and educational aspects of the program have been well accepted by the management, union, employees, and health and safety professionals who have participated.

Additional significant activities related to the ensuring of a safe and healthful work environment that involve the plant medical and safety staffs are medical surveillance and periodic workplace visits or audits.

Medical surveillance is the systematic collection, analysis, and dissemination of disease data on groups of workers or populations (see Chap. 3). Surveillance activities in the workplace include collection and analysis of data on the morbidity and mortality of workers and correlating these data with information concerning materials used in the workplace, exposure levels of workers to these materials, and safety data related to workplace accidents or employee complaints. Analysis of these data may help to determine if workplace control measures are adequate or to discover previously unrecognized problems that may be related to workplace exposures. To be effectively used in the ensuring of a safe and healthful workplace, the data should be routinely shared with the interested parties: management, labor, employees, and the scientific community.

Periodic workplace visits or audits by members of the medical and safety staffs are an integral part of an effective surveillance program. These visits are essential, for only by regular visits to the workplace can the health or safety professional have a complete understanding of effective job placement, the importance of ergonomics in the prevention of workplace injury and health problems, the roles of appropriate environmental controls and protective equipment in prevention programs, and the effectiveness of worker education programs.

TREATMENT AND REHABILITATION OF OCCUPATIONAL ILLNESSES AND INJURIES

Generally, workers' compensation regulations of the various states require employers to provide treatment and appropriate rehabilitative measures for work-related illnesses and injuries. Although the determination of work-relatedness may be difficult in some cases, it is important that prompt and appropriate treatment and rehabilitative measures be initiated meanwhile. This treatment can be rendered in a workplace medical department, in a nearby physician's office, or in a community outpatient medical facility or hospital. The best possible treatment is the most effective and least expensive in the long run.

Some arrangements should also be made to render temporary or interim medical treatment for non-work-related illnesses or injuries. It is also helpful to ensure that adequate long-term treatment for nonoccupational illnesses is being provided either by the worker's personal physician or by a physician appropriate to the worker's needs.

A major responsibility of the workplace medical department is to keep adequate and accurate medical records. These records are essential for legal reasons and important for epidemiologic purposes. The records must be kept in a manner that ensures the privacy of the workers and adequate access to the information as legally required.

HEALTH MAINTENANCE OR HEALTH PROMOTION PROGRAMS

Ill health, disability, impaired productivity, premature retirement, and death account for a huge cost to industry and the nation. Many of these costs are attributable to the so-called life-style diseases. For example, statistics reveal that alcoholism is the third most prevalent health problem in the United States, afflicting over 12 million people and costing society over $100 billion annually. Other drug abuse may cost the U.S. economy as much as another $50 billion annually. The annual cost of smoking-related illness is estimated to be $27 billion.

Health care expenditures account for more than 10 percent of the Gross National Product. Understandably employers have sought approaches to deal with these important and expensive issues. Although there may be considerable difference of opinion concerning terminology (health maintenance versus health promotion versus wellness versus employee assistance programs), there is little disagreement that an employer can have a positive effect on the health of the workforce by using programs of awareness, education, and behavior change.

The determinants of health behaviors are remarkably complex, and failure to be aware of them has caused some problems for behavior change practitioners. One thing is certain, however: Health promotion requires behavior change. This principle is equally applicable to accident prevention. A review article published in 1986 succinctly covers the current state of the art, including deficiencies in behavioral science understanding [3]. There are, however, a number of unanswered questions about behavior change that are basic, such as: (1) What factors prompt people to behave in ways known to be unhealthful? (2) How can efficient behavior-change methods be attractively and skillfully packaged, promoted, and disseminated? (3) How should programs be developed, organized, and coordinated? and (4) What should the goals of health behavior change programs be,

and who should decide what these goals are? Finally, the authors of the review believe that the rapid growth in behavior change technology has brought with it a sobering appreciation of the complexity of health promotion initiatives and the need for thoughtful blending of research and practice.

Despite our gaps in knowledge, several health promotion program elements that show reasonable promise for cost-effectiveness have been recommended [4]. These program elements, with comments on them, are listed below:

Blood Pressure Screening and Follow-Up

A blood pressure screening program is helpful in identifying employees with previously unknown hypertension or individuals whose hypertension is not adequately controlled by treatment. The secret of success for this type of program is similar to that for other screening programs. There must be referral for evaluation and appropriate treatment, and there must also be follow-up to ensure that treatment is maintained. A four-plant pilot program conducted jointly by a large company and a university and funded by the U.S. government has been reported [5]. Experience with that program amply documents the importance of follow-up.

Smoking Cessation

Smoking cessation programs conducted at the worksite can achieve long-term abstinence rates of 50 percent or greater. The average annual savings is estimated at $336 to $601 per employee who is successful in stopping smoking [6]. The cost of smoking cessation programs, even if fully subsidized by the employer, is considerably less than the potential annual savings for those who quit smoking.

Diet Modification

Diet modification programs are not only effective in weight control but also in lowering blood cholesterol levels. It is well known that the three most important risk factors in the genesis of coronary heart disease are cigarette smoking, high blood pressure, and elevated blood cholesterol. A recent consensus conference concluded that appropriate changes in diet will reduce blood cholesterol levels [7].

Employee Assistance Programs

Although there is a recent tendency to include other health promotion initiatives under this rubric, employee assistance programs traditionally have included counseling programs directed primarily toward alcohol and other substance abuse as well as emotional and other personal problems. There is ample documentation in the literature that these programs are cost-effective with some estimates ranging as high as a fivefold return on every dollar invested.

A special problem of relatively recent origin with regard to employee assistance programs relates to drug screening in the workplace. The American Occupational Medical Association recently developed and published guidelines on this subject [8]. Considerable controversy continues over various aspects of workplace drug-screening programs, even among a number of American Occupational Medical Association members [9]. Because drug screening is a large and complex subject, the reader should review the available literature before formulating a position on the desirability and scope of a workplace drug-testing program.

Auto Safety Programs

Programs aimed at improved driver behavior and increased use of seat belts have been shown to be effective in reducing the incidence and costs associated with injuries sustained in motor vehicle accidents.

A recent pilot study on seat belts in the author's company revealed that a 10 percent increase in seat belt use by employees would save the lives of three company employees each year, prevent injuries to 121 others, and save $2.75 million annually in medical insurance, disability claims, and train-

ing costs. A company-wide seat belt program was initiated, using education, incentives, and behavior modification techniques. This program resulted in an increase in seat belt use from 14 percent of employees who were using seat belts regularly when the program was initiated to 35 percent usage at the end of 1 year and 60 percent usage at the end of the second year.

This seat belt program was one of the first initiatives in a company program of health promotion that includes for employees, on a voluntary basis, the use of a health risk appraisal questionnaire with blood pressure and cholesterol screening to identify those health behaviors or physical abnormalities that have the potential for long-term adverse health consequences. The program has been developed in collaboration with the union and with input from employees. It is paid for by the company and participation in screening programs is on company time. The risk reduction programs are offered prior to, during, and after working hours depending on considerations at each location.

It is too soon to predict the outcome of the program, but, in addition to the increase in seat belt use, several observations can be made. There is great enthusiasm about the program by management, the union, and employees. Employee participation in screening programs varies from location to location, but overall, company participation is approximately 70 percent. Participation of at-risk employees in risk reduction programs has been excellent, and early risk reduction results have been encouraging.

Exercise

Exercise programs, either at the workplace or subsidized by the employer using community resources, are an important element in a well-rounded health promotion program. Although the data concerning cost-effectiveness are debatable, there is little question that a well-structured aerobic exercise program contributes significantly to an increased sense of well-being and perhaps even to increased employee morale and productivity.

Although the final answers on the aforementioned and other health promotion programs are not yet available, there is increasing evidence that these programs can affect adverse risk factors and probably contribute significantly to the prevention of the so-called life-style diseases. Another aspect of health promotion activities, which is receiving increased attention by management, is that these programs may well be most important in improving employee attitude or morale and may be helpful in improving productivity.

THE OCCUPATIONAL HEALTH AND SAFETY TEAM

To carry out an effective health and safety program, well-trained professionals are necessary. Before addressing the structure and organization of the workplace health and safety team, the follow-ing are reasons why an employer might wish to provide such services:

1. *Government regulations:* Without the incentive of government regulations, history has shown that most small employers do not sense the value of in-plant health and safety programs. Various governmental agencies at a local, state and federal level, primarily OSHA, set and enforce standards and regulations to ensure a safe and healthful workplace. Although many large employers initiated workplace health and safety programs prior to the enactment of OSHA, many other employers have initiated and maintained workplace health and safety programs in response to current or anticipated regulatory requirements.

2. *Pressure from organized labor:* In workplaces where workers are represented by a union, health and safety concerns are often given high priority

Fig. 34-1. Medical surveillance, screening programs, and a wide variety of other occupational health issues are discussed by health and safety committees. Committee meetings serve as forums for discussion of such issues among workers, management, and workplace health professionals. (Photograph by Earl Dotter.)

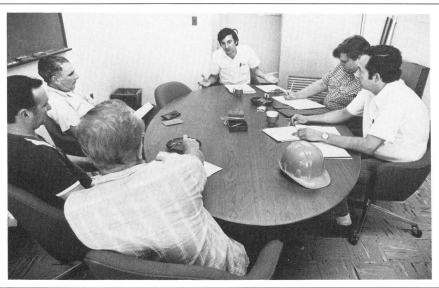

and may be dealt with through collective bargaining. The programs are most effective when the efforts of both the union and the employer are collaborative rather than adversarial (Fig. 34-1).

3. *Enlightened self-interest:* Effective workplace safety and health programs should reduce workers' compensation and medical care costs and increase productivity. Competitive pressures can be either incentives or disincentives. An employer can be encouraged to establish a workplace health and safety program because other employers in the same industry or geographic area are doing so. Conversely, in an intensely competitive environment, where cost reduction is the desired outcome, an employer may choose to provide a health and safety program in some manner other than in the workplace.

To be effective and adequately address the previously described program elements, a team including the talents of multiple professional disciplines is required. Although different employers have chosen various organizational structures to accommodate this team, all of the health and safety disciplines should be represented by this team. The author believes that in large companies with medical departments, the team should be headed by a physician and may include multiple other professionals, such as nurses, nurse practitioners, physician's assistants, safety engineers, industrial hygienists, toxicologists, epidemiologists, and others. In smaller workplaces where there may not be a physician closely identified with the health and safety program, a nurse or safety officer may more logically head the team. To function smoothly as a team, all of these professionals must interact with many other individuals, including representatives of management, labor, and community agencies.

The physician, to be the most effective team leader, should have ultimate loyalty to the employee/patient, as outlined in the American Occupational Medical Association Code of Ethics (see Chap. 13). Most workplace-based physicians have

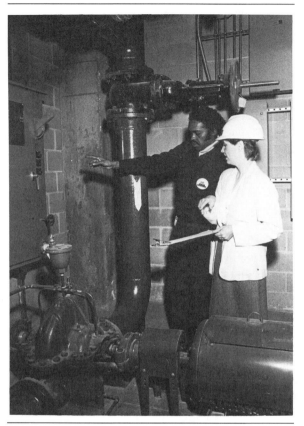

Fig. 34-2. In addition to regular duties, the occupational nurse performs walk-through inspections to detect health and safety hazards.

not had formal graduate education in occupational medicine and are not certified as specialists by the American Board of Preventive Medicine. Despite this fact, in recent years there have been increasing numbers of physicians selecting residencies in occupational medicine and increasing educational opportunities for other practicing physicians to improve their knowledge in this field (see Appendix B).

The role of the occupational health nurse is described in the box.

The key to the effectiveness of the workplace

OCCUPATIONAL HEALTH NURSING FUNCTIONS—Corinne J. Solomon

The first occupational health nurses (OHNs) were employed 100 years ago to teach sanitation and hygiene to workers' families and to perform first aid in quarrying operations, mines, and retail establishments. During World War I, their numbers increased as they provided health services in shipbuilding and other defense and manufacturing industries. Occupational health nursing remains the only specialized area of nursing practice focusing on preventing illness and injury and promoting wellness for workers and their families.

As the primary provider in almost 85 percent of occupational health services, the nurse sees employees during the employment process, throughout the workers' activities with the company, and after retirement. The position of the nurse in any industry dictates both a relationship with managers and employees and a responsibility for exercising independent judgment that are not typical of nursing in other settings.

OHNs may be designated "employee health nurses" in health care facilities. In addition to adhering to public health mandates affecting food-handlers and laboratory workers, these nurses coordinate preventive and educational activities relating to anesthetic gases, antineoplastic agents, communicable diseases, needle sticks or glass puncture wounds, slips, falls, and back injuries. They also are involved with patient and visitor safety.

In free-standing or hospital-based occupational health services, OHNs provide physical assessments and market the facilities' services to local industries.

OHNs with master's or higher degrees function independently in the role of consultants, educators, or managers.

OHN activities encompass all areas of employee health, including, but not restricted to, health maintenance; assessment and prevention of potential work and environmental hazards; the purchase, use, and care of personal protective equipment; health surveillance; absenteeism control; injury/illness management and accident reduction; safety awareness and disaster planning; health education and promotion; knowledge of health and safety statutes; counseling and stress reduction; and liaison with regulatory agencies, community resources, and insurance carriers. The quantity and quality of documentation required and generated is immense and must be managed and evaluated regularly.

OHNs have many opportunities for prevention through:

1. Recognizing that certain conditions or substances alter health.
2. Analyzing injuries and illnesses by type and location on a regular basis.
3. Evaluating working conditions, exposure, or potential for contact (Fig. 34-2).
4. Assessing whether remedies should be immediate or long-range.
5. Determining what resources are available.
6. Using health surveillance to compare deviations from expected norms or baselines.
7. Presenting information to management.
8. Educating supervisors and employees.
9. Observing behavioral or procedural changes in work areas.
10. Reevaluating conditions and work activities.

Occupational nurses and physicians work collaboratively toward development and maintenance of job descriptions, statements on confidentiality and employees' access to medical records, nursing protocols, and departmental budgets. In addition, OHN functions may include reviewing records and developing or revising health service policies and procedures in industries with part-time physicians.

The OHN plays a major role in Right-to-Know and hazard communication by interpreting Material Safety Data Sheets (MSDSs), describing potential health hazards, and explaining worker legal rights and duties to managers and other employees.

Nurses recognize that disaster planning involves more than first aid and CPR classes. Nursing functions include equipping "disaster" boxes with emergency supplies and materials for triage, evaluating egress for blind or wheelchair-bound workers, and drafting scenarios for regular drills involving local health care facilities. MSDSs are used in emergency treatment of employees and in communicating toxicologic information and emergency care to hospital personnel.

Today's OHNs are adept at utilization review and can identify a company's health costs and savings potential by reviewing data from records pertaining to absenteeism, workers' compensation, and long-term disability.

The nurse's scope of practice may include home visits or calls to monitor absent workers' health status, thereby promoting the OHN's role as a patient advocate in rehabilitation and management advisor for cost-containment.

Counseling is probably the least recognized OHN function. The nurse spends as much as 70 percent of the workday in health counseling and identifying workplace and family stressors, referring employees when necessary.

The OHN is uniquely qualified to provide clinical, technical, and preventive skills in the workplace using a holistic approach to both the facility and the employee as the "patient." Occupational health nursing incorporates a sound theoretical base with the necessary skills to meet today's demands to alter the impact of the workplace on worker health, the family, the community, and the environment.

Registered professional nurses who specialize in occupational health for 5 years are eligible to take the qualifying examination for board certification after meeting specified requirements and demonstrating current knowledge in occupational nursing. Currently, over 20 percent of practicing OHNs are entitled to use the Certified Occupational Health Nurse (COHN) designation.

health and safety program is expertise from the multiple scientific disciplines previously noted and described in greater detail (in Chaps. 5, 7, 8, and 9). A guide to professional staffing for various-sized workplaces is found in Table 34-1.

Workplaces with fewer than 1,000 employees usually require the services of a part-time physician. An additional physician and 1 to 2 nurses can be justified with worker population increments of 2,000. If physician's assistants are used, there must be supervision by a licensed physician. Paramedical personnel trained in cardiopulmonary resuscitation (CPR), first aid, and other related tasks can be effectively used in plants of all sizes in addition to full-time health care professionals.

Table 34-1. A guide to health care staffing by size of workforce

| Number of employees | No. of full-time health professionals | | |
	Physicians	Physician's assistants or nurse practitioners	Occupational health nurses
1–400	—	—	—
400–1,000	—	1	1–2
1,000–3,000	1	1	3
3,000–5,000	2	2	4

Source: Compiled by G Calvert in part from AL Knight and C Zenz. Organization and staffing. In C Zenz, ed. Occupational medicine: principles and practical applications. Chicago: Yearbook, 1975.

Finally, as an alternative to providing health and safety services at the workplace, there are many other possible methods. Many small companies have no in-plant health and safety expertise available. They rely on insurance companies or other sources for consultation and advice. Many of these companies also rely on community physicians or medical facilities to provide necessary health services. The options for providing health and safety programs for small plants depend, to some extent, on the community where the plant is located and the resources available. If the plant is remote or in a community with limited resources, it will need to be more self-sufficient with regard to health and safety services.

The National Institute for Occupational Safety and Health (NIOSH) had conducted two major national surveys as part of its hazard surveillance program. The National Occupational Hazard Survey (NOHS) was conducted from 1972 to 1974, and the National Occupational Exposure Survey (NOES) was conducted from 1981 to 1983. These two surveys permit the analysis of certain trends in the distribution of in-plant health and safety services as well as trends in patterns of employee exposures and control technology [10]. The results revealed that in the period between the surveys, there had been an increase in the proportion of plants that had (1) established a health unit at the facility (from 14% to 24%), (2) an employee designated to provide emergency medical treatment (from 48% to 57%), (3) at least one nurse on the payroll to provide care for employees (from 8% to 17%), and (4) a requirement that new employees have a medical examination (from 35% to 44%). The percentage of employees covered by these services had also increased.

In recent years, in an effort to reduce or control costs through headcount reductions, some companies who traditionally have had workplace health and safety personnel have begun to provide these services by contract. As a result, there has been an increase in the growth of community-, hospital-, and clinic-based occupational health programs. This growth has been enhanced by employers' desires to provide health promotion programs, many of which are also available in the community and often linked to the community clinics and hospitals. Although these sources may provide adequate health services, other health and safety disciplines, such as industrial hygiene, safety, toxicology, and epidemiology, are often underrepresented. Furthermore, the provider does not have an intimate knowledge of the workplace or a close working relationship with other important groups or individuals in the workplace. It remains to be seen whether this new development will be a satisfactory alternative to the traditional workplace health and safety program.

REFERENCES

1. American Medical Association. Scope, objectives, and functions of occupational health programs. Chicago: AMA, 1972.
2. National Safety Council. Accident facts. Chicago: NSC, 1985.
3. Best JA, Cameron R. Health behavior and health promotion. Am J Health Promotion 1986; 1:2.
4. Fielding JE. Preventive medicine and the bottom line. J Occup Med 1979; 21:79.
5. Foote A, Erfurt JC. Hypertension control at the worksite. N Engl J Med 1983; 308:14.
6. Kristein MM. How much can business expect to profit from smoking cessation. Prev Med 1983; 12:12.
7. Lowering blood cholesterol to prevent heart disease. Report of a consensus conference. JAMA 1985; 253:14.
8. American Occupational Medical Association. Drug screening in the workplace: ethical guidelines. J Occup Med 1986; 28:1240.
9. Atherly GRC, Bresnitz EA, Cullen M, et al. Letter to the editor. Drug screening: ethical guidelines. J Occup Med 1987; 29:300.
10. Seta JA, Sundin DS. Trends of a decade—a perspective on occupational hazard surveillance, 1970–1983. MMWR-CDC Surveillance Summaries 1985; 34:2SS–15SS.

BIBLIOGRAPHY

Fielding JE. Corporate health management. Reading, MA: Addison-Wesley, 1984.

An extensive review of the cost of ill health, problems with the health care system, methods of dealing with health care cost containment, and programs of disease prevention and health promotion.

Halperin WE, Schulte PA, Greathouse DG, Mason TJ, Prorok, PC, Costlow RD, eds. Conference on Medical Screening and Biological Monitoring for the Effects of Exposure in the Workplace. J Occup Med 1986; 28(8):543–788; 28(10):501–1126.

A summary of the proceedings of a federally sponsored, 3-day conference held in Cincinnati in 1984 covering the scientific issues related to biologic monitoring and medical screening as well as the legal, social, and ethical issues arising from such programs.

Howe HF. Organization and operation of an occupational health program. J Occup Med 1975; 17:360, 433, 528.

An in-depth discussion of how to develop an occupational health program. This three-part series is available in booklet form from the American Occupational Medical Association, 55 West Seegers Road, Arlington Heights, IL 60005.

Jackson G, ed. Substance abuse. Semin Occup Med 1986; 1:223–304.

An excellent compendium of articles on substance abuse in the workplace, with a particular emphasis on alternative approaches to recognition, management, prevention, and control.

Parkinson RS et al. Managing health promotion in the workplace. Palo Alto, CA: Mayfield, 1982.

An excellent collection of background papers, review of company programs, and guidelines for the development of health promotion programs in the workplace.

Schilling RSF, ed. Occupational health practice. 2nd ed. London: Butterworths, 1981.

A wealth of information on the functions, ethics, and programs of occupational health practice.

Tepper LB. The right to know, the duty to inform. J Occup Med 1980; 22:433.

An enlightening statement on the need for qualified health professionals to inform the workers, the management, and their colleagues about occupational and environmental hazards.

Walsh DC. Corporate physicians: between medicine and management. New Haven: Yale University Press, 1987.

A challenging insight into the context of the work of occupational physicians, the dilemmas they face in their corporate positions, and the routes that have been chosen in dealing with these dilemmas.

Zenz E, ed. Occupational medicine: principles and practical applications. Chicago: Yearbook, 1975.

An extensive review of the administrative, clinical, environmental, and psychosocial issues related to occupational medical practice.

35
Labor Unions and Occupational Health

Michael Silverstein

The history of industry and commerce has long been burdened with the loss of workers' lives. Events such as the Triangle Shirtwaist fire of 1911, the Gauley Bridge silicosis disaster of the 1930s, the Farmington Mine explosion of 1968, and the malignant legacy of past asbestos exposures have taught generations of workers that survival to retirement age cannot be taken for granted [1].

It was not until the Occupational Safety and Health Act (OSHAct) of 1970 that the right to a safe and healthful workplace was guaranteed by law (see Chap. 10). Working people, therefore, have turned to their unions and other organizations for protection from the chemical and physical hazards that frequently accompany the earning of a living.

Personal and union involvement in health and safety programs is a moral imperative for workers. It is also a practical necessity for occupational health professionals who seek to prevent job-related illness and injury. Just as clinical medicine cannot be practiced effectively without the participation of informed patients, occupational health and safety cannot be pursued successfully without the active involvement of the workers whose lives and health are at stake. Workers possess unique information about working conditions that is vital to the diagnostic process. Moreover, the health professional does not have the independent ability to intervene to correct problems on the job once they have been identified.

Many occupational health professionals have failed to recognize the potential for a mutually re-warding alliance with workers and their unions (see box), partly because of inadequate or misleading information generally available to health professionals about the role of unions and their commitment to health and safety—a problem this chapter addresses.

VEHICLES FOR WORKER INVOLVEMENT IN HEALTH AND SAFETY

Labor unions are the major organizations that represent and pursue the collective interests of workers in health and safety. In addition to assisting their members with day-to-day needs, unions have actively worked for legislative and regulatory remedies for health and safety problems. Therefore, although only about 20 percent of workers in the United States are unionized, their influence has extended far beyond the workplaces where their members are employed.

Labor unions represent workers who share common work (trade or craft unions, such as the International Brotherhood of Carpenters) or who work in a common industry (industrial unions, such as the United Steelworkers of America). Employees at a specific workplace may be organized into several different unions. At a construction site, there may be more than a dozen unions representing groups of workers in the various building trades, such as the International Brotherhood of Painters and Allied Trades.

At the individual workplace, unions are called

CHECKLIST FOR HEALTH AND SAFETY WORK WITH UNIONS

Health professionals providing health and safety services for a union-organized workplace cannot be fully effective until they establish a working relationship with unions based on trust and mutual respect. The following steps will help prepare health professionals for this:

1. Determine which union(s) represents workers. Identify the local union leaders (presidents or chairs) and key representatives, such as health and safety or benefits representatives. Identify the representatives of the international union (servicing representatives or business agents) who are assigned to work with the local leaders.

2. Find out what kind of help the international union provides the local union on health and safety problems. Is there a health and safety department? Who is its director? Does the international union have staff professionals, such as industrial hygienists, safety engineers, or health educators?

3. Determine whether the local union or the international union has arrangements with outside experts for help on health and safety, such as those at academic institutions, COSH groups, and the Workers Institute for Safety and Health (WISH).

4. Establish communications with local union leadership before specific problems arise. The first contact should be with the elected leaders of the local who can then make introductions to other key representatives. Ask about any outstanding issues of concern to the union.

5. Become knowledgeable about the nature of labor-management relations at the workplace. Read the collective-bargaining agreement with particular attention to any language on health and safety. Are there other written guidelines or procedures covering health and safety matters? For example, there should be a written respirator program under the terms of OSHA Standard 1910.134. How does the grievance procedure work for health and safety complaints? Does the union have the right to strike over health and safety? Is there a joint health and safety committee, a quality of work life program, or an employee assistance program?

6. Learn what procedures guard the confidentiality of workers with medical problems, and move immediately to strengthen them if they are inadequate.

7. Find out what types of health and safety training programs are provided for employees and seek to become directly involved with them.

8. Obtain and read copies of any health and safety studies that have been done at the workplace (industrial hygiene surveys, ventilation or other engineering studies, or medical surveillance or other epidemiologic reports). Make sure these have been made available to the union in accordance with legal requirements.

9. Visit the shop floor early and often. Establish a presence in the plant, independent of management or labor, but also be sure to tour the plant frequently while accompanied by union representatives. While observing jobs, be sure to talk with workers and listen carefully to their concerns.

local unions or *lodges*. These local unions are generally part of an international union. Most international unions in the United States are, in turn, affiliated with the American Federation of Labor-Congress of Industrial Organization (AFL-CIO), headquartered in Washington, DC, and composed of unions who represent over 13 million members. Several important unions, most notably the Teamsters and the United Mine Workers, are independent of the AFL-CIO. On a regional or city-wide basis, local unions may work together in a group called a *central labor council*.

Local unions and their internationals enter directly into collective bargaining with employers. The AFL-CIO and local labor councils do not generally engage in collective bargaining but rather focus on political action and other public policy initiatives on behalf of workers.

Relationships between employers and unions are governed by labor laws, including the National Labor Relations Act (Wagner Act, 1935), the Labor-Management Relations Act (Taft-Hartley Act, 1947), and the Labor-Management Reporting and Disclosure Act (Landrum-Griffin Act, 1959). These laws are designed to make employers bargain fairly with unions, to protect the rights of unions and union members in their relationships with employers, and to ensure democratic procedures and sound fiscal practices within unions. Labor law requires that employers bargain in good faith about concerns related to wages, hours, and conditions of employment. Bargaining must take place, therefore, over "conditions of employment" related to health and safety, such as the provision of ventilation, the use of personal protective equipment, or the operation of a plant medical clinic (Fig. 35-1).

Unions have represented their members on health and safety matters in four ways:

1. They bargain with employers for agreements aimed at improving working conditions. These agreements may include provisions for health and safety committees, union health and safety repre-

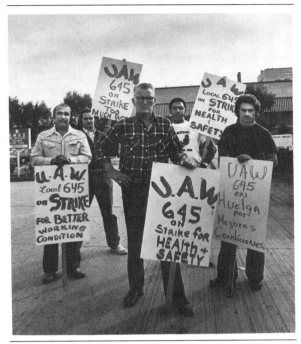

Fig. 35-1. Following the breakdown in local negotiations over health and safety conditions, a United Automobile Workers' local union went on strike at a California automobile assembly plant in an effort to secure improvements in the working environment. (Photograph by Robert Gumpert. Courtesy of United Automobile Workers.)

sentatives, rights to refuse unsafe work, environmental improvements, and grievance procedures for members to use in pressing specific complaints.

2. They provide technical assistance to members facing chemical or safety dangers. Many international unions have health and safety departments with professionals, such as industrial hygienists or safety engineers. Other unions secure technical aid from Committees on Occupational Safety and Health (COSH groups, see below), the Workers Institute for Safety and Health (WISH, a technical support group established by the Industrial Union Department of the AFL-CIO), academic programs, and government agencies.

3. They conduct educational and training programs so that members can better understand their legal and contractual rights and can more effectively recognize hazards and work for their elimination.

4. They work politically for laws, standards, and regulations designed to improve working conditions and worker health.

A number of organizations independent of the labor movement have been created by workers and sympathetic health professionals to educate and enlist the energies of workers on behalf of health and safety reforms and to apply pressure to employers, government agencies, and the scientific community. One of the earliest was the Workers' Health Bureau of America, which sought to assist labor unions with occupational health investigations, clinical services, education, and public policy agitation during the 1920s [2].

In the 1960s, the Black Lung Association (a coalition of mine workers and their families, union and community activists, and health professionals) used education, demonstrations, lobbying, and the media to raise awareness of the urgent need to eliminate the extreme hazards in the coal mines (Fig. 35-2). Special attention was focused on the risk of pneumoconiosis to underground coal miners. In conjunction with the United Mine Workers of America (UMWA), the Black Lung Association was instrumental in the passage of the federal Coal Mine Safety and Health Act of 1969 and later the Black Lung Benefits Reform Act. Dr. Lorin Kerr, director of the UMWA Occupational Health Department and for many years organized labor's only physician, was a major force in these proceedings. In a similar fashion, the Brown Lung Association and the Textile Workers Union (now the Amalgamated Clothing and Textile Workers Union) drew public attention to the hazards of byssinosis in the cotton textile industry and successfully pushed OSHA to promulgate its cotton dust standard in 1978.

In the past 15 years, the most important non-union support for health and safety has come from

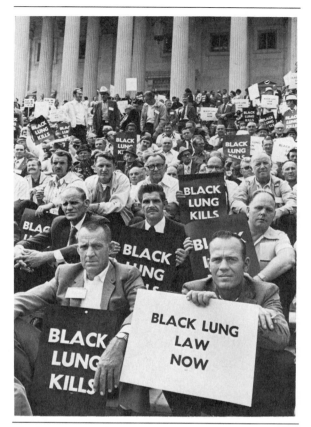

Fig. 35-2. Protest by union members that was part of the movement that led to the passage of the black lung legislation (Coal Mine Safety and Health Act) in 1969. (Photograph by Earl Dotter.)

the loose network of COSH groups. The Chicago area COSH group (CACOSH) was one of the early prototypes for these coalitions of local union activists with supportive health professionals, lawyers, and students. CACOSH generated excitement and action through worker education programs, provisions of technical support to local unions, and political pressure for workers' compensation reform and stronger OSHA enforcement. By the late 1970s, more than 25 COSH groups had developed across the country.

A significant outgrowth of the COSH groups

WORKERS USE RIGHT-TO-KNOW TO
WIN JOB SAFETY—Peter Dooley

Federal, state, and local Right-to-Know laws and regulations have prompted many workers and their unions to participate in health and safety on the job. This activism has been displayed in several ways.

Individual workers have become informed about some of the health and safety hazards they face on the job. An example occurred recently in a small machine shop in Michigan. An experienced tool grinder received labels on the stock he was working with that warned about the health hazards associated with grinding on metals, such as cobalt and beryllium. He questioned the adequacy of the current ventilation system. An industrial hygiene inspection verified that it was poorly designed and maintained. Changes are currently being implemented.

Workers are participating in health and safety programs by exercising their Right-to-Know. This has occurred in several areas. A union representative recently completed a class on the Right-to-Know and immediately requested to have a copy of her company's written program of compliance. After being denied her request, she produced a copy of the law and demanded it. On review, she found discrepancies in the written program. For instance, a "safety director" was designated to carry out compliance of the program, even though there was no such position at the plant. Following discussions with plant management, a new program was developed.

Another participant of Right-to-Know classes questioned his company's training and labeling program. After discussions in the joint health and safety committee, the company agreed to upgrade the labels by adding long-term chronic health effects and bringing in a union Right-to-Know training program to complement previous training.

Workers and unions are winning solutions to health and safety problems through the Right-to-Know. Warnings and information about chemical hazards have prompted new solutions to problems. For example, a workplace in Illinois is attempting to find safer substitutes for extensively used chlorinated hydrocarbons, such as 1,1,1-trichloroethane. It has had success in some areas using steam cleaning and other solvents as substitutes. A machining plant is experimenting with vegetable oils as lubricants to replace hazardous metalworking fluids. A large office recently stopped all use of its older duplicating machines because of concerns about methanol exposures. Many workers have discovered the correct type of gloves or respirators to be used with chemicals they handle.

As is evident by these examples, many workplaces have improved their health and safety programs by implementing effective Right-to-Know programs. Continuing efforts to improve the quality of Right-to-Know information and to educate workers and management about these programs is essential.

has been the Right-to-Know movement, initiated in the late 1970s by the Philadelphia area COSH group (PHILAPOSH). It brought national attention to the need for workers to have full and accurate information on the composition and the hazards of chemicals on their jobs. Following a tumultuous Philadelphia City Council hearing orchestrated by PHILAPOSH and the Delaware Valley Toxics Coalition, the nation's first local Right-to-Know ordinance was enacted in 1981. This city ordinance provided broad worker and community access to material safety data sheets (MSDSs) and other information on workplace chemicals (see box).

Under the leadership of Assistant Secretary of Labor and OSHA Director Dr. Eula Bingham,

OSHA was preparing to issue a federal Right-to-Know standard. When President Reagan replaced Bingham in 1981 with Florida businessman Thorne Auchter, OSHA moved to dismantle the Right-to-Know proposal. As unions and COSH groups continued their successful work on state and local Right-to-Know bills, industry groups reluctantly decided that it would be preferable to have a single, uniform regulation rather than the evolving patchwork of local provisions. OSHA responded with a new, weaker proposal.

When OSHA issued its Hazard Communication Standard in late 1983, it was very much a compromise regulation. Despite concern with weak parts of the standard, organized labor has concentrated on the provisions that require employers to provide training on hazard recognition and control for all employees. Many unions, through collective bargaining, have secured the right to participate directly in the development and delivery of this training, which would otherwise be a unilateral employer prerogative. There is reason to hope that the late 1980s will see a major burst in "shop-floor" health and safety activity, spurred by this new flow of information.

HEALTH AND SAFETY ISSUES OF IMPORTANCE TO WORKERS AND UNIONS

Union health and safety activities rest on a set of principles about rights and responsibilities in the workplace. Health professionals who intend to work with unions will be more effective if they understand and respect these premises.

Premise 1: Workers and their union representatives are entitled to participate fully in the development and implementation of health and safety policies and programs because their lives and well-being are directly affected by the decisions made.

This conviction about workplace democracy underlies worker demands for health and safety committees, union review of new technology and equipment, and access to technical information and reports. Worker involvement in health and safety has taken many forms. In a Vermont battery plant, for example, the United Automobile Workers (UAW) negotiated an agreement for medical examinations to be performed by an independently based physician mutually acceptable to the company and union. In an Oklahoma assembly plant, there is a full-time union representative to work on ergonomics programs, which previously had been a unilateral management activity. National collective-bargaining agreements with major automobile manufacturers provide for union representation on hazardous materials control committees.

Premise 2: All employees are equally entitled to safe working conditions and employers have an obligation, both legally and morally, to provide such conditions without resorting to discriminatory hiring and placement practices based on sex, ethnicity, genetic predispositions, or physical handicaps.

This premise means that the employer must make a good-faith effort to design or alter the job to fit the worker rather to limit jobs to those who are judged to be "fit." For example, the size and shape of tool handles should be adjustable so that workers of all sizes and shapes can work without fear of cumulative trauma disorders. Engineering controls and personal protective equipment should be used to reduce exposures sufficiently so that fertile or pregnant employees can work without discrimination. Return-to-work programs should be aimed at placing a worker back on the original job, even if the job must be adjusted to allow this (see Chaps. 9, 12, and 22).

This principle of equal opportunity has several corollaries. First, medical examination programs should be used to guide environmental interventions rather than to determine hiring and personnel decisions. Second, procedures should be established to permit an employee to refuse to work without penalty on a job that is honestly believed to be unsafe until appropriate investigations and corrections can be made. Third, in the event that all feasible protections have been built into a job and a medical examination determines that it is still unsafe for a specific worker, the employer should have a "medical removal protection" program that entitles a worker to an alternative placement without loss of seniority, earnings, or other employment rights and benefits.

Premise 3: Workers should not be asked to protect themselves from job hazards by employers who have not met their legal responsibility for making the workplace healthful and safe for all employees.

For example, personal respirators are not an acceptable alternative to local exhaust ventilation to reduce harmful chemical exposure. Workers should not be lectured to "be careful" around automated powered machinery by an employer who wants to substitute warning signs for mechanical enclosures that completely prevent worker entry into danger zones.

Premise 4: Workers have a fundamental need for and right to all information that is known to the employer, vendors, or suppliers about chemical and physical hazards on the job.

These needs exceed the provisions of the OSHA Hazard Communication Standard. For example, containers should be labeled with full chemical identities of all ingredients. Full disclosure of chemical ingredients should not be compromised by trade secret claims of chemical manufacturers.

Employers have argued that workers only need to be told how to protect themselves and can be provided this information without disclosure of detailed chemical data that is technically beyond worker comprehension. Unions respond that such policies are not only demeaning but also that workers cannot afford to defer vital judgments about their safety to company representative whose interests may conflict with their own. Many companies, for example, consider formaldehyde to be an irritant but deny that evidence is sufficient to treat it as a carcinogen. A data sheet that listed a formaldehyde resin merely as a "proprietary resin" with irritant properties would prevent workers from making an independent evaluation of risk and would seriously limit their ability to seek necessary protections.

Premise 5: Workers who have been subjects in scientific studies are entitled to full notification about the results along with advice and support services to help them cope with their problems if they were found to be at high risk.

Worker notification is a particularly serious problem for thousands of workers who are the surviving members of cohort studies that were conducted by employers, universities, and government agencies and were found at high risk of cancer mortality. Unless these survivors are notified, they will be unlikely to seek early diagnosis and treatment services, they will not have the opportunity to make informed choices about their remaining years, they will not be able to take prompt advantage of any forthcoming advances in cancer prevention, and they will be kept ignorant of the need for protections on the job if the high-risk conditions persist.

Premise 6: Workers who are temporarily or permanently disabled as a result of workplace injuries or illnesses deserve full, prompt compensation for any lost earnings and associated pain or suffering.

State compensation laws are antiquated. State-to-state differences in payment levels, diagnostic criteria, and filing and appeal procedures require substantial legislative reform including federal provisions that ensure equal treatment for all workers (see Chap. 11).

Premise 7: Workers should not work with chemicals that have not been adequately tested for toxicity. There is a need for a substantial increase in occupational health and safety research and a national commitment to apply the results of research to the workplace.

It is not acceptable to unions that thousands of potentially toxic chemicals are introduced into industrial use without adequate premarket toxicologic testing.

Premise 8: Workers need a combination of health and safety laws and collective bargaining agreements to achieve maximum protection on the job. Neither legislation nor contracts alone is sufficient.

Many serious health and safety problems are

not covered by OSHA standards and require direct agreements with employers. For example, there are no federal standards governing confined-space entry procedures or powered-machinery lockout procedures. Most OSHA health standards consist only of a permissible exposure limit (PEL) and contain no provisions for worker training, medical surveillance, process design, and work practices.

On the other hand, even the strongest union contracts can only reach their full potential in the context of well-designed labor and public health laws. The UAW, for example, recently worked with a major employer to develop two training programs for hourly employees. One was hazard communication training and the other was safety training for skilled trades workers. After the first year of implementation, 95 percent of eligible employees had received the hazard communication training, which was required by law, but less than 50 percent had received the skilled trades training, which was not required by law.

The box on page 545 provides an example of how workers can use OSHA and their collective bargaining relationship with the employer to solve health and safety problems.

Premise 9: OSHA standards can be counterproductive if they are obsolete. Vigorous efforts are needed to bring many existing standards in line with current scientific knowledge.

Almost all existing OSHA PELs for chemical exposure were adopted directly from the threshold limit value (TLV) list of the American Conference of Governmental Industrial Hygienists (ACGIH) in effect in 1968. Since that time the TLV list has been revised yearly on the basis of new knowledge, but most OSHA PELs have not changed. Most TLVs, which are only informal recommendations, are now much stricter than their corresponding OSHA-mandated PELs. The National Institute for Occupational Safety and Health (NIOSH) has also published numerous documents recommending more stringent PELs for dozens of chemicals.

The current situation is harmful to workers because most employers strongly resist demands that exposure levels be further reduced as long as the OSHA standards have been met, even though most scientists agree that many legal exposures, which are below the OSHA PEL, but above the ACGIH and NIOSH limits, are harmful.

Premise 10: Workers are entitled to strict protections of confidentiality and privacy when they participate in occupational medical programs. This premise is particularly important because a violation of confidentiality can result in discrimination or job loss.

All medical records should be maintained in locked files and restricted to the use of medical personnel unless authorized in writing by the employee or otherwise required by law. Unions strongly supported the passage of the OSHA Regulation on Access to Employee Exposure and Medical Records, which prohibits release of medical records to anyone without written authorization from the employee. However, this regulation makes it clear that personal air-sampling and biological-monitoring tests, such as blood lead tests, are measures of environmental conditions and are to be more widely available.

Unions support Principle 7 of the American Occupational Medical Association Code of Ethical Conduct, which permits physicians to counsel employers about the medical fitness of individuals to work but asks them not to provide the employer diagnoses or other clinical details [3] (see Chap. 13). There is a widespread perception among workers, however, that these guidelines are frequently violated by company physicians and nurses and that confidential medical information often ends up in the hands of supervisors and other management personnel. Substantial testimony was made to this effect during the public hearings on the OSHA access regulation.

UNION HEALTH AND SAFETY ACTIVITIES: EXAMPLES
Collective Bargaining
Prior to the passage of the OSHAct in 1970, collective-bargaining agreements typically contained general statements about health and safety. With

AN ILLUSTRATION OF RESOURCES WORKERS CAN USE TO SOLVE PROBLEMS

At an aircraft instrument plant in Massachusetts a vapor degreaser tank leaked a large pool of methylene chloride. Methylene chloride, which is used to clean oily equipment, is a highly volatile solvent. After being inhaled, it is converted to carbon monoxide in the blood and causes headache, dizziness, and, with prolonged exposure, unconsciousness and even death.

A worker at the plant, who was both a union shop steward and deputy chief of the plant's emergency crew, was requested to coordinate the emergency response to this leak. By the time he arrived at the scene, 50 people had left the building. He noted that the smell from the leaking solvent was overpowering, and that a few workers were ripping open 50-lb bags of an absorbent material and fabricating makeshift dams to contain the leak. There was no established emergency procedure for such a leak, and equipment and tools such as respirators and even brooms, which were necessary to respond to this emergency, were not available. Over the next 2 hours the leak was soaked up with approximately 300 pounds of the absorbent material, shoveled up, and hauled away. During this time the windowless plant was ventilated by opening the fire doors. Fortunately, no one was seriously injured.

Shortly after the accident, in response to a union complaint OSHA inspected the plant and cited the company for four "serious" violations of its regulations: failure to maintain the degreaser properly, locate eyewash and shower facilities near the tank, train workers in potential dangers of methylene chloride, and have clearcut emergency procedures and provide emergency crews with respirators and other necessary equipment. OSHA fined the company $2,240. The company contested these citations and appealed to the Occupational Safety and Health Review Commission, which has been es-

tablished by the Congress to hear such appeals. The union, in turn, exercised its right to participate in the appeals process.

Because there was an active and knowledgeable local union health and safety committee at this plant, and because OSHA had encouraged worker and union participation in the regulatory process, the union, with the support of the Solicitor of the U.S. Department of Labor, negotiated directly with the company. Management met several times with union officials over the next several months, and within 7 months after the accident a settlement had been reached that produced dramatic changes in the plant.

In exchange for reducing the four "serious" violations to two "non-serious" ones and the fine from $2,240 to $500, the company and the union agreed to the following: a detailed inspection and maintenance procedure for the vapor degreaser including air-supplied respirators for clean-out crew and backup; training of company medical personnel in recognizing symptoms of methylene chloride poisoning; informing present and new workers in the degreaser area of the health effects of methylene chloride; paying the workers who left the area during the emergency for time off the job (something that was originally denied); and installing a continuous monitor to measure airborne concentrations of methylene chloride near the degreaser. The monitor is equipped with a flashing light to indicate when methylene chloride levels represent a hazard (one-half the existing OSHA standard), and workers have been instructed to evacuate the area when this occurs. This spill evacuation procedure also requires that a trained emergency crew be established for all shifts.

Another result of this incident has been the realization by workers that they have the ability and expertise to stand up to the company in such situations and get results that improve conditions on the job. They have gained a great deal of confidence in the process and are prepared to continue their efforts to ensure the health and safety of their workplace.

This incident illustrates the variety of resources that workers can use to solve health and safety problems. In this case, there were two complementary resources: OSHA and the collective bargaining relationship with the employer. In the absence of the union, workers would not have had the organizational resources that enabled them to participate in the appeals process. With this relationship, the workers were able to negotiate with the employer, with OSHA encouragement, and achieve substantial changes on the job. Without the OSHA citation, little of this would have been possible. It also reinforces the point made earlier in this book that health professionals, in order to find out what is actually occurring on the job, must talk to workers.

Adapted with the assistance of Jim Weeks and Richard Youngstrom from R. Howard. Do-it-yourself safety. *In These Times* 5 (15):12, 1981.

---

the renewal of worker consciousness about health and safety in the late 1960s came the recognition that these agreements were insufficient and that stronger, more comprehensive contract language would be necessary to force employers to address serious hazards in a serious way. With a few unions leading the way, most notably the Oil, Chemical and Atomic Workers, a new generation of health and safety agreements began to emerge— often only in response to strike actions or other determined struggles between labor and management. The most fully developed agreements today address five areas:

1. *Responsibility.* The OSHAct states that employers have the legal obligation for maintaining a safe and healthful working environment. Union contracts often restate this employer obligation and amplify it by enumerating specific responsibilities such as providing appropriate medical examinations. The union role is typically expressed as a commitment to cooperate with and participate in programs aimed at fulfilling the employer's responsibility. The legal duty of the union is to represent its members fairly and fully with respect to the employer obligations and workers' rights spelled out in the contract. Courts have generally found that this duty does not mean that the union is responsible for the existence of unsafe conditions or the failure to correct them.

2. *Representation.* In many agreements, especially those that cover relatively small workplaces, it is part of the job of union stewards to handle health and safety matters along with their other duties. Some unions have been able to negotiate full-time positions for local union health and safety representatives in large plants appointed by the union and paid by the company. This representative receives special technical training, conducts investigations, and handles health and safety complaints (Fig. 35-3).

Many unions have bargained for joint health and safety committees to which the company and the union each appoint members. These committees are generally advisory in nature and have little authority to make environmental changes, enforce agreements, or shut down hazardous operations.

3. *Information and participation.* Some access to information is guaranteed by OSHA regulation, including the right of workers and union representatives under various circumstances to obtain MSDSs, industrial hygiene and biological monitoring results, the "OSHA 200" logs (of work-related injuries and illnesses that are maintained by employers), company medical records, and copies of any scientific analyses and reports prepared by or for the employer (see Chap. 10). Unions have bargained for agreements that incorporate these provisions and go beyond them. For example, some unions have won the right to review plans for the introduction of new processes or equipment so that potential health and safety problems

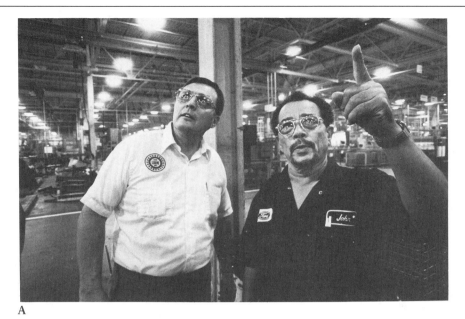

A

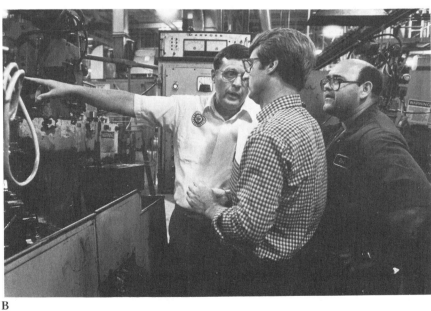

B

Fig. 35-3. A. A worker points out a faulty oil line in a grinder to the United Automobile Workers' health and safety representative (man in white shirt) in an Ohio automobile plant. Since 1973, most automobile plants have had full-time union health and safety representatives to assist workers in getting management to recognize and control hazardous conditions. B. The health and safety representative shows a supervisor (man in checked shirt) the dangling line that could get caught and cause a wheel to explode in the worker's face. The company agreed that the machine would not be used until the problem was corrected.
(Photographs by Russ Marshall. Courtesy of United Automobile Workers.)

can be identified and prevented before reaching the plant. Others have secured agreements to use air-monitoring equipment, to accompany company industrial hygienists during sampling, or to use the employer's computerized toxic materials data base.

Many unions have secured company agreement to provide training for employees in hazards recognition and control beyond that required by law. The most comprehensive agreements to date were reached in 1984 and 1985 between the UAW and General Motors (GM), Ford, and Chrysler. The centerpiece of these agreements is a fund for training activities, which is jointly administered by the company and the union. At GM, for example, 4 cents is put in this fund for every hour worked by a UAW member. The fund is used to develop training programs for skilled trades workers facing particularly dangerous risks, such as confined-space entry, and for local joint health and safety committees. While the funds do not pay for the employee hazard communication training required by law, the contracts do ensure that the training will include the union as a full participant in all phases of development and implementation.

4. *Grievance procedures.* Collective bargaining agreements invariably contain procedures for the union to follow when it believes the company has violated the rights guaranteed to members. Grievance procedures typically call for a series of meetings in which progressively senior management and union representatives attempt to settle a complaint. Some agreements establish special expedited procedures for health and safety complaints. In the event the parties find it impossible to agree, the contract will direct that disputes can ultimately be resolved by binding arbitration or by strike action.

5. *Environmental controls and other specific protections.* Some contracts go beyond general rights by specifying the way that particular problems will be handled. The company and union may agree that a new ventilation system will be installed, that a chemical will be eliminated, that

medical examinations will be offered, or that a research project will be undertaken.

Research

Unions have pressed employers, academic institutions, and government agencies to conduct high-quality occupational health research and to eliminate the inadequate and often self-serving research that has plagued the field for years. Two early leaders in this regard were the Oil, Chemical and Atomic Workers (OCAW) and the United Rubber Workers (URW).

During the 1970s, OCAW was aggressively engaged in nearly all elements of health and safety activity, including campaigns for better standards and enforcement, access to information for workers, and improved research. With an OSHA New Directions grant, OCAW was able to hire several health professionals who provided technical assistance to local unions and who worked to stimulate needed research on potential hazards faced by OCAW members. For example, OCAW was able to challenge research of dubious value being conducted by petrochemical companies and to press NIOSH for the improvement and expansion of its Health Hazard Evaluation and Industrywide Studies activities.

In 1970, the URW negotiated a research program of great vision and importance with the major tire manufacturers. Research funds were established with each employer contributing a sum of money, ranging from one-half to two cents for each hour worked by a URW member. These funds, under joint labor-management control, were used to support university research into the hazards of the rubber industry. A series of epidemiologic and industrial hygiene studies was conducted by two schools of public health. Valuable information emerged about the relationship between stomach cancer and leukemia and solvent exposures in the rubber industry. Most important, manuals were prepared with information about how to reduce exposures to the chemicals of likely danger.

In the 1980s, the UAW identified occupational health research as an area of major importance, expanding some of the earlier union initiatives. The UAW began to develop its own in-house epidemiololgy program. It established a mortality surveillance system, helped local unions undertake their own investigations, and completed a series of substantial mortality and morbidity studies [4, 5]. A number of work-related health risks were identified, including associations between stomach cancer and work with metalworking fluids, lung cancer and nonmalignant respiratory disease with foundry work, and cumulative trauma disorders with various assembly jobs.

In addition to this independent activity, the UAW reached a series of agreements on research with employers. In 1982, the UAW and GM agreed to establish an Occupational Health Advisory Board of six mutually acceptable university-based scientists to assist in the development of research activities. The board's first major task was to sponsor a competitive peer review process to consider proposals for a comprehensive investigation of the health effects of exposure to metalworking fluids. This process resulted in a contract to a school of public health for a major mortality, pulmonary function, and industrial hygiene investigation. In 1984, the UAW negotiated occupational health research funds with GM, Ford, and Chrysler totaling over $5 million for an initial 3-year period. Areas receiving support include the health effects of solvent and polymer systems, health and industrial hygiene surveillance for foundry workers, engineering controls for cutting fluids, and mortality surveillance systems.

OSHA Standards

Unions have consistently been the chief advocates for more protective OSHA standards, pressuring successive generations of OSHA administrators who have moved slowly on their own (and in some cases not at all). The history of the early OSHA standards (lead, vinyl chloride, asbestos, benzene, arsenic, and cotton dust) reveals that unions played a vital role at every step. They petitioned for emergency action, participated in public hearings, went to court to stop administrative delays, and filed complaints when employers failed to implement the provisions of new standards. For example, the regulatory agenda set by unions for the 1987 to 1991 period includes standards on formaldehyde, methylene chloride, wood dust, grain dust, field sanitation, and power lockout. Unions have also supported the notion of "generic" standard-setting, which would regulate large groups of similar materials, such as chlorinated solvents or pesticides, at one time rather than the current inefficient and time-consuming substance-by-substance approach (see Chap. 10).

Legislation

Unions were deeply involved in activities necessary to secure passage of the federal Coal Mine Health and Safety Act in 1969 and OSHAct in 1970. Since then, much union energy has gone toward implementing these acts, protecting them from erosion, and supplementing the statutory protections with collective-bargaining protections. However, there is still a need for additional legal protection for workers.

High-Risk Worker Notification. There are thousands of workers who were included in epidemiologic studies and, as a result, are known to be at high risk for the eventual development of occupational diseases. With rare exceptions, government agencies and academic institutions have simply filed away the lists of cohort members, and the workers at risk have not been notified of their status. To remedy this situation unions have supported establishing procedures for the notification of workers at high risk and developing medical surveillance and related support programs for these workers and their families. During 1986, those legislative initiatives were actively opposed by employer groups and by the Federal Office of Management and Budget and the Department of Health and Human Services. Although no legislation was enacted in 1987, NIOSH has begun notification activities with regard to its own studies and legislative debate is expected to continue.

Workers' Compensation Reform. Workers' compensation laws are generally recognized to be outmoded and flawed. Award levels for lost wages and benefits are inadequate. Many states limit compensation to acute injuries and exclude occupational illnesses or cumulative trauma from coverage. In states where illnesses are covered, statutes of limitations are sometimes written so that most affected workers are excluded from benefits. State-to-state inconsistencies have resulted in harmful inequities. A worker may be compensated at a rate of 80 percent of lost wages in one state whereas a worker suffering a similar illness from the same cause in another state may receive only one-half as much award or may be denied benefits altogether. Unions have supported proposals for state and federal laws that would provide uniform and improved compensation protection for the victims of occupational illness and injury (see Chap. 11).

Liability Law. Because compensation laws have proven inadequate, sick and injured workers have looked elsewhere for help. Although compensation laws are "exclusive remedies" and exempt employers from additional liability, it has been possible for victims of chemical and physical hazards to file suit against third parties, such as the manufacturers of defective equipment or the formulators of dangerous chemicals. The success of some plaintiffs, particularly those suffering the effects of past asbestos exposure, has generated a fierce backlash by the insurance industry. There have been numerous proposals to limit liability by placing caps on the amounts awarded to victims for pain and suffering, by establishing more restrictive statutes of limitations, and by creating more narrow criteria for causation. Unions have been active in each new legislative session, supporting proposals designed to preserve the ability of workers to

seek just awards for the effects of negligent exposure to harmful conditions.

REFERENCES
1. Cherniack M. The Hawk's Nest incident: America's worst industrial accident. New Haven, CT: Yale University Press, 1986.
2. Rosner D, Markowitz G. Safety and health on the job as a class issue: the workers' health bureau of America in the 1920s. Science and Society 1984; 48: 466–82.
3. Code of Ethical Conduct for Physicians Providing Occupational Medical Services. Chicago: American Occupational Medical Association, 1976.
4. Silverstein M, Maizlish N, Park R et al. Mortality among workers exposed to coal tar pitch volatiles and welding emissions: an exercise in epidemiologic triage. Am J Public Health 1985; 75:1283–7.
5. The case of the workplace killers: a manual for cancer detectives on the job. Detroit: United Automobile Workers, 1981.

BIBLIOGRAPHY
AFL-CIO. Manual for Shop Stewards. Washington, DC.: American Federation of Labor and Congress of Industrial Organizations, 1984.
  A basic guide for union representatives, including information about rights and responsibilities.
Babson S. Working Detroit: the making of a union town. New York: Adama, 1984.
  An excellent chronicle of workers and unions in America's industrial heartland.
Cherniack M. The Hawk's Nest incident: America's worst industrial disaster. New Haven, CT: Yale University Press, 1986.
  A historical and epidemiologic reconstruction of the scandalous epidemic of acute silicosis among workers building the Hawk's Nest Tunnel 50 years ago to provide hydroelectric power for a Union Carbide Corporation plant in Gauley Bridge, West Virginia.
Deutsch S, ed. Theme issue: occupational safety and health. Labor Studies, 6:1981.
  A collection of articles providing more details about several of the subjects covered in this chapter, including health and safety committees, collective bargaining, COSH groups, and workplace democracy.
McAteer JD. Miner's manual: a complete guide to health and safety protection on the job. Washington, DC.: Crossroads, 1981.

A good example of a health and safety training publication designed with rank-and-file workers in mind.

Melkin D, Brown M. Workers at risk: voices from the workplace. Chicago: The University of Chicago Press, 1984.

A powerful series of first-person accounts by workers faced with chemical hazards on the job.

Page J, O'Brien M. Bitter wages. New York: Grossman, 1973.

The best discussion available about the origins of the OSHAct, including substantial material about the political activity of labor unions in health and safety during the pre-OSHA era.

Rashke R. The killing of Karen Silkwood: the story behind the Kerr-McGee plutonium case. Boston: Houghton Mifflin, 1981.

An investigative reporter's probe into the tangled story of union activism, radiation hazards, the nuclear fuel industry, liability law, and, in the view of some, murder.

Stein L. The Triangle fire. New York: Carroll & Graf, 1962.

A historical recreation of a workplace disaster that was linked to industry negligence and that led to important health and safety reforms in the early twentieth century.

36
Occupational Health in Selected Developing Countries

David Michaels, René Mendes, David C. Christiani, and Gu Xue-qi

In this textbook, occupational health programs and other activities are discussed largely in the context of how they operate or are performed in the United States. It is important to realize, however, that occupational health programs and activities differ from nation to nation because of differences in political structure, organization of health care delivery, level and type of economic development and attendant occupational health hazards, availability of financial resources and professional personnel, and other factors.

Information on occupational health activities in other developed nations can be readily found in various publications [1, 2]. There is, however, very little information available concerning the organization and delivery of occupational health services and prevention activities in developing nations. For this reason occupational health in two settings, Latin America and China, are discussed here to illustrate variations that exist in addressing the needs to reduce workplace hazards and to prevent occupational disorders when information on distribution of hazards and prevalence of disease is sparse or non-existent and resources for control of risks are severely limited. Further reading is suggested for a more detailed consideration of the strengths and weaknesses of different options.

Appendix C provides some additional information, specifically on three international organizations that provide various services for and various types of information on occupational health and safety in both developing and developed nations.

Latin America
David Michaels and René Mendes

Latin America has rapidly industrialized in the past few decades. The size of the region's manufacturing sector, for example, quadrupled from 1960 to 1980. In contrast, the extractive industries, such as mining and agriculture, traditionally the most important sector of the Latin American economy, increased at a much slower rate and now contribute only one-half as much as manufacturing to the region's gross domestic product.

The Latin American workforce is one of the fastest growing in the world, doubling every 25 years: in 1960, it had 67 million workers; in 1980, 112 million; and by the year 2000, it will have almost 200 million. Its nature has changed, reflecting the new economic order. The percentage of the workforce employed in agricultural activities is decreasing throughout Latin America (Table 36-1), and rapid urbanization is occurring in virtually every country in the region [3]. Many more rural dwellers have been forced to leave the countryside than can be absorbed by the growing manufacturing and service sectors, causing urban unemployment and underemployment to become one of Latin America's most pressing problems [4].

Much of Latin America's industrial growth has occurred in industries in which workers are exposed to significant health hazards. Many countries in the region, most notably Mexico, Colombia, Venezuela, Peru, Brazil, and Argentina, have developed their own "heavy" industrial concentra-

Table 36-1. Percentage of work force employed in agriculture, industry, and service, 1965 and 1980, in selected Latin American countries

Country	Agriculture		Industry*		Service	
	1965	1980	1965	1980	1965	1980
Argentina	18	13	34	34	48	53
Bolivia	54	46	20	20	26	34
Brazil	48	31	20	27	31	42
Colombia	45	34	21	24	34	42
Cuba	33	24	25	29	41	48
Ecuador	55	39	19	20	26	42
El Salvador	59	56	16	14	25	30
Guatemala	64	57	15	17	21	26
Mexico	50	37	22	29	29	34
Nicaragua	57	47	16	16	27	38
Panama	46	32	16	18	38	50
Peru	50	40	19	18	31	42
Venezuela	30	16	24	28	47	56

*Industry category is composed of manufacturing, mining, construction, and utilities (electricity, water, and gas).
Source: Excerpted from *World Bank Development Report: 1986.* Copyright © 1986 by The International Bank for Reconstruction and Development/The World Bank. Reprinted by permission of Oxford University Press, Inc.

tions, producing steel, automobiles, tires, chemicals, and other durable goods. Mexico City and São Paulo, the industrial hubs of Mexico and Brazil, are the two largest cities of the hemisphere, each having more than 15 million inhabitants, with populations of greater than 25 million predicted by the end of the century.

AGRICULTURAL TRANSFORMATION AND RURAL HEALTH

Throughout Latin America, large portions of arable land have been reallocated, often forcibly, changing from production for local consumption to export-oriented agriculture. This reallocation has been accompanied by the concentration of land holdings in the hands of a small number of agribusiness firms and wealthy individuals as well as by major alterations in the methods used to produce these crops. To obtain employment harvesting crops, which are in areas where many do not live, a significant portion of Latin American workers have become seasonal migrants, following the harvest cycles. One study estimates that over 40 percent of Central American workers are now migrant farm workers. The health effects of these trends include increased malnutrition, endemic parasite infestation, other infectious disease, and work injuries. Seasonal migration also is directly related to increases in alcoholism, stress-related complaints, and sexually transmitted diseases, in addition to having an important detrimental impact on family structure and educational opportunity [5].

This agricultural transformation has also been accompanied by greatly increased use of pesticides. Since 1972, world pesticide consumption has, on average, increased 5 percent per year, with some countries in Latin America experiencing an even sharper rise. Many of the most hazardous pesticides are commonly used throughout the less-developed countries; approximately one-third of U.S. pesticide exports to Latin America are products prohibited for use in the United States because of their extreme toxicity (see Chap. 33).

Much of the rural population of Latin America

receives little or no training in the safe handling of these extremely dangerous substances (Fig. 36-1). One study found that three-fourths of the Central American workers employed in cultivating cotton, a crop that uses numerous toxic pesticides, were not sufficiently literate to read pesticide use instructions or warnings; almost none of the workers in that study had access to protective clothing. Virtually all the workers lived within 100 meters of the cotton fields, many in temporary housing with no walls for protection from pesticides sprayed from airplanes. Workers and their families often washed in irrigation channels containing pesticide residues, resulting in increased exposures.

The incidence of pesticide poisoning among Latin American agricultural workers appears to be quite high, although there are few systematic studies on this subject. During the years 1971 through 1976, for example, there were 17,183 cases of pesticide intoxication reported in El Salvador and Guatemala alone. Certain agricultural groups are apparently at greater risk of pesticide exposures; a study of agricultural fumigators in Colombia found that 34 percent had depressed cholinesterase levels, a sign of significant exposure to organophosphate pesticides.

Potentially hazardous levels of environmental pesticide pollution are now ubiquitous throughout Latin America, much of it attributable to widespread pesticide contamination of water and food. As a result of DDT use throughout Guatemala, a Guatemalan suckling infant consumes daily be-

Fig. 36-1. Disposal of empty pesticide containers in Venezuelan farmlands is an unsolved problem. (Photograph courtesy of Gustavo Molina.)

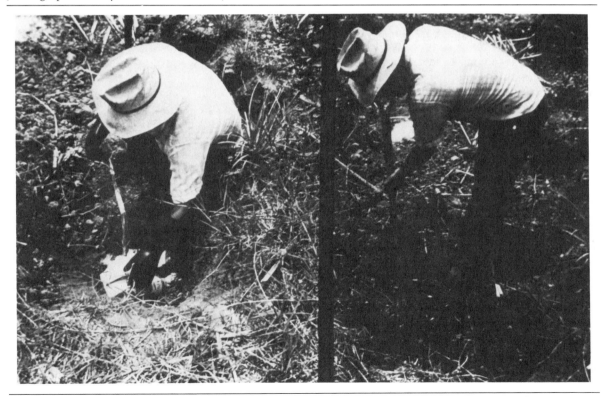

tween 7 and 244 times the maximum daily DDT intake that is legally permitted in the United States and advocated by the World Health Organization (WHO) and the Food and Agriculture Organization (FAO). The organochloride pesticide residue found in adipose tissue of Mexicans, as well as of residents of other Latin American countries, is far greater than pesticide residue present in adipose tissue of North Americans or Europeans. Ironically, some pesticides exported to Central America return to the United States through residues in imported agricultural products, particularly beef and coffee [6].

OCCUPATIONAL ILLNESS
IN LATIN AMERICA

The epidemiologic literature concerning the effects of occupational exposures in Latin America is limited, consisting primarily of cross-sectional studies that measure only the prevalence of a particular disease or health effect in a segment of the exposed population at one point in time. While studies of this sort are inadequate to investigate many types of occupationally related chronic disease, the striking results of these studies demonstrate that occupational disease is a large and growing problem in Latin America. They also suggest that current social, economic, and environmental conditions may result in even greater occupational disease risks for Latin American workers than for their counterparts in developed countries. A few examples illustrate this phenomenon:

The current U.S. standard for lead exposure mandates immediate medical removal of a worker from lead exposure when blood lead equals or exceeds 50 μg per dl. In a recent study, 71 percent of workers in two Medellin, Colombia, battery factories were found to have blood lead levels of more than 50 μg per dl, with one individual having a level of 180 μg per dl. At one of the plants, 13 of the 14 employees exceeded the 50 μg per dl removal level. In addition, symptoms consistent with lead exposure, including abdominal colic,

nausea, and muscle pain, were reported by over 70 percent of the workers in the study [7].

A cohort of 8,500 underground miners, primarily involved in the mining of tin, was studied by the Bolivian National Institute of Occupational Health. Although most (73%) had worked fewer than 15 years in the mines, over 40 percent of the miners suffered from either silicosis or silicotuberculosis [8].

In 1981, Nicaraguan physicians conducted an investigation into neurologic disease in mercury-exposed workers employed in a transnationally owned Managua chloralkali plant; of 152 exposed workers, 56 (37%) exhibited symptoms of mercurialism [9].

In a review of 3,440 adult male tuberculosis patients hospitalized in the southeastern part of Brazil, investigators found 119 (3.5%) with silicotuberculosis. Applying this rate of disease to all adult male hospital admissions for tuberculosis and considering the tuberculosis frequency in Brazilian silicotics (3.3%), it was estimated that, in 1977, there were 20,000 persons with silicosis in southeastern Brazil alone [10].

THE DOUBLE BURDEN
OF UNDERDEVELOPMENT

Toxicologic evidence suggests that the health effects of exposure to hazardous chemicals are increased by nutritional deficiencies common in Latin America. Low-protein diets, for example, increase the susceptibility of exposed individuals to the toxic effects of three widely employed pesticides—carbaryl, malathion, and parathion—as well as to several heavy metals. Similarly, the risk of lead-exposed workers developing anemia is greatly increased if they also suffer from hookworm infection. Vitamin-enriched diets have been shown to protect laboratory animals exposed to certain heavy metals, solvents, and pesticides [11].

Children and young people make up a large and apparently growing percentage of the workforce in many developing countries. In recent years, researchers have begun to document the increased susceptibility of children and adolescents to the health effects of toxic substances, particularly those that affect the development of the reproductive system. Prominent among these substances are pesticides, to which many of the children employed in agricultural work are exposed [12].

In addition, children and adolescent workers are at greater risk for work-related injuries than adult workers are.

SOCIAL AND TECHNICAL BARRIERS TO CONTROLLING WORKPLACE HAZARDS

Although occupational safety and health research and law enforcement structures equivalent in function to those of developed countries exist throughout Latin America, they are, in general, extremely ineffectual. With a few important exceptions, Latin American workplace inspectors have little ability to monitor occupational hazards and even less ability to mandate hazard abatement.

Engineering controls of toxic exposures are almost unknown in smaller Latin American factories and are grossly inadequate in other workplaces (Fig. 36-2). Few standards are applied to limit workplace exposures; in most of the region's countries, the standard-setting process is either just beginning or has not yet begun. In those nations where standards regulating work practices or toxic exposure exist, they are often not enforced, primarily because of political and economic reasons and because of a lack of trained inspectors.

The chronically elevated unemployment and underemployment rates throughout Latin America undoubtedly contribute to the continued existence of occupational health hazards. In many countries, unemployment insurance, social security, and income maintenance programs are virtually nonexistent for the unemployed and for those working in marginal sectors of the economy. The tens of millions of Latin American workers with jobs are understandably more concerned with maintaining

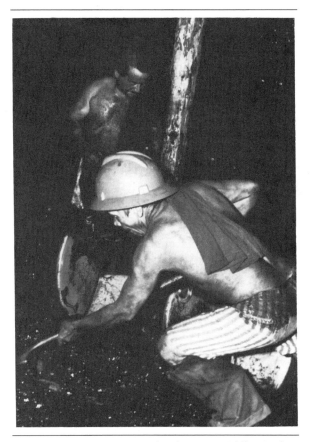

Fig. 36-2. Coal miner in Colombia in a middle-sized operation. There is little mechanization. Workers labor in hot and humid conditions.
(Photograph courtesy of Gustavo Molina.)

their jobs to feed themselves and their families than with the possible health effects of toxic exposures.

There are few programs in Latin America to train health and safety technicians who can serve as government inspectors or as safety specialists in the private and academic sectors. Most Latin American subsidiaries of major transnational chemical and electronic manufacturers have no trained industrial hygienists on their staffs; comparable factories operated by their parent companies in industrialized nations would employ one or more hygienists to monitor and control hazardous exposures.

Adequate personal protective equipment is also a rarity in developing nations. Recent study of Colombian industries revealed that workers in lead battery factories and foundries were using no respiratory protection at all—or only cloth scarves. When appropriate respirators are used, incorrect cartridges are commonly employed, and respirator cartridges are changed infrequently.

THE EXPORT OF HAZARDOUS INDUSTRIES

Several U.S.-based economists and public health experts have documented the flight of dangerous industries, such as the benzidine-based dye and asbestos textile industries, from the more-regulated environments of the developed countries. By shifting hazardous production processes to less-developed countries, where little or no environmental regulation exists, these manufacturers avoid investing capital in equipment necessary to control hazardous exposures. As a result of lower wages, taxes, energy costs, and capital investment, profits are substantially higher. The postulated effect of this trend is that workers in the less-developed countries are exposed to disease-producing levels of toxic substances, and unemployment increases in the developed countries. The final products of the relocated industries are then exported back to the industrialized countries.

While the extent of this practice is not known, several U.S. studies have shown that the cost of health and safety regulation does not significantly contribute to a manufacturer's decisions to relocate production facilities; of greater importance are the markedly lower wages, benefits, and taxation structures of most less-developed countries and the absence or lack of power of trade unions. Furthermore, virtually all U.S. manufacturing firms that have been reported to have closed as a result of health and safety regulation were fi-

nancially marginal firms that would have had to cease operating even if environmental regulations did not exist [13].

RECENT TRENDS AND FUTURE DIRECTIONS

In recent years there has been a marked increase in occupational safety and health activities in Latin America. In Colombia, for example, the Institute of Social Security (ISS) has initiated a national program of occupational safety and health education and technical assistance, funded by the allocation of 5 percent of all injury and illness insurance payments made by employers. Since the program's inception in 1981, several hundred professional and paraprofessional ISS employees have attended 6-month intensive education programs. Increased resources are being allocated to occupational health services in Brazil as well, where the federal and state governments have added inspectors and focused greater attention on occupational health.

Many trade unions are working actively to improve the conditions in which their members work. Demanding safer jobs, these unions have waged numerous, although often unpublicized, health and safety campaigns, sometimes involving long and bitter strikes. Worker organizations also have begun to collaborate with the public health community in addressing safety and health issues. For example, several São Paulo-area unions, including those representing textile, metal, and electrical workers, employ full-time physicians to educate their members about safety and health hazards and to provide technical and clinical consultation services. Although these developments are likely to contribute to improvement of working conditions, they affect only a small portion of the Latin American workforce: those belonging to progressive trade unions.

In general, Latin American governments appear likely to continue to adopt, with limited modifications, the occupational health regulations and structures existing in Western developed countries. In many cases, this action may be neither appropriate nor effective. Even a large staff of inspectors is unlikely to have the ability—because of lack of time and resources—to conduct comprehensive inspections of all potentially hazardous workplaces. In addition, political and economic factors further reduce the effectiveness of many Latin American governmental health and safety programs. Given these considerations, implementing massive worker education programs is more likely to contribute to improved working conditions than enlarging staff of governmental inspection programs.

In the area of standard-setting, the development of a uniform, international set of permissible exposure levels would be extremely useful. Few developing countries have the resources to undertake the toxicologic and epidemiologic studies that serve as the necessary basis for exposure standards. Internationally accepted standards are less likely to be compromised by local economic interests and are more likely to be based on solid scientific data. Until these standards are developed, however, multinational corporations could be required to limit workplace exposure to the levels permissible in the countries where the parent companies are based or to the lowest level permissible in any country in which they operate.

More broadly, there are practical goals that occupational health programs in developing countries, in Latin America or elsewhere, should aim to achieve. One of these goals is that occupational health—art, science, and especially commitment—must be present at all levels of delivery within the health care system. Workers' health cannot depend exclusively on specialists in occupational medicine, industrial hygiene, toxicology, or ergonomics, particularly where there is a very large "informal" sector of workers who do not have any in-plant health services. This sector constitutes the vast majority of workers in developing countries, including workers in agriculture, small industries, and construction, as well as casual laborers.

A second practical goal is the inclusion of workers in all facets of occupational health. Their participation, through their trade unions, is important in (1) discussion of occupational health problems, (2) planning and organizing strategies for prevention and control, (3) surveillance of risks, and (4) enforcement of laws and regulations.

REFERENCES

1. Ashford NA. Foreign experience and its relevance for the United States. In Crisis in the workplace. Cambridge, MA: MIT Press, 1976.
2. Elling RH. The struggle for worker's health: a study of six industrialized countries. Farmingdale, NY: Baywood, 1986.
3. World Bank Development Report: 1986. New York: Oxford University Press, 1986.
4. Tockman VE. The unemployment crisis in Latin America. Int Labour Rev 1984; 123:585–97.
5. Laurell A. Mortality and working conditions in agriculture in underdeveloped countries. Int J Health Serv 1981; 11:3–20.
6. Bull D. A growing problem: pesticides and the Third World poor. London: Oxfam, 1982.
7. Gacharná MG, Ruiza F, Herrera A, et al. Prevalencia de plomo corporal correlacion clinico-epidemiologica en trabajadores de dos industrias y en sus contractos. Boletin de Investigationes 1976; 2:10–24.
8. Pinell LF. Frequency of silicosis and silicotuberculosis among mine workers in Bolivia: an epidemiologic study. Bull Int Union Against TB 1976; 51:577–82.
9. Hassan A, Velasquez E, Belmar R, et al. Mercury poisoning in Nicaragua: a case study of the export of environmental and occupational health hazards by a multinational. Int J Health Serv 1981; 11:221–6.
10. Mendes R. Estudo epidemiológico sobre a silicose pulmonar na regiào sudeste do Brasil, através de inquérito em pacientes internaos em hospitais de tisiologia. Rev Saúde Públ (S. Paulo) 1979; 13:7–19.
11. Lee DHK, Kotin P, eds. Multiple factors in the causation of environmentally induced disease. New York: Academic, 1972.
12. Hunt VR, Smith MK, Worth D, eds. Environmental factors in human growth and development. Banbury Report 1982; 11:3–541.
13. Duerksen C. Environmental regulation of industrial plant setting: how to make it work better. Washington, DC.: Conservation Foundation, 1983.

BIBLIOGRAPHY

Bull D. A growing problem: pesticides and the Third World poor. London: Oxfam, 1982.
An excellent source of information on the effects of

pesticide use in less-developed countries and the United States.

Ives J, ed. The export of hazard: transnational corporations and environmental control issues. Boston: Routledge & Kegan Paul, 1985.
Several important aspects of the debate on the export of hazardous industries to less-developed countries are discussed in this recent collection.

Lappe RM, Collins J, Kinley D. Food first: beyond the myth of scarcity. Boston: Houghton Mifflin, 1977.
A well-written introduction to the global food system, focusing on agribusiness and pesticides in the world economy.

Mendes R. Salud ocupacional: un area prioritaria en la salud de los trabajadores. Bol of Sanit Panam 1982; 93:506–21.
An important Spanish-language introduction to the topic.

Michaels D, Barrera C, Gacharna MG. Economic development and occupational health in Latin America: new directions for public health in less developed countries. Am J Public Health 1985; 75:536–43.
A recent overview of occupational health in Latin America: much of the material in this chapter is adapted from this article.

The People's Republic of China

David C. Christiani and Gu Xue-qi

China, the world's largest developing country, is striving to accomplish unprecedented modernization, in which science and technology play a crucial role. Occupational health in China can be understood in the context of three determinants: (1) China's current level of development, in particular that of industry, public health, and medicine; (2) the tasks that China has defined as critical to its future development; and (3) its available resources.

BACKGROUND

China has emerged from a period of intense and thorough self-examination of its economic and political institutions and their ability to solve the serious problems related to modernization. The Chinese have had remarkable success in achieving the basics of governing, feeding, clothing, and housing the world's largest national population. However, the population has almost doubled in 30 years and the economy has not expanded fast enough to raise the standard of living beyond basic necessities for all, or to provide employment for the vastly increased population of urban youth.

Since 1979, major reforms in economic management have taken place, including transference of financial planning and management responsibilities to local levels, expansion of joint venture with foreign businesses, resurgence of the collective and cooperative industry, and (limited) private business expansion. Emphasis has been placed on developing a plan for economic development, which recognizes both the limits of China's resources and the need to improve the standard of living. Light industry and agriculture have therefore expanded rapidly over the decade.

Collectives have also grown rapidly over the past decade, representing an alternative to state and private ownership. The collectives generally produce light industrial and consumer goods and provide services. They are cooperatively run by small groups; sometimes a whole village starts a business with its own capital or government loans. The participants take their own business risks, pay taxes, and divide profits among themselves. About one-fourth of the industrial workforce now works in collective industry. These enterprises provide employment for many working-age youth. Since the collectives are not state-owned, the workers may lack many of the benefits that state factory and state farm workers may enjoy and may have suboptimal working conditions.

The growth of private enterprise businesses in the mid-1980s has also been notable. These businesses are established by an individual or a family, using private capital or government loans. The government has encouraged such private ventures by permitting persons taking the business risk to pay retainer fees to their state employers to reserve their job. While the business venture is too new to realize much return, the worker retains the health, education, and other benefits provided by the state employer. If the venture fails, the worker may return to the previous job, which is reserved for as long as the retainer fee is paid. There are about one-half million workers in such private enterprise businesses, not including household production in the countryside.

A developing country with limited capital attempting modernization by the year 2000 has intensified occupational health problems. Furthermore, the same superstructural problems that hamper China's overall modernization may also affect efforts to modernize its occupational health activities and policies. In the past, when China has been faced with limited technology, it has attempted to overcome this limitation by using its vast labor power. However, modernization presents problems not easily solved by labor power alone. Providing a healthful work environment is one of these problems.

MAJOR OCCUPATIONAL HEALTH PROBLEMS

Before 1949, the health problems most prevalent in China were similar to those of other developing countries: primarily infectious diseases and malnutrition. Tremendous social progress since then has resulted in morbidity and mortality patterns that are beginning to resemble those of developed nations. Industrialization has been rapid since the 1950s and has received an extra boost since 1976. Thus, it is not surprising that occupational and environmental health problems are becoming more visible. Chinese health officials identify their current major occupational health problems as occupational lung disease, industrial chemical poisoning, pesticide poisoning, heavy metal poisoning, physical hazards, and occupational cancer. Each of these categories is now examined.

Occupational Lung Diseases

Pneumoconioses. Coal worker's pneumoconiosis (CWP) and silicosis are prevalent, as coal is the major energy source in China. Many rock and coal miners are exposed to high silica concentrations. The true prevalence of silicosis and coal worker's pneumoconiosis is unknown. Cases of acute silicosis and silicotuberculosis are still fairly commonly seen. A large number of workers are disabled with these diseases. However, incidence rates are expected to drop in the larger industries, since dust control measures are being introduced. Outbreaks of acute silicosis have occurred in rural workers who have moved from agricultural work to stone cutting and quarrying.

Asbestosis has been documented mainly in the asbestos textile and friction products industry. Asbestosis prevalence in a large asbestos products factory in Shanghai in 1980 was 20 percent and its incidence 1.5 percent per year. Prevalence was highest in those workers who worked in small asbestos plants in the 1950s before moving to the large plant. Many cases seen today are due to exposure in the distant past.

Organic Dust-Induced Lung Diseases. Byssinosis and chronic bronchitis in cotton textile workers are currently under investigation. Byssinosis was described in China in the early 1960s and field surveys for byssinosis have been done. Cotton dust-related diseases, however, are a relatively new area of research in China. As China is the world's largest cotton consumer and its cotton textile industry continues to expand, Chinese colleagues are pursuing research on both the problems and the solutions of cotton dust exposure.

Hypersensitivity pneumonitis (including "farmer's lung") has been described in East China among farm workers exposed to moldy hay. Preliminary reports reveal that about 6 percent of these workers have acute symptoms, and 15 percent of those with acute symptoms have nodular opacities on chest x-ray. Detailed epidemiologic, physiologic, and immunologic work is now being performed. Respiratory abnormalities among grain dust-exposed workers are also being investigated. Recent investigations of grain and mushroom workers have also been undertaken.

Respiratory disease in tea workers has been researched in China for many years.

Industrial Chemicals

The chemical industry has expanded rapidly in China, resulting in relatively new workplace exposures such as vinyl chloride, polytetrafluoroethylene (PTFE), decaborane, acrylonitrile, acrylamide, styrene, and toluene diisocyanate. Cases of acute and chronic poisoning by these and other chemicals have been documented by factory industrial hygiene and medical services, as well as by referral hospitals and institutes.

Benzene is still a widely used solvent, although it is gradually being replaced by such compounds as toluene, xylene, and kerosene. Chinese scientists have done much research on benzene. Techniques such as sister chromatid exchange (SCE) and cell inhibition are used in the evaluation of benzene and other solvents.

Compounds used in the growing plastics and synthetic fiber industries have been examined for their potential toxicity, for biologic indicators of exposure, and maximum allowable concentration of exposure. For example, "polymer fume fever" and pneumonitis induced by PTFE pyrolysis products were discovered in the polymer industry soon after PTFE was introduced. After animal studies on the effects of exposure revealed pulmonary edema and nodular lung infiltrates at relatively low levels of exposure, maximum allowable concentrations (MACs) were then proposed for the principal pyrolysates.

Epidemiologic studies of carbon disulfide exposure have also been done. With expansion of the viscose rayon industry, the potential for carbon disulfide exposure has increased. (Viscose rayon production began in the 1960s and has expanded over the past 15 years.) Recently, studies have been performed investigating the cardiovascular and neurobehavioral effects of chronic low-level, 10 ppm time-weighted average (TWA) carbon disulfide exposure.

Pesticide Poisoning

More than 80 percent of China's huge population lives and works in the countryside; hence pesticide exposure is a serious occupational hazard, and control of pesticide poisoning is a major priority. For example, in the 1960s organophosphate poisoning occurred in Shanghai's 10 rural counties whose total population then was approximately 3.6 million and where the main agricultural products are rice, cotton, vegetables, and fruit. When the organophosphates demeton-o and parathion were introduced, acute poisonings occurred, with rates as high as 130 cases per ton of pesticides used. Within 3 years after an effective control program was instituted, the rate used dropped to less than two cases per ton of pesticides used. Research has been performed on serum cholinesterase activity, percutaneous absorption of radioactive-labeled pesticides, and MACs for a variety of pesticides in use. Work is now proceeding on the carcinogenicity and teratogenicity of organophosphates and other pesticides.

Heavy Metal Poisoning

Cases of heavy metal poisoning have been discovered among workers regularly exposed to heavy metals, such as lead, mercury, cadmium, and manganese. Lead poisoning illustrates this problem in its historical context.

Lead poisoning has been a research priority in China for approximately 40 years. Between 1949 and 1959, 38 scientific papers were published in China on lead poisoning, compared with a total of 6 before 1949. From 1950 to the present, more than 1,100 papers have been published and more than 69,000 workers examined. During the 1950s, air concentrations of inorganic lead fumes and dust were found to be as high as 41 mg per cubic meter, with prevalence rates of clinical lead poisoning approaching 100 percent in primary smelters and storage battery plants. In the same decade, the newly developed network of public health "epidemic prevention" stations attacked the problem in both industries and average air-borne lead dust levels were reduced in that decade to 0.16 mg per cubic meter. Today many large plants (except in primary smelting) are reported to have air levels close to the MAC.* Cases of lead poisoning are still seen but are concentrated mainly in the smelting, storage battery, and lead-mining industries. Severe cases are reportedly rare in large factories while data from small collective factories in Shanghai County reveal an average clinically evident lead poisoning prevalence of 8.5 percent per year over the past 10 years. Most of these cases were in asymptomatic workers who had high blood lead levels. Usually, such asymptomatic workers are not only removed from further exposure, but also often hospitalized and treated with chelation.†

Physical Hazards

Noise is a major problem, particularly in plants not yet modernized, such as most textile mills. Company managers, staff, and workers are all concerned about health problems induced by noise (and vibration) and are actively seeking effective controls. No data are available on the prevalence of hearing loss among textile mill, shipyard, or other noise-exposed workers, but site visits to older cotton and silk mills have roughly estimated noise levels at 95 to 110 decibels, the loudest measurements being in weaving and spinning areas. Research on hearing loss will become a major effort in textile and other industries.

Hot environments are also a problem, particularly in southeast China, which has very hot and humid summers.

Occupational Cancer

Cases of occupational cancer have been reported in industries in which it has been found in other countries. In 1982, the Ministry of Public Health launched a nationwide epidemiologic survey of occupational cancer. Eight known carcinogens then in use were targeted: asbestos, vinyl chloride, benzidine dyes, benzene, chromates, bischloromethylether (BCME), arsenic, and coal tar derivatives. Laboratory investigations of these and other carcinogenic and mutagenic substances are underway. Tests for mutagenicity, such as the Ames test and cell cultures, are among those being used.

Occupational and environmental cancer research is beginning in China. Active discussions and debates over the most appropriate epidemiologic techniques and laboratory evaluations are taking place in Chinese research institutes and schools of public health.

CONTROL OF OCCUPATIONAL HAZARDS

China's strategy for control of occupational hazards includes seven parts: (1) setting of occupational health standards (MACs); (2) engineering controls; (3) personal protective equipment (PPE) and personal hygiene; (4) worker education; (5) preventive diagnosis; (6) professional training; and (7) worker's compensation.

Occupational Health Standards

Immediately following "Liberation" in 1949, the Chinese began systematic occupational health activities by passing several workplace safety and hygiene laws and adopting a number of Soviet occupational health standards. Short courses were organized for workers and professionals. By 1953, some 20,000 workers had been trained as workplace inspectors, and by 1958, a foundation for occupational health practice was established with regulations (actually "guidelines" since they were not enforceable by law), inspectors, research insti-

---

*The latest MAC for lead, set in 1979, is 0.33 mg per cubic meter for lead fume and 0.05 mg per cubic meter for lead dust.
†Chelation for asymptomatic patients is at variance with practices in the developed countries and is apparently done to speed return to work. This practice is currently under review in China and some other developing countries.

tutes, worker and professional training programs, and worker's compensation provisions.

China is now establishing its own occupational health standards. As of 1987, more than 150 standards had been set, serving as guidelines for departments of occupational health and medicine in the epidemic prevention stations and in the factory clinics. The Ministry of Public Health has proposed that the standards become law, and enforcement procedures are being studied.

The general approach to occupational health standards is to develop a performance standard—setting a maximum allowable concentration (MAC) for each hazardous substance and requiring industry to attain the MAC by engineering controls.

The procedure for setting a standard is as follows: Data are presented to the National Standards Committee and to a standing committee of scientists, many of whom also hold government positions. Data must include a thorough review of both national and international literature, as well as original laboratory and epidemiologic research done in China. Recommendations for standards are expected to consider the feasibility of control defined in light of China's current level of technology; this means first examining what success industries in China have had in controlling a particular hazard and then setting the standard accordingly. For example, in revising the MAC for silica dust, the committee reviewed techniques and industrial hygiene data from an East China factory that retrofitted its plant and attained levels of 1 mg per cubic meter, one-half the previous MAC. Since this factory proved that such a level could be attained in China, the new silica MAC was set at 1 mg per cubic meter. Consideration is now being given to control technology that is soon to be within reach.

Engineering Controls

Engineering controls are employed in two ways: fitting newly constructed factories with modern control technology and retrofitting older plants with appropriate control technology.

An example of the former is a cotton textile mill in Shanghai's satellite town, Wu Song. This yarn preparation and spinning mill began production in 1982. Most of the production equipment was imported, but the physical facility and dust control system were designed before construction. The dust control system consisted of efficient dust capture from enclosed machines and in several filtration steps, of captured air before recirculation. The dust was carried to a central room where, along with waste cotton, it was compressed and bagged. Total dust concentrations were quite low. Noise in this plant was well controlled by use of plastic spindles, and quiet, energy-efficient motors, and machine enclosures.

The problem of retrofitting old plants with effective hazard control technology exists in China as it does elsewhere. An example of effective retrofitting is a chemical fiber factory in Shanghai. This factory, which produces viscose rayon, began operation in the 1960s, when workers and staff knew little about the hazards of carbon disulfide, a catalyst in the production process. Between 1963 and 1967, 19 workers were diagnosed as having

Fig. 36-3. Concern for control of cotton dust has led to retrofitting with local exhaust ventilation. This cotton mill in Shanghai, China, is undergoing installation of such apparatus. (Photograph by David Christiani.)

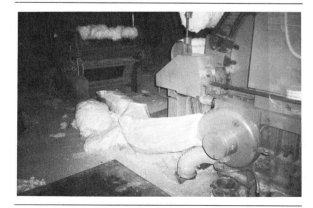

acute or chronic carbon disulfide poisoning. An aggressive control program was devised in 1972 to lower exposure by installing appropriate local and general exhaust systems and replacing existing reactors with leak-proof vessels (Fig. 36-3). The exhaust capture system recovered approximately half of the carbon disulfide vapor. Finally, independently ventilated isolation booths were built for workers after the point of carbon disulfide introduction on the production line.

Airborne carbon disulfide levels after implementation of this control measure averaged 10 mg per cubic meter (3 ppm)–8-hour TWA. With the success of this and other chemical fiber factories, the MAC in China for carbon disulfide is now 10 mg per cubic meter (3 ppm). The medical staff and workers' union at this plant have reported that there has not been a case of carbon disulfide poisoning in their plant since 1974.

Personal Protective Equipment

Realizing that personal protective equipment (PPE) never should be the principal method of occupational hazard control, Chinese occupational health professionals nevertheless are placing increasing importance on PPE devices. China is a poor country; retrofitting of old factories and modernization of whole industries will take time. Whether the rapid expansion of cooperative factories, which have even less capital than state factories, will lead to an overreliance on PPE remains to be seen. In fact, until recently, not enough attention has been paid to PPE, except in rural areas where pesticide exposure has been a serious problem and where barrier creams and foot/leg protection have been reported to reasonably control pesticide poisoning in rice fields.

Worker Education

Training workers to recognize health hazards, early symptoms of disease, and proper work and hygiene practices is done in at least three ways. First, the epidemic prevention centers prepare educational materials for the factories in their area. Second, the occupational medicine section of a

factory's medical services department provides education on specific hazards of their industry. Third, an occupational health educational magazine, *Labor Protection (Laodong Baohu)*, is published by the Ministry of Labor and Personnel is Beijing and distributed to workers by labor unions. With the decentralization of farming under the economic reforms, more individuals now apply pesticides on state and individuals farms; this increase in exposure will present a challenge to the Chinese to educate the general population effectively regarding the hazards and control of pesticide exposures.

Preventive Diagnosis

The Chinese view early detection of occupational disease, for prompt treatment or removal from further exposure, as the second line of prevention. Factory-based medical services in urban areas provide primary care as well as occupational medical services. In rural areas, with the assistance of the epidemic prevention stations, rural medical services are now integrating occupational health services into the primary care system.

Although occupational medicine services in urban industrial areas differ from those in the countryside, in both cases the role of the epidemic prevention station is the key to understanding medical and public health services. The epidemic prevention stations (literal translation, "anti-epidemic stations") are located in every Chinese province and in the three independent municipalities (Beijing, Tianjin, and Shanghai). A central station in each of these areas is connected with branch stations in every city district and rural county. In the early 1950s, some of these centers developed sections on occupational health, using the newly developed network of relationships among the centers, hospitals, neighborhood health stations, and factory health services.

The Shanghai Municipal Epidemic Prevention Center has one of the more-developed occupational health sections, collecting all case reports of occupational disease from branch stations and clinics throughout Shanghai municipality. The center has a laboratory and industrial hygiene sampling section capable of performing biological assays for workplace contaminants. Usually, the branch stations do sampling in factories that do not have their own occupational medicine and industrial hygiene services.

The occupational health section also provides worker and professional education and instructs company medical personnel on the keeping of industrial hygiene records.

Finally, the occupational health department of the epidemic prevention center conducts epidemiologic research, often in cooperation with an academic department of a school of public health or institute.

PROFESSIONAL TRAINING

There are professionals and paraprofessionals involved in occupational health care at all levels of direct service. They include college, medical school and public health school graduates; "middle medical doctors"; midwives; laboratory technicians; and rural paramedics (formerly "barefoot doctors").

Occupational health training for nurses is new in China and is likely to become an important aspect of occupational health professional training. Occupational health training for primary health care professionals is also a high priority in China. As in most countries, the occupational health training of clinicians is weak, but in recent years there has been increased emphasis on teaching preventive medicine to medical students. Within the preventive medicine curriculum for future practitioners, occupational medicine occupies an important part. In addition to didactic lectures, during internship all students do a 1-month rotation at a field center practicing occupational medicine. A two-volume primer on the clinical aspects of occupational health is used for intensive short-course training of professionals and for independent study and reference. A review text on occupational health for clinicians has also been published. Several domestic and international journals are published on occupational health and industrial hygiene.

RECENT TRENDS

Since the early 1980s, increasing scientific exchange between foreign and Chinese occupational health professionals has afforded excellent opportunities for both groups to examine and learn from each other. One result of such long-term relations is the ability to describe changes. Since 1981, advances in occupational health in China have been seen in at least five areas:

1. *Coordination of industrial hygiene and occupational health research.* As is commonly the case elsewhere, practical industrial hygienists (ventilation engineers, air-monitoring personnel, and safety specialists) come from engineering schools and technical institutes, whereas occupational health specialists (research industrial hygienists, toxicologists, and epidemiologists) are trained in medical universities with schools of public health. Practicing industrial hygienists are based in the factories and the Ministry of Labor and Personnel; practicing occupational health specialists are employed in industrial workplaces or anti-epidemic centers. Research occupational health specialists, on the other hand, work in schools of medicine or public health or in the Institute of Occupational Medicine of the Chinese Academy of Preventive Medicine. Historically, there has been little communication among these sectors. However, there appears to be increasing recognition of the value of cooperation between industry and academia. For example, Shanghai Medical University now provides training in public health education, including occupational health, to the staffs of anti-epidemic centers in rural Shanghai County and adjacent provinces. In several regions, universities and industry cooperate to do research on health effects and hazard controls for exposures to coal, carbon disulfide, silica, and noise.

2. *Emphasis on epidemiology as a tool for occupational health research.* Most Chinese research on toxic chemical substances has been either experimental animal toxicologic work, based on the Soviet model, or clinical case studies. Since the 1970s, and especially in the 1980s, the number of professionals and students receiving training in epidemiology and conducting epidemiologic research on a wide variety of occupational hazards has notably expanded. There is increasing emphasis on the role of epidemiologic data in standard settings. Integrated risk assessment of pesticide toxicity has been proposed to incorporate animal toxicology data with toxicokinetic studies on workers and farmers exposed during application. In many ways epidemiologic methods are particularly suited for use in China because the working populations tend to be large, workers do not change jobs frequently, and the relatively stable structure of work, coupled with virtually universal and systematic provision of health care services, facilitate record keeping and longitudinal surveillance. However, workplace epidemiology could be hindered if recent economic changes encourage some workers to bypass the health care system.

3. *Laboratory pretesting of toxic substances.* In vitro mutagenicity tests, such as the Ames and sister chromatid exchange tests, as well as animal toxicity tests for new compounds, are being utilized in testing of chemicals before they are used. For new chemicals, the goal is to complete a thorough toxicologic evaluation before they are introduced into production and application. Substances already in use are studied epidemiologically after appropriate review of the international toxicology literature. Some occupational health scientists hope to incorporate fairly sophisticated risk assessment techniques, including economic cost-benefit analysis, into the future evaluations.

4. *Regulation and standard setting.* In the past few years large state-owned enterprises have highlighted the difficulties inherent in enforcing occupational health and safety standards when one branch of the government is supposed to regulate the other. In some instances, the realities of the modernization drive contradict the ideals of the socialist system. Despite this conflict, there are signs of progress on the legislative and enforcement fronts. A recent law established a Ministry of Environmental Protection with jurisdiction over solid waste, air, and water pollution. New factories must receive approval from this ministry for their pollution control measures, including waste disposal, before opening. Factories already in existence are required to clean up air or water emissions, as determined by the ministry; a provision exists for levying fines against those who do not cooperate with ministry recommendations.

Chinese public health scientists express hopes that a similar and equally comprehensive law governing industrial health and safety will be enacted soon. In the meantime, a 1984 regulation permits the enforcement of health and safety recommendations by local anti-epidemic centers. It provides for fines against factories and factory managers (50,000 Yuan plus 20% of the manager's wages*) when consultation by the center is refused and workers are harmed by identifiable overexposures.

In addition to the occupational standards, the criminal code has been invoked for managers shown to be negligent. This happened in the cases of an oil rig accident during a storm in 1981 and a shoe-manufacturing process that exposed young rural workers to extremely high concentrations of benzene vapors.

5. *Onsite workplace hazard prevention.* Primary health care has been delivered at the worksite for many years—a benefit for occupational health because work-related illness and injury may be being detected more often as a result. Within the past few years, some Chinese industries have incorporated occupational health prevention services into workplace clinics to provide a more complete system of prevention and care. Engineering controls, such as local and general ventilation systems, machine guarding, or ergonomically de-

*Exchange rate in 1988, 3.71 Yuan = 1 U.S. dollar.

signed seating, are implemented in selected areas of some of the large, state-owned factories. These controls are still generally lacking in most of the smaller industries. Administrative controls such as rest breaks, safety "buddies" and job rotation are commonly used in heavy industry. Provision and instruction of PPE is also beginning in these industries, though generally PPE is underused.

Occupational health professionals in universities and in the ministries of health as well as labor and personnel recognize the importance of worker health and safety training. Labor unions cooperate with them to educate workers primarily on materials handling and personal protection. Some unions organize health and safety committees that generally work with factory managers to teach health, safety, and birth control and to monitor in-plant accident rates. Although safety posters frequently decorate the walls of both heavy and light industry, few people appear to be specifically trained to carry out effective educational programs. Worker education in most factories is often the responsibility of the trade union, plant physician, or a staff member of the anti-epidemic center; however, in some locations the school of public health trains an employee of the Ministry of Labor and Personnel to undertake educational programs in the local factories.

Despite limitations, there is evidence that on-site control measures have been effective, for example, in reducing the incidence and severity of acute pesticide poisonings, at least in the Shanghai area. In one agricultural district, from 1981 to 1983, the number of people occupationally exposed to pesticides (primarily in applications) increased by 159 percent to 326 million, and the amount applied increased by 206 percent to 10,086 tons. During the same period, however, the cumulative incidence of pesticide poisoning dropped from 7.1 percent to 0.2 percent, and the mortality rate dropped from 4.4 to 0.1 deaths per 100,000 per year. These marked improvements have been attributed to training in safe practices, increased use of full-body protection during pesticide application, and substitution of less toxic compounds for the previously widely used parathion.

BIBLIOGRAPHY

Christiani DC. Occupational health in the People's Republic of China. Am J Public Health 1984; 74:58–64.

Gu XQ, Liang YX. Standard setting for occupational health in clinics. Occupational Health Bulletin. Shanghai, People's Republic of China: World Health Organization Collaborating Center for Occupational Health, School of Public Health, Shanghai Medical University, 1985: 27–33. Vol. 1.

Quinn MM, Punnett L, Christiani DC, Levenstein CH, Wegman DH. Modernization and trends in occupational health in China, 1981-85. Am J Ind Med 1987; 12:499–506.

Wegman DH, Christiani DC, Quinn MM, Levenstein C, Levy BS, Gu XQ, He FS, Xue SZ, Lu PL, Liang YX (guest editors). Problems of modernization and occupational health in the People's Republic of China. Scand J Work Environ Health [suppl 4] 1985; 11.

Appendixes

A
Some Illustrative Toxins and Their Effects

Compiled by Howard Frumkin and Updated by James Melius

The tables on pages 572–586 list various toxins and their effects.

METALS AND METALLIC COMPOUNDS

Agent	Exposure	Route of entry	System(s) affected	Primary manifestation	Aids in diagnosis*	Remarks
Arsenic	Alloyed with lead and copper for hardness; manufacturing of pigments, glass, pharmaceuticals; by-product in copper smelting; insecticides; fungicides; rodenticides; tanning	Inhalation and ingestion of dust and fumes	Neuromuscular	Peripheral neuropathy, sensory> motor	Arsenic in urine	
			Gastrointestinal	Nausea and vomiting, diarrhea, constipation		
			Skin	Dermatitis, finger and toenail striations, skin cancer, nasal septum perforation		
			Pulmonary	Lung cancer		
Arsine	Accidental by-product of reaction of arsenic with acid; used in semiconductor industry	Inhalation of gas	Hematopoietic	Intravascular hemolysis: hemoglobinuria, jaundice, oliguria or anuria	Arsenic in urine	
Beryllium	Hardening agent in metal alloys; special use in nuclear energy production; metal refining or recovery	Inhalation of fumes or dust	Pulmonary (and other systems)	Granulomatosis and fibrosis	Beryllium in urine (acute) Beryllium in tissue (chronic) Chest x-ray Immunologic tests (such as lymphocyte transformation) may also be useful	Pulmonary changes virtually indistinguishable from sarcoid on chest x-ray

Metal	Uses / Industry	Route of Entry	System	Effects	Laboratory Aids	Comments
Cadmium	Electroplating; solder for aluminum; metal alloys, process engraving; nickel-cadmium batteries	Inhalation or ingestion of fumes or dust	Pulmonary Renal	Pulmonary edema (acute) Emphysema (chronic) Nephrosis	Urinary protein	Also a respiratory tract carcinogen
Chromium	In stainless and heat resistant steel and alloy steel; metal plating; chemical and pigment manufacturing; photography	Percutaneous absorption, inhalation, ingestion	Pulmonary Skin	Lung cancer Dermatitis, skin ulcers, nasal septum perforation	Urinary chromate (questionable value)	
Lead	Storage batteries; manufacturing of paint, enamel, ink, glass, rubber, ceramics, chemical industry	Ingestion of dust, inhalation of dust or fumes	Hematologic Renal Gastrointestinal Neuromuscular CNS Reproductive	Anemia Nephropathy Abdominal pain ("colic") Palsy ("wrist drop") Encephalopathy, behavioral abnormalities Spontaneous abortions (?)	Blood lead Urinary ALA Zinc protoporphyrin (ZPP); free erythrocyte protoporphyrin (FEP)	Lead toxicity, unlike that of mercury, is believed to be reversible, with the exception of late renal and some CNS effects.

*Occupational and medical histories are, in most instances, the most important aids in diagnosis.

573

Agent	Exposure	Route of entry	System(s) affected	Primary manifestation	Aids in diagnosis	Remarks
Mercury Elemental	Electronic equipment; paint; metal and textile production; catalyst in chemical manufacturing; pharmaceutical production	Inhalation of vapor; slight percutaneous absorption	Pulmonary CNS	Acute pneumonitis Neuropsychiatric changes (erethism); tremor	Urinary mercury	Mercury illustrates several principles. The chemical form has profound effect on its toxicology, as is case for many metals. Effects of mercury highly variable. Though inorganic mercury poisoning is primarily renal, elemental and organic mercury poisoning are primarily neurologic. These responses are difficult to quantify, so dose-response data are generally unavailable. Classic tetrad of gingivitis, sialorrhea, irritability, and tremor is associated with
Inorganic		Some inhalation and GI and percutaneous absorption	Pulmonary Renal CNS	Acute pneumonitis Proteinuria Variable	Urinary mercury	
Organic	Agricultural and industrial poisons	Efficient GI absorption, percutaneous absorption, and inhalation	Skin CNS	Dermatitis Sensorimotor changes, visual field constriction, tremor	Blood and urine mercury, but ? sensitivity	

						Comments
						both elemental and inorganic mercury poisoning; the four signs not generally seen together. Many effects of mercury toxicity, especially those in CNS, are irreversible.
Nickel	Corrosion-resistant alloys; electroplating; catalyst production; nickel-cadmium batteries	Inhalation of dust or fumes	Skin Pulmonary	Sensitization dermatitis ("nickel itch") Lung and paranasal sinus cancer		
Zinc oxide*	Welding by-product; rubber manufacturing	Inhalation of dust or fumes that are freshly generated		"Metal fume fever," (fever, chills, and other symptoms)	Urinary zinc (useful as an indicator of exposure, not for acute diagnosis)	A self-limiting syndrome of 24–48 hours, with apparently no sequelae
HYDROCARBONS Benzene	Manufacturing of organic chemicals, detergents, pesticides, solvents, paint removers; used as a solvent	Inhalation of vapor; slight percutaneous absorption	CNS Hematopoietic Skin	Acute CNS depression Leukemia, aplastic anemia Dermatitis	Urinary phenol	Note that benzene, as with toluene and other solvents, can be monitored via its principal metabolite.

*Zinc oxide is a prototype of agents that cause metal fume fever. See box in Chap. 19 for more complete list.

Agent	Exposure	Route of entry	System(s) affected	Primary manifestation	Aids in diagnosis	Remarks
Toluene	Organic chemical manufacturing; solvent; fuel component	Inhalation of vapor, percutaneous absorption of liquid	CNS Skin	Acute CNS depression Chronic CNS problems, such as memory loss (see Chap. 25) Irritation, dermatitis	Urinary hippuric acid	
Xylene	A wide variety of uses as a solvent; an ingredient of paints, lacquers, varnishes, inks, dyes, adhesives, cements; an intermediate in chemical manufacturing	Inhalation of vapor; slight percutaneous absorption of liquid	Pulmonary Eyes, nose, throat CNS	Irritation, pneumonitis, acute pulmonary edema (at high doses) Irritation Acute CNS depression	Methylhippuric acid in urine, xylene in expired air, xylene in blood	
Ketones Acetone Methyl ethyl ketone (MEK) Methyl n-propyl ketone (MPK) Methyl n-butyl ketone (MBK) Methyl isobutyl ketone (MIBK)	A wide variety of uses as solvents and intermediates in chemical manufacturing	Inhalation of vapor, percutaneous absorption of liquid	CNS PNS Skin	Acute CNS depression MBK has been linked with peripheral neuropathy Dermatitis	Acetone in blood, urine, expired air (used as an index for exposure, not for diagnosis)	The ketone family demonstrates how a pattern of toxic responses (that is, CNS narcosis) may feature exceptions (that is, MBK peripheral neuropathy).

	Uses/Sources	Route	Organ System	Effects	Laboratory Test	Comments
Formaldehyde	Widely used as a germicide and a disinfectant in embalming and histopathology, for example, and in the manufacture of textiles, resins, and other products	Inhalation	Skin Eye Pulmonary	Irritant and contact dermatitis Eye irritation Respiratory tract irritation, asthma	Patch testing may be helpful for dermatitis.	Recent animal tests have shown it to be a respiratory carcinogen. Confirmatory epidemiologic studies are in progress.
Trichloroethylene (TCE)	Solvent in metal degreasing, dry cleaning, food extraction; ingredient of paints, adhesives, varnishes, inks	Inhalation, percutaneous absorption	Nervous Skin Cardiovascular	Acute CNS depression Peripheral and cranial neuropathy Irritation, dermatitis Arrhythmias	Breath analysis for TCE	TCE is involved in an important pharmacologic interaction, Within hours of ingesting alcoholic beverages, TCE workers experience flushing of the face, neck, shoulders, and back. Alcohol may also potentiate the CNS effects of TCE. The probable mechanism is competition for metabolic enzymes.

Agent	Exposure	Route of entry	System(s) affected	Primary manifestation	Aids in diagnosis	Remarks
Carbon tetrachloride	Solvent for oils, fats, lacquers, resins, varnishes, other materials; used as a degreasing and cleaning agent	Inhalation of vapor	Hepatic Renal CNS Skin	Toxic hepatitis Oliguria or anuria Acute CNS depression Dermatitis	Expired air and blood levels	Carbon tetrachloride is the prototype for a wide variety of solvents that cause hepatic and renal damage. This solvent, like trichloroethylene, acts synergistically with ethanol.
Carbon disulfide	Solvent for lipids, sulfur, halogens, rubber, phosphorus, oils, waxes, and resins; manufacturing of organic chemicals, paints, fuels, explosives, viscose rayon	Inhalation of vapor, percutaneous absorption of liquid or vapor	Nervous Renal Cardiovascular Skin Reproductive	Parkinsonism, psychosis, suicide Peripheral neuropathies Chronic nephritic and nephrotic syndromes Acceleration or worsening of atherosclerosis; hypertension Irritation; dermatitis Menorrhagia and metorrhagia	Iodine-azide reaction with urine (nonspecific since other bivalent sulfur compounds give a positive test); CS_2 in expired air, blood, and urine	A solvent with unusual multisystem effects, especially noted for its cardiovascular, renal, and nervous system actions.
Stoddard solvent	Degreasing, paint thinning	Inhalation of vapor, percutaneous absorption of liquid	Skin CNS	Dryness and scaling from defatting; dermatitis Dizziness, coma, collapse (at high levels)	A mixture of primarily aliphatic hydrocarbons, with some benzene derivatives and naphthenes.	

Substance	Uses/Exposure	Route	Target Organs	Effects	Comments
Ethylene glycol ethers Ethylene glycol monoethyl ether (cellosolve) Ethylene glycol monoethyl ether acetate (cellosolve acetate) Methyl- and butyl-substituted compounds such as ethylene glycol monomethyl ether (methyl cellosolve)	The ethers are used as solvents for resins, paints, lacquers, varnishes, gum, perfume, dyes, and inks; the acetate derivatives are widely used as solvents and ingredients of lacquers, enamels, and adhesives. Exposure occurs in dry cleaning, plastic, ink, and lacquer manufacturing, and textile dying, among other processes.	Inhalation of vapor, percutaneous absorption of liquid	Reproductive, CNS, renal, liver Hematopoietic CNS	Pancytopenia Fatigue, lethargy, nausea, headaches, anorexia, tremor, stupor (due to encephalopathy)	Ethylene glycol ethers, as a class of chemicals, have been shown in animals to have adverse reproductive effects, including reduced sperm count and spontaneous abortion, as well as CNS, renal, and liver effects. Effects primarily associated with ethylene glycol monomethyl ether (methyl cellosolve)
Ethylene oxide	Used in the sterilization of medical equipment, in the fumigation of spices and other foodstuffs, and as a chemical intermediate	Inhalation	Skin Eye Respiratory tract Nervous system	Dermatitis and frostbite Severe irritation; possibly cataracts with prolonged exposure Irritation Peripheral neuropathy	Recent animal tests have shown it to be carcinogenic and to cause reproductive abnormalities. Epidemiologic studies indicate that it may cause leukemia in exposed workers.

Agent	Exposure	Route of entry	System(s) affected	Primary manifestation	Aids in diagnosis	Remarks
Dioxane	Used as a solvent for a variety of materials, including cellulose acetate, dyes, fats, greases, resins, polyvinyl polymers, varnishes, and waxes	Inhalation of vapor, percutaneous absorption of liquid	CNS	Drowsiness, dizziness, anorexia, headaches, nausea, vomiting, coma		Dioxane has caused a variety of neoplasms in animals. Dioxane should not be confused with "dioxin" (2,3,7,8-trichlorodibenzo-*p*-dioxin), a contaminant of the chlorphenoxy herbicide 2,4,5-T (2,4,5-trichlorophenoxyacetic acid). Dioxin has several adverse health effects, including neuropathy, birth defects, chemical hepatitis, and possibly cancer.
			Renal	Nephritis		
			Liver	Chemical hepatitis		

Substance	Uses/Source	Route of Entry	Organs Affected	Effects	Tests	Comments
Polychlorinated biphenyls (PCBs)	Formerly used as a dielectric fluid in electrical equipment and as a fire retardant coating on tiles and other products. New uses were banned in 1976, but much of the electrical equipment currently used still contains PCBs	Inhalation, ingestion, skin absorption	Skin Eye Liver	Chloracne Irritation Toxic hepatitis	Serum PCB levels for chronic exposure	Animal studies have demonstrated that PCBs are carcinogenic. Epidemiologic studies of exposed workers are inconclusive.

IRRITANT GASES

Note: The less water-soluble the gas, the deeper and more delayed its irritant effect (see Chaps. 14 and 21).

Substance	Uses/Source	Route of Entry	Organs Affected	Effects	Tests	Comments
Ammonia	Refrigeration; petroleum refining; manufacturing of nitrogen-containing chemicals, synthetic fibers, dyes, and optics	Inhalation of gas	Upper respiratory tract	Upper respiratory irritation		Also irritant of eyes and moist skin
Hydrochloric acid	Chemical manufacturing; electroplating; tanning; metal pickling; petroleum extraction; rubber, photographic, and textile industries	Inhalation of gas or mist	Upper respiratory tract	Upper respiratory irritation		Strong irritant of eyes, mucous membranes, and skin

Agent	Exposure	Route of entry	System(s) affected	Primary manifestation	Aids in diagnosis	Remarks
Hydrofluoric acid	Chemical and plastic manufacturing; catalyst in petroleum refining; aqueous solution for frosting, etching, and polishing glass	Inhalation of gas or mist	Upper respiratory tract	Upper respiratory irritation		In solution, causes severe and painful burns of skin and can be fatal
Sulfur dioxide	Manufacturing of sulfur-containing chemicals; food and textile bleach; tanning; metal casting	Inhalation of gas, direct contact of gas or liquid phase on skin or mucosa	Middle respiratory tract	Bronchospasm (pulmonary edema or chemical pneumonitis in high dose)	Chest x-ray, pulmonary function tests*	Strong irritant of eyes, mucous membranes, and skin
Chlorine	Paper and textile bleaching; water disinfection; chemical manufacturing; metal fluxing; detinning and dezincing iron	Inhalation of gas	Middle respiratory tract	Tracheobronchitis, pulmonary edema, pneumonitis	Chest x-ray, pulmonary function tests	Chlorine combines with body moisture to form acids, which irritate tissues from nose to alveoli.
Fluorine	Uranium processing; manufacturing of fluorine-containing chemicals; oxidizer in rocket fuel systems	Inhalation of gas	Middle respiratory tract	Laryngeal spasm, bronchospasm, pulmonary edema	Chest x-ray, pulmonary function tests	Potent irritant of eyes, mucous membranes, and skin

	Sources/Uses	Route	Effects	Diagnostic Tests	Comments
Ozone	Inert gas-shielded arc welding; food, water, and air purification; food and textile bleaching; emitted around high-voltage electrical equipment	Inhalation of gas	Lower respiratory tract	Delayed pulmonary edema (generally 6–8 hours following exposure)	Chest x-ray, pulmonary function tests	Ozone has a free radical structure and can produce experimental chromosome aberrations; it may thus have carcinogenic potential.
Nitrogen oxides	Manufacturing of acids, nitrogen-containing chemicals, explosives, and more; byproduct of many industrial processes	Inhalation of gas	Lower respiratory tract	Pulmonary irritation, bronchiolitis fibrosa obliterans ("silo filler's disease"), mixed obstructive-restrictive changes	Chest x-ray, pulmonary function tests	
Phosgene	Manufacturing and burning of isocyanates, and manufacturing of dyes and other organic chemicals; in metallurgy for ore separation; burning or heat source near trichloroethylene	Inhalation of gas	Lower respiratory tract	Delayed pulmonary edema (delay seldom longer than 12 hours)	Chest x-ray, pulmonary function tests	

*PFTs are useful aids in diagnosis of irritant effects if the patient is subacutely or chronically ill.

583

Agent	Exposure	Route of entry	System(s) affected	Primary manifestation	Aids in diagnosis	Remarks
Isocyanates TDI (toluene diisocyanate) MDI (methylene di-phenyldiiso-cyanate) Hexamethylene diisocyanate and others	Polyurethane manufacture; resin-binding systems in foundries; coat-ing materials for wires; used in certain types of paint	Inhalation of vapor	Predomi-nantly lower re-spiratory tract	Asthmatic reaction and accelerated loss of pulmo-nary function	Chest x-ray, pulmonary function tests	Isocyanates are both respiratory tract "sensitiz-ers" and irri-tants in the conventional sense (see Chap. 21).

ASPHYXIANT GASES

Agent	Exposure	Route of entry	System(s) affected	Primary manifestation	Aids in diagnosis	Remarks
Simple as-phyxiants: nitrogen, hy-drogen, meth-ane, and others	Enclosed spaces in a variety of in-dustrial settings	Inhalation of gas	CNS	Anoxia	O_2 in environ-ment	No specific toxic effect; act by displacing O_2

Chemical asphyxiants

Agent	Exposure	Route of entry	System(s) affected	Primary manifestation	Aids in diagnosis	Remarks
Carbon monoxide	Incomplete com-bustion in foun-dries, coke ovens, refiner-ies, furnaces, and more	Inhalation of gas	Blood (Hemo-globin)	Headache, dizzi-ness, double vi-sion	Carboxy-hemoglobin	
Hydrogen sulfide	Used in manufac-turing of sulfur-containing chemicals; produced in pe-troleum pro-duction; by-product of petroleum product use; decay of or-ganic matter	Inhalation of gas	CNS / Pulmonary	Respiratory center paralysis, hypo-ventilation Respiratory tract ir-ritation	PaO_2	

Cyanides	Metallurgy, electroplating	Inhalation of vapor, percutaneous absorption, ingestion	Cellular metabolic enzymes (especially cytochrome oxidase)	Enzyme inhibition with metabolic asphyxia and death	SCN⁻ in urine	
PESTICIDES Organophosphates: malathion, parathion, and others		Inhalation, ingestion, percutaneous absorption	Neuromuscular	Cholinesterase inhibition, cholinergic symptoms: nausea and vomiting, salivation, diarrhea, headache, sweating, meiosis, muscle fasciculations, seizures, unconsciousness, death	Refractoriness to atropine; plasma or red cell cholinesterase	As with many acute toxins, rapid treatment of organophosphate toxicity is imperative. Thus, diagnosis is often made based on history and a high index of suspicion rather than on biochemical tests. Treatment is atropine to block cholinergic effects and 2-PAM (2-pyridine-alsoxine methiodide) to reactivate cholinesterase.
Carbamates: carbaryl (Sevin) and others		Inhalation, ingestion, percutaneous absorption	Neuromuscular	Same as organophosphates	Plasma cholinesterase; urinary 1-naphthol (index of exposure)	Treatment of carbamate poisoning is the same as that of organophosphate poisoning except that 2-PAM is contraindicated.

Agent	Exposure	Route of entry	System(s) affected	Primary manifestation	Aids in diagnosis	Remarks
Chlorinated hydrocarbons: chlordane, DDT, heptachlor, chlordecone (Kepone), aldrin, dieldrin, uridine		Ingestion, inhalation, percutaneous absorption	CNS	Stimulation or depression	Urinary organic chlorine, or *p*-chlorophenyl acetic acid	The chlorinated hydrocarbons may accumulate in body lipid stores in large amounts.
Bipyridyls: paraquat, diquat		Inhalation, ingestion, percutaneous absorption	Pulmonary	Rapid massive fibrosis, only following paraquat ingestion		An interesting toxin in that the major toxicity, pulmonary fibrosis, apparently occurs only after ingestion

B
Training and Career Opportunities

Howard Frumkin, Howard Hu, and Patricia Hyland Travers

EDUCATION AND TRAINING

Few medical schools and training programs teach occupational health in anything more than a cursory fashion. The same is true for most nursing schools and other clinically oriented health professional schools in the United States.

In the 1970s, however, training opportunities began to expand for both students and professionals. This trend, with support from government, labor, and industry, reflected a growing recognition of the importance of occupational health. Although federal budget cuts in the 1980s have dampened this trend, many opportunities remain.

Some medical and nursing schools have now developed formal courses, and others include occupational health in their basic science and clinical curricula, often as the result of student efforts. Many students find it easier to incorporate occupational health into existing courses, rather than to add extra courses to already crowded schedules. Advice and examples of curricular materials may be found in the *Directory of Educational Resources and Training Opportunities in Occupational Health,* a publication of the Association of Teachers of Preventive Medicine (ATPM) Occupational Health Committee that is periodically updated (for a copy, contact Association of Teachers of Preventive Medicine, 1030 15th Street, NW, Washington DC 20005 telephone 202-682-1698).

Students can also participate in full-time structured programs that include occupational health field work. In such programs students learn the fundamentals of recognizing occupational disease, occupational history taking, and work process analysis. They visit various worksites and conduct health evaluations, sometimes designing and implementing specific projects. Several universities offer such field programs; these are described in the ATPM directory.

Students can also participate in a wide variety of extracurricular activities, many of which are acceptable for elective credit by medical schools. Examples include work with public interest organizations, labor unions, companies, and academic research groups.

Those who seek training at the postgraduate level will find a variety of opportunities available. A good source for information on current training programs is the Division of Training at NIOSH (513-533-8225). The most complete programs are located at the NIOSH Educational Resource Centers (ERCs). As of 1988, there were 14 ERCs in the United States aiming to provide full- and part-time academic career training, cross-training of occupational health and safety practitioners, mid-career training in the field of occupational safety and health, and access to relevant courses for students pursuing various degrees. The ERCs are located in:

4. Illinois (University of Illinois)

5. Maryland (Johns Hopkins School of Hygiene and Public Health)

6. Massachusetts (Harvard School of Public Health; Boston University; University of Massachusetts Medical School)

7. Michigan (University of Michigan)

8. Minnesota (University of Minnesota; St. Paul-Ramsey Medical Center)

9. New York/New Jersey (Mt. Sinai School of Medicine; New York University; Hunter College; City College of New York; Robert Wood Johnson Medical School)

10. North Carolina (University of North Carolina; North Carolina State University; Duke University)

11. Ohio (University of Cincinnati)

12. Texas (University of Texas; Texas A&M University)

13. Utah (University of Utah; Utah State University)

14. Washington (University of Washington)

ERCs have developed core areas of instruction for graduate and postgraduate students and continuing education programs for professionals. Areas of study include epidemiology and biostatistics, toxicology, industrial hygiene, safety and ergonomics, policy issues, administration, and clinical occupational medicine. Many ERCs are located at schools of public health, where they draw on the strength of departments in related disciplines. Emphasis is placed on training occupational physicians, industrial hygienists, occupational health nurses, and other professionals to work as a team in preventing occupational disease and accidents.

The schools of public health that house ERCs, and many others as well, offer masters and doctoral programs that focus on occupational health. Some medical students earn master of public health (M.P.H.) or equivalent degrees during medical school elective time or during time off from medical school. Interested professionals may enroll in public health programs after completing other professional study; some have done so after many years of practice.

Both occupational health specialists and nonspecialists can seek continuing education credits in occupational health by attending appropriate seminars and short courses. These are frequently offered by ERCs. Another source is the American Occupational Medical Association, through both its national office and its regional affiliates. Announcements appear in its *Journal of Occupational Medicine* and other journals in the field.

Finally, physicians—and a few nonphysicians—who seek full-time on-the-job training may join a 2-year program administered by NIOSH in conjunction with the Epidemic Intelligence Service (EIS) of the Centers for Disease Control (CDC). Members of this program may work with the Division of Surveillance, Hazard Evaluations, and Field Studies in Cincinnati, the Appalachian Laboratory for Occupational Safety and Health in Morgantown, West Virginia, or the CDC headquarters in Atlanta, learning occupational disease epidemiology through rigorous field studies, data analyses, and seminars. Information may be obtained from NIOSH, Centers for Disease Control, Atlanta, GA 30333.

CAREER OPPORTUNITIES

The following is an overview of career opportunities available to professionals in occupational health with personal examples of career pathways.

Physicians Employed by Companies

Industry has traditionally provided the lion's share of employment in occupational medicine. Those employed by companies have responsibilities in three general areas: prevention and early detection of occupational disease and injury; diagnosis and treatment of occupational disease and injury (emphasizing return of workers to their jobs); and diagnosis and treatment of nonoccupational disease or injury in emergency situations or when community resources are unavailable (see Chap. 34).

The American Occupational Medical Association (AOMA) has listed some specific duties of the company physician in meeting these responsibilities:

1. Preplacement examinations
2. Periodic health examinations and screening surveys
3. Immunization of employees
4. Provision of consultative services to other company units
5. Inspection of workplace environmental conditions
6. Close cooperation with community physicians
7. Cooperation with public health authorities and community health agencies
8. Education of employees
9. Assistance in epidemiologic surveillance of populations at risk
10. Medical surveillance related to the use of personal protective equipment
11. Maintenance of confidential occupational medical records
12. Assistance in interpretation and development of government regulations
13. Assistance in controlling illness-related job absenteeism
14. Determination of consumer health hazards from company products
15. Employee training in first-aid procedures
16. Employee counseling and education in health matters
17. Review of food handling and sanitary practices in in-plant feeding facilities
18. Consultation with management regarding employees' symptoms or physical limitations not under treatment by the medical department
19. Research in pertinent areas

Physicians who work at the upper management level are more involved in questions of policy, whereas those at the plant level are more involved in clinical duties. David C. Logan, M.D., M.P.H.,

BOARD CERTIFICATION
IN OCCUPATIONAL HEALTH
FOR PROFESSIONALS

Physicians may pursue board certification in occupational medicine. Eligibility is based on academic training, clinical training, and practical experience. A current list of approved academic and field-training programs and criteria for board certification may be obtained from the American Board of Preventive Medicine (contact Stanley R. Mohler, M.D., Secretary-Treasurer, Department of Community Medicine, Wright State University School of Medicine, P.O. Box 927, Dayton, OH 45401).

Certification for industrial hygienists is based on academic preparation, experience, and written examinations. Further information, including a list of suitable training programs, may be obtained from the American Board of Industrial Hygiene, 4600 West Saginaw, Suite 101, Lansing MI 48917 (telephone: 517-321-2638).

Certification for industrial safety professionals is also based on academic preparation, experience, and written examinations. Further information, including a list of training programs, may be obtained from the Board of Certified Safety Professionals, 208 Burwash Avenue, Savoy IL 61874 (telephone: 217-359-9263).

The designation of Occupational Health and Safety Technologist is a new joint certification offered by the American Board of Industrial Hygiene and the Board of Certified Safety Professionals (BCSP). Further information may be obtained from the BCSP.

Board certification is available for occupational health nurses and requires passing a written examination, five years of occupational health nursing practice, letters of reference, and 75 contact hours of continuing education. Information on board certification can be obtained by contacting the American Board of Occupational Health Nursing, Inc., 2210 Wilshire Boulevard, Suite 771, Santa Monica, CA 90403; (telephone: 213-450-4468).

Clinical Toxicologist for the Mobil Oil Corporation, writes:

I provide guidance and technical assistance to the company on issues pertaining to the health and safety of our processes and products. One of my responsibilities is to review the company's existing medical surveillance programs in accord with current medical knowledge. In addition, I am called upon to develop medical department procedures to ensure compliance with company standards for workplace and product safety and the medical requirements of OSHA and other federal and state regulations. Another important responsibility is to respond to customer and employee concerns regarding the health and safety of our operations. Recent inquiries have included questions on the safety of video display terminals and the use of contact lenses in our various work environments.

My office works very closely with environmental affairs, toxicology, industrial hygiene, and product safety professionals in performing risk assessments, setting internal exposure standards, planning our toxicology testing programs, providing recommendations concerning the medical information to be included on labels and material safety data sheets, and evaluating adverse effect allegations received by the company. Recent areas of review have included the potential toxicity of ceramic fiber insulation and the thermal degradation products of plastics commonly referred to as "blue haze." I participate as a member of the company's Product Safety Emergency Response Team and in disaster preparedness activities of the company.

My group has also had a role in developing a process for evaluating the reproductive risks of our operations, which includes a computerized reproductive health citations data base. Over the past 3 years, we have coordinated reviews at various company locations to evaluate potential reproductive health risks that exposures at these facilities might pose to our male and female employees.

Providing assistance to attorneys in our Office of General Counsel has become another important responsibility. Along with other physicians in our department, I am frequently called upon to review medical records related to lawsuits against the company and to provide recommendations and opinions regarding the medical complaints involved. Neurobehavioral effects related to solvents are currently a prominent area of activity.

As a member of the Corporate Medical Director's Office, I also contribute to policy development, program planning and the administration of the Medical Department. For example, my office has helped in developing the Medical Department role in the company's Alcohol and Drug Control Program, which has become a model for other companies. One important activity in this area has been to review the laboratory-testing methods used in our program to ensure the accuracy and reliability of alcohol and drug screening test results. We have also developed a medical department information paper, entitled "Control of Drug Abuse in the Workplace."

Finally, I represent the company in outside professional organizations and teaching activities. I am a member of the AOMA Committee on Occupational and Clinical Toxicology and a member of the American Petroleum Institute (API) Neurobehavioral Task Force. I have participated on a federal advisory panel to address reproductive health hazards in the workplace and have lectured in the AOMA Basic Curriculum in Occupational Medicine.

Company physicians may face conflicts of interest arising from their dual responsibilities to both company interests and worker health (see Chap. 13).

Physicians Employed by Labor Unions

Physicians employed by labor unions work closely with other members of their unions' health and safety departments. Their job responsibilities are generally less well defined and more flexible than those of company physicians and nurses. Responsibilities may include worker education, health hazard evaluation, participation in contract negotiations, research, and maintenance of disease registries.

Health providers employed by labor unions may function as worker advocates. This perspective is described by one union physician, Dr. Michael Silverstein of the United Auto Workers union (UAW), as follows:

The basic thrust of the union's health and safety program is to identify hazardous plant conditions and eliminate them before damage has been done to workers' health. In situations of uncertainty, the benefit of the doubt goes to the worker. In other words, it is assumed that an exposure or condition is hazardous until and unless we can demonstrate otherwise.

Dr. Silverstein described his work as follows:

I spend my time doing basically four types of things, as do the other members of the health and safety department. First, we respond to requests for service and assistance from local unions. This may involve inspecting a plant to identify hazards and to recommend protective measures. It may involve design of a medical screening program, review of industrial hygiene or toxicologic data, interviews with local union members about signs and symptoms, or liaison work with OSHA and NIOSH. We are in the process of developing an in-house epidemiologic program so that we can respond more systematically and promptly to local unions who feel their members may be suffering excessive job-related mortality.

Second, we have an active educational program within the union. This involves a variety of classes and training programs as well as the development of educational materials on health and safety issues.

Third, the health and safety staff takes an active role in collective bargaining concerning specific issues in which we have particular expertise. Most union contracts include guarantees to members of certain rights to health and safety protection of various types.

Fourth, our staff plays a role in defining and implementing the union's public posture and activity in the area of health and safety. This includes work on health and safety legislation, OSHA standard setting, and workers' compensation reform.

Within this framework, I have found myself able to apply a substantial portion of my medical skills and resources to a diversified set of problems in a manner that has been professionally challenging and politically satisfying. I fall among those who approach occupational medicine as a public health discipline rather than an internal medicine specialty. I would rather spend time with an industrial hygienist or ventilation engineer working out protective strategies than with a pathologist identifying end-stage disease. When I consult with oncologists, my inclination is to discuss primary prevention and early detection rather than treatment regimens.

(See also Dr. Silverstein's Chap. 35.)

Federal Government Physicians

Physicians work with NIOSH and have worked with OSHA, assisting in the functions of these two agencies (see Chaps. 4 and 10). Since NIOSH is primarily a research agency, its medical staff is devoted primarily to research. This research may take the form of health hazard evaluations or field investigations under the Division of Surveillance, Hazard Evaluations and Field Studies, or it may involve basic scientific or epidemiologic investigation at one of the NIOSH research facilities.

Dr. Paul Seligman has worked in that division, in both the Hazard Evaluation Program and in the Surveillance Branch. He writes:

During my time at Hazard Evaluation I visited worksites with the following problems: (1) two outbreaks of phytophotodermatitis in grocery workers; (2) carpal tunnel syndrome and other cumulative trauma disorders (CTD) of the wrist in machine operators in the bookbinding and wire die industries and among police transcribers; (3) breast cancer and spontaneous abortion clusters among women exposed to radiofrequency heat sealers in the manufacture of loose-leaf binders; (4) lead and arsenic exposures in a copper smelter; (5) health effects among fire fighters exposed to polychlorinated biphenyls (PCBs) and PCB pyrolysis products during a dumpsite fire; (6) skin sensitization and restrictive lung disease in workers exposed to hard metals in the manufacture of hardened blade tips; (7) control of ethylene oxide (EtO) exposures in hospitals; (8) acute neuropathy and cataracts in EtO-exposed workers in the manufacture of hospital supplies; (9) an assessment of carboxyhemoglobin levels in workers exposed to methylene chloride in the electronics industry; (10) health effects from exposure to chlordane following a misapplication; and (11) eye irritation associated with use of soft contact lenses among university biochemists.

Other than field investigations, I responded to numerous telephone calls and letters from workers and/or their families requesting information and advice concerning workplace exposures and their potential health effects. On occasion, I answered requests for information from the press, other governmental agencies, or Congress.

I then moved to the Surveillance Branch, where I study workers' compensation claims in Ohio, as a source for describing the epidemiologic characteristics of occupational lead poisoning, skin disease, cumulative trauma disorders, and work-related violent crime injuries. Work in surveillance has offered me the opportunity to learn how to use data sets to create surveillance systems for the identification and follow-back of companies with lead exposure, skin disease, or cumulative trauma problems, and to generate hypotheses relating disease outcomes with industries at high risk. This work is very satisfying in that it allows me to work in the area where policy planning, epidemiology, and health overlap.

Dr. Seligman counts as the advantages of his job: the NIOSH mission to promote worker safety and health, the access to workplaces for study purposes, the variety of problems he confronts, the freedom and responsibility it entails, the opportunity for interdisciplinary collaboration, and the opportunity to publish. He notes that work at NIOSH offers little opportunity for clinical practice.

Other federal agencies that employ physicians may also become involved in occupational health issues. For example, a medical epidemiologist at the National Cancer Institute might study mortality patterns among certain occupational groups, or a staff physician at the Office of Technology Assessment of the U.S. Congress might review the health effects of certain occupational exposures.

State and Provincial Government Physicians

Some states and provinces that are active in occupational health and safety regulation employ physicians. In some cases, physicians work in environmental health or cancer prevention programs and naturally become involved with issues of occupational safety and health.

Dr. Rose Goldman, one of two occupational hygiene physicians for Massachusetts, describes her work as follows:

The Division of Occupational Hygiene inspects workplaces and assists employers and employees in correcting health hazards and improving working conditions. It also publishes recommended exposure limits and safe practice bulletins. I participate in worksite health hazard evaluations, conduct small-scale epidemiologic projects, perform educational activities, answer telephone inquiries, and supervise a full-time occupational hygiene nurse who surveys health programs in industrial plants.

For workplace evaluations, I work with an industrial hygienist to assess health hazards and evaluate workers. We usually make recommendations to eliminate or diminish the hazard; sometimes we recommend a program of ongoing medical surveillance. For example, in evaluating workers at a sewage treatment plant with possible lead and chromate exposure, I administered brief questionnaires, performed physical examinations, and obtained blood analyses for chromium and lead. We were able to determine that the current control measures usually limited exposure and protected workers, but that in a few parts of the work process additional control measures were warranted.

The opportunity for plant access provides the potential to perform epidemiologic surveys, such as a recent survey of automobile radiator repair shops and workers for lead poisoning. Previous state occupational hygiene physicians in Massachusetts have performed important studies of the health effects of beryllium, cadmium, toluene diisocyanate (TDI), lead, and talc, which have often led to important preventive measures.

I also educate employers and employees daily on hazardous exposures and control measures, update and write the medical aspects of safe practice guides and material safety data sheets, supervise medical residents and industrial hygiene students learning about worksite evaluations, and participate in preparing state regulations and proposed statutes. I am also a member of a state interagency task force that is developing methods for surveillance and intervention of occupational health problems.

Although a strong national program is integral to controlling workplace hazards, state agencies perform additional important functions: they provide services more readily to local small plants not covered by OSHA, respond quickly to emergencies, provide enforcement on problems not covered by OSHA, help employers comply with OSHA standards, and respond to complaints.

Occupational Medicine in the Community Setting

A growing number of opportunities to practice occupational medicine can be found in clinical settings in the community. In some cases occupational medical clinics exist as independent contractors that sell to client companies such services as preplacement and return-to-work evaluations, drug screening, and trauma care. Alternatively, some clinical occupational medicine units exist as parts of hospital staffs, usually within departments of medicine or family practice. Dr. John Davis, Chief of Occupational Health at Norwood Hospital in Norwood, Massachusetts, reports that both community hospitals and local industries have an interest in such arrangements, the former, in part, to increase revenues and the latter to cope with regulatory demands and workers' compensation costs. Dr. Davis indicates that a wide range of options may be available in the community hospital setting, including (1) extension of emergency services that triage the injured worker, (2) extension of employee health services, (3) development of free-standing occupational health departments, and (4) development of satellite sites.

Dr. Davis reports that his clinical practice is a combination of general internal medicine and office orthopedics. He performs "complex injury management," evaluates patients for insurance companies, manages an active executive health and wellness program, and establishes medical surveillance programs on a consultative basis, subcontracting with industrial hygiene and clinical laboratory facilities when appropriate. He notes that one potential controversy is that some community physicians might feel threatened by an occupational medicine service if they have been previously performing such duties on an informal basis.

Nurses in Occupational Health

Occupational health nursing has undergone a metamorphosis since its beginnings in the late 1800s, when nurses were employed by industries to care for ailing workers and their families. Attention in the field of occupational health nursing has shifted from a narrow focus on communicable disease, maternal and child health issues, and emergency treatment of injured workers to a much broader focus today. Presently, the occupational health nurse (OHN) applies public health principles to meet the needs of workers in an ever-changing work environment. The focus of the OHN has thus expanded to include integration of many areas, including epidemiology, industrial hygiene, environmental health, toxicology, safety, management, health education, early disease detection, disease prevention, health promotion, and health and environmental surveillance.

The American Association of Occupational Health Nurses (AAOHN) defines occupational health nursing as:

. . . the application of nursing principles in conserving the health of workers in all occupations. It emphasizes prevention, recognition, and treatment of illnesses and injuries and requires special skills and knowledge in the fields of health education and counseling, environmental health, and human relations.

Most OHNs work for company medical departments. The OHN, whether employed as a single health care provider at a small plant or as a member of a multidisciplinary health unit, must balance ethical and clinical responsibilities to employees with ethical and administrative responsibilities to management. This balance requires the OHN to assist management in providing a safe and healthful work environment through disease prevention and health promotion activities. Some of the responsibilities include the daily operation of a comprehensive health care program; development of treatment and surveillance protocols; keeping informed about health and safety legislation; maintenance of a toxic substance list; identification of high-risk areas; clinical intervention, including delivery of health care and counseling services; record keeping; liaison with managers, workers, and health and safety colleagues; and implementation of health-related programs on a primary, secondary, and tertiary level. (See P. Travers. *A Comprehensive Guide for Establishing an Occupational Health Service.* New York: AAOHN, 1987. Available from AAOHN, 50 Lenox Pointe, Atlanta, GA 30324; 1-800-241-8014.)

Judy H. Manchester, R.N., manager of nursing and health services for the GTE Products Corporation, writes:

I am responsible for overseeing nursing functions and health services for approximately 150 locations throughout the United States, Canada, Puerto Rico, Haiti, and Central America. My responsibilities include performing audits of health services throughout the company, developing policy, arranging for continuing education, and apprising the nurses who report to me of current events in medicine, legislation, health care delivery, and other fields as they relate to employee health and safety. I act as a resource, consultant and liaison among health services and other areas of the company, and as an advocate for the nurses.

I find the field of occupational health very exciting. In no other area of nursing does one need such a broad base of nursing knowledge or have such a varied role. In no other area of nursing does one have such a captive audience in which to promote health and wellness, or such an opportunity to express individualism and creativity within a practice.

Opportunities for OHNs also exist in other sectors, such as organized labor and government. Maxine Garbo, R.N., M.S., works in the Right-to-Know Program of the Division of Occupational Hygiene of the Massachusetts Department of Labor and Industries. This program assists Massachusetts employers in complying with the state's Right-to-Know law through plant visits and hazard reviews. Ms. Garbo writes of her work:

Because of my work experience and training as a nurse, I have assumed some unique responsibilities. One of these is a file that contains articles and studies on substances and occupations with known or suspected reproductive hazards and on related policy issues. We receive and respond to phone calls from women who are pregnant or are contemplating pregnancy (and from other workers). They want information on the substances with which they work or on the policies related to their jobs.

Education and research comprise a large share of what I do as an OHN. This includes outreach to other OHNs regarding the Right-to-Know law. Possible work-related symptoms in an office building and occupationally related reproductive hazards are subjects of two epidemiologic projects on which I've worked. I also research information for the reproductive hazards section for material safety data sheets.

Much of my work is done in collaboration with industrial hygienists and other occupational health professionals in our division with whom I work.

(See box in Chap. 34 for more on occupational health nursing.)

Industrial Hygiene
The practice of industrial hygiene includes the recognition, evaluation, and control of occupational hazards. Most industrial hygienists are employed directly by companies; however, many are also employed by government agencies concerned with regulation, independent consulting groups, and academic institutions. A few are also employed by labor unions. The following is an account by an industrial hygienist that reflects the breadth of opportunities in this field. Barbara Plog, an industrial hygienist with the Labor Occupational Health Program, Northern California Occupational Health Center, University of California at Berkeley, writes:

My job as an industrial hygienist involves the development and implementation of education and training programs on all aspects of industrial hygiene for workers, their representatives, managers, and members of labor-management health and safety committees. This work has included training programs that address basic hazard recognition procedures, hearing conservation, dust exposures (silica and asbestos), chemical exposures, hazardous waste, OSHA standards, ventilation, control measures used in the workplace, ergonomics, and manual materials handling. I also teach in university courses for occupational and environmental health sciences students and in continuing education courses for occupational health professionals at a NIOSH educational resource center. I have trained contractors and workers in asbestos abatement techniques at an EPA asbestos training center.

The creation of written materials has been a key part of my career. I have written a number of slide and videotape training programs and a series of guidebooks on various industrial hygiene topics. I am the editor of the third edition of the *Fundamentals of Industrial Hygiene*, a basic textbook in the field.

Providing technical assistance to workers, managers, and the general public has also been a part of my work. Acting as a technical resource is a large part of industrial hygienists' work, whether they work for industry, labor, academic institutions, or the government.

My career as an industrial hygienist reflects a heavy emphasis on writing and teaching. Many industrial hygienists may find themselves also performing a training and education function, but as a smaller part of their jobs. They may be in the field, performing sampling and evaluations much of the time. These evaluations may cover a wide range of chemical and physical workplace health hazards. Some industrial hygienists specialize in one particular hazard. For example, health physicists specialize in ionizing radiation while other industrial hygienists may specialize in hearing conservation and noise control technologies or in asbestos abatement work.

Governmentally employed industrial hygienists run the gamut from those employed in more administrative program development, training, and education jobs to compliance officers who inspect and evaluate worksites.

Industrial hygienists who work for private industry may work mainly as field hygienists, performing daily sampling and evaluation; as trainers and program developers; or as program administrators. The typical job incorporates all of these functions, depending upon the size of the company.

Industrial hygienists in academic organizations typically divide their time between teaching and research functions. Some are program administrators.

The field of industrial hygiene is exciting and challenging. It draws upon many other disciplines (chemistry, biology, toxicology, epidemiology, occupational medicine, health physics, engineering, and health edu-

cation) to meet its goal of protecting the health of workers.

The industrial hygiene field, in general, is described in Chap. 7. Further information on specific educational requirements can be obtained by contacting sources listed in the box on p. 590.

Academic Occupational Health

Many occupational health specialists have faculty appointments at schools of medicine, nursing, public health, or other disciplines. Often these are part-time appointments that complement clinical appointments or employment in other settings.

Academic positions in occupational health entail the same types of duties as do other faculty posts, including research and publication, classroom and clinical teaching, outside consulting, and patient care. Faculty members may specialize further, depending on their interests and training. Many collaborate with statisticians, epidemiologists, toxicologists, and others in their research and with clinicians from other fields in their clinical duties. Specific job responsibilities are variable and are often largely defined by the individual.

Dr. Linda Rosenstock, Director of the University of Washington Occupational Medicine Program, writes:

Academic medicine is traditionally described as demanding productivity in three areas: clinical service, teaching, and research. Increasingly, administrative activities are added responsibilities even for junior faculty. Although these expectations may be viewed as overly demanding in some disciplines, they add to the variety and challenge of working in the emerging academic field of occupational medicine. My colleagues and I have responsibility for teaching medical students in the basic science years and providing elective opportunities to them in the clinical years. Residents in internal medicine, family medicine, and occupational medicine also rotate through our program, participating in clinical and research activities and interacting with a multidisciplinary staff of physicians, industrial hygienists, and nurses. Other trainees are also involved, including students in industrial hygiene and occupational nursing.

Our main objective, determining whether an individual's health problem is work-related, is largely carried out in a consultative clinic setting. Here, patients are referred for evaluation by themselves or by physicians, unions, companies, and workers' compensation and other agencies. After our review of medical records and available information about exposures, each patient undergoes a comprehensive interview eliciting information about work and exposure history, a physical examination, and appropriate laboratory tests. It is against this background that a determination about the individual's medical condition and its relation to workplace factors is made. Often this task is relatively straightforward, but sometimes in the process we recognize unexpected or new associations between the workplace and health.

Probably in no other field is there this same potential for discovering and detecting new etiologies and syndromes. But, regardless of the complexity of evaluating disease and its cause in an individual, we are always thinking about the implications of our findings in terms of prevention—for the individual in terms of returning to the workplace and for others who may be similarly affected or at risk.

This process—from initial evaluation to diagnosis and follow-through—is, I think, the most rewarding part of clinical occupational medicine. In our setting all aspects of a patient's situation are discussed by the entire staff in case conferences; these discussions are open and sometimes heated, recognizing that occupational diseases have not only medical, but also social, economic, legal, and political components.

Scholarly investigation and research are also fundamental to our activities and often brought about by problems encountered in the clinic. Occasionally, this leads to basic "bench" research, but the objectives of such inquiry—to provide new knowledge—can also be achieved by describing individual cases or clusters of cases, or by undertaking population-based studies to answer predetermined questions systematically.

In sum, our work is diverse. I think I can speak for others in our program as well as in other academic settings in saying that we bring a collaborative spirit to all these activities, that they are largely enjoyable (and often fun), and rewarding. It is an opportunity and challenge to work in an evolving field, to be humble in recognizing what we do not know, to be vigilant about opportunities to broaden knowledge, and to recognize that in occupational health we are dealing with the social context of disease, a context that is central to the recognition, determination of causation, and prevention of occupational diseases.

Dr. Arthur Frank, Professor and Chairman of the Department of Preventive Medicine and Environmental Health at the University of Kentucky College of Medicine, also describes teaching, research, patient care, and administration as his four duties. He writes:

As an academic occupational health physician, I see to it that our medical students get a reasonable amount of occupational health in their curriculum (with all the usual constraints and competing educational needs). I have started a masters program, on which to base a new residency program in occupational medicine. Patient care activities are in many ways similar to traditional occupational medicine, and patients are seen in the university occupational medicine clinic. In addition, the department operates occupational health programs for several companies in such fields as coal mining and electronics repair, and I have served as medical consultant to Toyota Motor Manufacturing, U.S.A., Inc., as it builds a major new facility near Lexington. My busy program of work at the university is supplemented by regional and national activities; I serve as a board member of several national organizations and as a consultant to NIOSH.

Academic occupational medicine is clearly a viable option for those entering the field and will continue to be a "growth" area for physicians for many years.

C
Other Sources of Information

Compiled by Marianne Parker Brown and Daniel E. Kass

The following resources can be obtained or contacted for additional health and safety information:

GENERAL RESOURCES

1. Emergency Services

Listed below are telephone numbers to call for technical, medical, regulatory, or reporting information in the event of an exposure-related problem or medical emergency.

CHEMTREC
(800) 424-9300

24-hour hotline operated by the Chemical Manufacturers' Association relays information to manufacturers about a spill involving their products or employees and will rapidly determine for the caller the contents of a spilled container and suggest appropriate action for containment.

National Response Center
(800) 424-8802

First federal point of contact for reporting of and guidance on oil and hazardous spills. 24-hour hotline relays information to regulatory and response agencies and immediately contacts appropriate regional or state coordinators to respond to the spill.

NIOSH "Hot Line"
1-800-35-NIOSH

Provides technical assistance on workplace hazards.

OSHA Technical Support Services
(202) 523-7031

Central number for federal OSHA provides rapid technical support and will notify, in the event of a significant medical emergency, the OSHA Salt Lake City Medical Response Team. Also provides phone number for regional technical support offices for further assistance.

Poison Control Centers

Each state or region has a 24-hour poison control center offering expert emergency medical information and referrals. Centers are listed on the inside cover of local phone directories. They can also be reached by dialing 911 and asking for the Poison Control Center or by calling the National Response Center, listed before.

Tox-Center
(800) 227-6476 (U.S.)
(800) 682-9000 (California only)

Responds to nationwide calls, providing 24-hour, immediate information on toxic incident containment and control, sampling, protective measures for on-scene personnel, evaluation, and medical treatment advice.

2. Guides, Catalogs, and Directories

NIOSH Publications Catalog (6th ed., 1986)
    4676 Columbia Parkway, Cincinnati, OH
    45226

List of all NIOSH publications, including criteria documents, manuals, reports, health hazard evaluations, and others.

OSHA Publications and Audiovisual Programs (1986)
OSHA Office of Information, U.S. Department of Labor, Room N-3637, Washington, DC 20210

List of available OSHA educational materials oriented toward workers and managers; some copies available in Spanish.

A Directory of Educational Opportunities in Occupational Health for Health Science Students

Published in 1987 by the Association of Teachers of Preventive Medicine and NIOSH. Contact NIOSH, Division of Training, 4676 Columbia Parkway, Cincinnati, OH 45226.

A Resource Guide to Worker Education Materials in Occupational Safety and Health, Vols. 1 and 2. Washington, DC.: OSHA, 1982.

Listing of materials produced by citizen organizations, college and university labor education programs, and labor unions.

3. Films and Other Audiovisuals

American Labor, Nos. 25/26, 29. American Labor Education Center (ALEC), 1984 and 1985.

Annotated listings of over 50 health and safety audiovisuals and their distributors. Includes films produced by universities, federal agencies, nonprofit organizations, and labor unions. Reprints available from: ALEC, 1835 Kilbourne Place, NW, Washington, DC 20010.

BNA Communications Safety Catalog, Bureau of National Affairs, 9439 Key West Avenue, Rockville, MD 20850

Distributes several hundred safety films and videos, including a Right-to-Know package and a new Hazardous Waste Management Series for purchase or rental.

Films and Video Tapes for Labor; Film Division, AFL-CIO Department of Education, 815 16th Street, NW, Washington, DC 20006

Lists 26 films and videos on occupational health and safety, including training on regulations, workers' rights, and union strategies. For rental only.

Media Resource Catalog; National Audiovisual Center of the National Archives and Records Administration, 8700 Edgeworth Drive, Capitol Heights, MD 20743

Includes 155 health and safety training programs developed by 28 federal agencies. Materials include films, videos, slide and tape shows, and audio cassettes. For purchase only.

Film and Video Finder; Access Innovations, Inc. (1987); NICEM, P.O. Box 40130, Albuquerque, NM 87196

Exhaustive compilation, categorized by subject and title. Available at most research libraries. Also accessed on-line through *Dialogue Computer Network.*

Audiovisual Material Catalogue (1987); NIOSH, 4676 Columbia Parkway, Cincinnati, OH 45226

Describes the 14 NIOSH-produced films available either for purchase or copying.

OSHA Audiovisual Programs; OSHA Office of Information, U.S. Department of Labor, Room N-3637, Washington, DC 20210

Listing of over 40 films, videos, slide/tape shows, and cassettes for purchase or rental.

Management Training Catalog; International Film Bureau, 332 South Michigan Avenue, Chicago, IL 60604.

Lists dozens of films available for purchase or rental in 16-mm or videotape format. These internationally produced films are available in many languages.

Audiovisual Resources in Occupational Safety and Health: An Evaluative Guide (1985); Oryx Press, 2214 North Central Encanto, Phoenix, AZ 85004

Critically reviews scores of audiovisual training materials in the field. Information on the availability of these materials is also included.

ORGANIZATIONS

1. Federal Government

National Institute for Occupational Safety and Health (NIOSH)

Main Offices

Building 1, Room 3007, D-35, Centers for Disease Control, Atlanta, GA 30333

Robert A. Taft Laboratories, 4676 Columbia Parkway, Cincinnati, OH 45226

Appalachian Laboratory for Occupational Safety and Health, 944 Chestnut Ridge Road, Morgantown, WV 26505

NIOSH Regional Offices

In 1986, NIOSH consolidated the number of regional offices from 10 to 3. The 3 regional offices now cover 20 states. West Virginia is covered by the Morgantown office and the remaining 29 states are handled by the Cincinnati office (see addresses above).

Boston Regional Office (CT, MA, ME, NH, RI, and VT), JFK Federal Building, Room 1401, Boston, MA 02203

Atlanta Regional Office (AL, FL, GA, KY, MS, NC, SC, and TN), 101 Marietta Tower, Atlanta, GA 30323

Denver Regional Office (CO, MT, ND, SD, UT, and WY), Federal Building, Room 1185, 1961 Stout Street, Denver, CO 80294

Occupational Safety and Health Administration (OSHA)

Main Office

U.S. Department of Labor, 200 Constitution Avenue, NW, Washington, DC 20210

OSHA Regional Offices

Region I (CT, MA, ME, NH, RI, and VT), 16-18 North Street, 1 Dock Square Building, 4th floor, Boston, MA 02109

Region II (NJ, NY, Puerto Rico, and Virgin Islands), 1 Astor Plaza, Room 3445, 1515 Broadway, New York, NY 10036

Region III (DC, DE, MD, PA, VA, and WV), Gateway Building, Suite 2100, 3535 Market Street, Philadelphia, PA 19104

Region IV (AL, FL, GA, KY, MS, NC, SC, and TN), 1375 Peachtree Street, NE, Suite 587, Atlanta, GA 30367

Region V (IL, IN, MI, MN, OH, and WI), 230 South Dearborn Street, 32nd floor, Room 3244, Chicago, IL 60604

Region VI (AR, LA, NM, OK, and TX), 525 Griffin Square Building, Room 602, Dallas, TX 75202

Region VII (IA, KS, MO, and NE), 91 Walnut Street, Room 406, Kansas City, MO 64106

Region VIII (CO, MT, SD, ND, UT, and WY), Federal Building, Room 1554, 1961 Stout Street, Denver, CO 80294

Region IX (AZ, CA, HI, NV, American Samoa, Guam, and Pacific Trust Territories), P.O. Box 36017, 450 Golden Gate Avenue, San Francisco, CA 94102

Region X (AK, ID, OR, and WA), Federal Office Building, Room 6003, 909 First Avenue, Seattle, WA 98174

2. *State Agencies*

States with approved plans are listed below. Unless indicated, plans cover public and private workers.

Alaska Department of Labor, P.O. Box 1149, Juneau, AK 99802

Industrial Commission of Arizona, 800 West Washington, Phoenix, AZ 85007

California Department of Industrial Relations Cal-OSHA, 525 Golden Gate Avenue, San Francisco, CA 94102 (public sector only)

Connecticut Department of Labor, 200 Folly Brook Boulevard, Wethersfield, CT 06109

Hawaii Department of Labor and Industrial Relations, 825 Mililani Street, Honolulu, HI 96813

Indiana Department of Labor, 1013 State Office Building, 100 North Senate Avenue, Indianapolis, IN 46204

Iowa Department of Employment Services, Division of Labor Services, 307 East 7th Street, Des Moines, IA 50319

Kentucky Labor Cabinet, U.S. Highway 127 South, Frankfort, KY 40601

Maryland Division of Labor and Industry, Department of Licensing and Regulation, 501 St. Paul Place, Baltimore, MD 21202

Michigan Department of Labor (for safety matters), 7150 Harris Drive, Box 30015, Lansing, MI 48909

Michigan Department of Public Health (for health matters), 3500 North Logan Street, Box 30035, Lansing, MI 48909

Minnesota Department of Labor and Industry, 444 Lafayette Road, St. Paul, MN 55101

Nevada Department of Industrial Relations, Division of Occupational Safety and Health, Capitol Complex, 1370 South Curry Street, Carson City, NV 89710

New Mexico Environmental Improvement Division, Health and Environment Department, P.O. Box 968, Santa Fe, NM 87504-0968

New York Department of Labor, One Main Street, Brooklyn, NY 11201 (Public sector only)

North Carolina Department of Labor, 214 West Jones Street, Shore Building, Raleigh, NC 27603

Oregon Workers' Compensation Department, Labor and Industries Building, Salem, OR 97310

Puerto Rico Department of Labor and Human Resources, Prudencio Rivera Martinez Building, 505 Munoz Rivera Avenue, Hato Rey, Puerto Rico 00918

South Carolina Department of Labor, 3600 Forest Drive, P.O. Box 11329, Columbia, SC 29211-1329

Tennessee Department of Labor, 501 Union Building, Suite "A," 2nd floor, Nashville, TN 37219

Utah Industrial Commission, Utah Occupational Safety and Health, 160 East Third South, P.O. Box 5800, Salt Lake City, UT 84110-5800

Vermont Department of Labor and Industry, 120 State Street, Montpelier, VT 05602

Virgin Islands Department of Labor, Box 890, Christiansted, St Croix, Virgin Islands 00820

Virginia Department of Labor and Industry, P.O. Box 12064, Richmond, VA 23241-0064

Washington Department of Labor and Industries, General Administration Building, Room 334 - AX-31, Olympia, WA 98504

Wyoming Department of Occupational Health and Safety, 604 East 25th Street, Cheyenne, WY 82002

3. Other Federal Agencies

Agency for Toxic Substances and Disease Registry (ATSDR), ATSDR-Chamblee, 1600 Clifton Road, Atlanta, GA 30333

U.S. Public Health Service agency that implements the health-related sections of the "Superfund" Act and its amendments and the Resource Conservation and Recovery Act (RCRA). Involved in the areas of: emergency response, health assessments, health effects research, literature inventory/dissemination, exposure and disease registries, toxicologic profiles, health professional training, and worker health; and maintains a list of toxic waste sites closed to the public.

Environmental Protection Agency (EPA), 401 M Street, SW, Washington, DC 20460

Responsible for assessment and control of air and water pollution, solid waste management, pesticides, radiation, noise, toxic substances, and other environmental problems.

Mine Safety and Health Administration (MSHA), Ballston Towers #3, 4015 Wilson Boulevard, Arlington, VA 22203

Regulates health and safety in the mining industry.

National Cancer Institute (NCI), National Institutes of Health, Public Health Service, U.S. Department of Health and Human Services, Bethesda, MD 20205

Has published and distributes the annotated bibliography *Cancer Information in the Workplace* and free educational materials. Supports various types of research related to occupational cancer hazards, including epidemiologic studies, carcinogenesis assays of industrial chemicals, and, recently, worker education programs. A new occupational cancer branch within the institute will focus on applied prevention programs for workers to minimize potential hazards.

National Institute of Environmental Health Sciences (NIEHS), National Institutes of Health, Public Health Service, U.S. Department of Health and Human Services, P.O. Box 12233, Research Triangle Park, NC 27709

Principal federal agency for biomedical research on the effects of chemical, physical, and biologic environmental agents on human health and well-being. Supports and conducts basic research focused on the interaction between humans and potentially hazardous agents. Through its research, it provides an essential knowledge base on the impact of environmental factors on human health in order to aid those agencies charged with devising and instituting control or therapeutic measures.

National Toxicology Program (NTP), M.D. B2-04, Box 12233, Research Triangle Park, NC 27709

Established in 1978 to develop scientific information needed to determine the toxic effects of chemicals and to develop better, faster, and less expensive test methods.

Nuclear Regulatory Commission (NRC), Washington, D.C. 20555

Regulates the commercial use of nuclear materials and issues licenses for such use.

4. Professional Organizations in the United States

Aerospace Medical Association, Washington National Airport, Washington, DC 20001

Publishes a monthly journal, *Aviation, Space, and Environmental Medicine,* concerned with promoting a safe environment for individuals in air and space operations, including ground support personnel. Considers toxic hazards and environmental effects of and protection from heat, cold, acceleration, vibration, noise, and altitude.

American Association of Occupational Health Nurses (AAOHN), 50 Lenox Pointe, Atlanta, GA 30324

Professional organization of registered nurses engaged in occupational health nursing. Major activities are the following: formulating and developing principles and standards of occupational health nursing practice; promoting, by means of publications, conferences, continuing education courses, and symposia, educational programs designed specifically for the occupational health nurse; and impressing on managers, physicians, and others the importance of integrating occupational health nurse services into employee activities.

American Cancer Society (ACS), 90 Park Avenue, New York, NY 10016

Voluntary health organization, in part, funds research projects on occupationally related cancer.

American College of Preventive Medicine (ACPM), 1015 15th Street, NW, Suite 403, Washington, DC 20005

National society of public health and preventive medicine physicians. Sponsors workshops and conferences, serves as a clearinghouse for continuing medical education and information of interest to physicians in these fields, and helps shape national preventive policy and legislation.

American Conference of Governmental Industrial Hygienists (ACGIH), 6500 Glenway Avenue, Cincinnati, OH 45211

Organization of occupational health professionals who work at governmental agencies and educational institutions and who are engaged in occupational health services, consultation, enforcement, research, or education. Publishes information for all occupational health workers to assist them in providing more adequate health services for workers. Publications include specific health protection symposia proceedings and listings of threshold limit values (TLVs) for over 600 chemical and physical agents and their rationale.

American Industrial Hygiene Association (AIHA), 475 Wolf Ledges Parkway, Akron, OH 44311

Professional organization of industrial hygienists and allied specialists. Publishes *AIHA Journal* and extensive literature on all phases of industrial hygiene. Promotes information on career opportunities in industrial hygiene.

American Lung Association (ALA), 1740 Broadway, New York, NY 10019

In addition to supporting and participating in occupational health programs, the ALA offers literature and films on occupational lung diseases, chronic obstructive pulmonary disease, TB, adult and pediatric lung diseases, air conservation, and smoking. Publishes *American Review of Respiratory Disease*. Its medical section is the American Thoracic Society. Local branches conduct a variety of activities directed at a more limited geographic area.

American Medical Association, Department of Environmental, Public, and Occupational Health, 535 North Dearborn Street, Chicago, IL 60610

Conducts programs, prepares monographs, reviews, and comments on federal documents and proposed regulations; responds to professional and public queries on occupational medical and health issues. These activities are designed to attract, motivate, and educate physicians; encourages and supports medical societies; assists governmental agencies and allied health organizations; and informs the public. Extensive literature available.

American Medical Student Association (AMSA), Task Force on Occupational and Environmental Health, 1910 Association Drive, Reston, VA 22091

Publishes a quarterly newsletter, develops and publicizes educational materials, and facilitates student participation in occupational and environmental health projects.

American National Standards Institute (ANSI), 1430 Broadway, New York, NY 10018

Coordinates the voluntary development of national standards. Serves as a clearinghouse and information center for national and international safety standards.

American Occupational Medical Association (AOMA), 55 West Seegers Road, Arlington Heights, IL 60005

Largest society in the United States of physicians in industry, government, and academia who promote the health of workers through clinical practice, research, and teaching. Cosponsors with AAOHN the annual American Occupational Health Conference each spring; conducts other educational programs; and publishes the monthly *Journal of Occupational Medicine,* the *AOMA Report, the AOMA Self Assessment Program in Occupational Medicine,* and other materials.

American Public Health Association (APHA), Occupational Health and Safety Section, 1015 15th Street, NW, Washington, DC 20005

Presents numerous sessions at annual APHA meeting each fall, develops public policy statements on occupational health and safety issues, and publishes a newsletter. Develops links between occupational health and public health.

American Society for Safety Engineers (ASSE), 1800 East Oakton, Des Plaines, IL 60018

Publishes *Professional Safety.* Supports safety professionals for accident, injury, and illness prevention.

Association of Teachers of Preventive Medicine (ATPM), 1030 15th Street, NW, Washington, DC 20005

Promotes and supports teaching of preventive medicine, including occupational medicine, in medical schools.

The Ergonomics Society, Department of Human Sciences, University of Technology, Loughborough, Leics., LE11-3TU, Great Britain

Original society for ergonomics, which has special interest in industrial ergonomics. Publishes *Ergonomics* and *Applied Ergonomics* and holds annual meeting.

Human Factors Society, P.O. Box 1369, Santa Monica, CA 90406

Professional organization of ergonomics and human factors professionals. Holds annual meeting and its technical groups hold regular meetings. Publishes *Human Factors* and the proceedings of the annual meeting. Its Industrial Ergonomics Technical Group is of special interest.

National Safety Council (NSC), 444 North Michigan Avenue, Chicago, IL 60611

Offers occupational health training programs and literature, use of health and safety library services, and free telephone consultation with experts in safety, industrial hygiene, and occupational health.

Society for Occupational and Environmental Health (SOEH), 1341 G Street, NW, Washington, DC 20005

Actively seeks to improve the health quality of the workplace by holding open forums that focus public attention on scientific, social, and regulatory problems.

5. Occupational Health Clinics
Association of Occupational and Environmental Clinics (AOEC), P.O. Box 5214, Takoma Park, MD 20812-0214

Recently formed organization of clinics to aid in identifying, reporting, and preventing occupational/environmental health hazards nationwide; to increase communication among such clinics concerning issues of patient care; and to provide data for occupational/environmental research projects.

6. Committees on Occupational Safety and Health (COSH Groups)
COSH groups are grassroots voluntary advocacy organizations consisting of health professionals,

legal professionals, and labor representatives who work to improve health and safety in the workplace through education and policy change.

National Clearinghouse
Alice Hamilton Center for Occupational Safety and Health, 801 Pennsylvania Avenue, SE, Suite 303, Washington, DC 20003

Serves as a clearinghouse for COSH groups around the United States. It may be contacted for general information on COSH activities.

ALASKA
Alaska Health Project, 417 West 8th Avenue, Anchorage, AK 99501

CALIFORNIA
BACOSH (San Francisco Bay Area COSH), c/o LOHP, Institute of Industrial Relations, University of California, 2521 Channing Way, Berkeley, CA 94720
LACOSH (Los Angeles COSH), 2501 South Hill Street, Los Angeles, CA 90007
SacramentoCOSH, c/o Fire Fighters Local #522, 3101 Stockton Boulevard, Sacramento, CA 95820
SCCOSH (Santa Clara Center for Occupational Safety and Health), 304 West Hedding, San Jose, CA 95110

CONNECTICUT
ConnectiCOSH (Connecticut COSH), 425 Washington Avenue, New Haven, CT 06473

ILLINOIS
CACOSH (Chicago COSH), 33 East Congress Expressway, Suite 723, Chicago, IL 60605

MAINE
Maine Labor Group on Health, Inc., Box V, Augusta, ME 04330

MARYLAND
MaryCOSH (Maryland COSH), 325 East 25th Street, Baltimore, MD 21218

MASSACHUSETTS
MassCOSH (Massachusetts Coalition for Occupational Safety and Health)
Eastern Office: 625 Huntington Avenue, Boston, MA 02115
Western Office: 458 Bridge Street, Springfield, MA 01103

MICHIGAN
SEMCOSH (Southeast Michigan COSH), 1550 Howard Street, Detroit, MI 48216

NEW YORK
ALCOSH (Allegheny COSH), 210 West 5th Street, Jamestown, NY 14701
CNYCOSH (Central New York COSH), 615 West Genessee Street, Syracuse, NY 13204
NYCOSH (New York COSH), 275 Seventh Avenue, 25th floor, New York, NY 10001
ROCOSH (Rochester COSH), 502 Lyell Avenue, Suite #1, Rochester, NY 14606
WNYCOSH (Western New York COSH), 450 Grider Street, Buffalo, NY 14215

NORTH CAROLINA
NCOSH (North Carolina Occupational Safety and Health Project), P.O. Box 2514, Durham, NC 27705

OHIO
ORVCOSH (Ohio River Valley COSH), 35 East 7th Street, Suite 200, Cincinnati, OH 45202

PENNSYLVANIA
PHILAPOSH (Philadelphia Project in Occupational Safety and Health), 3001 Walnut Street, 5th Floor, Philadelphia, PA 19104

RHODE ISLAND
RICOSH (Rhode Island COSH), 340 Lockwood Street, Providence, RI 02907

TENNESSEE
TNCOSH (Tennessee COSH), 705 North Broadway, Room 212, Knoxville, TN 37917

WISCONSIN

WISCOSH (Wisconsin COSH), 1334 South 11th Street, Milwaukee, WI 53204

CANADA

WOSH (Windsor Occupational Safety and Health Project), 1109 Tecumseh Road East, Windsor, Ontario N8W 2T1, Canada

7. University Labor Education Programs

Some universities have labor education programs that focus on occupational safety and health. They are also good sources for written and audiovisual materials designed for workers. This list is not comprehensive.

University of California, Berkeley, Labor Occupational Health Program (LOHP), 2521 Channing Way, Berkeley, CA 94720

University of California, Los Angeles (UCLA), Labor Occupational Safety and Health (LOSH) Program, 1001 Gayley Avenue, 2nd floor, Los Angeles, CA 90024

Cornell University, Division of Extension and Public Service, New York State School of Industrial Relations, Ithaca, NY 14850

Ohio State University, Labor Education and Research Service, 1810 College Road, Columbus, OH 43210

University of Wisconsin-Extension School for Workers, 1 South Park Street, # 701, Madison, WI 53706

8. Industry-Sponsored Advisory and Research Groups

American Petroleum Institute, 1220 L Street, NW, Washington, DC 20005

Conducts research programs on occupational health and industrial hygiene aspects of all phases of the petroleum industry. These projects may result in manuals or guides or in research reports, which are available to interested parties.

American Welding Society, 550 Northwest LeJeune Road, P.O. Box 351040, Miami, FL 33135

Offers seminars and home-study courses designed specifically to relate welding and cutting operations to plant environmental safety and health.

Chemical Industry Institute of Toxicology (CIIT), P.O. Box 12137, 6 Davis Drive, Research Triangle Park, NC 27709

Examines toxicologic problems arising from the manufacture, handling, use, and disposal of commodity chemicals. Acquires, interprets, and disseminates technical information and test data. Assists in training toxicologists and scientists in related fields.

Chemical Manufacturers Association, 2501 M Street, NW, Washington, DC 20037

Publishes monthly newsletter, *ChemEcology*. Has a committee that deals with occupational safety and health matters. Has over 200 member companies. Sponsors projects and occasionally publishes educational materials.

Chlorine Institute, 2001 L Street, NW, Washington, DC 20037

Promotes safety in manufacturing and handling of chlorine products. Provides educational materials to over 200 member companies and to the public.

Industrial Health Foundation, 34 Penn Circle West, Pittsburgh, PA 15206

Conducts engineering plant visits to review industrial hygiene and health and safety aspects, publishes extensive abstracts, performs short-term toxicology studies, conducts training courses in occupational health and safety, and performs analytical testing of environmental and biologic samples.

International Lead-Zinc Research Organization, 2525 Meridian Parkway, P.O. Box 12036, Research Triangle Park, NC 27709

Conducts occupational and environmental health research on such subjects as pediatric lead absorption, occupational lead and cadmium exposure, and biologic interactions. Publishes annual lead/cadmium research digest.

Joint Labor Management Committee of the Retail Food Industry, 2120 L Street, NW, Washington, DC 20037

Studies and recommends programs to provide safe working conditions and to protect employees in all phases of retail food operations from exposure to hazardous working conditions.

Plastics Education Foundation, 14 Fairfield Drive, Brookfield, CT 06805

Provides audiovisual materials, including films and videotapes, on occupational health and safety in plastics and manufacturing industries.

9. Labor-Oriented Advisory/Research Groups

American Labor Education Center (ALEC), 1835 Kilbourne Place, NW, Washington, DC 20010

Provides education and educational materials to workers about health and safety. Publishes bimonthly American Labor, which often highlights health and safety issues.

Center for Occupational Hazards, 5 Beekman Street, New York, NY 10038

National clearinghouse for research and information on health hazards in the arts, including the visual arts and crafts, theater, and museum conservation. Has lecture and consultation program, art hazards newsletter, and an art hazards information center.

Environmental Defense Fund, 1616 P Street, NW, Washington, DC 20036

Toxic Chemicals Programs seeks to establish public policy that minimizes or eliminates the use of toxic chemicals. Past actions have related to both occupational and general consumer exposure to toxic chemicals and have involved DDT, endrin,

chlordane/heptachlor, 2,4,5-T, asbestos, benzene, TRIS, and hair dye chemicals.

Environmental Policy Institute, 218 D Street, SE, Washington, DC 20003

Advisory group working with professionals, community members, and grassroots organizations to raise the level of awareness on the hazards, proper handling, and transportation of chemicals and toxic wastes.

Health Research Group, Public Citizen, 2000 P Street, NW, Suite 708, Washington, DC 20036

Public interest group that studies many subjects, including occupational health hazards, and disseminates information to the working public. Has numerous publications and other informational resources that are of value to medical students and physicians. In certain circumstances, it can also investigate specific hazardous situations.

Highlander Research and Education Center, Box 370, Route 3, New Market, TN 37820

Major labor education center, which among other things, conducts educational conferences on occupational safety and health for labor activists, health science students, and others.

Labor Institute for Education and Research, 853 Broadway, Room 2007, New York, NY 10003

Specializes in developing economic analyses of the problems workers face and presents them in easy-to-understand language from the workers' point of view. Has produced a 24-minute slide/tape show that examines the economic roots of occupational hazards and is in the process of preparing materials on the economic feasibility of making the workplace safer and healthier.

Labor Safety and Health Institute, 377 Park Avenue South, New York, NY 10016

Has published a handbook for local unions on control of workplace hazards and an occupational safety and health workbook. Maintains a library on job safety and health information.

Scientists' Institute for Public Information (SIPI), 355 Lexington Avenue, New York, NY 10017

Publishes *Environment and Sipiscope,* containing information on environmental hazards. Past articles have been on subjects including asbestos, fibrous glass, pesticides, and polychlorinated biphenyls (PCBs). Other published materials also available.

Women's Occupational Health Resource Center (WOHRC), 117 St. John's Place, Brooklyn, NY 11217

Helps working women, unions, management, health professionals, and government policymakers become aware of women's occupational health needs. Publishes a bimonthly newsletter, fact sheets, and fact packs on specific occupational health hazards and policies. Answers requests for technical information and specialized computer bibliographies and conducts a speakers bureau.

Workers' Institute for Safety and Health (WISH), 1126 16th Street, NW, Washington, DC 20036

Labor-supported organization that provides technical, scientific, and educational services in occupational health and safety to unions. Responds to requests for information.

Working Women Educational Fund, 614 Superior Avenue, NW, Cleveland, OH 44113

National association that works to win rights and respect for women office workers. Engaged in a specific effort to address health and safety problems of office workers with research and education.

10. International Organizations

International Commission on Occupational Health (ICOH), c/o Luigi Parmeggiani, M.D., 10, Avenue Jules-Crosnier, CH-1206 Geneva, Switzerland

International scientific society that fosters scientific progress, knowledge, and development of all aspects of occupational health on an international basis. Holds a triennial international congress, maintains scientific committees, and collects and disseminates information on occupational health.

International Labour Organization (ILO), CH-1211, Geneva 22, Switzerland

Focuses on the prevention of occupational accidents and diseases; promotion of safety, health, and well-being in all occupations; and identification and elimination of problems of working environments. Involvement in occupational safety and health is articulated in its International Programme for the Improvement of Working Conditions and Environment (PIACT). Modes of action include adoption of international conventions and recommendations, the establishment of model codes of practices, convening of tripartite meetings, collection and dissemination of information (including the *Encyclopedia of Occupational Health and Safety),* and technical cooperation.

World Health Organization (WHO), Environmental Health Division, 1211 Avenue Appia, Geneva 27, Switzerland

Offers a wide range of services in occupational health and safety, including publishing documents and sponsoring a variety of educational programs.

11. Labor Organizations

The following list of labor organizations is not all-inclusive but includes some of those with the most active health and safety departments.

American Federation of Labor and Congress of Industrial Organizations (AFL-CIO), 815 16th Street, NW, Washington, DC 20006

Confederation of labor unions serving as their advocate in health and safety matters. The Building and Construction Trades Department, AFL-CIO, is housed in the same offices and works extensively on health and safety for unions in those industries.

American Federation of Government Employees, 1325 Massachusetts Avenue, NW, Washington, DC 20005

American Federation of State, County and
Municipal Employees (AFSCME), 1625 L
Street, NW, Washington, DC 20036

Communication Workers of America (CWA),
1925 K Street, NW, Washington, DC 20005

International Brotherhood of Painters and Allied
Trades, United Unions Building, 1750 New
York Avenue, NW, Washington, DC 20006

International Chemical Workers Union (ICWU),
1655 West Market Street, Akron, OH 44313

International Union of Automobile, Aerospace
and Agricultural Implement Workers (UAW),
8000 East Jefferson Avenue, Detroit, MI 48214

Oil, Chemical and Atomic Workers International
Union (OCAW), P.O. Box 2812, Denver,
CO 80201

Service Employees International Union (SEIU),
2020 K Street, NW, Washington, DC 20006

United Mine Workers of America (UMWA), 900
15th Street, NW, Washington, DC 20005

Index

Index

I
Work and Health